Pediatric Education

for Prehospital Professionals

FIFTH EDITION

AF901484

American Academy of Pediatrics

DEDICATED TO THE HEALTH OF ALL CHILDREN®

THE AMERICAN ACADEMY OF PEDIATRICS®

PEPP

Pediatric Education for Prehospital Professionals™

American Academy of Pediatrics Publishing Staff

Jeff Mahony, *Senior Director, Professional and Consumer Publishing*
Annika Hawkinson, *Editorial Assistant*
Jason Crase, *Senior Manager, Production and Editorial Services*
Leesa Levin-Doroba, *Production Manager, Practice Management*
Shawn Viane, *Production Manager, Professional/Clinical Publications*
Soraya Alem, *Manager, Digital Publishing*
Emily Slayden, *Marketing Manager, Professional Resources*

Published by the American Academy of Pediatrics
345 Park Blvd
Itasca, IL 60143
630/626-6000
www.aap.org

The American Academy of Pediatrics is an organization of 67,000 primary care pediatricians, pediatric medical subspecialists, and pediatric surgical specialists dedicated to the health, safety, and well-being of all infants, children, adolescents, and young adults.

While every effort has been made to ensure the accuracy of this publication, the American Academy of Pediatrics does not guarantee that it is accurate, complete, or without error.

The recommendations in this publication do not indicate an exclusive course of treatment or serve as a standard of medical care. Variations, taking into account individual circumstances, may be appropriate.

Statements and opinions expressed are those of the authors and not necessarily those of the American Academy of Pediatrics.

Any websites, brand names, products, or manufacturers are mentioned for informational and identification purposes only and do not imply an endorsement by the American Academy of Pediatrics (AAP). The AAP is not responsible for the content of external resources. Information was current at the time of publication.

The persons whose photographs are depicted in this publication are professional models. They have no relation to the issues discussed. Any characters they are portraying are fictional.

The publishers have made every effort to trace the copyright holders for borrowed materials. If they have inadvertently overlooked any, they will be pleased to make the necessary arrangements at the first opportunity.

This publication has been developed by the American Academy of Pediatrics. The contributors are expert authorities in the field of pediatrics. No commercial involvement of any kind has been solicited or accepted in the development of the content of this publication. Disclosures: Dr Ann Dietrich has disclosed a nonfinancial relationship as an associate medical director with EPC. Dr Kory Lane has disclosed a financial relationship as a board member with NAEMSE and a financial relationship as an author with ITLS. Any other disclosures were reviewed and determined not relevant to the work related to *Pediatric Education for Prehospital Professionals*, 5th Edition. Disclosures are reviewed and mitigated through a Conflict of Interest process that consists of reviewing pertinent information which is then used to decide what action is required to maintain content integrity. There may be instances where no action is necessary. This process has been approved by the AAP Board of Directors.

Every effort has been made to ensure that the drug selection and dosages set forth in this publication are in accordance with the current recommendations and practice at the time of publication. It is the responsibility of the health care professional to check the package insert of each drug for any change in indications or dosage and for added warnings and precautions.

Every effort is made to keep *Pediatric Education for Prehospital Professionals,* 5th Edition, consistent with the most recent advice and information available from the American Academy of Pediatrics.

Please visit www.aap.org/errata for an up-to-date list of any applicable errata for this publication.

Special discounts are available for bulk purchases of this publication. Email Special Sales at nationalaccounts@aap.org for more information.

Printed in the United States of America

5-331/0926 1 2 3 4 5 6 7 8 9 10

MA1200
ISBN: 978-1-61002-846-2
eISBN: 978-1-61002-847-9

Cover design by Michael Chang

Publication design by Peg Mulcahy

The American Academy of Pediatrics gratefully acknowledges the generous support of Laerdal Medical toward the publication of *Pediatric Education for Prehospital Professionals,* 5th Edition.

Library of Congress Control Number: 2025933468

American Academy of Pediatrics Reviewers

American Academy of Pediatrics Board of Directors
Committee on Infectious Diseases
Committee on Medical Liability and Risk Management
Committee on Pediatric Emergency Medicine
Council on Child Abuse and Neglect
Council on Children With Disabilities
Council on Injury, Violence, and Poison Prevention
Neonatal Resuscitation Program Steering Committee
Section on Cardiology and Cardiac Surgery
Section on Child Death Review and Prevention
Section on Clinical Pharmacology and Therapeutics
Section on Emergency Medicine
Section on Endocrinology
Section on Neonatal-Perinatal Medicine
Section on Neurology
Section on Transport Medicine

Pediatric Education for Prehospital Professionals Steering Committee

Jennifer F. Anders, MD, FAAP
Associate Editor, *Pediatric Education for Prehospital Professionals,* 5th Edition
Associate Professor of Pediatrics
The Johns Hopkins University School of Medicine
Baltimore, MD
Associate State Medical Director for Pediatrics
Maryland Institute of Emergency Medical Services Systems
Baltimore, MD

Kathleen Adelgais, MD, MPH, FAAP, FAEMS
Liaison, National Association of EMS Physicians
Professor, Pediatrics and Emergency Medicine
Department of Pediatrics
University of Colorado School of Medicine
Aurora, CO

Jermaine Clayborne, MSN, APRN, NEA-BC, NNP-BC, CCRN-Neonatal, CCRN-Adult, CFRN, FP-C of Virginia
Liaison, Emergency Nurses Association
Director
University of Virginia Health Medical Transport Network
Charlottesville, VA

Rehman Chowdhry, MD, FAAP
Attending Neonatologist
Neonatal Transport Director
Associate Professor of Pediatrics
Department of Pediatrics, Division of Neonatology
Albany Medical Center
Albany, NY

Marshal Cloud
Liaison, International Association of Fire Fighters
Fire-Based EMS Specialist
International Association of Fire Fighters
Washington, DC

Susan Fuchs, MD, FAAP, FACEP
Coeditor, *Pediatric Education for Prehospital Professionals,* 5th Edition
Professor of Pediatrics
Northwestern University Feinberg School of Medicine
Attending Physician, Division of Emergency Medicine
EMS Medical Director
Ann & Robert H. Lurie Children's Hospital of Chicago
Chicago, IL

Kevin Joles
Liaison, International Association of Fire Chiefs
Chair, International Association of Fire Chiefs—Emergency Medical Services Section
Division Chief, Emergency Medical Services
Olathe Fire Department
Olathe, KS

Rudy Kink, MD, FAAP
Chair, Pediatric Education for Prehospital Professionals Steering Committee
Section on Transport Medicine Liaison
Professor of Pediatrics
University of Tennessee Health Science Center
Medical Director, Pedi-Flite
Department of Emergency Medicine
Le Bonheur Children's Hospital
Memphis, TN

Mike McEvoy, PhD, NRP, RN, CCRN
Coeditor, *Pediatric Education for Prehospital Professionals,* 5th Edition
EMS Coordinator
Saratoga County
Ballston Spa, NY
Nurse Clinician, Adult & Pediatric Cardiac Surgical Intensive Care Units
Albany Medical Center
Albany, NY
Chief Medical Officer
West Crescent Fire Department
Halfmoon, NY
Board Chair
National Registry of Emergency Medical Technicians
Columbus, OH

Vishal Naik, MD, MEd, FAAP
Medical Director, Center for Transport Medicine
Ann & Robert H. Lurie Children's Hospital of Chicago
Assistant Professor of Pediatrics
Northwestern University Feinberg School of Medicine
Chicago, IL

Karen J. O'Connell, MD, Med, FAAP
Professor of Pediatrics
Professor of Emergency Medicine
The George Washington University School of Medicine and Health Sciences
Children's National Hospital
Washington, DC

Megan Petrucelli, MSN, RN, EMSI, CEN, CPEN
National Association of State EMS Officials Liaison
Program Coordinator, Connecticut Emergency Medical Services for Children
Yale New Haven Health System
Cromwell, CT

Beth Spurlin, MD, FAAP, PhD, MBA
American College of Emergency Physicians Liaison
Associate Professor of Pediatrics
University of Louisville School of Medicine
Louisville, KY

Carlene Thornton, EdD, NRP
Liaison, National Association of EMS Educators
Education Content Director
National Association of EMS Educators
Pittsburgh, PA

Theresa A. Walls, MD, MPH, FAAP
Associate Professor of Clinical Pediatrics
Perelman School of Medicine
University of Pennsylvania
Attending Physician
The Children's Hospital of Philadelphia
Philadelphia, PA

AAP STAFF

Erica Kane, MPH, CHES
Manager, First Responder & Lay Provider Initiatives

Karen Kostakis
Clinical Skills Training Assistant

Jessica Weglarz, MBA
Senior Director, Clinical Skills Training

Contributors

EDITORS

Susan Fuchs, MD, FAAP, FACEP
Coeditor, *Pediatric Education for Prehospital Professionals,* 5th Edition
Professor of Pediatrics
Northwestern University Feinberg School of Medicine
Attending Physician, Division of Emergency Medicine
EMS Medical Director
Ann & Robert H. Lurie Children's Hospital of Chicago
Chicago, IL

Mike McEvoy, PhD, NRP, RN, CCRN
Coeditor, *Pediatric Education for Prehospital Professionals,* 5th Edition
EMS Coordinator
Saratoga County
Ballston Spa, NY
Nurse Clinician, Adult & Pediatric Cardiac Surgical Intensive Care Units
Albany Medical Center
Albany, NY
Chief Medical Officer
West Crescent Fire Department
Halfmoon, NY
Immediate Past Board Chair
National Registry of Emergency Medical Technicians
Columbus, OH

Jennifer F. Anders, MD, FAAP
Associate Editor, *Pediatric Education for Prehospital Professionals,* 5th Edition
Associate Professor of Pediatrics
The Johns Hopkins University School of Medicine
Baltimore, MD
Associate State Medical Director for Pediatrics
Maryland Institute for Emergency Medical Services Systems
Baltimore, MD

CONTRIBUTORS

Kathleen Adelgais, MD, MPH, FAAP, FAEMS
Professor, Pediatrics and Emergency Medicine
Department of Pediatrics
University of Colorado School of Medicine
Aurora, CO

Aaron Bates, NRP
Director, Emergency Medical Technician Program
Contra Costa College
San Pablo, CA

Debra L. Bell, MS, CCEMTP, EMT-T, NJ-CEM
Paramedic, Field Training Officer and Educator
Inspira Health Emergency Medical Services
Richland, NJ

T.J. Bishop, AS, NRP, NCEE
Assistant Chief
San Juan Island EMS
Friday Harbor, WA

Elizabeth Blizzard, BA, NRP, FP-C, CCP-C
Advanced Life Support Educator
Capital Health
Pennington, NJ

Archana Reddy Bongurala, MD, FAAP
Pediatrician
Omni Family Health
Bakersfield, CA

Jonathan P. Carolla, BSc, NRP, FPC
Education Coordinator—EMS & Critical Care/Flight Paramedic
Penn State Health Life Lion
Hershey, PA

Theresa Censoplano, MS, RN, NRP
Registered Nurse and Paramedic
Ascension St. Thomas Emergency Medical Services
Nashville, TN

Alexandra Cheetham, MD, MEd, FAAP
Assistant Professor of Pediatrics
Cincinnati Children's Hospital Medical Center, Division of Emergency Medicine
University of Cincinnati College of Medicine
Cincinnati, Ohio

Tabitha Cheng, MD
Director of Prehospital Education and Research
Harbor-UCLA Medical Center
Torrance, CA

Rehman Chowdhry, MD, FAAP
Attending Neonatologist
Neonatal Transport Director
Associate Professor of Pediatrics
Department of Pediatrics, Division of Neonatology
Albany Medical Center
Albany, NY

Chris Coughlin, PhD, NRP
Program Director, Paramedic Studies
Contra Costa College
San Pablo, CA

Sean Davis, MSEd, CIC, NRP, FESI-2
Director of Public Safety
Auburn Career Center
Concord, OH

Ann Dietrich, MD, FAAP, FACEP
Division Chief, Pediatric Emergency Medicine
Department of Emergency Medicine
Prisma Health
Greenville, SC
Clinical Professor of Pediatrics and Emergency Medicine
University of South Carolina School of Medicine
Columbia, SC

Tyler Diettert, NREMTP, EC
Lieutenant Firefighter and Paramedic
Prince William County Fire & Rescue System
Prince William, VA

H. Joel Dishroon, PM, IC
Captain, Training Officer
CHI Memorial Hospital Emergency Medical Services
Chattanooga, TN

Shea Duerring, MD, NRP, FAAP, FACEP, FAEMS
Associate Professor
The University of Alabama at Birmingham
Birmingham, AL

John A. Erbayri, MS, NRP, CHSE
Manager
Center for Life Support Education and Outreach
Academy for Resuscitation of Children
Outreach Center for Expertise in Pediatric Emergency Readiness and Training (ExPERT)
Children's Hospital of Philadelphia
Philadelphia, PA

Claire Gahm, MD, MPH, FAAP
Assistant Professor of Pediatric Emergency Medicine, EMS and Global Health
Children's Hospital Colorado
Aurora, CO

Michael K. Kim, MD, FAAP
Associate Professor of Emergency Medicine & Pediatrics
BerbeeWalsh Department of Emergency Medicine
University of Wisconsin–Madison
Madison, WI

Rudy Kink, MD, FAAP
Professor of Pediatrics
University of Tennessee Health Science Center
Medical Director, Pedi-Flite
Department of Emergency Medicine
Le Bonheur Children's Hospital
Memphis, TN

Kory Lane, MEd, NRP, FP-C, CCP-C, NCEE
Director/Instructor, Emergency Medical Services
Piedmont Community College
Roxboro, NC

Kayla Long, DO, MS, MAPP, FACEP, FAEMS
EMS Physician
Centra Health
Forest, VA

Franscesca Miquel-Verges, MD
Professor
University of Arkansas for Medical Sciences
Arkansas Children's Hospital
Little Rock, AR

Amy Mitchell-Van Steele, PharmD, FPPA
Senior Clinical Pharmacy Specialist, Women and Children
Albany Med Health System
Albany Medical Center
Albany, NY

Tyler Molleur, MSN, RN, CEN, TCRN, CPEN, CTRN, CFRN, AEMT
Clinical Assistant Professor
University of Vermont
Burlington, VT

Maggie Coen Murphy, BS, EMT-P
Ambulance Commander—Retired
Chicago Fire Department
Chicago, IL

Vishal Naik, MD, MEd, FAAP
Medical Director, Center for Transport Medicine
Ann & Robert H. Lurie Children's Hospital of Chicago
Assistant Professor of Pediatrics
Northwestern University Feinberg School of Medicine
Chicago, IL

Karen J. O'Connell, MD, MEd, FAAP
Professor of Pediatrics
Professor of Emergency Medicine
The George Washington University School of Medicine and Health Sciences
Children's National Hospital
Washington, DC

Dawn Poetter, Oregon Paramedic
Oregon State Paramedic
Oregon EMS Education Foundation
Hillsboro, OR

Robert Sharkey, EMT-P, IC
Performance Improvement Coordinator and Instructor
United Ambulance Service
Lewiston, ME

Michael J. Stoner, MD, FAAP
Professor of Pediatrics
University of Central Florida, College of Medicine
Orlando, FL
Chief, Emergency Medicine and Urgent Care
Nemours Children's Hospital
Orlando, FL

Matthew R. Streger, Esq, MPA, NRP
Attorney
Keavney & Streger, LLC
Princeton, NJ

Hoi See Tsao, MD, MPH
Assistant Professor of Pediatric Emergency Medicine
Department of Pediatrics
UT Southwestern Medical Center
Dallas, TX

Theresa A. Walls, MD, MPH, FAAP
Associate Professor of Clinical Pediatrics
Perelman School of Medicine
University of Pennsylvania
Attending Physician
The Children's Hospital of Philadelphia
Philadelphia, PA

Evelyn Wilson, EdD, NRP, NCEE
Program Director, Emergency Medical Care
Teaching Associate Professor
College of Health and Human Sciences
Western Carolina University
Cullowhee, NC

Contents

Preface

***Pediatric Education for Prehospital Professionals,* 5th Edition: Written by EMS for EMS**

We are excited to present *Pediatric Education for Prehospital Professionals* (*PEPP*), 5th Edition, the gold standard in pediatric emergency care, designed to equip prehospital professionals with the knowledge and skills they need. As always, the content within this manual has been meticulously crafted by a dedicated team of emergency medical services clinicians and physicians, each bringing extensive expertise in prehospital care.

The foundations of PEPP were established in the 1990s, with their origins in state EMS for Children programs in California and Washington. Dr Ron Dieckmann in San Francisco, CA, conceived of the Pediatric Assessment Triangle (PAT) and wrote substantial portions of the early textbooks and student manuals. In southern California, Dr Marianne Gausche-Hill created the California Pediatric Airway Project, and Dr Dena Brownstein developed the Washington Pediatric Prehospital Care Project. On the groundwork laid by these early ventures, the American Academy of Pediatrics instituted the first National Steering Committee for PEPP in 1998, with Dr Dieckmann as its chairperson. For almost 3 decades, PEPP has remained the premier pediatric educational program for EMS clinicians. We acknowledge the lasting impact of prior leaders and are inspired by the fresh energy of many new contributors.

PEPP, 5th Edition, is at the heart of the PEPP course and has undergone a complete update and revision, featuring numerous exciting additions and enhancements to ensure its relevance and effectiveness in the ever-evolving field of emergency medical services.

What's New in the Fifth Edition

- **New Chapters:** Covering neurological emergencies, infectious disease, environmental and endocrine emergencies, and toxicology
- **Updated Procedures:** Including new push-pull fluid administration procedure
- **Enhanced Medication Formulary:** Now featuring additional medications
- **Family-Centered Care:** A renewed focus on this vital aspect of pediatric emergency treatment
- **Updated Visuals:** With refreshed images to improve understanding and application

We trust that these updates will make *PEPP*, 5th Edition, an even more dynamic, innovative, and flexible resource, better meeting your ongoing education needs in the field.

Susan Fuchs, MD, FAAP, FACEP
Mike McEvoy, PhD, NRP, RN, CCRN
Jennifer F. Anders, MD, FAAP

Acknowledgments

Photo Shoot Acknowledgments

We would like to thank the following institutions for their collaboration on the photo shoot for this project. Their assistance is greatly appreciated.

- Carol Stream Fire District Carol Stream, IL
- Le Bonheur Children's Hospital Memphis, TN

CHAPTER 1

Pediatric Assessment

Maggie Coen Murphy, BS, EMT–P
Vishal Naik, MD, MEd, FAAP

LEARNING OBJECTIVES

1. Describe Pediatric Education for Prehospital Professionals (PEPP) as a program that meets national education priorities in the emergency care of children.
2. Discuss the special challenges for the prehospital professional in pediatric assessment.
3. Recognize the key features of prearrival preparation and the scene size-up.
4. Differentiate the 3 elements of the Pediatric Assessment Triangle (PAT).
5. Describe the important pediatric considerations for each step in the hands-on airway-breathing-circulation (ABC) sequence of the primary assessment.
6. Discuss guidelines for when to stay on scene and treat, and when to immediately transport an ill or injured child, including appropriate mode of transport.
7. Recognize clinical situations requiring pain assessment and management.
8. Outline the unique considerations in the additional assessment of a child, including history taking, secondary assessment, monitoring devices, and ongoing reassessment.

CASE STUDY 1

A 9-year-old unhelmeted boy rode his bicycle out of his driveway into the path of an oncoming car. According to witnesses, the car was moving about 25 mph (40 kph), the victim was struck and thrown approximately 15 ft (4.5 m), and he was unconscious for 1 minute. On your arrival, the child is crying and anxious but responds appropriately to questions. He is complaining that his stomach hurts. The child has no abnormal airway sounds, grunting, flaring, or retracting. His skin is pale. The respiratory rate is 30 breaths/min, there are equal breath sounds with good air exchange, and the pulse oximetry reading is 98% on room air. His heart rate is 140 beats/min, and his blood pressure is 80/40 mm Hg. Capillary refill time is 4 seconds.

1. How badly injured is this child, and which physiological process requires your emergent attention?
2. Should this child's pain be treated?

Introduction

Caring for a critically ill or injured infant or child is one of the most stressful duties of the prehospital professional. Key history may be unreliable or unknown because the patient may be too young to have descriptive language, or the child may be afraid and unable to accurately recount the key events. The caregiver may be sobbing, frightened, and anxious for reassurance. Examination may be limited because of the child's small size and resistance to hands-on evaluation. **Vital signs** may be deceptive because of normal age-based variations and the difficulty in obtaining them accurately. It is the job of the prehospital professional to bring comfort to the child, caregiver, or family and to bring order to the chaos on scene. The prehospital professional must conduct an accurate assessment and deliver effective emergency treatment to the child.

The Pediatric Education for Prehospital Professionals (PEPP) course, developed by the American Academy of Pediatrics (AAP), provides the core cognitive knowledge and skills to prepare EMS clinicians for comprehensive assessment and management of any ill or injured infant and child. PEPP materials are designed to meet the national emergency medical services (EMS) education standards for all levels of emergency medical provider, as established by the US Department of Transportation's National Highway Traffic Safety Administration (NHTSA). Therefore, some of the terminology previously used in PEPP (general, initial, and additional assessment) has been modified to reflect the national EMS core content and the Definitions and Assessment Approaches for Emergency Medical Services for Children document.

Effective emergency care of children involves many professionals inside and outside of the hospital setting. Two of the most important concepts for comprehensive and high-quality prehospital pediatric emergency care are teamwork and prevention. Teamwork involves professionals working together to develop and implement comprehensive clinical services, professional education, and appropriate administrative oversight specifically for children.

Prevention involves professionals recognizing the limitations of an emergency care system oriented toward treatment after an illness or injury occurs and working to change potentially dangerous conditions before an event of this type occurs. Of all community activities that can improve children's overall health and well-being, prevention of acute injury and illness is by far the most cost-effective. "Making a difference," as described in detail in Chapter 19, involves new roles for EMS clinicians in injury and illness prevention, in their professional day-to-day duties, and as part of their activities as community leaders and health advocates.

TIP

A pediatric emergency care coordinator (PECC) can act as a liaison between EMS agencies and the hospital setting. Agency PECCs can help with protocol development, pediatric case reviews, agency pediatric quality assurance/quality improvement (QA/QI), ensure the presence of adequate pediatric supplies, assist in injury prevention activities, help promote family-centered care, identify local pediatric trends, and coordinate with emergency departments (EDs).

Accurate assessment of a child with an illness or injury requires special knowledge and skills. For patients of all ages, the prehospital professional's evaluation includes 4 steps: (1) scene size-up; (2) use of the **Pediatric Assessment Triangle (PAT)**; (3) primary assessment using the Airway, Breathing, Circulation, Disability (neurological status), and Exposure (skin/temperature) (ABCDE) assessment, vital signs, and pulse oximetry; and (4) **secondary assessment**, including a focused history, focused examination, monitoring devices, ongoing reassessment of physiological status, and response to treatment. The primary and secondary assessments have well-defined components that follow the same sequence used for adult patients. However, all 4 steps in the primary assessment have important pediatric modifications. The tertiary assessment includes laboratory and radiologic tests that can include point-of-care laboratory tests in the prehospital setting, but these are usually performed in the ED.

Summary of Assessment Flowchart

This chapter introduces a flowchart (below) that reflects the sequence of pediatric assessment taught by the PEPP course. The flowchart reinforces the interconnecting relationships of the different assessment components. Sometimes the assessment sequence must be stopped after the primary assessment to allow the prehospital professional to treat potentially life-threatening problems and initiate transport. For example, when a child has a critical injury, the secondary assessment must be deferred until after the child has been resuscitated and stabilized.

Reassessment, however, is required in every case to monitor response to treatment, guide further interventions, and assist with transport and triage decisions. Monitoring devices such as a pulse oximeter or end-tidal CO_2 monitor and bedside glucose checks may provide valuable adjunctive data to confirm and guide treatment in the prehospital setting.

Scene Size-Up

↓

Pediatric Assessment Triangle (PAT)

↓

Primary Assessment
Hands-on ABCDEs
Vital Signs
Pulse Oximetry
Transport Decision: Stay or Go

↓

Secondary Assessment
History Taking
Physical Examination
Monitoring Devices
Ongoing Reassessment

Scene Size-Up

On the way to the scene, prepare mentally to approach and treat an infant or child, and to interact with a distressed family. This means planning for a pediatric scene size-up, pediatric equipment and medication requirements, and age-appropriate assessment. All pediatric equipment and medications should be routinely checked, as they are less often used by most EMS clinicians and it is easy to forget their application. The information from dispatch on age and sex of the child, location of the scene, and chief complaint or mechanism of injury (or both) is the basis for prearrival preparation.

At the scene, begin the size-up by looking for possible safety threats to the EMS clinicians, child, caregiver, and/or bystanders. Examples of safety threats include spilled toxins, open containers of alcohol, drug paraphernalia, weapons, or fire. The child may be a safety threat if they have an infectious disease, such as **varicella** or **meningococcemia**, which may require the prehospital professional to don personal protective equipment.

TIP

On the way to the scene, mentally rehearse your approach to the assessment and treatment of an infant or a child and the expected interaction with a caregiver or family. Dispatch information, when available, about the child's age can be helpful to mentally prepare for age-appropriate developmental considerations and for anticipating equipment and medication requirements for assessment and treatment.

Evaluating the setting includes an inspection of the physical environment and watching family–child or caregiver–child interactions (**FIGURE 1-1**). For example, documenting observations of dangerous scene conditions and inappropriate statements from caregivers greatly assists child protective services if the child is later determined to be a victim of child maltreatment. On the scene, be like a sponge; soak up as much useful information as possible. Also, ensure scene safety for both your team and the child.

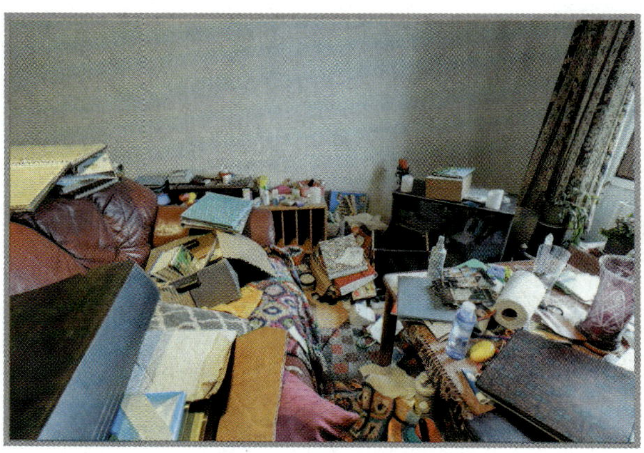

FIGURE 1-1 Environmental assessment.

The Pediatric Assessment Triangle

After the scene size-up, begin an assessment of the child, which must have a developmentally appropriate approach. This assessment includes a visual and auditory general impression of the child and uses the PAT as a standardized method to gather this information.

Rapid assessment is essential to determine the level of acuity and urgency for treatment and transport. Ask yourself, "Is the patient sick or not sick?" In the case of a child who is a victim of trauma with a known mechanism of injury, or of a child with a clear-cut complaint of pain in a specific anatomical location, the assessment may be straightforward. Still, careful evaluation is needed to identify less obvious, but potentially serious, injuries or **physiological** instability. For a child with an illness, the assessment may be much trickier. The prehospital professional must elicit information on the onset, duration, severity, and progression of symptoms, often from a child who cannot accurately provide such history. Moreover, illness complaints may be vague and less specific to an anatomical region. Whether the child has an injury or

Scene Size-Up
↓
Pediatric Assessment Triangle (PAT)
↓
Primary Assessment
Hands-on ABCDEs
Vital Signs
Pulse Oximetry
Transport Decision: Stay or Go
↓
Secondary Assessment
History Taking
Physical Examination
Monitoring Devices
Ongoing Reassessment

illness, the PAT helps to identify physiological instability, direct resuscitation priorities, and determine the timing of transport.

DEVELOPING A GENERAL IMPRESSION: THE PAT

The PAT is an easy tool to use during the rapid assessment of any child (**FIGURE 1–2**). It allows the prehospital professional to develop a first general impression of the patient's status with only visual and auditory clues. By using the PAT at the point of first contact with the patient, the prehospital professional can immediately establish a level of severity, determine urgency of need for life support, and identify the general type of physiologic problem. Continued use of the PAT gives the prehospital professional a way to track response to therapy and determine timing of transport. It also allows for communication among medical professionals about the child's physiological status and for accurate radio reporting.

There are 3 components of the PAT that together reflect the child's overall physiological status: (1) appearance, (2) work of breathing, and (3) circulation to the skin. The PAT is based on listening and seeing and does not require a stethoscope, blood pressure cuff, cardiac monitor, or pulse oximeter. The PAT should be completed in less than 30 seconds and is designed to organize a time-honored process of "across the room assessment," an intuitive process that experienced pediatric providers do instinctively.

> **TIP**
> Use the PAT at the point of initial contact with every child, regardless of age or presenting complaint.

> **TIP**
> The elements of the PAT incorporate auditory and visual clues that should be obtained from "across the room," without appearing threatening to an already anxious child.

Together, the physical characteristics of the PAT provide an accurate initial picture of the child's underlying cardiopulmonary status and level of consciousness. Although the PAT does not necessarily lead to a diagnosis, it identifies the general category of the physiological problem and establishes urgency of need for treatment or transport. The PAT does not replace traditional vital signs and the essentials of airway, breathing, and circulation (the ABCs), which are part of the primary assessment in the next phase of the physical evaluation.

The patient characteristics emphasized by the 3 arms of the PAT did not originate with PEPP. Experienced pediatric health care providers developed these characteristics to share the intuitive assessment skills needed to obtain a rapid first general impression of ill or injured children. What is unique about the PAT is its systematic approach to making, integrating, and communicating these observations. The PAT is the cornerstone of the PEPP course. Use

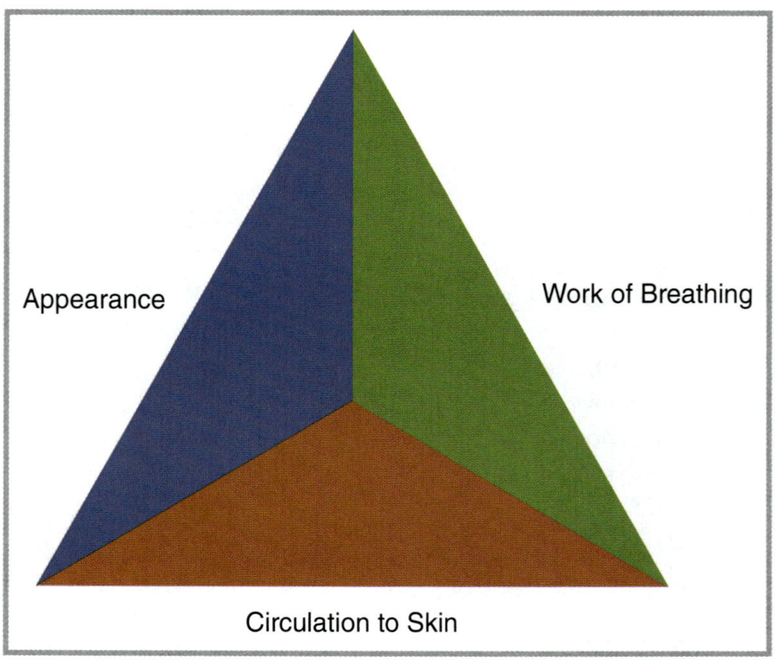

FIGURE 1–2 Pediatric Assessment Triangle (PAT).

TABLE 1–1 Characteristics of Appearance: The "Tickles" (TICLS) Mnemonic

Component	Characteristic Features
▪ Tone	Is the child moving or vigorously resisting examination? Do they have good muscle tone? Or are they limp, listless, or flaccid?
▪ Interactiveness	How alert is the child? How readily does a person, object, or sound distract them or draw their attention? Will they reach for, grasp, and play with a toy or examination instrument, such as a penlight? Or are they uninterested in playing or interacting with the caregiver?
▪ Consolability	Can they be consoled or comforted by the caregiver? Or is their crying or agitation unrelieved by gentle reassurance?
▪ Look/Gaze	Does the child fix their gaze on a face? Or is there a "nobody home," glassy-eyed stare?
▪ Speech/Cry	Is the child's speech or cry strong and spontaneous? Or is it weak, muffled, or hoarse?

the PAT in every encounter with every child. Over time, it will become an indispensable and spontaneous method of making a rapid initial "sick or not sick" assessment of ill or injured children of all ages.

Appearance

Characteristics of Appearance. The child's general appearance is the most important factor in determining the severity of the illness or injury, the need for treatment, and the response to therapy. Appearance reflects the adequacy of ventilation, oxygenation, **brain perfusion**, body **homeostasis**, and **central nervous system (CNS)** function. There are many characteristics of appearance; the most important are summarized in the "tickles" (TICLS) mnemonic: tone, interactiveness, consolability, look/gaze, and speech/cry (**TABLE 1–1**).

CAUTION

In assessing patients with mild to moderate illness or injury, numerical "scoring" methodologies and severity scales for levels of consciousness are rarely useful. These classical neurological evaluation systems work best in patients with severe injury or illness as a tool to monitor for changes in children with serious brain dysfunction.

Identifying abnormal appearance is a better way to detect subtle abnormalities in behavior than the conventional **"alert, verbal, painful, unresponsive" (AVPU) scale** or the Pediatric Glasgow Coma Scale (GCS) for neurological evaluation. Most children with mild to moderate illness or injury are "alert" on the AVPU or "15" on the Pediatric GCS. Children with an abnormal appearance must be assumed to have a potentially serious underlying problem.

Therefore, assessing a child's appearance is the most useful first thing to do in evaluating every pediatric patient.

TIP

Never ignore the pale infant, the "nobody-home stare," or the infant who does not respond appropriately to stimulation.

Techniques to Assess Appearance. Assess the child's appearance from the doorway. This is step 1 in the PAT. Techniques for assessment of a conscious child's appearance include observing from a distance; allowing the child to remain in the caregiver's lap or arms; using distraction tools, such as bright lights or toys, to measure the child's ability to interact; and kneeling down to be at eye level with the child. An immediate "hands-on" approach may cause agitation and crying and may complicate the assessment. Unless a child is unconscious or obviously critically ill, get as much information as possible by observing the child before touching the child or taking vital signs.

One example of a child with a normal appearance is an infant who holds themself upright in the caregiver's arms, makes good eye contact, and has good color (**FIGURE 1–3**). An example of an infant or child with a worrisome appearance is one who makes poor eye contact with the caregiver or prehospital professional and is pale and listless (**FIGURE 1–4**).

An abnormal appearance may have many causes including the following: inadequate oxygenation, ventilation, or brain perfusion; systemic abnormalities, such as poisoning, infection, or **hypoglycemia**; or acute or chronic brain injury. Regardless of the cause,

TIP

The child's general appearance is the single most important feature when assessing severity of illness or injury, need for treatment, and response to therapy.

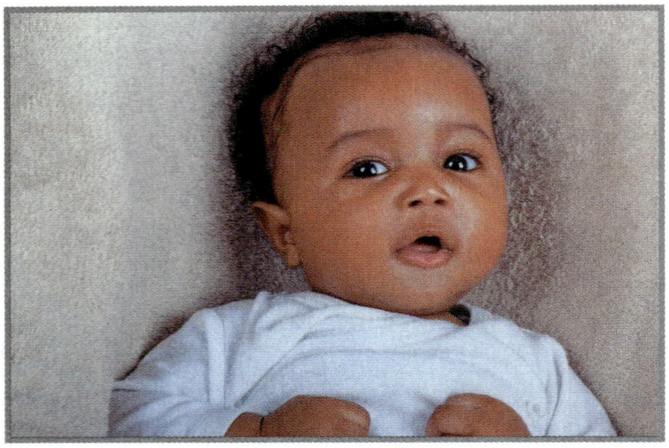

FIGURE 1–3 Good eye contact in a child is normal and a sign of a good appearance.

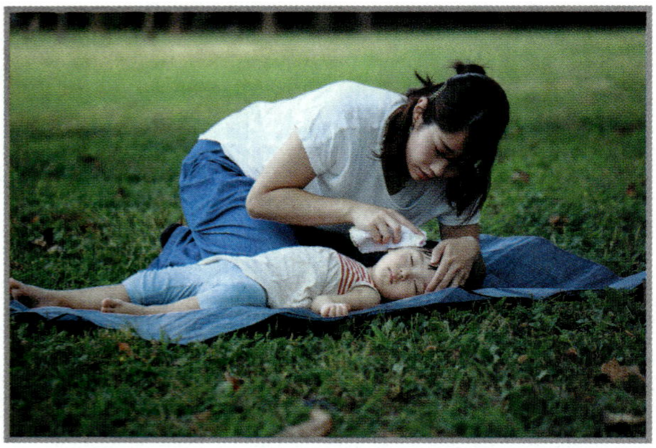

FIGURE 1–4 A limp, pale child unable to make eye contact or a child with retractions may be critically ill or injured.

> **CAUTION**
> **Although an alert, interactive child is usually not critically ill, there are some exceptions to the reliability of general appearance as an indicator of stable cardiopulmonary and neurological function. The most common exceptions are ingestions with delayed physiological effects and blunt injury with slow internal bleeding.**

a child with a grossly abnormal appearance is seriously ill or injured and needs immediate life support efforts to increase oxygenation, ventilation, and perfusion.

Although an alert, interactive child is usually not critically ill, there are some cases in which a child may have life-threatening problems despite an initially normal appearance. Toxicologic or traumatic emergencies are good examples:

1. A child with acetaminophen, iron, or **cyclic antidepressant** overdose may not show symptoms immediately after ingestion. Despite their normal appearance, the child may develop deadly complications in the coming minutes or hours.
2. A child with blunt trauma and solid organ injury may be able to maintain adequate **core perfusion**, despite internal bleeding, by increasing cardiac output and systemic vascular resistance; therefore, the child may appear normal during the primary assessment. However, when these **compensatory mechanisms** fail, the child may acutely "crash," with rapid progression to **hypotensive (decompensated) shock**. Pallor may be the only finding on the PAT that suggests impending disaster.

A benign appearance should never justify a denial of transport. However, depending on the chief complaint, a normal appearance usually means that a transport with lights and siren is not necessary. Follow your system protocol(s) with regard to the use of lights and sirens.

Age differences are associated with important developmental differences in psychomotor and social skills. "Normal" appearance and behavior vary by age group, as discussed in Chapter 2. Children of all ages engage with their environment: newborns do this through energetic sucking and crying; older infants by smiling or tracking a light; toddlers through physical exploration; and adolescents through speech. Knowledge of normal child development through the age groups should guide the assessment of appearance and result in more accurate treatment and transport decisions. Although appearance reflects the severity of illness or injury, it does not identify the cause. Appearance is the "screening" portion of the PAT. The other elements of the PAT (work of breathing and circulation to the skin) provide more specific information about the type of physiological derangement, while giving additional clues about severity.

Work of Breathing

Characteristics of Work of Breathing. In children, **work of breathing** is a more accurate indicator of oxygenation and ventilation than respiratory rate or breath sounds on auscultation, the standard measures of breathing effectiveness in adults. Work of breathing reflects the child's attempt to compensate for abnormalities in oxygenation and ventilation, and it is a proxy for the effectiveness of gas exchange. This component of the PAT requires listening carefully for abnormal airway sounds and looking for signs of increased breathing effort. It is another "hands-off" evaluation method that does not require a stethoscope or pulse oximeter. **TABLE 1–2** summarizes the key characteristics of work of breathing.

TABLE 1–2 Characteristics of Work of Breathing

Characteristic	Features to Look For
Abnormal airway sounds	Snoring, muffled or hoarse speech, stridor, grunting, wheezing
Abnormal positioning	Sniffing position, tripoding, refusing to lie down
Retractions	Supraclavicular, intercostal, or substernal retractions of the chest wall; head bobbing in infants
Flaring	Flaring of the nares on inspiration

Abnormal Airway Sounds. Examples of abnormal airway sounds that can be heard without a stethoscope are snoring, muffled or hoarse speech, stridor, grunting, and wheezing. Abnormal airway sounds provide information about the physiology and anatomical location of the breathing problem.

Upper Airway. Snoring, muffled or hoarse speech, and stridor suggest an upper airway obstruction. Snoring or gurgling occurs when the **oropharynx** is partially obstructed by the tongue and soft tissues. Muffled or hoarse speech reflects inflammation of the **glottis** or **supraglottic** structures. **Stridor** is a high-pitched sound heard on inspiration, or during inspiration and expiration, reflecting an obstruction at the level of the glottis or subglottic trachea. All of these sounds reflect abnormal airflow through partially obstructed upper airway structures. Obstruction of the upper airway passages can occur in a variety of illnesses and injuries, including croup, foreign body aspiration, and bacterial upper airway infections, or as a result of bleeding or edema.

Lower Airway. Abnormal lower airway sounds that may be heard during the PAT include **grunting** and **wheezing**. Grunting is a sound produced by partial closure of the glottis on the end of expiration. Grunting is a form of auto positive end-expiratory pressure, a way to distend lower respiratory tract air sacs (**alveoli**) to promote maximum gas exchange. Grunting involves exhaling against a partially closed glottis. This short, low-pitched sound is best heard at the end of the exhalation and is easily mistaken for whimpering.

Grunting is often present in children with moderate to severe hypoxia, and it reflects poor gas exchange caused by obstruction in the lower airways and alveoli. Conditions that cause hypoxia and grunting are **pneumonia**, **pulmonary contusion** (bruising of the lungs), and **pulmonary edema** (a build-up of fluid in the lungs).

Wheezing is the result of movement of air across partially blocked small airways. At first, wheezing usually occurs during exhalation and can be heard only by **auscultation** of the chest with a stethoscope. As the airway obstruction increases and breathing requires more work, wheezing is often present during inhalation and exhalation. With more obstruction, wheezing may be audible without a stethoscope. Finally, if respiratory failure develops, work of breathing may diminish and the wheezing may not be heard at all. The most common cause of wheezing in childhood is **asthma**, although wheezing may also be associated with **bronchiolitis** (a viral respiratory infection in infants, typically not responsive to albuterol) and lower airway foreign body aspiration.

TIP

Abnormal airway sounds can provide excellent information about breathing effort, type of breathing problem, location of the breathing problem, and potential degree of hypoxia.

Visual Signs of Increased Work of Breathing. There are several useful visual signs of increased work of breathing. These signs reflect an increased breathing effort by the child to improve oxygenation and ventilation. The presence of certain physical features, such as abnormal positioning, retractions, and nasal flaring, reflects overall illness or injury severity. Abnormal positioning is usually evident from the doorway. There are several types of abnormal postures that can indicate the child is struggling to improve airflow. A child who is in the **sniffing position** is trying to align the axes of the airways to improve patency and increase airflow (**FIGURE 1–5**). This position is usually the result of severe upper airway obstruction. The child who lifts their chin attempting to swallow could indicate a foreign body. The child who refuses to lie down, or who leans forward on outstretched arms (**tripoding**), is creating optimal mechanical positioning to use accessory muscles of respiration (**FIGURE 1–6**). The sniffing position and tripoding are abnormal and indicate airway obstruction, increased work of breathing, and severe respiratory distress.

Retractions are physical signs of increased work of breathing. Retractions represent the recruitment

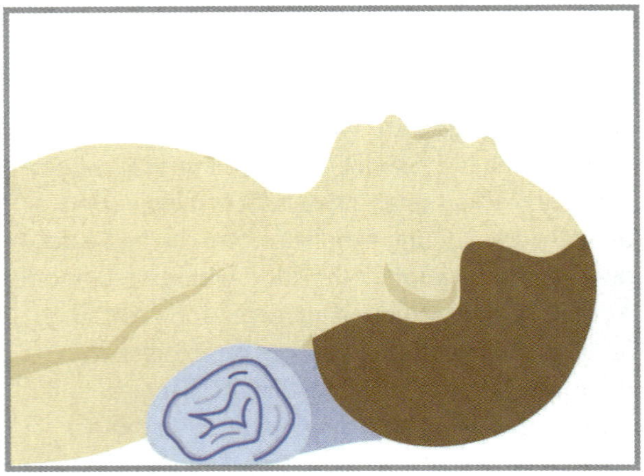

FIGURE 1-5 The sniffing position opens up the airways to improve patency.

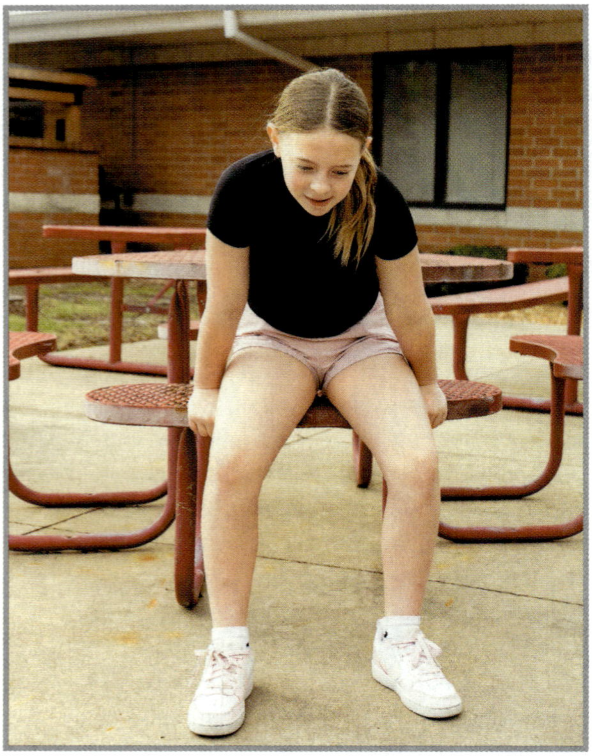

FIGURE 1-6 The abnormal tripod position indicates the patient's attempts to maximize accessory muscle use.

of accessory muscles of respiration to provide more "muscle power" to move air into the lungs in the face of airway or lung disease or injury. To optimally observe retractions, expose the child's chest. Retractions are a more useful measure of work of breathing in children than in adults, because a child's chest wall is less muscular and the inward excursion of skin and soft tissue between the ribs is more apparent. Retractions may be in the **supraclavicular** area (above the clavicle), the **intercostal** area (between the ribs), or the **substernal** area (under the sternum), as illustrated in **FIGURE 1-7**. Another form of accessory muscle use seen only in infants is "**head bobbing**," which is the use of neck muscles to assist breathing during times of severe hypoxia. The infant extends the neck as they inhale and then allows the head to fall forward as they exhale.

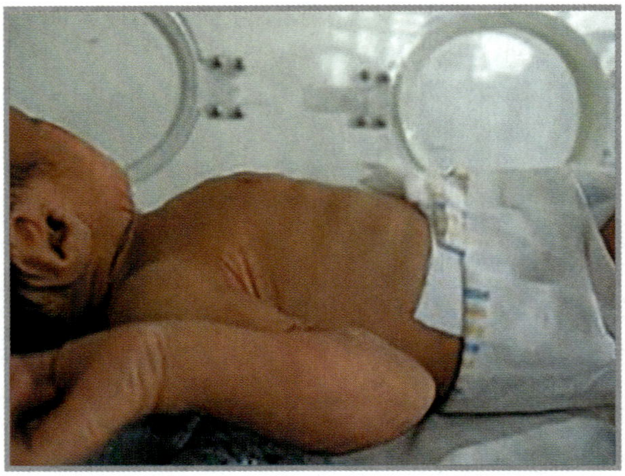

FIGURE 1-7 Retractions indicate increased work of breathing and may occur in the supraclavicular, intercostal, and substernal areas.

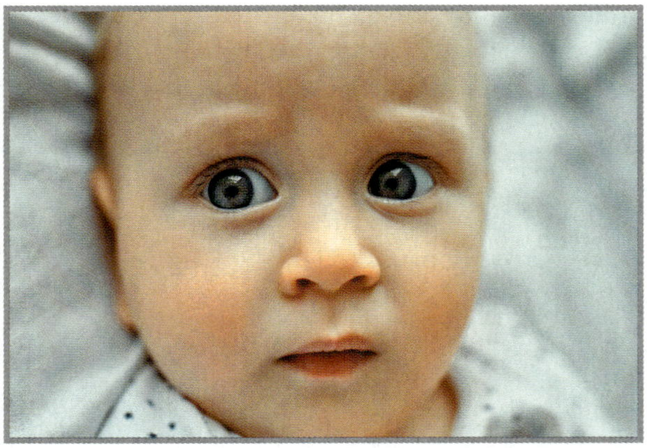

FIGURE 1-8 Nasal flaring indicates increased work of breathing and moderate-to-severe hypoxia.

Nasal flaring is another sign of increased work of breathing (**FIGURE 1-8**). **Nasal flaring** is the exaggerated opening of the nostrils during labored inspiration and indicates moderate to severe hypoxia. It reflects the child's extra effort to breathe during **hypoxic stress**, usually caused by such conditions as croup, pneumonia, asthma, bronchiolitis, or pulmonary contusion.

TIP

Head bobbing is a form of accessory muscle use specific to infants and is indicative of increased work of breathing.

Assessment of Work of Breathing. Begin the assessment by listening carefully from a distance for abnormal airway sounds. Next, look for key physical signs. Note if the child has an abnormal posture, most notably the sniffing position or tripoding. Next, have the caregiver uncover the chest of the child for direct inspection, or have the child undress on the caregiver's lap. Look for intercostal, supraclavicular, and substernal retractions, and note if there is head bobbing in infants. After examining for retractions, inspect for nasal flaring. This stepwise process is critical for gathering accurate information. After an infant or child begins to cry, assessment of work of breathing becomes more difficult.

Children may have increased work of breathing because of abnormalities anywhere in their upper or lower airways, alveoli (air sacs), **pleura** (membrane surrounding the lungs and lining the walls of the pleural cavity), or chest wall. The type of abnormal airway sounds gives an important clue to the anatomical location of the illness or injury process, whereas the number and type of physical signs of increased work of breathing help in determining the degree of physiological stress.

Combining assessment of appearance and work of breathing can also help establish the severity of the child's illness or injury. A child with a normal appearance and increased work of breathing is in respiratory distress. An abnormal appearance and increased work of breathing suggest respiratory failure. An abnormal appearance and abnormally decreased work of breathing imply impending respiratory arrest.

Circulation to Skin

Characteristics of Circulation to Skin. The goal of rapid circulatory assessment is to determine the adequacy of cardiac output and core perfusion or perfusion of the vital organs. The child's appearance is one indicator of brain perfusion, but abnormal appearance may be caused by other conditions unrelated to circulation, such as hypoxia, hypoglycemia, brain injury, or intoxication. For this reason, other signs of adequacy of perfusion must be added to the evaluation of appearance to assess the child's true circulatory status.

An important sign of **core perfusion** is circulation to the skin. When cardiac output is inadequate, the body shuts down circulation to nonessential anatomical areas, such as the skin and mucous membranes, to preserve blood supply to the most vital organs (brain, heart, and kidneys). Therefore, circulation to the skin reflects the overall status of core circulation. **Pallor**, **mottling**, and **cyanosis** are key visual indicators of reduced circulation to the skin and mucous membranes. **TABLE 1–3** summarizes these characteristics.

TABLE 1–3 Characteristics of Circulation to Skin

Characteristic	Features to Look For
Pallor	White or pale mucous membrane coloration caused by inadequate blood flow
Mottling	Patchy skin discoloration caused by vasoconstriction or vasodilation
Cyanosis	Bluish discoloration of skin and mucous membranes

Pallor may be the first sign of poor skin or mucous membrane perfusion; it may be the only visual sign apparent in a child with compensated shock and indicates reflex peripheral vasoconstriction to shunt blood away from the skin to the core. Pallor may also be a sign of anemia or hypoxia. Mottling is another sign of inadequate skin perfusion, reflecting vasomotor instability (abnormal blood vessel tone) in the capillary beds of the skin. Mottled skin has patchy areas of **vasoconstriction** (pallor) mixed with areas of **vasodilatation** (cyanosis or erythema). Mottling may also be a normal physiological response in a child exposed to cold environmental temperatures.

Cyanosis is blue discoloration of the skin and mucous membranes. It is the most extreme visual indicator of poor perfusion or poor oxygenation. Do not confuse **acrocyanosis** (blue hands and feet in a newborn or infant less than 2 months of age) with true cyanosis.

Acrocyanosis is a normal finding when a young infant is cold, and it reflects **vasomotor** instability rather than hypoxia or shock. True cyanosis is a late finding of respiratory failure or **shock**. A hypoxic child is likely to show other physical abnormalities long before turning blue. These abnormalities may include abnormal appearance with agitation or lethargy and increased work of breathing. A child in shock may also have pallor or mottling. Never wait for cyanosis to begin treatment with supplemental oxygen. However, the presence of cyanosis is always a critical sign that requires immediate intervention with breathing support.

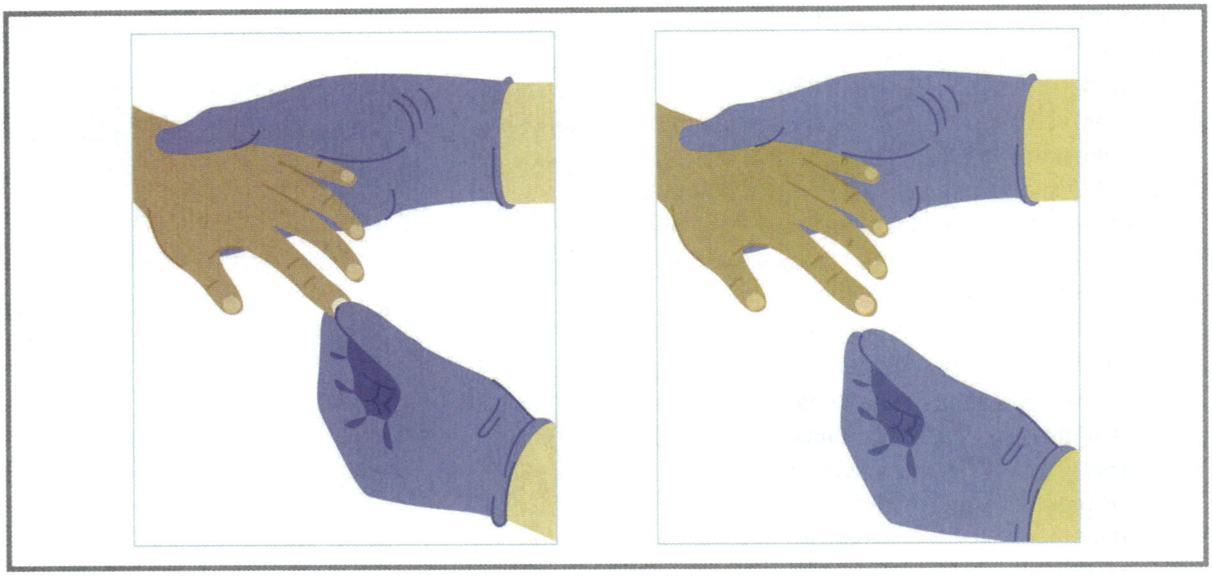

FIGURE 1–9 In dark-skinned children, circulation to the skin is sometimes more difficult to assess, and the lips, mucous membranes, and nail beds may be the best places to look for pallor or cyanosis.

Abnormal circulation to the skin, in combination with an abnormal appearance, suggests shock. However, the abnormalities in appearance in early phases of compensated shock may be subtle, and some children may remain alert. As perfusion worsens and compensatory mechanisms fail, appearance becomes abnormal, reflecting inadequate delivery of oxygen and glucose to the brain. Another clue to the presence of shock is **effortless tachypnea**, or **tachypnea** without signs of increased work of breathing. Effortless tachypnea is a reflex mechanism that allows the body to blow off carbon dioxide to compensate for the metabolic **acidosis** caused by poor peripheral perfusion (**lactic acidosis**). **Hypocarbia** (low blood CO_2 levels) generates a respiratory alkalosis and helps to restore normal pH (blood acid–base balance). Effortless tachypnea is different from the rapid and labored respirations that are present with illnesses and injuries associated with airway or lung pathology.

Assessment of Circulation to Skin. To begin the assessment, be sure the child is exposed long enough for visual inspection but not long enough to become cold. A cold child may have normal core perfusion but abnormal circulation to the skin. Cold circulating air temperature is the most common reason for misinterpretation of skin signs, and an exposed young infant may become hypothermic quickly, even at normal ambient temperatures.

Inspect the skin and mucous membranes for pallor, mottling, and cyanosis. Look at the face, chest, abdomen, and extremities, and then inspect the lips for cyanosis. In dark-skinned children, circulation to the skin is sometimes more difficult to assess, and the lips, mucous membranes, and nail beds are the best places to look for pallor or cyanosis (**FIGURE 1–9**). Combining assessment of appearance and circulation to the skin can also help establish the severity of the child's illness or injury. A child with a normal appearance and poor circulation to the skin is possibly cold. An abnormal appearance and circulation to the skin suggests the child is in shock.

Using the PAT to Evaluate Severity and Illness or Injury. The PAT provides a general impression of the pediatric patient. The intent is to provide a standardized approach to the "general impression" and an immediate picture of the child's physiological status. By combining the 3 components of the PAT, the prehospital professional should be able to answer 3 critical questions: (1) How severe is the child's illness or injury? (2) What is the most likely physiological abnormality? (3) What is the urgency of the need for treatment? This information helps the prehospital professional select the most important actions: how fast to intervene, what type of general and specific treatments to give, and how rapidly to transport.

The 3 elements of the PAT work together and allow a rapid assessment of the child's overall physiological stability. For example, if a child is interactive and pink but has mild intercostal retractions, the prehospital professional can take time to approach the child in a developmentally appropriate manner to complete the primary assessment. However, if the child is limp, with unlabored rapid breathing and pale or mottled skin, shock is likely. In this case, the prehospital professional must move rapidly through the primary assessment and begin resuscitation. A child who has an abnormal appearance, but normal work of breathing and normal circulation to skin, probably has a primary brain dysfunction or a major metabolic or systemic problem, such as **postictal state**, **subdural hemorrhage**, **concussion**, intoxication, hypoglycemia, or **sepsis**.

The PAT has 2 important advantages. First, it allows the examiner to quickly obtain critical information about the child's physiological status before touching or agitating the child. Second, the PAT helps set priorities for the rest of the hands-on primary assessment. The PAT takes only seconds, it helps to identify the need for lifesaving interventions, and it assists in the transition into the next phase of hands-on physical assessment.

The 3 components of the PAT (appearance, work of breathing, and circulation to the skin) can be assessed in any sequence, unlike the ordered ABCDEs of resuscitation discussed next.

TIP

By combining the 3 components of the PAT, the prehospital professional can answer 3 critical questions: (1) How sick or injured is the child? (2) What is the most likely physiological abnormality? (3) What is the urgency of need for treatment?

Scene Size-Up

↓

Pediatric Assessment Triangle (PAT)

↓

Primary Assessment

Hands-on ABCDEs

Vital Signs

Pulse Oximetry

Transport Decision: Stay or Go

↓

Secondary Assessment

History Taking

Physical Examination

Monitoring Devices

Ongoing Reassessment

Primary Assessment

HANDS-ON ABCDEs

The primary assessment continues the process of identifying life-threatening conditions using an ordered hands-on physical evaluation of the ABCDEs. It provides a prioritized sequence of life-support interventions to reverse critical physiological abnormalities. As in adults, there is a specific order for treating life-threatening problems as they are identified, before moving to the next step. The steps are the same, but there are important pediatric differences in anatomy, physiology, and signs of distress. The components of ABCDE assessment are as follows:

1. Airway
2. Breathing
3. Circulation
4. Disability
5. Exposure

AIRWAY

Assess the continued patency of the airway. The PAT may identify the presence of an airway obstruction based on the presence of abnormal airway sounds. However, the loudness of the stridor or wheezing is not necessarily related to the amount of airway obstruction. For example, children with asthma in severe distress may have little or no wheezing. Similarly, children with an upper airway foreign body below the **vocal cords** may have minimal stridor. Abnormal positioning and retractions provide further information about the degree of obstruction, as does the quality of air entry on auscultation during the hands-on assessment.

If the airway is open, ensure that the chest rises with each breath. If a child has assumed a position that maximizes their ability to maintain a spontaneously open airway, allow the child to remain in that position of comfort. If gurgling is present, there may be mucus, blood, or a foreign body in the mouth or upper airway. Oropharyngeal suctioning of mucus or blood, or removal of a visible foreign body, very often restores patency. If the airway is totally obstructed, advanced life support (ALS) interventions are necessary. Advanced life support interventions may also be necessary if the child's mental status does not support a sustained open airway.

BREATHING

Respiratory Rate. Verify the respiratory rate per minute by counting the number of chest rises in

30 seconds, then doubling that number. Interpret the respiratory rate carefully. Normal infants may show "periodic breathing" or variable respiratory rate with short (< 10 seconds) periods of apnea. Therefore, counting for only 10 to 15 seconds may give a falsely low respiratory rate.

The significance of respiratory rates may be confusing. Rapid respiratory rates may simply reflect high fever, anxiety, pain, or excitement. Normal rates, however, may occur in a child who has been breathing rapidly with increased work of breathing for some time and is now becoming fatigued. Finally, interpretation requires knowledge of normal values for age (**TABLE 1–4**).

> **TIP**
> "Red flag" respiratory rates are less than 20 breaths/min for children younger than 6 years and less than 12 breaths/min for children between 6 and 18 years of age.

Serial assessment of respiratory rates may be especially useful, and the trend is sometimes more accurate than any single value. A sustained increase or decrease in respiratory rate is usually significant.

Pay close attention to extremes of respiratory rate. A very rapid respiratory rate (> 60 breaths/min for any age), especially with abnormal appearance or marked retractions, indicates respiratory distress and possibly respiratory failure. An abnormally slow respiratory rate is always worrisome because it might mean respiratory failure. Red flags are respiratory rates less than 20 breaths/min for children younger than 6 years of age and less than 12 breaths/min for children between 6 and 18 years of age. A normal respiratory rate alone never guarantees adequate oxygenation and ventilation. The respiratory rate must be interpreted along with appearance, work of breathing, and air movement.

TABLE 1–4 Normal Respiratory Rate for Age

Age	Respiratory Rate (Breaths/Min)
Infant (birth–12 mo)	30–60
Toddler (1–3 y)	24–40
Preschooler (3–5 y)	22–34
School-aged child (6–12 y)	18–30
Adolescent (13–18 y)	12–16

Scene Size-Up
↓
Pediatric Assessment Triangle (PAT)
↓
Primary Assessment
Hands-on ABCDEs
Vital Signs
Pulse Oximetry
Transport Decision: Stay or Go
↓
Secondary Assessment
History Taking
Physical Examination
Monitoring Devices
Ongoing Reassessment

In a crying infant or child, it is often difficult to obtain an accurate respiratory rate. Have the parent/caregiver hold the child and lift their clothing. This can allow you to count abdominal excursions ("belly breathing").

PULSE OXIMETRY

Oxygen Saturation. Pulse oximetry is an excellent tool to assess how well a child is oxygenating. **FIGURE 1–10A** illustrates a pulse oximeter and an example of a probe. Infants and younger children may better tolerate a wraparound probe, which is placed around the toe or foot (**FIGURE 1–10B** shows the clip-on oximeter), and is better tolerated than a clip-on probe. Covering the extremity with a blanket, sock, or towel may also help improve tolerance of the probe. A pulse oximetry reading above 94% saturation on room air indicates good oxygenation. Be careful not to underestimate respiratory distress in a child with a reading above 94%. Sometimes the child can compensate for hypoxia by significantly increasing work of breathing and respiratory rate, and pulse oximetry may not reflect the true severity or urgency of the respiratory problem. As with any other measurement, interpret pulse oximetry in the context of the "big picture," including work of breathing, appearance, and circulation.

> **TIP**
> Infants and younger children may better tolerate a wraparound probe, which is placed around the toe or foot, rather than a clip-on probe.

Covering the extremity with a blanket, sock, or towel may also help improve tolerance of the probe.

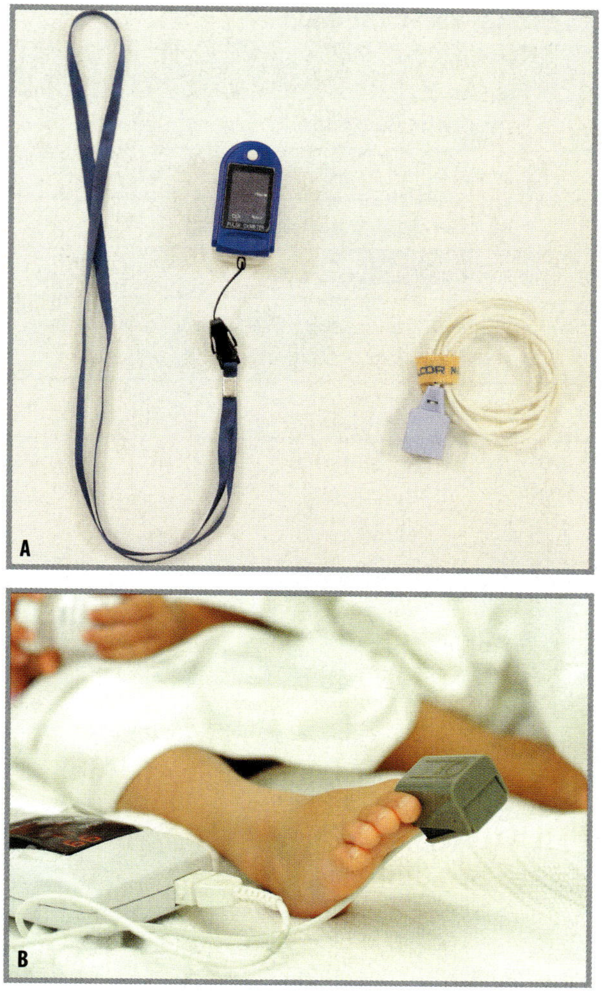

FIGURE 1–10 **A.** Pulse oximeter and probe. **B.** Pulse oximetry is an excellent tool for assessing the effectiveness of oxygenation.

> **TIP**
>
> The accuracy of a pulse oximetry reading is impacted by decreased body temperature, skin pigmentation, movement, nail polish, poor circulation, and intravenous dyes.

Although pulse oximetry is quite helpful in identifying a child with moderate respiratory distress, it can also help identify the child in respiratory failure. When the pulse oximetry reading is below 90% saturation in a child on 100% oxygen by a nonrebreathing mask, this usually represents respiratory failure requiring **assisted ventilation**. However, sometimes a child in severe respiratory distress or early respiratory failure may maintain measured oxygen saturation by increasing work of breathing and respiratory rate. This child may not appear to be critically ill according to pulse oximetry alone. Again, interpret pulse oximetry together with the rest of the assessment to accurately evaluate the degree of respiratory distress or failure.

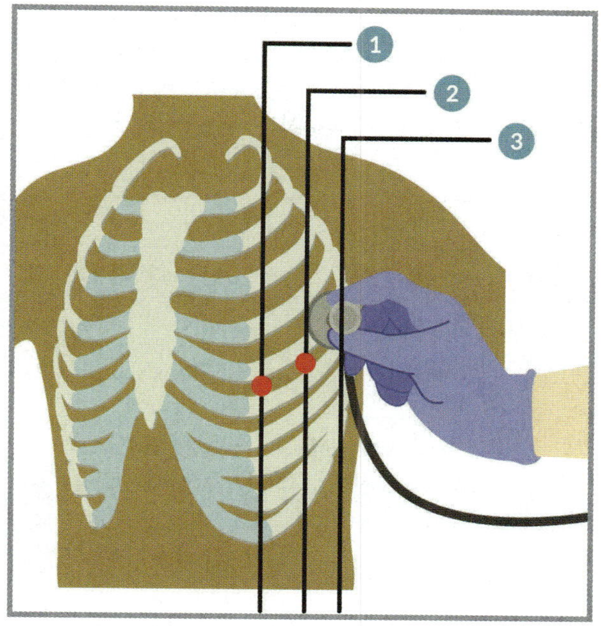

FIGURE 1–11 Listen for air movement over the midaxillary line. 1. Midclavicular line, 2. Anterior axillary line, 3. Midaxillary line.

Auscultation. Listen with a stethoscope over the midclavicular and **midaxillary lines** during inhalation and exhalation to hear abnormal lung sounds, such as **crackles** and wheezing (**FIGURE 1–11**). **Inspiratory** crackles indicate disease in the alveoli (air sacs) themselves. Often, crackles are not heard on auscultation, even when the child has a pathologic condition, such as pneumonia. The younger the child, the more difficult it is to appreciate abnormal sounds during auscultation. Expiratory wheezing indicates lower airway obstruction. Auscultation also helps evaluate the volume of air movement and effectiveness of work of breathing. A child with increased work of breathing and poor air movement may be in impending respiratory failure.

TABLE 1–5 lists abnormal breath sounds, their causes, and common examples of associated disease processes.

CIRCULATION

> **CAUTION**
>
> **Be careful not to underestimate respiratory distress in a child with a pulse oximetry reading above 94%. This child may be using increased work of breathing and tachypnea to compensate for serious hypoxic stress.**

The PAT provides important visual clues about circulation to the skin. Information obtained from the hands-on evaluation of heart rate, pulse quality, skin temperature, capillary refill time, and

TABLE 1–5 Interpretation of Abnormal Breath Sounds

Sound	Cause	Examples
Stridor	Upper airway obstruction	Croup, foreign body aspiration, retropharyngeal abscess
Wheezing	Lower airway obstruction	Asthma, foreign body, bronchiolitis
Expiratory grunting	Inadequate oxygenation	Pulmonary contusion, pneumonia, drowning
Inspiratory crackles	Fluid, mucus, or blood in airway	Pneumonia, pulmonary contusion
Absent breath sounds despite increased work of breathing	Severe airway obstruction (upper or lower airway)	Physical barrier to transmission of breath sounds, foreign body, severe asthma, hemothorax, pneumothorax, pleural fluid, pneumonia

TABLE 1–6 Normal Heart Rate for Age

Age	Heart Rate (Beats/Min)
Infant (birth–12 mo)	100–160
Toddler (1–3 y)	90–150
Preschooler (3–5 y)	80–140
School-aged child (6–12 y)	70–120
Adolescent (13–18 y)	60–100

blood pressure provides further information on the adequacy of perfusion.

Heart Rate. Methods used to assess adult circulatory status (heart rate and blood pressure) have important limitations in children. First, normal heart rate varies with age, as noted in **TABLE 1–6**. Second, tachycardia may be an early sign of hypoxia or poor perfusion, but it may also reflect fever, anxiety, pain, and excitement. As with respiratory rate, interpret heart rate within the context of the overall history, PAT, and primary assessment. A trend of increasing or decreasing heart rate may be quite useful: It may suggest worsening hypoxia or shock or improvement after treatment. When hypoxia or shock becomes critical, the heart rate falls, leading to frank bradycardia. **Bradycardia** indicates critical hypoxia or ischemia. With tachycardia greater than 180 beats/min, an electronic monitor is necessary to accurately determine heart rate.

> **TIP**
>
> A rapid initial respiratory rate may simply reflect high fever, anxiety, pain, and/or excitement and not any real physiological or anatomical problem. Noting a trend of an abnormal respiratory rate or heart rate is more useful for indicating true pathology.

Pulse Quality. Feel the pulse to ascertain pulse quality. Normally, the brachial pulse is palpable

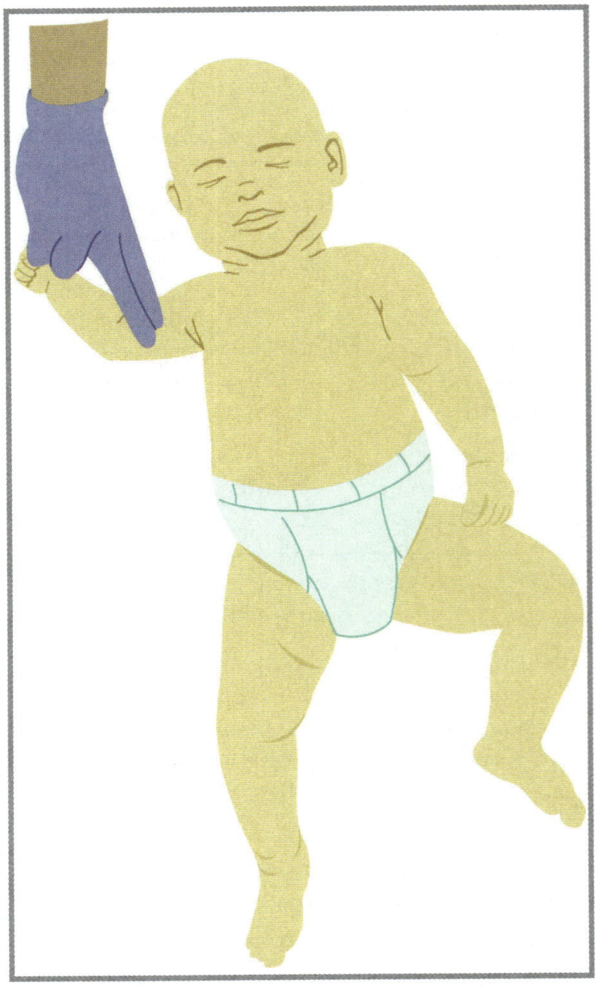

FIGURE 1–12 The anatomical position of the brachial pulse is in the medial aspect of the antecubital fossa.

in the medial aspect of the **antecubital fossa** (**FIGURE 1–12**). Note the quality as either weak or strong. If the brachial pulse is strong, the child is probably not hypotensive. If a peripheral pulse cannot be felt, attempt to find a central pulse. Check the femoral pulse in infants and young children or the carotid pulse in an older child or adolescent. If there

CASE STUDY 2

A 3-year-old girl was found face down in the family swimming pool. She was under water for no more than 1 minute but required cardiopulmonary resuscitation by the mother to get her breathing again. On arrival of EMS, the child is alert, pink, and clinging to her mother.

Respirations appear regular and nonlabored. When you examine her further, she screams and fights you. Her respiratory rate is 26 breaths/min, but you are unable to obtain a blood pressure or heart rate or assess lung sounds. The mother is sobbing and frightened.

1. How useful is the PAT in evaluating severity of illness and urgency of need for care?
2. How is the PAT different from the ABCDEs in the primary assessment?

is no pulse, or the pulse is low (<60 beats/min) and the child is symptomatic with poor circulation, start cardiopulmonary resuscitation (CPR) (see Chapter 5 for more information).

TIP

Interpret heart rate in the context of the overall history, PAT, and entire physical assessment.

Skin Temperature and Capillary Refill Time. Next, do a hands-on evaluation of circulation to the skin. Although children with normal circulation may have cool hands and feet, the skin should be warm above the wrists and ankles. With decreasing perfusion, the extremities become cooler proximally. Check capillary refill time in a fingertip, toe, or heel or on the pads of the fingertips. Normal capillary refill time is less than 2 to 3 seconds. The value of measuring capillary refill time is controversial for several reasons: the peripheral perfusion baseline may vary from child to child; environmental factors, such as cold room temperature, may complicate interpretation; and it may be difficult for the prehospital professional to accurately count seconds under critical circumstances. The capillary refill time is just 1 element in the assessment of circulation. It must be evaluated in the context of the PAT and other perfusion characteristics, such as heart rate, pulse quality, and blood pressure.

Signs of circulation to the skin (skin temperature, capillary refill time, and pulse quality) are helpful tools to assess a child's circulatory status, especially when performed consecutively on a child who is not cold.

CONTROVERSY

The value of capillary refill time is controversial. Peripheral perfusion may be variable in some children, and such environmental factors as ambient temperature may have a strong influence on capillary refill time.

Blood Pressure. Blood pressure determination and interpretation may be difficult in children because of the lack of patient cooperation, confusion about proper cuff size, and problems remembering normal values for age. **FIGURE 1-13A** illustrates the different sizes of blood pressure cuffs, and **FIGURE 1-13B** demonstrates the technique for getting a correct blood pressure in the arm or thigh. *Always use a cuff with a width of two-thirds the length of the upper arm or thigh.* For patients 3 years or younger, technical difficulties reduce the value of a blood pressure in the field. When shock is suspected in this age group based on other assessments (eg, history, mechanism, PAT), consider attempting blood pressure once on scene, but do not

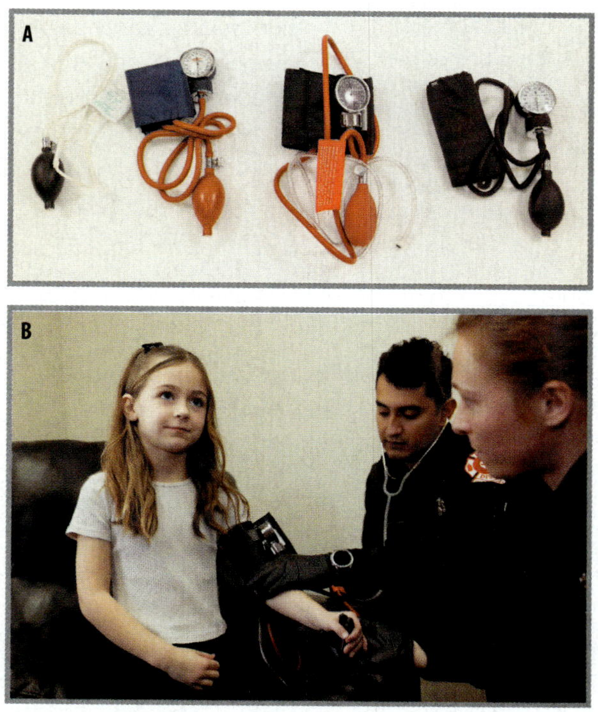

FIGURE 1-13 **A.** There are several different blood pressure (BP) cuff sizes: neonatal, infant, child, and adult. **B.** To obtain an accurate BP reading, use a cuff that is two-thirds the length of the child's upper arm.

delay treatment or transport. In a child who is clearly unstable (requiring assisted ventilation, absent radial or femoral pulses), begin immediate resuscitation and delay blood pressure until child is in a more stable condition. For patients in stable condition who are older than 3 years, try one blood pressure measurement in the field, then move on to the rest of the assessment.

TIP

For patients younger than 3 years of age, the value of obtaining a blood pressure in the field may be outweighed by the technical difficulties of getting an accurate measurement. Focus on immediate resuscitation in a child with an unstable airway, tachycardia, and poor perfusion or absent radial or femoral pulses, and delay blood pressure until the child's condition stabilizes.

For children older than 1 year, an easy formula for determining the lower limit of acceptable blood pressure by age is as follows: minimal systolic blood pressure should be greater than $70 + (2 \times \text{age in years})$. For example, a 2-year-old child with a systolic blood pressure of 65 mm Hg is hypotensive. **TABLE 1–7** shows approximate normal minimal systolic blood pressure values for different ages. High blood pressure is usually not a clinical problem for children in the field. Assume that a blood pressure is within normal limits if an infant or young child is agitated, is crying, has pink skin, and has easily palpable peripheral pulses. In a patient with this clinical profile, do not delay transport to obtain a blood pressure. Remember, a normal blood pressure measurement may be misleading. Although a low blood pressure definitely indicates hypotensive shock, a "normal" blood pressure frequently exists in children with compensated shock.

CAUTION

Do not depend on blood pressure readings to diagnose shock. A "normal" blood pressure frequently exists in compensated shock.

TABLE 1–7 Minimum Systolic Blood Pressure by Age

Age	Minimal Systolic Blood Pressure (mm Hg)
Newborn (birth-1 mo)	>60
Infant (1 to 12 mo)	>65
Toddler (1–3 y)	>70
Preschooler (3–5 y)	>75
School-aged child (6–12 y)	>80
Adolescent (13–18 y)	>90

Note that a widening pulse pressure (systolic pressure minus diastolic pressure) may occur secondary to increased intracranial pressure and early septic shock; a narrowing pulse pressure may be seen early in hypovolemic shock.

DISABILITY

Assessment of disability, or neurological status, involves quick evaluation of the 2 main parts of the CNS: the **cerebral cortex** and the **brainstem**. First assess neurological status, which is controlled by the cerebral cortex, by looking at appearance as part of the PAT, then assess the level of consciousness using the AVPU scale (**TABLE 1–8**). Evaluate the brainstem by checking the responses of each pupil to a direct beam of light. A normal pupil constricts after a light stimulus. Pupillary response may be abnormal in the presence of drugs, ongoing seizures, hypoxia, or **impending brainstem herniation**. Next, evaluate motor activity. Look for symmetric movement of the extremities, seizures, posturing, or **flaccidity**.

CAUTION

Neither the AVPU scale nor the Pediatric GCS allows assessment of restless or agitated behavioral states.

AVPU Scale. The AVPU scale is a standardized method of assessing the level of consciousness in all patients. It helps categorize motor response based on simple responses to stimuli. The patient is either alert, responsive to verbal stimuli, responsive only to painful stimuli, or unresponsive.

Abnormal Appearance and the AVPU Scale. Assessment of appearance using the PAT provides different information than assessment using the AVPU scale. A child with an altered mental status on the AVPU scale always has an abnormal appearance in the PAT, because such a child almost always has a serious or critical condition. However, a child with a mild to moderate illness or injury may be alert on the AVPU scale, but have an abnormal appearance in the PAT. Assessing appearance using the PAT may provide an earlier indication of the presence of serious illness and injury.

The accuracy of the AVPU scale is controversial, and it has a few important limitations. Its ability to predict the extent of neurological compromise has not been well tested in children. Its scope is limited

TABLE 1–8 AVPU Scale

Category	Stimulus	Response Type	Reaction
Alert	Normal environment	Appropriate	Normal interactiveness for age
Verbal	Simple command or sound stimulus	Appropriate or inappropriate	Responds to name; nonspecific or confused
Painful	Pain	Appropriate, inappropriate, or pathologic	Withdraws from pain or sound or motion without purpose or localization of pain; posturing
Unresponsive	—	—	No perceptible response to any stimulus

in the evaluation of children with restless or agitated states. The scale only addresses decreased levels of responsiveness, a problem common to all of the current prehospital methods for disability assessment. However, it is easy to remember (there are no numbers to recall) and to use. The more complicated Pediatric GCS involves memorization and numerical scoring, tasks that may be hard to remember and apply in critical situations (**TABLE 1–9**). Recent data suggest that the much simpler-to-administer motor component of the GCS alone may be adequate for mental status evaluation in the field. The motor categories of the GCS from lowest point value to highest are (1) no response, (2) **extensor posturing**, (3) flexor posturing, (4) withdrawing, (5) **localizing**, and (6) obeying instructions (as age-appropriate). Like the AVPU scale, the GCS does not address degrees of neurological disability in children who are restless, agitated, or combative.

> **TIP**
>
> Hypoglycemia is a common cause of mental status changes in infants and school-aged children owing to lack of fat/glycogen stores. The "D" in the hands-on ABCDEs can also be used to signify "dextrose" as a memory trigger to check for hypoglycemia while in the field.

EXPOSURE

Proper exposure of the child is necessary for completion of the primary physical assessment. The PAT requires that the caregiver remove part of the child's clothing to allow careful observation of the face, chest wall, and skin. Completing the ABCDE components of the primary assessment may require further exposure to fully evaluate physiological function, anatomical abnormalities, and unsuspected injuries. Pay attention to the need for privacy, even for prepubescent children, when possible. Be careful to avoid heat loss, especially in infants, by covering the child up as soon as possible. Infants and younger children have a larger body-surface-to-body-weight ratio and are at a greater risk of rapidly losing body heat when left exposed. Cold stress in critically ill or injured patients can increase metabolic demands, worsen the effects of hypoxia and hypoglycemia, and adversely affect the response to resuscitative efforts.

Scene Size-Up
↓
Pediatric Assessment Triangle (PAT)
↓
Primary Assessment
Hands-on ABCDEs
Vital Signs
Pulse Oximetry
Transport Decision: Stay or Go
↓
Secondary Assessment
History Taking
Physical Examination
Monitoring Devices
Ongoing Reassessment

The Transport Decision: Stay or Go?

After completing the PAT and the hands-on ABCDEs and beginning resuscitation as necessary, the prehospital professional must make a crucial decision: Should they immediately transport the child to the ED, or should they continue with the additional assessment and treatment on scene? Should they transport the child, or is there a more

TABLE 1–9 Pediatric Glasgow Coma Scale

Score	Child	Infant
Eyes		
4	Opens eyes spontaneously	Opens eyes spontaneously
3	Opens eyes to speech	Opens eyes to speech
2	Opens eyes to pain	Opens eyes to pain
1	No response	No response
= Score (Eyes)		
Motor		
6	Obeys commands	Spontaneous movements
5	Localizes	Withdraws to touch
4	Withdraws	Withdraws to pain
3	Flexion	Flexion (decorticate)
2	Extension	Extension (decerebrate)
1	No response	No response
= Score (Motor)		
Verbal		
5	Oriented	Coos and babbles
4	Confused	Irritable cry
3	Inappropriate words	Cries to pain
2	Incomprehensible words	Moans to pain
1	No response	No response
= Score (Verbal)		
= Total Score (Eyes, Motor, Verbal). Scores will range from 3 to 15.		

Adapted from James HE, Anas NG, Perkin RM. *Brain Insults in Infants and Children*. Grune & Stratton; 1985.

appropriate mode of transport available (eg, aeromedical services, pediatric specialty transport teams)? Should the child be transported to a local community hospital for either treatment or stabilization, or does the child need to go directly to a trauma center or pediatric specialty hospital? This decision process is different for each child and for each EMS system. Although vital signs and pulse oximetry are listed in the primary assessment, the transport decision can be made if the EMS clinician determines the need for expedited transport after using the PAT and evaluating the ABCDEs.

TIP

Deciding when to go and when to stay is different for each child and for each EMS system.

TIP

If the child is physiologically unstable, defer or omit history taking and physical examination on scene and perform en route.

EXPECTED BENEFITS OF TREATMENT

The time it takes to reach definitive care in the hospital has a major effect on the outcomes of children with serious injuries. The time it takes to reach hospital care may also significantly affect the outcomes of children with certain medical illnesses. For example, a child in cardiogenic shock benefits most from rapid transport to definitive care, because the hospital is the best place for lifesaving treatments of this rare and complex condition.

However, some critically ill children benefit from basic life support (BLS) and ALS treatment on scene. For example, for a child who is seizing, early treatment with a benzodiazepine is the best hope to get the seizure under immediate control and avoid additional **anticonvulsant** administration and advanced airway management. A child with an anaphylactic reaction requires an intramuscular (IM) epinephrine injection from an autoinjector or drawn up by a BLS or an ALS provider. A nasal spray formulation of epinephrine is also available for children over 30 kg, as allowed by local protocols and availability. Similarly, the risk of brain injury is decreased if glucose is administered to the unconscious child with diabetes at the time the prehospital professional recognizes hypoglycemia with a bedside test.

EMS SYSTEM REGULATIONS

The decision to stay or go often is defined by EMS system regulations about treatment and transport. For example, some systems allow EMS clinicians to treat a child in cardiopulmonary arrest with ALS interventions until either the resuscitation is successful or death is declared. Other systems require transport after initial resuscitation is under way, with the decision to discontinue efforts left to the ED staff.

COMFORT LEVEL

Whenever a prehospital professional believes that the illness or injury requires a higher level of care, it is best to initiate transport quickly. Moreover, whenever the prehospital professional feels uncomfortable with a critical intervention, it is best to transport and attempt the intervention on the way to the ED, rather than on scene. For example, a child with hypotensive (decompensated) shock usually deserves 1 attempt at vascular access on scene, then fluid administration on the way to the ED. The time spent on multiple intravenous attempts on scene might be better spent in transporting the child to definitive care, where the underlying cause of shock can be more appropriately addressed. On the other hand, for a child in cardiac arrest, begin CPR, and defibrillate if indicated, prior to transport.

TRANSPORT TIME

The time to the nearest ED is another key factor. A shorter transport time ordinarily supports a shorter scene time. For example, if a child has ingested a potentially lethal poison, immediate transport is prudent if the ED is close by because of the complications related to delay of definitive care. However, if transport time is long, consider initiating treatment on scene.

Emergency medical services clinicians should also consider the pediatric capabilities of the area EDs compared to the criticality of the patient's condition. Although pediatric patients are best served at pediatric hospital EDs, the criticality of the patient's condition may prompt the EMS clinician to transport a pediatric patient in critical condition to the closest ED for stabilization before being transported to a pediatric hospital. Knowing the pediatric readiness/capabilities of the community ED may also determine which ED is the most appropriate for the child.

Summary of Primary Assessment

The components of the pediatric primary assessment include the PAT, the ABCDEs, immediate resuscitation needs, and transport decision. The PAT is the basis for the general impression. It includes evaluation of the characteristics of appearance, work of breathing, and circulation to the skin and uses clues obtained by looking and listening from across the room. The primary assessment includes a hands-on evaluation of pediatric-specific indicators of cardiopulmonary or neurological abnormalities. Although vital signs can be useful in the primary assessment, they can also be misleading. They must be interpreted in the context of age and the overall general and primary assessments. Interventions may be necessary at any point in the ABCDE sequence. After determining the ABCDEs, another crucial decision is whether to stay on scene and begin treatment or transport immediately. The type of clinical problem, the expected benefits of earlier transport, the local EMS policies, the prehospital professional's comfort level, and the transport time are all important elements in the transport decision.

TIP

Always perform reassessment to track problems and monitor response to treatment.

Scene Size-Up

↓

Pediatric Assessment Triangle (PAT)

↓

Primary Assessment

Hands-on ABCDEs

Vital Signs

Pulse Oximetry

Transport Decision: Stay or Go

↓

Secondary Assessment

History Taking

Physical Examination

Monitoring Devices

Ongoing Reassessment

Secondary Assessment: History Taking

History taking has 2 objectives and should be performed for both medical and trauma patients:

1. To obtain a complete description of the main complaint
2. To determine the mechanism of injury or circumstances of the illness

If the child seems to be physiologically unstable according to the primary assessment, the prehospital professional may decide to transport immediately and defer the history and secondary assessment. If the child's condition is stable and the scene is safe, the prehospital professional should obtain a thorough history and complete the secondary assessment on the scene and before transport. In contrast to the primary assessment, which focuses on physiological problems that may be immediately life-threatening, this secondary assessment focuses on anatomical abnormalities, which are rarely life-threatening.

A history should be obtained from the caregiver of the pediatric patient or from the caregiver and the older child or adolescent. In some cases, it may be helpful to interview the adolescent separate from the caregiver; many adolescents are hesitant to disclose information about drug use or sexual activity (as it relates to the current illness or injury) in front of their caregiver. The history provides important information that assists the prehospital professional in analyzing assessment findings. The SAMPLE mnemonic may be used to elicit information: Signs and Symptoms, Allergies, Medications, Past medical problems, Last food or liquid, and Events leading up to this illness or injury (**TABLE 1-10**).

Children with special health care needs often require additional history collection, but the type of history necessary depends on the underlying illness or condition. The use of an **emergency information form (EIF)** can be extremely helpful in obtaining critical information about these patients. More information about children with special health care needs can be found in Chapter 12.

If a child has an apparently minor condition (eg, low-grade fever, feeding difficulties, fussiness, minor trauma), be careful not to overlook clues to possible serious underlying conditions. Ingestions, metabolic problems, and systemic infections may present with nonspecific findings in infants and toddlers. Consider child maltreatment when the physical findings are not logically related to the complaint leading to the call or if the history is implausible or changes.

TABLE 1-10 Pediatric SAMPLE Components

Component	Explanation
Signs and symptoms	Onset and nature of symptoms of pain or fever Age-appropriate signs of distress
Allergies	Known drug reactions or other allergies
Medications	Exact names and doses of ongoing drugs Timing and amount of last dose Timing and dose of analgesics or antipyretics
Past medical problems	History of pregnancy, labor, delivery Previous illness or injuries Immunizations
Last food or liquid	Timing of the child's last food or drink, including bottle or breastfeeding
Events leading to the injury or illness	Key events leading to the current incident Fever history

Scene Size-Up
↓
Pediatric Assessment Triangle (PAT)
↓
Primary Assessment
Hands-on ABCDEs
Vital Signs
Pulse Oximetry
Transport Decision: Stay or Go
↓
Secondary Assessment
History Taking
Physical Examination
Monitoring Devices
Ongoing Reassessment

Physical Examination

Often, this portion of the assessment is not possible because of transport and treatment priorities. Sometimes it is unnecessary because the problem has been fully evaluated in earlier phases of the assessment or the complaint and history are minor or well localized (eg, minor laceration or twisted ankle).

If the child with traumatic injuries is in stable condition on scene and does not need resuscitation after the primary assessment, or if the child is on the way to the hospital but does not require ongoing treatment, perform a detailed secondary assessment. This physical evaluation must include all anatomical areas affected and builds on the findings of the primary assessment and history taking.

Use the toe-to-head sequence for the detailed secondary assessment of infants, toddlers, and preschoolers. This approach allows the prehospital professional to gain the child's trust and cooperation and increases the accuracy of the physical findings. Ask for the assistance of the caregiver in the assessment. Note the following special anatomical characteristics of children when performing the secondary assessment.

GENERAL OBSERVATIONS

Observe the clothing for any unusual odors or for stains that might suggest a poison. If poisoning is suspected, remove soiled or dirty clothing and save it, and wash the child's skin with soap and water.

SKIN

Observe the skin carefully for rashes and bruising patterns that may suggest maltreatment, as discussed in Chapter 13. Look for bite marks; straight line marks from cords or straps; pinch marks; or hand, belt, or buckle pattern bruises. Patterned injuries, or those with a geometric shape, are often indicative of abuse. Inspect for **nonblanching petechial** or **purpuric** lesions (which may indicate severe infections), and look for any new lesions that develop during transport.

HEAD

The younger the infant or child, the larger the head is in proportion to the rest of the body (**FIGURE 1–14**). This disproportionate size increases the risk of experiencing head injury with deceleration, such as in motor vehicle crashes. Look for bruising, swelling, and **hematomas**. Significant blood can be lost between

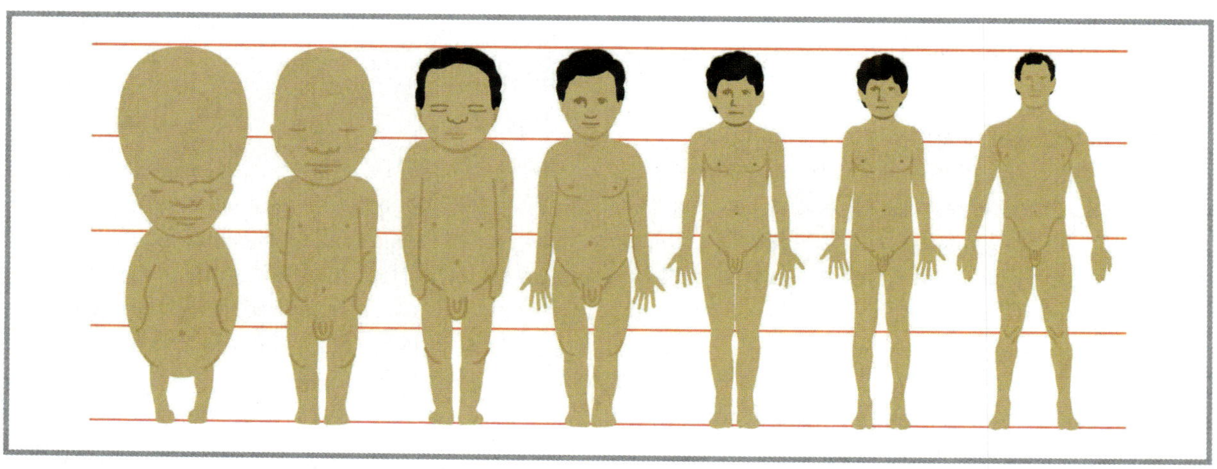

FIGURE 1–14 The relationship of the head to the body changes with advancing age.

Modified from McKinney ES, James SB, Murray SS Ashwill JW, eds. Maternal-Child Nursing. 3rd ed. Saunders; 2009

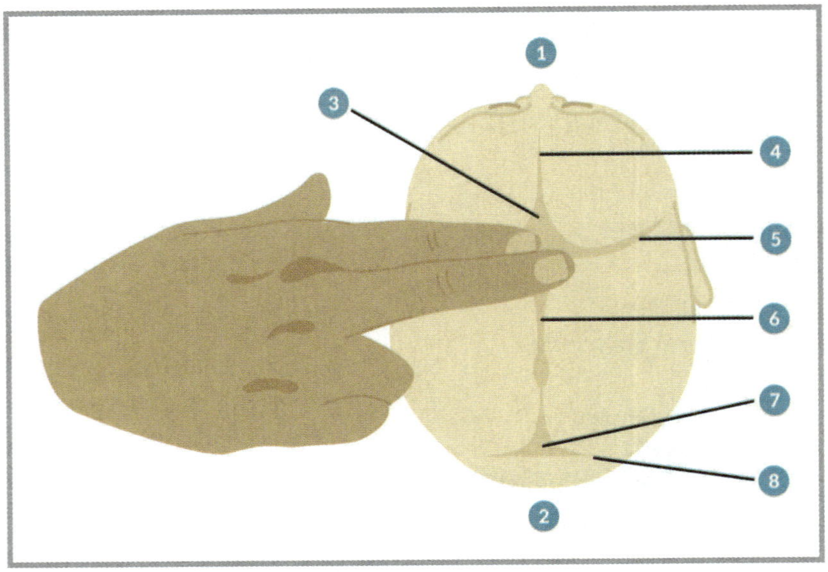

FIGURE 1–15 The anterior fontanelle of the infant is a window to the CNS. 1. Anterior, 2. Posterior, 3. Anterior fontanelle, 4. Metopic suture, 5. Coronal suture, 6. Sagittal suture, 7. Posterior fontanelle, 8. Lambdoid suture.

the skull and scalp of a small infant. Assessment of the anterior **fontanelle** in infants younger than 9 to 18 months can provide helpful information (**FIGURE 1–15**). If possible, the fontanelle should be assessed with the infant in a sitting position, and when not crying. A bulging and **nonpulsatile fontanelle** suggests elevated intracranial pressure caused by **meningitis**, **encephalitis**, or **intracranial** bleeding. A sunken fontanelle suggests dehydration.

EYES

A thorough evaluation of pupil size, reaction to light, and symmetry of **extraocular** muscle movements may be difficult to perform in infants. Gently rocking infants in the upright position often gets them to open their eyes. A colorful distracting object can then be used to help assess eye movements.

NOSE

Young infants preferentially breathe through their noses, so nasal congestion with mucus can cause marked respiratory distress. Gentle bulb or catheter suction of the nostrils may bring relief (**FIGURE 1–16**). In a trauma patient, leaking blood (**rhinorrhea**) or **cerebrospinal fluid (CSF)** suggests a **basilar skull fracture**.

EARS

Look for any drainage from the ear canals (**otorrhea**). Bruises to the ear pinna, especially in a nonambulatory child, may suggest inflicted trauma. Leaking blood or CSF suggests a basilar skull fracture. Check for bruises behind the ear or **Battle sign**, another indicator of basilar skull fracture. The presence of **pus** may indicate an ear infection or perforation of the eardrum (tympanic membrane).

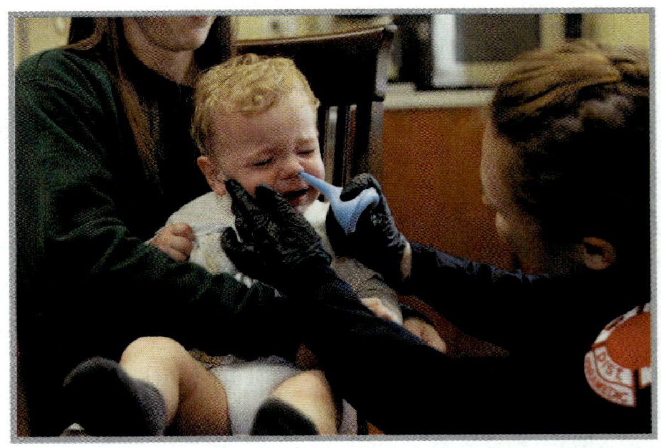

FIGURE 1–16 Gentle bulb suction may bring relief to the infant.

MOUTH

In the trauma patient, look for active bleeding and loose teeth. In nonambulatory children, mouth trauma such as tears to the **frenulum** may be a sign of inflicted trauma. Note the smell of the breath. Some ingestions are associated with identifiable odors, such as **hydrocarbons**. Acidosis, as in **diabetic ketoacidosis**, may impart a sweet or "fruity" smell to the breath.

NECK

Examine the **trachea** for **edema** or bruising. Listen with a stethoscope over the trachea at the midline

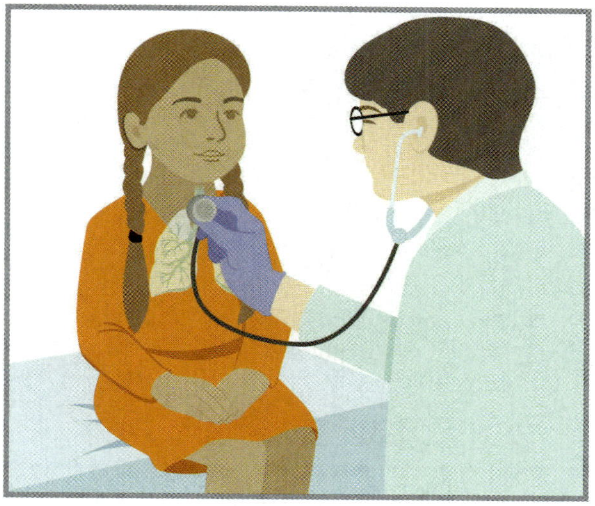

FIGURE 1–17 Listen at the trachea to determine the origin of abnormal airway sounds.

(**FIGURE 1–17**). This is a quick and easy way to differentiate between very proximal airway obstruction (usually mucus in the nose) and true wheezing or stridor. The neck should also be assessed for a tracheal shift or **jugular venous distension (JVD)**. These are classic signs of tension pneumothorax, but occur late in the physiological process. Jugular venous distension may not be present if there are other injuries present that have led to hypovolemia. Assess for neck tenderness.

The use of spinal motion restriction is an area of ongoing debate and review. The National Association of State EMS Officials (NASEMSO) currently recommends spinal motion restriction for children with neck pain, an inability to move the neck, focal neurological deficit, altered mental status, high-risk mechanism (ie, high-speed motor vehicle collision, diving), torso trauma, or a predisposing condition.

CHEST

Reexamine the chest for penetrating injuries, lacerations, bruises, or rashes. If the child is injured, feel the **clavicles** and every rib for tenderness or deformity.

BACK

Inspect the back for lacerations, penetrating injuries, bruises, or rashes.

ABDOMEN

Inspect the abdomen for any bruising, swelling, deformities, or rashes. Multiple bruises or bruises in different stages of healing on the chest or abdomen may be associated with inflicted injury. In the trauma patient, redness or bruising under the site of protective straps, or "seat belt sign," may be apparent. A "handlebar" mark may also be present if a child had contact with the handlebar of a bicycle during an accident. Both seat belt marks and handlebar injuries are associated with significant internal injuries. Also, inspect the abdomen for **distension**. Gently palpate the abdomen, and watch closely for guarding or tensing of the abdominal muscles, which may suggest infection, obstruction, or **intra-abdominal** injury. Note any tenderness or masses. If an infant or toddler has been crying for a prolonged period of time, or if a child's respiratory effort has been supported with a bag-mask device, this may also lead to abdominal distension because of air that has been pushed into the stomach.

EXTREMITIES

Assess for **symmetry**. Compare both sides for color, warmth, size of joints, and tenderness. Put each joint through a full range of motion while watching the eyes of the child for signs of pain; understandably, if there is obvious deformity of the extremity suggesting a fracture, this technique should not be used, and the extremity should be splinted. If there is a suspected fracture present, assess for a pulse, capillary refill, motor function, and sensation distal to the injury. Fractures in nonambulatory children should raise suspicion regarding inflicted trauma.

ADDITIONAL VITAL SIGNS

Although pulse and respirations have been assessed in the primary assessment, they may or may not have been formally counted and recorded because of circumstances of resuscitation or brevity of transportation. It is important to obtain and record these vital signs to assess and monitor the child's changing condition. When resuscitation is necessary, pulse and respirations should be monitored frequently, but recording additional vital signs may be deferred until the child has stabilized or the transportation is completed.

ASSESSMENT OF PAIN

It is easy for the prehospital professional to ignore, underestimate, or misinterpret the signs and symptoms of pain in infants and young children. Children are much less likely to receive effective pain medications than adults. Studies have demonstrated reluctance by all levels of emergency care personnel to administer medications to children for control of pain and anxiety. The younger the child,

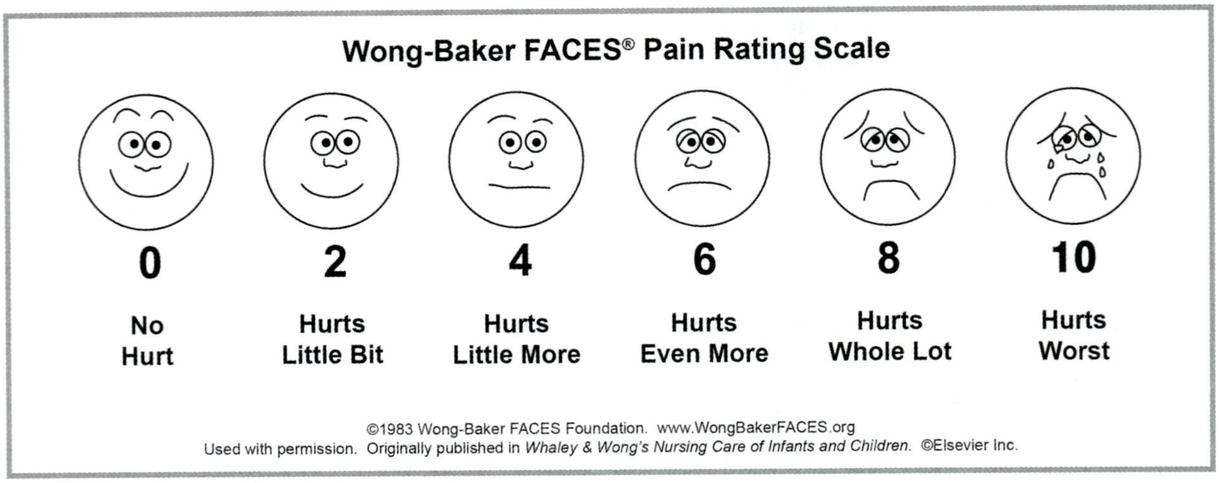

FIGURE 1–18 Wong-Baker FACES Pain Rating Scale for self-assessment of pain.

Wong-Baker FACES Foundation (2019). Wong-Baker FACES® Pain Rating Scale. Retrieved with permission from http://www.WongBakerFACES.org.

the less likely the child will receive effective **analgesia** and **anxiolysis**. This is also true for Black and Hispanic children of all ages. However, adult and pediatric experience has validated the effectiveness of analgesia in the prehospital setting to decrease pain without causing respiratory depression or interference with the accuracy of the physical assessment.

Pain is present with most types of injuries and with many illnesses. Inadequate treatment of pain has many adverse effects on the child and family. Pain itself causes significant morbidity and misery for the child and family or caregivers and interferes with the prehospital professional's accurate assessment of physiological abnormalities. Children who do not receive appropriate analgesia are more likely to have exaggerated pain responses to subsequent painful procedures. Even neonates have demonstrable chronic changes in pain perception when they are subjected to painful procedures without the benefit of analgesia. Posttraumatic stress is also more common among children who experience pain during acute illness and injury and do not receive pharmacological relief. Hence, just as with adults, it is essential to carefully assess pain in all children and to consider effective methods to provide relief from suffering when appropriate.

Local EMS protocols now require that EMS clinicians assess and manage pain as a part of the secondary assessment. Indeed, evaluation of pain has become a new vital sign in patients of all ages, including children. Appropriate pain management relieves distress of the child and family or caregivers and facilitates communication, physical assessment, and ease of transport.

Assessment of pain must take into consideration the developmental age of the patient. The ability to recognize pain improves as the age of the child increases. For example, in a preverbal infant, crying and agitation unrelieved by being held by the caregiver may be caused by hunger, hypoxia, or pain. In infants, further assessment is essential to identify sources of pain before administration of analgesia. In contrast, verbal children older than 3 years of age are usually quite vocal about pain. Therefore, in older children, pain scales using pictures of facial expressions (Wong-Baker FACES Scale) or **visual analog scores (VAS)** may be helpful in assessing the need for pharmacologic relief of pain. **FIGURE 1–18** illustrates the Wong-Baker FACES Scale. Although such "self-report" scales have not yet been extensively used in the prehospital environment, they have been validated in other settings to provide an immediate evaluation of intensity of pain and to monitor response to treatment.

There is much overlap between the management of fear and anxiety and the management of pain in infants and young children. Many nonpharmacological and pharmacological methods relieve anxiety and reduce the perception of pain, as summarized in **TABLE 1–11**. Remaining calm and providing quiet, professional reassurance to caregivers and the child are the first important steps. A calm caregiver helps to make the child calm and more at ease. Distraction techniques may be extremely helpful in reducing pain. Many EMS clinicians learn to use toys, "magic tricks," or engaging stories to provide distraction. Some EMS systems have developed a "toolbox" with distraction equipment to facilitate pain relief (**FIGURE 1–19**). Keeping the caregiver with the child and sometimes holding the child are also useful strategies.

TABLE 1–11 Methods of Providing Prehospital Analgesia and Anxiolysis

Nonpharmacological
Calm manner
Caregiver assistance through presence or holding
Distraction techniques with "toolbox" of toys
Ice
Visual imagery
Pacifier
Music
Splinting of fractures
Pharmacological
Morphine
Fentanyl
Midazolam
Ketamine
Nitrous oxide
Benzodiazepines
12%–25% sucrose for neonates
Acetaminophen
Ibuprofen (do not use ibuprofen in infants < 6 months old)

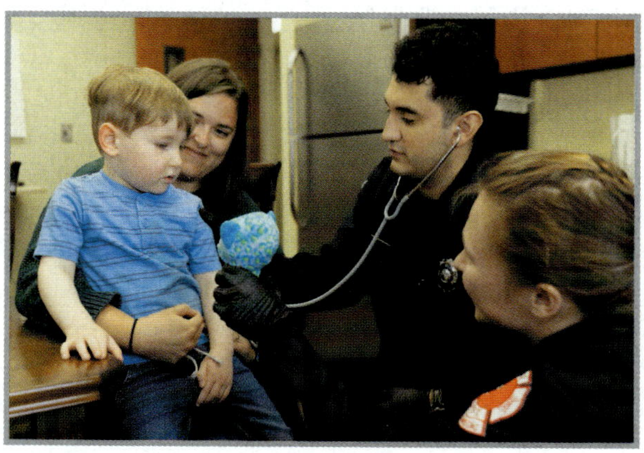

FIGURE 1–19 Use distraction techniques to help reduce the child's pain.

TIP

Pain is often considered an additional vital sign. Pain management can help relieve distress of the child and family, greatly facilitate communication and physical assessment, assist in timely provision of necessary interventions, and ease the transport process.

CONTROVERSY

Although "self-report" pain scales have not yet been extensively used for pediatric patients in the prehospital environment, they have been validated in other clinical settings. They can help provide an immediate evaluation of pain intensity, and they can aid in monitoring response to treatment.

In older children, visual imagery techniques can often be helpful. Ask the child where they would most prefer to be at the present time, then assist the child in closing their eyes and visualizing a more tranquil or enjoyable environment. Music is also an effective distraction.

Pharmacologic methods for reducing pain are also a standard of prehospital care. Opiates, benzodiazepines, ketamine, and nitrous oxide are available to EMS clinicians in many EMS systems. **Intramuscular** medications are less effective because children fear needles, and the injection site pain may last for days. Analgesic and anxiolytic drugs may be easily delivered through inhalation techniques, by the **transmucosal** (eg, sublingual, intranasal, and rectal) route, or by the **transdermal** route. Several techniques, such as inhaled nitrous oxide, intranasal fentanyl, intranasal midazolam, and rectal diazepam, have had excellent success in prehospital pediatric care.

Intravenous delivery provides the most effective and most controllable or **titratable** method. A downside is that it does involve establishing vascular access, which, like the IM route, is usually painful. Also, the child's response to pain and anxiolytic medication is sometimes unpredictable and must be carefully weighed against unwanted side effects. Medications to reduce pain also cause sedation and can result in respiratory depression, bradycardia, **hypoxemia**, **hypotension**, and even loss of protective airway reflexes. Occasionally, anxiolytic drugs cause a paradoxical worsening of agitation.

TIP

Analgesic and anxiolytic drugs may be easily delivered through inhalation, transmucosal (eg, intranasal, sublingual, rectal), or transdermal routes. Several techniques, such as inhaled nitrous oxide, intranasal fentanyl, intranasal midazolam, inhaled naloxone, and rectal diazepam, have had excellent success in prehospital pediatric care.

CASE STUDY 3

You are called to the home of a 1-month-old boy who stopped breathing and turned blue, according to his babysitter. He reportedly had a fever all day. The infant is lying supine; his skin is pale and mottled. When touched, the infant becomes extremely irritable and exhibits a high-pitched screeching cry. When left alone, he appears lethargic and poorly responsive. There is no abnormal positioning and there are no abnormal airway sounds, stridor, nasal flaring, or grunting. The infant's color is pale. The respiratory rate is 60 breaths/min and unlabored. The heart rate is 200 beats/min. His peripheral pulses are weak and his extremities are cool to the touch. Capillary refill time is approximately 5 seconds.

1. Does this infant's appearance suggest a serious problem?
2. Is this infant in shock?

Assessment of pain has become a "vital sign," and management of pediatric pain and anxiety must be a routine part of field care in all EMS systems. This entails a thorough understanding of available nonpharmacological techniques, medications, potential medication contraindications and complications, and management of those complications.

Scene Size-Up
↓
Pediatric Assessment Triangle (PAT)
↓
Primary Assessment
Hands-on ABCDEs
Vital Signs
Pulse Oximetry
Transport Decision: Stay or Go
↓
Secondary Assessment
History Taking
Physical Examination
Monitoring Devices
Ongoing Reassessment

Additional Monitoring Devices

The prehospital professional can perform some types of specific testing in the field, such as rapid glucose determinations, point-of-care lactate testing, 12-lead electrocardiogram monitoring, waveform capnography, and other specialty testing available based on local protocols.

Scene Size-Up
↓
Pediatric Assessment Triangle (PAT)
↓
Primary Assessment
Hands-on ABCDEs
Vital Signs
Pulse Oximetry
Transport Decision: Stay or Go
↓
Secondary Assessment
History Taking
Physical Examination
Monitoring Devices
Ongoing Reassessment

Ongoing Reassessment

Perform reassessment of all patients to gauge the response to treatment and to track the progression of identified physiological and anatomical problems. New problems may also be identified on reassessment. Data from the reassessment will guide ongoing treatment. The elements in the reassessment are as follows:

1. The PAT
2. The ABCDEs with repeat vital signs
3. Assessment of positive anatomical findings
4. Review of the effectiveness and safety of treatment

The elements in the reassessment are also the basis for determination of an appropriate transport destination and for accurate, pediatric-specific radio or telephone communications with medical oversight or the ED.

RADIO REPORTING

Proper radio reporting promotes a seamless transfer of care from the prehospital setting to the ED, maximizing the ability of all clinicians to provide efficient and effective care. A good radio report transmits vital data completely and concisely, highlighting pediatric-specific information to allow the ED team to best prepare for the patient's arrival. If available, provide the ED with the patient's weight, as reported by the caregiver or as obtained by means of a length-based resuscitation tape. For a step-by-step explanation, see **Procedure 1, Field Reporting**.

Summary

After the primary assessment, and before beginning any necessary resuscitative efforts, the prehospital professional must determine the severity of the illness or injury and make a decision regarding mode and timing of transport. If additional evaluation is appropriate, perform a detailed history and secondary assessment either on scene or on the way to the ED. These additional phases of assessment are not indicated if there is an acute life-threatening or limb-threatening problem that requires the prehospital professional's ongoing attention. The secondary assessment is more for the detection of anatomical problems than for evaluation of physiological abnormalities. Always perform reassessments to observe the patient's response to interventions and to guide changes in treatment, transport, and triage. Diagnostic testing refers to laboratory and radiographic evaluation to determine causation and mainly occurs after arrival in the ED and during hospitalization for admitted patients.

CASE STUDY ANSWERS

CASE STUDY 1

Beware of the pale child! Consider any child who has experienced significant trauma and is pale at the scene to have significant blood loss until proven otherwise. Children are able to compensate for blood loss and hypovolemia through catecholamine surges, which cause tachycardia and peripheral vasoconstriction. These reflexes inhibit the circulation to the skin and result in a pale patient. Although this child could have had a significant head injury based on the mechanism of injury, the level of consciousness is normal; therefore, the initial issue needing emergent attention is hemorrhagic shock. Abdominal injuries with blunt trauma to the liver or spleen can result in significant internal bleeding without external signs of injury. Many children with internal bleeding do not have abdominal tenderness. Indicators of suspected hemorrhagic shock are tachycardia, weak pulses, and delayed capillary refill, and a late sign is a decrease in the blood pressure (80 mm Hg/palp). This child requires timely transport to a trauma center with pediatric capabilities. Delay vascular access until the child is en route to the hospital.

This child is also clearly in pain. However, weigh the benefits of pharmacologic therapy to relieve pain against the potential for circulatory collapse, delay in transport, and the need to effectively assess appearance. Use opiate analgesics, such as morphine, in patients with suspected compensated hemorrhagic shock cautiously because of morphine's vasodilatory effect.

At the hospital, the patient was found to have a liver laceration and pancreatic injury. He was admitted to the pediatric intensive care unit (PICU). He did not require surgery and was discharged a few days later.

CASE STUDY 2

The PAT is an accurate tool to evaluate severity of illness or injury and to determine the urgency of providing lifesaving care. Upon arrival at the scene of this patient, it is quite reassuring to find the toddler alert, pink, and with nonlabored respirations. Her vigorous responses make it difficult to perform the conventional ABCDE assessment. Because this child clearly has no serious immediate cardiorespiratory problems, is alert and awake, and fights your examination, history-taking and secondary assessment can occur. However, the prehospital professional should transport every infant or child who has had a submersion injury to a hospital for observation of progression of symptoms.

Continued

CASE STUDY ANSWERS—cont'd

Still, the findings on the PAT allow the prehospital professional to slow the pace and get more information while on the scene. There is no need for immediate resuscitative interventions, and the prehospital professional can avoid the risk of "lights and siren" transport.

Any time there is an unwitnessed submersion event, consider that a traumatic injury may be present. The usual mechanism of a toddler pool drowning involves falling less than 3 ft (1 m) into a body of water. In this scenario, it is unlikely that she has sustained a significant head or spinal injury. Furthermore, if she is moving his neck without apparent discomfort while in her mother's arms, but then vigorously screams and fights when you attempt to examine her, it is unlikely that spinal motion restriction will be helpful (and may prove more harmful and distressing than not). Local protocols govern this decision. Although treatment and transport of this patient are not emergent, ongoing assessment during transport is necessary. Pulmonary complications of submersion, primarily hypoxia, may have a delayed presentation.

At the hospital, the chest radiograph was clear, so the patient was observed for 6 hours, had no increased respiratory distress, and was discharged home.

CASE STUDY 3

Any infant who has a brief, resolved, unexplained event and who reportedly stopped breathing or turned blue deserves EMS transport, regardless of their appearance on your arrival. In this case, the need for urgent treatment and transport is obvious. One of the PAT indicators of shock in this infant is altered appearance. Although that finding could be due to causes other than poor brain perfusion (eg, infection, trauma, toxins, hypoxia), the presence of effortless tachypnea and pale, mottled skin supports the diagnosis of shock. Alternating lethargy and irritability may progress to unresponsiveness as perfusion worsens.

The hands-on examination confirms the suspicion of shock. This patient's heart rate is rapid at 200 beats/min, with weak peripheral pulses, cool extremities, and delayed capillary refill. Even without a blood pressure, the abnormal appearance and skin findings suggest that he should be treated for hypotensive shock. Although the cause of shock is unknown, treatment of any type of hypotensive shock includes vascular access and 20-mL/kg boluses of crystalloid fluid. Make 1 attempt at vascular access on scene and then rapidly transport this patient to definitive care. Reassess his response to therapy frequently en route.

The glucose level was 75 mg/dL. The patient received another fluid bolus in the emergency department. The head computed tomographic scan was negative but he was found to have meningitis, so was admitted and treated with IV antibiotics.

Suggested References

TEXTBOOKS

Aehlert B. *Mosby's Comprehensive Pediatric Emergency Care.* Elsevier; 2012

American Academy of Orthopaedic Surgeons. *Emergency Care and Transportation of the Sick and Injured.* 11th ed. Jones & Bartlett Learning; 2016

American Academy of Pediatrics and the American College of Emergency Physicians. *APLS: The Pediatric Emergency Medicine Resource.* 5th ed. Jones & Bartlett Learning; 2012

American Heart Association and American Academy of Pediatrics. *Pediatric Advanced Life Support Provider Manual.* American Heart Association; 2020

Anne M, Agur A, Dalley A. *Grant's Atlas of Anatomy.* 16th ed. Lippincott Williams & Wilkins; 2024

Bledsoe B, Porter R, Cherry R. *Essentials of Paramedic Care.* Prentice Hall; 2007

Zitelli B, McIntire S, Nowalk AJ, eds. *Zitelli and Davis' Atlas of Pediatric Physical Diagnosis.* 7th ed. Elsevier; 2017

ARTICLES

Callahan JM, Baldwin S, Bodnar C, et al; Committee on Pediatric Emergency Medicine; Council on Clinical Information Technology; Council on Children and Disasters; American College of Emergency Physicians,

Pediatric Emergency Medicine Committee. Access to critical health information for children during emergencies: emergency information forms and beyond. *Pediatrics*. 2023;151(3):e2022060970. doi:10.1542/peds.2022-060970

Fernández A, Ares MI, Garcia S, Martinez-Indart L, Mintegi S, Benito J. The validity of the pediatric assessment triangle as the first step in the triage process in a pediatric emergency department. *Pediatr Emerg Care*. 2017;33(4): 234–238. doi:10.1097/PEC.0000000000000717

Fernandez A, Benito J, Mintegi S. Is this child sick? Usefulness of the Pediatric Assessment Triangle in emergency settings. *J Pediatr (Rio J)*. 2017;93(Suppl 1):60–67. doi:10.1016/j.jped.2017.07.002

Fleming S, Gill PJ, Van den Bruel A, Thompson M. Capillary refill time in sick children: a clinical guide for general practice. *Br J Gen Pract*. 2016;66(652):587–588. doi:10.3399/bjgp16X687925

Fuchs S, Terry M, Adelgais K, et al. Definitions and assessment approaches for emergency medical services for children. *Pediatrics*. 2016;138(6):e20161073. doi:10.1542/peds.2016-1073

Harris M, Lyng JW, Mandt M, et al. Prehospital pediatric respiratory distress and airway management interventions: an NAEMSP position statement and resource document. *Prehosp Emerg Care*. 2022;26(Supp1):118–128. doi:10.1080/10903127.2021.1994675

Hoffmann F, Schmalhofer M, Jehner M, Zimatschek S, Grote V, Reiter K. Comparison of the AVPU scale and the Pediatric GCS in prehospital setting. *Prehosp Emerg Care*. 2016;20(4):493–498. doi:10.3109/10903127.2016.1139216

Owusu-Ansah S, Moore B, Shah MI, et al; American Academy of Pediatrics, Committee on Pediatric Emergency Medicine, Section on Emergency Medicine, EMS Subcommittee, Section on Surgery. Pediatric readiness in emergency medical services systems. *Pediatrics*. 2020;145(1):e20193308. doi:10.1542/peds.2019-3308

OTHER RESOURCE

Prehospital Pediatric Readiness Project. Prehospital Pediatric Readiness Project Toolkit. Accessed March 18, 2024. https://emscimprovement.center/domains/prehospital-care/prehospital-pediatric-readiness/pprp-toolkit

CHAPTER 2

Using a Developmental Approach

Tyler Diettert, NREMTP, EC
Vishal Naik, MD, MEd, FAAP

LEARNING OBJECTIVES

1. **Discuss the communication challenges in handling the emotional responses of a family with a child who is ill or injured.**
2. **Provide family-centered care.**
3. **List the expected changes in vital signs with advancing age.**
4. **Describe key growth and developmental characteristics for the following groups: infants, toddlers, preschoolers, school-aged children, adolescents, and children and youth with special health care needs.**
5. **Explain unique anatomical and physiological characteristics that influence assessment of children in each group.**

Introduction

Infants and children constitute a small percentage of all patients seen in an emergency medical services (EMS) system. An even smaller percentage require advanced life support. EMS clinicians must become comfortable with pediatric-specific information to promote success while interacting with this special patient population. Because of the unique anatomical, physiological, and developmental differences in children, EMS clinicians must be well-versed in normal developmental changes in infants and children. To successfully complete a pediatric patient assessment, the provider must be able to incorporate an understanding of how a child's physical growth and psychosocial development relate to their condition.

In addition to knowing the growth and developmental characteristics of the different age groups, the EMS clinician must be aware of special considerations when assessing children and youth with special health care needs (CYSHCN). Sometimes the chronological age of the CYSHCN does not correspond with their developmental stage, and physical growth may not reflect emotional maturity.

Caring for a child also includes caring for the family. Caregivers, friends, and siblings may be present,

CASE STUDY 1

You receive a 9-1-1 call about a fussy infant. On your arrival, a crying mother meets you at the door with her 2-week-old daughter in her arms. The infant is crying inconsolably. She has no retractions, but her skin is mottled on both the trunk and the extremities. Her arms and legs are cool. The mother tells you that the baby has been fussy all day and vomiting all her feedings, and the mother thinks her stomach looks big.

1. What are the steps to assess and treat this child, and how will you address the mother's concerns?
2. What are the worrisome findings in this infant?

in addition to parents. Each person may have a different response to the child who is ill or injured, and the prehospital professional must be prepared to care for the entire "extended" family of friends and relatives. Communication skills are often as important as assessment and treatment skills in establishing an atmosphere of trust and comfort. Creating such an atmosphere requires that the EMS clinicians display a confident and professional attitude toward children's care and use age-appropriate pediatric skills. Communication skills become especially important in the event of a mass-casualty incident or natural disaster (see Chapter 16).

This chapter addresses age-specific growth characteristics and assessment techniques for physiologically stable children from infancy to adolescence, and for CYSHCN. Chapter 1 addresses general assessment techniques for the acutely ill or injured child, and Chapter 12 expands the discussion on CYSHCN.

Pediatric Calls and Response From Family and Providers

Every family responds differently when a child is ill (**FIGURE 2-1**). Having an ill child places immense pressure on the family unit. Common responses are presented in **TABLE 2-1**. Providers should focus on delivering family-centered care. This approach emphasizes the partnership between health care providers and families in the evaluation, planning, and delivery of care. It is based on the understanding that the family is the child's primary source of strength and support. This approach can lead to improved health outcomes and enhanced patient safety, and it fosters better communication. In this strategy, listening is imperative. Although some caregivers' responses may seem too emotional or illogical, listen to their concerns. *Acting as an advocate for proper care allows the EMS clinician to best approach the pediatric patient.* Caregivers usually know the patient best and can provide vital information that allows the EMS interaction to be successful. The EMS clinician needs to build rapport with the family by respecting their familiarity and expertise with the patient, while providing emergency care to the best of their abilities.

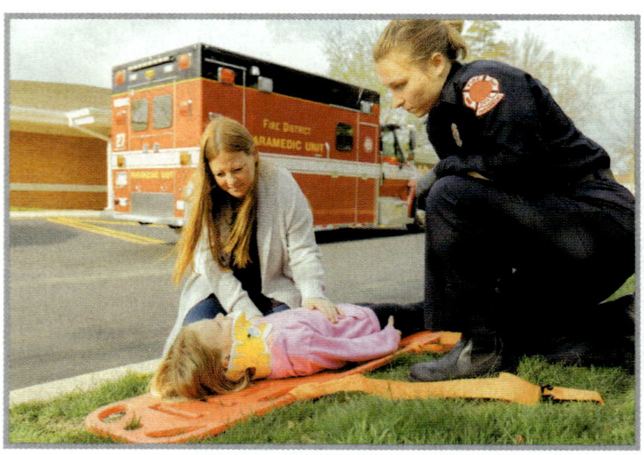

FIGURE 2-1 Every family responds differently to a child's illness or injury.

TABLE 2-1 Common Responses of Caregivers to Acute Illness or Injury in a Child

Response	Description
Disbelief	Caregivers may be struggling with a child's illness or injury. They may seem too calm or unconcerned.
Guilt	Caregivers may be horrified that they were unable to recognize the serious nature of their child's condition or that they were unable to prevent an injury. They may focus their attention on what should have been done, rather than on the child's immediate situation.
Anger	Caregivers may show their concern as anger, and they may direct their anger at the EMS clinician. Caregivers may become hostile when the EMS clinician makes efforts to stabilize their child. They may attempt to refuse transport.
Physical symptoms	Caregivers may have tachycardia, nausea, headache, chest pain, sweaty palms, dry mouth, or hyperventilation.

TIP

A family's response to a child's illness or injury is influenced by the child's developmental level, previous experience with the medical system, coping strategies, and culture; availability of support systems; and the nature of the emergency.

EMS clinicians, similar to family members, may respond emotionally to a pediatric patient. In addition, EMS clinicians may experience any of the emotional responses outlined in **TABLE 2-1**. Acting in a calm, professional manner gains trust from the family or caregivers and helps the EMS crew to establish control of a potentially emotional situation. This approach also allows the providers to gain as much valuable information as possible from the family or caregivers, which ultimately helps to triage the patient to the correct emergency department or include the most accurate differential diagnosis as part of the patient assessment.

The best way to reduce provider stress related to patient interactions is to remain current with pediatric patient assessment and treatment standards. Being familiar with the currently stocked pediatric equipment and medications, as well as their locations, can also decrease stress while interacting with an ill child. Because of the limited number of pediatric calls, being well-versed via review and hands-on training (ie, simulation) with the pediatric devices on an EMS unit becomes increasingly important.

TIP

Any provider can experience difficult emotions after a stressful pediatric call. EMS clinicians should seek professional help from a licensed mental health professional when unresolved stress results from these interactions.

Communication With the Child and Family or Caregiver

To effectively approach infants and children, EMS clinicians should account for developmental information as it relates to the patient assessment at hand. Each pediatric patient has a distinct personality that can impact the EMS clinician's ability to obtain pertinent assessment information. Calling 9–1–1 is often a stressful situation for the patient and family. Approaching the patient gently and at their eye level is important to initiating communication with the child. The best policy is to be honest with a child, because distrust can interfere with obtaining important information about the situation at hand. Observing the patient's behavior can provide clues to age-specific actions. Providers may also be able to pick up nonverbal clues from across the room as they approach the patient.

In addition to communication with the pediatric patient, communication with the caregiver or family is also important. Children seek clues from their parents regarding safety. Infants and children never make for a single-patient EMS call. The family and caregivers must be treated as therapeutic allies because their involvement can provide necessary information to properly handle the situation. Whenever possible, the pediatric patient and family or caregiver should be kept together. A successful pediatric patient interaction includes information gathering from family and primary caregivers. Effective communication is the cornerstone of effective prehospital care. For those with limited English proficiency, use of interpreter services via phone or video may be needed.

TIP

Communication skills are often as important as assessment and treatment skills.

Vital Signs at Different Life Stages

A common challenge in evaluating infants and children is determining when vital signs are normal according to the age of the patient. Respiratory rate, heart rate, blood pressure, and temperature all change with age. The presence or absence of fever, anxiety, or pain and the child's activity level also affect vital signs. In ill or injured children, the EMS clinician must distinguish the impact of these outside influences on vital signs from changes caused by pathologic processes. Chapter 1 presents key physical characteristics and assessment techniques that assist the EMS clinician in separating a "sick" child from a "not sick" child.

RESPIRATORY RATE

Although normal values for vital signs vary with age, there are a variety of physiological or anatomical bases for these changes. The normal range of respiratory rate slows with age because of an increase in the number of **alveoli** and increasing lung volume and lung compliance with physical growth. **TABLE 2–2** lists the normal respiratory rate for age.

At times, there is a problem with accurate counting of the rate, especially if the count is done in

TABLE 2–2 Normal Respiratory Rate for Age

Age	Respiratory Rate (Breaths/Min)
Infant (birth–12 mo)	30–60
Toddler (1–3 y)	24–40
Preschooler (3–5 y)	22–34
School-aged child (6–12 y)	18–30
Adolescent (13–18 y)	12–16

a 15-second interval. In infants, observe and count **abdominal excursions** (belly breathing) for 30 seconds to obtain an accurate respiratory rate. As a child grows, breathing becomes less dependent on abdominal muscles and the diaphragm and more dependent on the chest muscles. Observing **thoracic excursions** (movement of the chest wall) for 15 to 30 seconds provides an accurate respiratory rate in an older child. Use of accessory muscles to breathe, such as intercostal and subcostal muscles, is never normal when examining a child for normal respirations.

TIP

In infants, observe abdominal excursions and count the rate for 30 to 60 seconds to obtain an accurate respiratory rate.

HEART RATE

The baseline heart rate of infants and children slows with age, reflecting increasing control of the heart rate by the **vagus nerve**. The vagus nerve transmits **cholinergic impulses**, which slow the beating of the heart. **TABLE 2–3** lists normal heart rates for age.

TABLE 2–3 Normal Heart Rates for Age

Age	Heart Rate (Beats/Min)
Infant (birth–12 mo)	100–160
Toddler (1–3 y)	90–150
Preschooler (3–5 y)	80–140
School-aged child (6–12 y)	70–120
Adolescent (13–18 y)	60–100

In addition, by 2 years of age, a **circadian rhythm** in the heart rate is present, seen in a decline of 10 to 20 beats/min while the child is asleep. One confusing factor in assessing a child's heart rate during different phases of the sleep-wake cycle, or during different phases of respiration, is that the child's rhythm is more irregular than an adult's. This **sinus arrhythmia** is more prominent in toddlers to school-aged children and is caused by immature vagus nerve control (**FIGURE 2–2**).

BLOOD PRESSURE

A child's **blood pressure** increases with age (**TABLE 2–4** lists minimum systolic blood pressure values for age). A quick formula for the *minimum systolic blood pressure in a child 1 year and older is greater than 70 + (2 × age in years)*. The measured blood pressure is affected by equipment size. A cuff that is too small gives falsely elevated readings, whereas one that is too large gives readings that are too low. To measure blood pressure in the legs, the patient should be prone if possible. An appropriately sized cuff should be placed mid-thigh with the stethoscope placed over the popliteal artery. The systolic blood pressure in the legs is usually 10% to 20% higher than that in the arms. If **diastolic pressure** cannot be **auscultated**, obtain a systolic pressure by palpating the pulse as the cuff deflates. This value is approximately 10 mm Hg lower than an auscultated pressure because of the relative insensitivity of **palpation** in appreciating initial pulsations as the cuff is deflated.

TEMPERATURE

Body temperature also varies with age and site of measurement. Fever is equal to or greater than 38.0°C (100.4°F). Newborn temperatures are often higher than

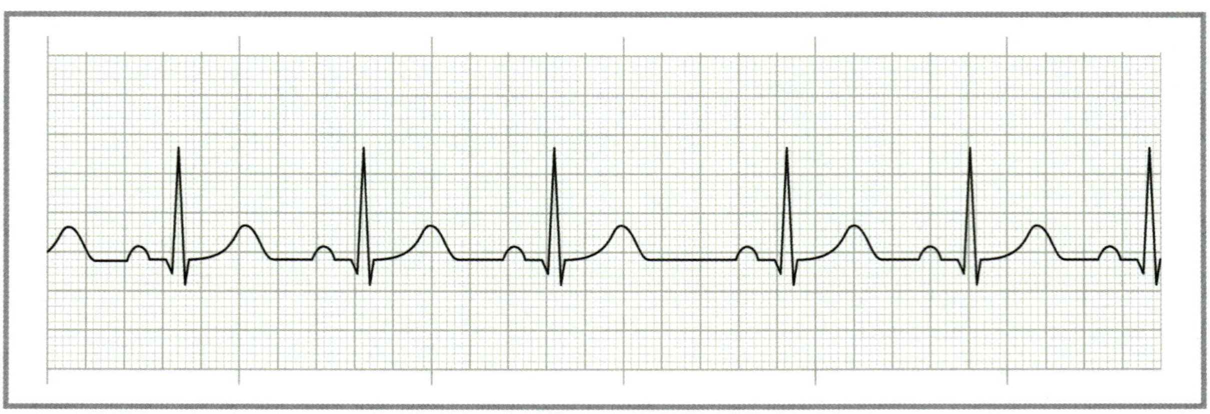

FIGURE 2–2 Electrocardiogram (ECG) of a sinus arrhythmia.

TABLE 2–4 Minimal Systolic Blood Pressure Values for Age

Age	Minimal Systolic Blood Pressure (mm Hg)
Newborn (birth–1 mo)	>60
Infant (1–12 mo)	>65
Toddler (1–3 y)	>70
Preschooler (3–5 y)	>75
School-aged child (6–12 y)	>80
Adolescent (13–18 y)	>90

those of older children, averaging 37.5 °C (99.5 °F) regardless of the measurement method during the first 6 months after birth. After 3 years of age, the temperature falls to below 37.2° C (99 °F), and finally to 36.7 °C (98 °F) by 11 years of age. A circadian rhythm to body temperature also develops by 5 years of age. This results in a lower temperature at night and a higher temperature during the day. In infants, when a recorded temperature is important to the assessment and the child is stable, ask the caregiver to obtain a rectal temperature. A rectal temperature is the accepted standard for infants. A **tympanic temperature** may be acceptable in older children (> 1 year), but may not be accurate depending on the caregiver's technique. Temperature may also be obtained with temporal artery thermometers. These devices use infrared technology to measure temperature in the superficial temporal artery. If obtained with good technique, these devices are quite accurate. An **axillary temperature** is approximately 1 °C (2 °F) lower than the rectal temperature. Normal body temperature decreases with increasing distance from the central circulation.

GROWTH RATES

Physical growth of infants and children includes body (somatic) growth and organ system growth. Skeletal and muscular growth has 2 spurts, the first from birth to 4 years of age and the second in adolescence (ages 9–14 for girls, ages 10–16 for boys). Brain, spinal cord, and nerve growth occurs maximally in the first few years and reaches adult proportions by 10 years of age.

The presence or absence of key secondary sex characteristics, especially pubic hair, marks a physiologic turning point for children. Genital growth begins at about 8 years of age in girls and 9 years of age in boys, but there is significant variation. When children have visible pubic hair, they have usually attained adult physiology.

Anatomical Changes

NECK AND AIRWAY

The neck is short in infancy and elongates during childhood because of vertebral growth. As this occurs, anatomical landmarks also change in shape, size, and location. The **epiglottis** changes from a U-shape to the longer and thinner adult structure (**FIGURE 2–3**). It also moves in location from the level of the C1 vertebra to the C3 vertebra as the child's

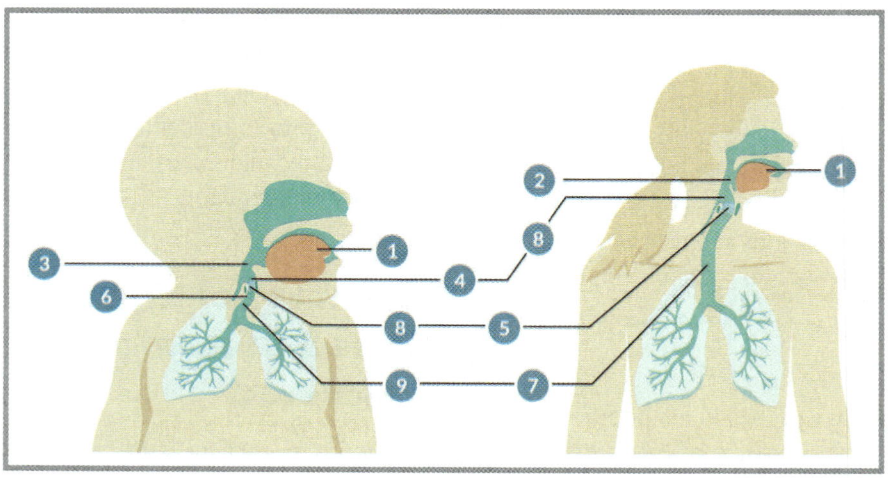

FIGURE 2–3 Differences between the child and adult airways. 1. Tongue, 2. Lower epiglottis, 3. U-shaped and more floppy epiglottis, 4. Vocal cord, 5. Cricoid ring, 6. More anterior and higher airway, 7. Trachea, 8. Narrowest area.

height increases. At birth, the **larynx** is only one-third the adult size. It becomes wider and longer until 3 years of age and undergoes another growth spurt during puberty. At birth, the **trachea** is one-third the adult length and increases 300% in circumference by puberty.

> **TIP**
> Contrary to prior belief, the airway of an infant is *not* funnel shaped. It has been confirmed that the airway is cylindrical, similar to that of an adult. This means that cuffed endotracheal tubes should be used in most infant intubations. (Continue to use uncuffed endotracheal tubes in newborn intubations.)

CHEST AND LUNGS

At birth, the chest wall is round (anteroposterior [AP] diameter equals lateral diameter). As the infant grows, it flattens out (lateral growth exceeds AP growth). Because an infant's chest wall is thin, heart and lung sounds are transmitted throughout the chest. Breath sounds are often audible on inspiration and expiration (**bronchovesicular**). In addition, secretions present anywhere in the respiratory tract are often heard throughout the chest. In an infant, respirations are mainly abdominal because of the greater role of the **diaphragm** in breathing mechanics. By 6 years of age, breathing becomes more thoracic in origin because of the development of chest wall musculature.

The lung tissue itself also changes with age. At birth, an infant has only 8% of the number of alveoli in adults. The number of alveoli increases until 8 years of age, after which they increase in size but not in number.

HEART

At birth, the right **ventricle** is the same size as the left ventricle, a function of the demands of fetal circulation. This accounts for the right axis deviation seen on **electrocardiograms (ECGs)** in infants. However, the left ventricle quickly grows in size and muscle mass and greatly outsizes the right ventricle with age. The left ventricle reaches adult proportions of 2:1 by 1 year of age.

ABDOMEN

A newborn infant has a protuberant abdomen for numerous reasons: The liver is relatively large, the stomach is more horizontal, and the lungs expand downward with a movement of the diaphragm. There is also less coverage of the abdominal solid organs (liver and spleen) by mature abdominal muscles. The stomach capacity increases from 30 to 90 mL at birth, to 210 to 360 mL by 1 year of age, and to 500 mL by 2 years of age. It assumes a more vertical position and reaches an adult volume of 750 to 900 mL during childhood. The abdomen also seems protuberant in toddlers because of a normal lumbar **lordosis** (curvature) of the spine. The abdomen becomes more **scaphoid** (flat) in school-aged children.

MUSCULOSKELETAL SYSTEM

In infants and young children, new longitudinal bone growth occurs in secondary centers of **ossification** at the end of the long bones, in **vertebral bodies**, and in the **cranium (physeal plates)**. These **cartilaginous growth plates** are relatively weak and are vulnerable to fractures exclusive to childhood. Bone growth ends with the ossification of the growth cartilage and union of the **epiphysis** and **diaphysis**. Growth in children is asymmetrical, with the lower extremities, especially the **distal extremities** (eg, feet), growing before puberty and the trunk during puberty.

Muscle growth includes an increase in the size of muscle cells. There is a spurt in the number of muscle cells at 2 years of age, with a maximal increase during puberty. The proportion of muscle mass to body weight changes during childhood, going from 1:5 at birth to 1:3 in adolescence.

NERVOUS SYSTEM

The growth of the nervous system occurs rapidly during infancy. It is 25% of the adult size at birth, 50% by 1 year of age, 80% by 3 years of age, and 90% by 7 years of age. This includes the growth of **glial cells**, **dendrites**, and **synaptic connections**. This growth is associated with a rapid increase in fine motor, gross motor, and language skills of infants and toddlers. These changing competencies impact the type of assessment techniques appropriate for evaluating children of different ages.

Summary of Changes in Vital Signs and Anatomy Through Childhood

Vital signs are useful for assessment but are sometimes difficult to obtain and difficult to interpret. Not only do normal vital signs change significantly with age, but respiratory and heart rates are especially sensitive to **adrenaline** release because of fear, pain, anxiety, cold, or high activity level. Other anatomical changes in the airway, chest, heart, abdomen, musculoskeletal system, and nervous system occur throughout childhood and require adaptations in assessment techniques.

Infants

DEVELOPMENTAL CHARACTERISTICS

Neonates range in age from birth to 28 days. They do not elicit interactive behavior, and therefore communicate predominantly by crying, though they are able to recognize their mother's voice. Neonates are physiologically immunodeficient. Infants are aged 1 month to 12 months, and their development varies dramatically by age in months. Infants are vulnerable and have a limited number of behaviors (**FIGURE 2–4**). Infants younger than 2 months spend most of their time sleeping or eating. They are not yet able to tell the difference between parents and other caregivers or strangers. They need to be kept warm, dry, and fed. They experience the world through their bodies. Being held, cuddled, or rocked soothes the infant. Hearing is also well-developed at birth, and calm and reassuring talk is often helpful.

Infants between 2 and 6 months of age are more active, which makes them easier to evaluate. They spend more time awake, they begin to make eye contact, and they recognize caregivers. Healthy infants in this age group have a strong suck, active extremity movement, and a vigorous cry. They may follow a bright light or toy with their eyes or turn their heads toward a loud sound or the caregiver's voice.

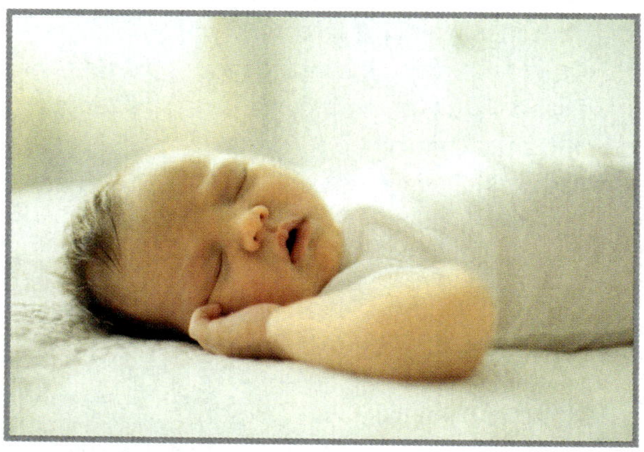

FIGURE 2–4 Infants are vulnerable, with a limited number of behaviors.

Between the ages of 6 and 12 months, most infants learn to talk or babble, sit unsupported, reach for toys, move objects from one hand to another, and put things in their mouths. At approximately 1 year of age, most infants start to scoot or crawl, pull themselves to a standing position, "cruise" on furniture, and possibly start to walk.

At 7 to 8 months, infants show a clear preference for their parents or caregivers, and by the age of 9 to 10 months demonstrate stranger anxiety, making separation of the child and caregiver for the purposes of assessment or transport especially problematic. They are most easily comforted by their parent or by a familiar adult. **TABLE 2–5** summarizes anatomical and physiological differences that are important in the assessment and care of the infant.

TABLE 2–5 Anatomical and Physiological Features of Infants

▪ Infants are nose breathers for the first several months after birth. Obstruction of the nose from secretions, blood, or edema may cause respiratory distress.
▪ The muscles of the infant's chest wall are not yet developed, and the abdominal muscles are the main muscles used for breathing. "Belly breathing" is normal in infants and may become exaggerated as breathing becomes more rapid.
▪ Retractions are easily seen in the infant with respiratory distress.
▪ A faster metabolic rate increases the need for oxygen and nutrients.
▪ Because of immature temperature regulation and high body surface-to-mass ratio, infants are at risk of experiencing heat loss and hypothermia if left undressed.
▪ The head is large in proportion to the body (**FIGURE 2–5**) and may be a potential source of significant heat loss.

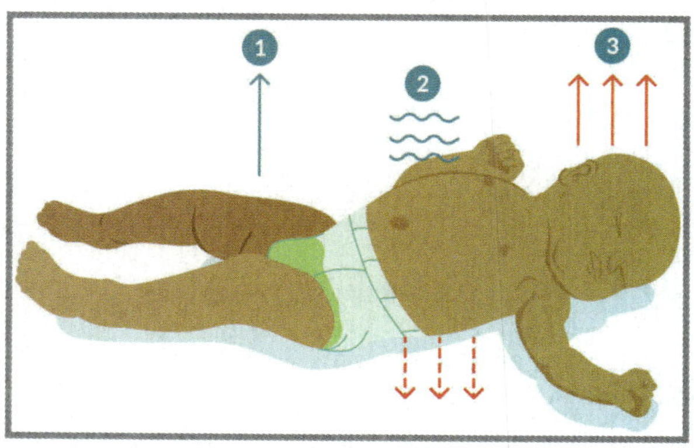

FIGURE 2–5 The infant's head is disproportionately large compared with older children and adults. The head may be a source of significant heat loss. 1. Evaporation, 2. Convection, 3. Radiation.

> **TIP**
> An infant younger than 3 months of age who is reported to be fussier than usual, feeding poorly, or sleeping excessively, or who has a temperature greater than 38 °C (100.4 °F), must be evaluated by a physician.

The infant's capacity to interact with the environment is limited, and signs and symptoms of illness are not always easy to appreciate. Because of these factors, always take seriously the caregiver's perception that "something is wrong." *A neonate or infant in the first 3 months after birth who is reported to be fussier than usual, feeding poorly, or sleeping excessively, or who has a temperature greater than 38 °C (100.4 °F), must be evaluated by a physician*. It is important to find out if there has been a recent history of trauma, how the infant was acting before the event, and if the infant has been healthy since birth. Find out if the infant was born at term and if there were any problems during pregnancy, labor, delivery, or immediately after the birth.

In the first few months after birth, excessive irritability or sleeping, fever, and poor feeding may be symptoms of a serious illness, such as **sepsis** or **congenital heart disease**. **Apnea** is a common chief complaint in the infant. Periods of apnea may be a sign of infection, heart disease, seizure activity, head injury, or a metabolic problem such as **hypoglycemia**. As the infant grows older and the behavioral repertoire expands, making the "sick" versus "not sick" decision becomes potentially easier.

Common Conditions in Infants

- Viral syndromes (vomiting and diarrhea)
- Respiratory problems
- Fever
- Ear infections
- Sudden unexpected infant death syndrome (SUIDS)
- Child maltreatment

Assessment of the Infant

Conduct the assessment of the infant using the following principles:

- Obtain the name of the patient, and use it while interacting with them.
- Obtain the normal disposition of the patient, and compare it with the current behavior being displayed. Any acute change in disposition should be noted and relayed during the transfer-of-care report. Communicate using a confident but smiling face directed at the infant.
- Ask the caregiver to hold the infant while the EMS clinician completes the assessment. Unless the infant requires a lifesaving intervention, the infant is better assessed in the arms of someone with whom they are familiar (**FIGURE 2-6**).
- Observe, auscultate, and palpate, in that order, to get the most information with the least amount of stress to the infant.
- Approach the infant slowly and calmly, because loud voices and quick movements may frighten them.
- Squat down or sit at "baby level."
- Observe the interaction of the infant with the caregiver. At age 7 to 8 months, infants may begin to show stranger anxiety.
- A comfortable environment is important. An infant who is happily snuggled in a caregiver's arms may become fussy and cry when unwrapped and placed on cold sheets.
- If the infant begins to cry, a pacifier, blanket, or favorite toy may help to calm them. Avoid feeding an infant who is seriously ill or injured.
- Perform the assessment according to the infant's activity level. For example, if the infant is calm, obtain the respiratory rate and auscultate lung sounds at the beginning of the assessment.
- Make nonthreatening physical contact first, such as touching an extremity to assess warmth and capillary refill. Perform the most upsetting parts of the examination last.
- Use a warmed stethoscope and warm hands and handle the infant gently. Avoid doing anything potentially painful or distressing until the assessment is nearly complete. It is difficult to assess heart and lung sounds or to palpate the abdomen when the infant is crying.
- Consider offering the infant a toy as a distraction.
- Assess motor strength by hand grasp strength and head control.
- In the older infant who may have stranger anxiety, ask the caregiver to remove the baby's clothing. Remove one item of clothing at a time, and then replace it, if possible, to avoid heat loss and hypothermia.

> **CAUTION**
> **The older infant is fearful of separation and develops stranger anxiety. Approach slowly and assess the infant while the infant being held by the caregiver.**

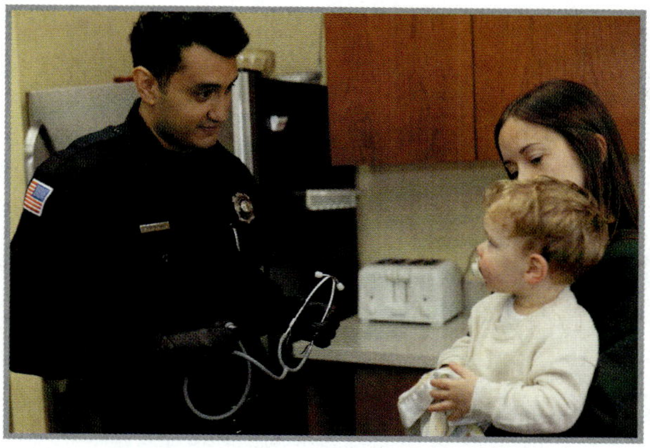

FIGURE 2-6 Approaching an infant: Observe the infant in the caregiver's arms before palpating or auscultating.

Toddlers

DEVELOPMENTAL CHARACTERISTICS

Toddlers (ages 1–3 years) experience rapid changes in growth and development. Developmentally, it is a critical time in brain development and learned behaviors. By approximately 18 months of age, toddlers are able to run, feed themselves, play with toys, and communicate with others. They begin making their own decisions and asserting their independence. The "terrible 2" stage actually begins at about 1 year of age and often lasts into the 3rd year. Toddlers are mobile and opinionated and may be terrified of strangers. They are illogical by nature and intensely curious, but lack a sense of danger. Problem-solving is concrete because toddlers cannot reason abstractly. Learning is done by trial and error, with little anticipation of consequences. Toddlers are playful, magical thinkers and are tremendously self-centered. They understand ownership and label things (eg, toys) as "mine."

Language capabilities vary widely. Some toddlers utter only single words, whereas others may speak in paragraphs. They often understand what is being said, even if they cannot respond with words. Older toddlers may remember earlier experiences with doctors or nurses, such as vaccinations or stitches, and be fearful about being examined.

The toddler's anatomy and physiology are much like the infant's, notably a large head and use of abdominal muscles to breathe. **Thermoregulation** is better, and limb muscles are more developed.

Common Ailments in Toddlers

- Viral syndromes (vomiting and diarrhea)
- Respiratory problems
- Febrile seizures
- Ear infections
- Child maltreatment
- Unintentional ingestions
- Open wounds

CAUTION
Do not separate the older infant or toddler from the caregiver.

Assessment of the Toddler

Conduct the assessment of the toddler using the following principles:

- Obtain the name of the patient, and use it while interacting with them.
- Obtain the normal disposition of the patient, and compare it with the current behavior being displayed. Any acute change in disposition should be noted and relayed during the transfer-of-care report.
- Approach the toddler slowly, and keep physical contact to a minimum until the child is familiar with you. Watch the toddler's activity level and behavior as you approach.
- Communicate with the toddler using a confident but friendly tone of voice.

CASE STUDY 2

You respond to a call for a 2-year-old who is having respiratory difficulty. On your arrival, you hear a barking cough from the child's room. When you enter, the child is sitting up in bed; he starts to cry and hides behind his mother. With crying, his breathing becomes noisier, and he becomes more anxious. Even though he has pajamas on, you can see suprasternal retractions.

His skin is pink. His parent states he was fine today, but suddenly woke up during the night "gasping for air."

1. Is this appropriate behavior for this child?
2. How can you assess this child without making him more upset?

- Sit or squat and use a quiet, soothing voice. Allow the toddler to remain on the caregiver's lap.
- Use play and distraction tools, such as a penlight or teddy bear, to help with the assessment (**FIGURE 2-7**). Introduce equipment slowly, and encourage the toddler to hold it.
- Talk to the toddler, preferably about themself. Admire their clothes; ask about pets or recent events. The toddler is the center of their universe.
- Give the toddler limited choices, such as "Do you want me to listen to your belly or your heart first?" This provides the toddler with a sense of control.
- Avoid questions that the toddler can answer with "no."
- Use simple, concrete terms. Provide a lot of reassurance and praise.
- Perform the most critical parts of the assessment first, working from toe to head, with the head and neck last.
- Ask for caregiver assistance with the assessment. The toddler is often less upset if the caregiver removes the toddler's clothes or administers oxygen.
- If necessary, ask the caregiver to gently palpate the toddler's extremity to test for pain.
- Do not expect toddlers to sit still and cooperate. Be flexible, but thorough.
- In certain situations, examining the toddler may be extremely difficult. If the child is alert but resists the examination, determine the need for transport based on history. Use of lights and sirens during transport may increase the toddler's level of fear.

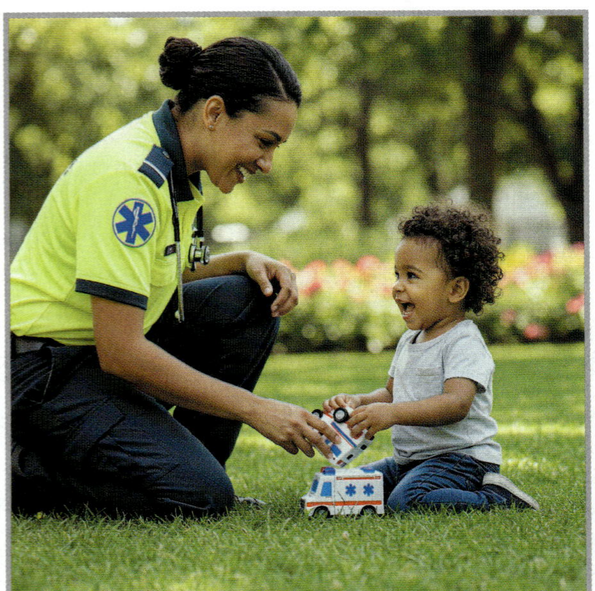

FIGURE 2-7 Approaching a toddler: Offer a toy or distraction tool to help with the assessment.

Preschoolers

DEVELOPMENTAL CHARACTERISTICS

Preschoolers (ages 3–5 years) are creative, illogical, and literal thinkers (**FIGURE 2-8**). They are not always able to distinguish between fantasy and reality, and they have many misconceptions about illness, injury, and bodily functions. For example, a preschooler might think of a cut as "my insides leaking out." If you tell a preschooler you are going to take their pulse, they may ask, "Where are you going to take it and will I get it back?" Common fears for this age group include body mutilation, loss of control, death, darkness, and being left alone. Attention span is short. It is always best to be honest about painful procedures. Information should be told as close to the procedure as possible to avoid miscommunication and increased anxiety. Preschool patients can be easily distracted by caregivers or friendly EMS clinicians. Positively rewarding these patients can help them maintain a good memory about interacting with EMS.

Common Ailments in Preschoolers

- Unintentional ingestions
- Respiratory problems

TIP

Preschoolers are creative thinkers who fear the loss of control. Explain procedures in simple terms, allow them to handle equipment, and assess from toe to head.

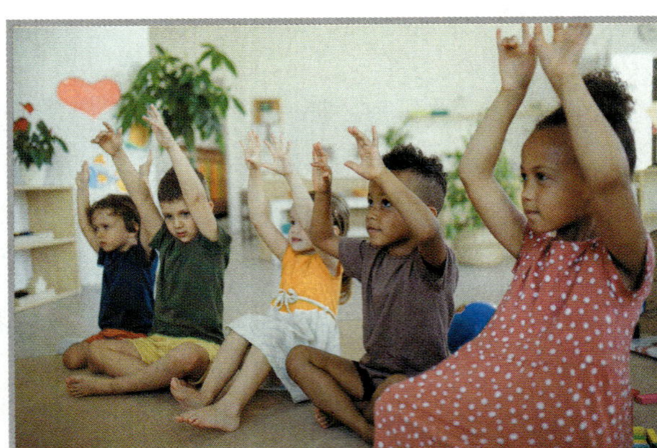

FIGURE 2-8 Preschoolers are creative and illogical thinkers.

- Febrile seizures
- Viral syndromes (vomiting and diarrhea)
- Open wounds
- Child maltreatment

Assessment of the Preschooler

Conduct the assessment of the preschooler using the following principles:

- Obtain the name of the patient, and use it while interacting with them.
- Obtain the normal disposition of the patient, and compare it with the current behavior being displayed. Any acute change in disposition should be noted and relayed during the transfer-of-care report.
- Use simple terms to explain procedures.
- Choose words carefully, using language that is age-appropriate and that does not induce fear.
- Clarify any apparent misconceptions.
- Use dolls or puppets, if available, to explain what you are doing.
- When appropriate, allow the child to handle equipment (**FIGURE 2-9**). Allow the patient to help.
- Set limits on behavior—for example, "You can cry or scream, but don't bite or kick."
- Praise good behavior.
- Use games or distraction tools. Ask them to name their favorite toy or color.
- Use dressings or bandages freely.
- Focus on and carry out one thing at a time.

School-Aged Children

DEVELOPMENTAL CHARACTERISTICS

School-aged children are talkative, analytical, and able to understand the concept of cause and effect (**FIGURE 2-10**). They feel a sense of accomplishment as they acquire new skills. Their knowledge of how bodies work may be sketchy, and they have limited ability to gauge the seriousness of a particular illness or injury. With a careful choice of words, they can understand simple explanations about their bodies, and they like to be involved in their own care.

Common fears include separation from parents and friends, loss of control, pain, and physical disability. School-aged children are often afraid to talk about their feelings and may be unable to put their feelings into words. As they become more mobile and more independent, they begin to take more risks. They live in the present. Belonging and peer group support are important.

The anatomy and physiology of a child are similar to an adult's by about 8 years of age.

Common Conditions in School-Aged Children

- Poisonings/ingestion
- Respiratory problems
- Fractures (eg, sports injuries)
- Open wounds
- Viral syndromes (vomiting and diarrhea)

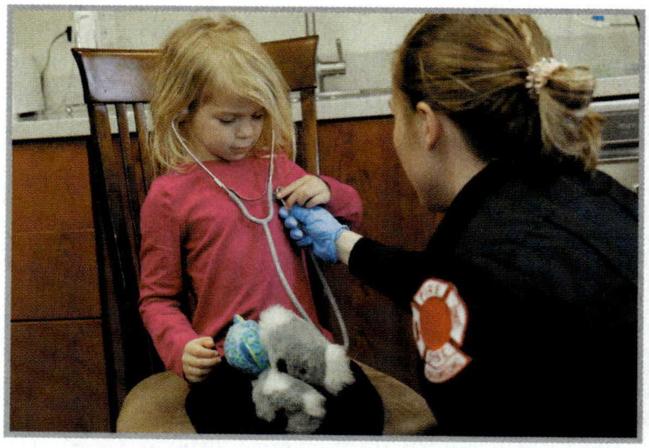

FIGURE 2-9 When approaching a preschooler, allow the child to handle the equipment.

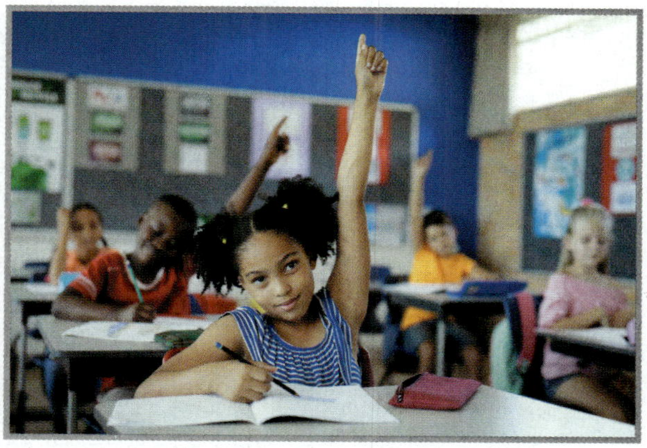

FIGURE 2-10 School-aged children are talkative, analytical, and able to understand the concept of cause and effect.

Assessment of the School-Aged Child

Conduct the assessment of the school-aged child using the following principles:

- Obtain the name of the patient, and use it while interacting with them.
- Obtain the normal disposition of the patient, and compare it with the current behavior being displayed. Any acute change in disposition should be noted and relayed during the transfer-of-care report.
- Speak directly to the child, and then include the caregiver. Be careful not to offer too much information.
- Anticipate the child's questions and fears, and discuss them immediately.
- Explain in simple terms what is wrong and how it will affect them. For example, when speaking to a 5-year-old, you may explain, "Your arm bone is broken, but the doctor will be able to fix it good as new. We'll give you some medicine in your arm to help stop it from hurting so much."
- Explain procedures immediately before doing them. Never lie to a child, telling the child that something will not hurt or that you are almost finished if this is not true. Remember that the child may not ask questions, even if they have real concerns.
- Ask the older school-aged child if they would like the caregiver to be present.
- Provide privacy. Children in this age group are modest. Expose the child for physical assessment as necessary, and cover them up when done.
- If physical restraint is necessary to complete a procedure or to guarantee the safety of the child or crew, tell the child what is going to happen and then do it.
- Do not negotiate unless the child really has a choice. For example, it is okay to ask the child if they would like the intravenous (IV) line in the right or left hand, but not to ask if it is okay to start an IV when it must be done.
- Let the child be involved in their own care. Children in this age group are afraid of being out of control (**FIGURE 2-11**).
- Reassure the child that being ill or injured is not a punishment.
- Praise the child for cooperating. Be careful not to be irritable if the child does not cooperate.

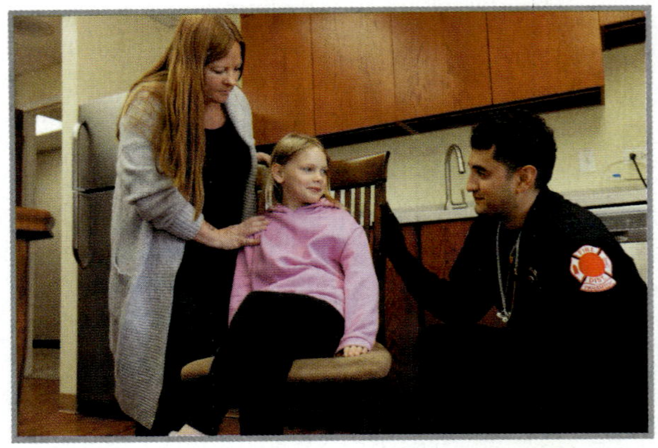

FIGURE 2-11 Approaching a school-aged child: Let the child be involved in their own care.

- The physical assessment can usually be done in the head-to-toe format.

Adolescents

GROWTH AND DEVELOPMENTAL CHARACTERISTICS

Adolescents sometimes seem to share some characteristics of toddlers: They are very mobile but may lack common sense. However, adolescents are rational, understand cause and effect, and are able to express themselves with words. Adolescence is a time of experimentation and risk-taking behaviors (**FIGURE 2-12**). Adolescents often believe they are immune to danger, that they are "indestructible." They gradually shift from relying on family to relying on friends for psychological support and social development.

- Adolescents struggle with independence, loss of control, body image, sexuality, and peer pressure. Anything that makes them different from their peers causes anxiety. Psychosomatic complaints are common in this age group. They may have mood swings or depression and when ill or injured may act younger than their age, leaving a scared child in an adult body.
- Respect is an important part of the relationship and interaction with the adolescent patient, as it may enable an opportunity to gain information needed to provide the appropriate care in a short time. An example may be a situation in which there is the need to determine use of drugs and which drug may have been used. Most toxicology drug screens detect only a small number of common drugs used, but not drugs

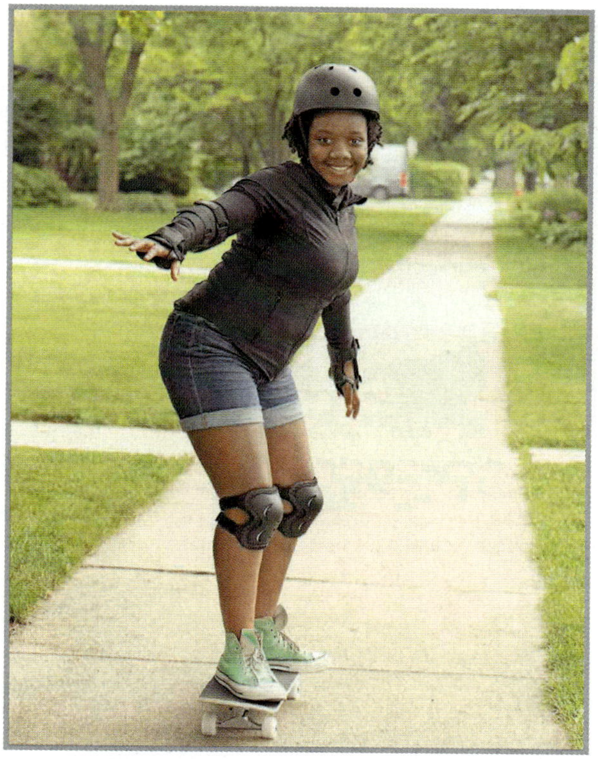

FIGURE 2–12 Adolescence is a time of experimentation and risk-taking behaviors.

such as synthetic marijuana. An adolescent may be able to guide you in the right direction if there is a trusting relationship developed in a short period.

> **TIP**
>
> Adolescents struggle with independence, loss of control, body image, sexuality, and peer pressure. Provide concrete information, respect their privacy, and speak to them directly.

Common Conditions in Adolescents

- Poisonings/drug ingestion
- Respiratory problems
- Fractures (eg, sports injuries)
- Open wounds
- Mental health/behavioral concerns

Assessment of the Adolescent

Conduct the assessment of the adolescent using the following principles:

- Obtain the name of the patient, and use it while interacting with them.

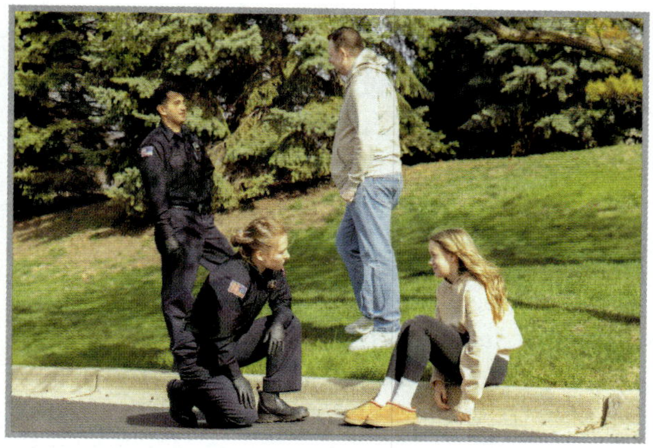

FIGURE 2–13 Approaching an adolescent: Speak to them directly.

- Obtain the normal disposition of the patient, and compare it with the current behavior being displayed. Any acute change in disposition should be noted and relayed during the transfer-of-care report.
- Provide accurate information about the illness or injury, normal body functions, and interventions. Explain what you are doing and why.
- Encourage the patient to ask questions and to be involved in their own care.
- Show respect. Speak directly to the adolescent. Do not turn to the caregiver for initial information (**FIGURE 2–13**).
- Obtain consent for treatment from a parent/caregiver if the patient is not old enough.
- Respect the adolescent's modesty, privacy, and confidentiality unless it places them at risk.
- Be honest and nonjudgmental.
- Do not be misled by the adolescent's size or make assumptions about their comprehension of events. Adolescents may misinterpret the seriousness of the situation. They may also have many fears about permanent injury, disfigurement, or "being different" as a result of the illness or injury. Give adolescents accurate information, and anticipate their questions or fears.
- Avoid becoming frustrated or angry if the adolescent does not talk or is uncooperative.
- Enlist the adolescent's friends to help persuade the adolescent to cooperate with the assessment or treatment if they resist.
- Be mindful of their modesty.

Children and Youth With Special Health Care Needs

GROWTH AND DEVELOPMENTAL CHARACTERISTICS

Approximately 15% of children and youth have special health care needs. They have, or are at risk of developing, chronic conditions that require additional health and support services. About 1% have medical complexity, which is a state in which an individual has multiple chronic health conditions that interact with each other, resulting in significant challenges in their health care management. When working with **children and youth with special health care needs (CYSHCN)**, it is important to consider developmental age, rather than chronological age. Information about the patient should be obtained from caregivers. If an EMS clinician does not fully understand the child's medical or developmental history, *it is better to be honest than to feign understanding and potentially place the patient at risk.* Children and youth with special health care needs may have any type of chronic condition that affects health, normal growth, or development. This may include physical disability, developmental or learning disability, technological dependency, or chronic illness. The developmental or learning disability may include mental impairment, difficulties in communication, sensory impairment, or limitations in physical activity. The child who is technology dependent may have a home **ventilator**, **tracheostomy**, **gastric feeding tube**, or long-term IV device. Specific categories of patients and methods of assessment and treatment are discussed in Chapter 12.

The number of children in the community with special needs is growing. EMS clinicians must be familiar with the conditions and types of technology used in assessing and treating CYSHCN. These children may require transport and care for exacerbation of their illness or for an unrelated illness or injury.

Unique aspects related to children with special needs include the following:

- Baseline vital signs may be outside the age-appropriate values.
- Weight may be significantly higher or lower than expected.
- Standard prehospital quick-reference guides may be inaccurate.
- The child may have a limited ability to endure respiratory distress or shock.
- The child may not have an age-appropriate understanding of the immediate medical problem.
- The child may have communication issues.
- Be alert for a latex allergy.

CAUTION

Do not assume that a child with a physical disability is cognitively impaired. Always ask the caregiver to clarify the child's normal level of functioning and interaction.

TIP

Even if a disabled child cannot talk or interact, show your respect by introducing yourself, explaining what you are doing, and providing verbal reassurance.

TIP

When treating a child with special health care needs, ask the parents/caregivers if they have a "go bag" of supplies that may aid in treatment, and bring this bag to the hospital.

Assessment of Children and Youth With Special Health Care Needs

Conduct the assessment of CYSHCN using the following principles:

- Obtain the name of the patient, and use it while interacting with them.
- Check for any medical alert or allergy jewelry.
- Obtain the normal disposition of the patient, and compare it with the current behavior being displayed. Any acute change in disposition should be noted and relayed during the transfer-of-care report. Include the impressions of the caregiver in chart documentation. Ask the caregiver what they think of the child's condition, activity, and behaviors. Find out if the caregiver believes that the child is "not acting right."
- Get a careful history from the caregiver. The caregiver can provide detailed information about the child's medical history, medications, and current complaints. The caregiver is also aware of how best to approach the child and of typical responses and behaviors.
- Ask about the presence of any special equipment.
- Approach the child with a developmental delay gently, and use techniques appropriate to their

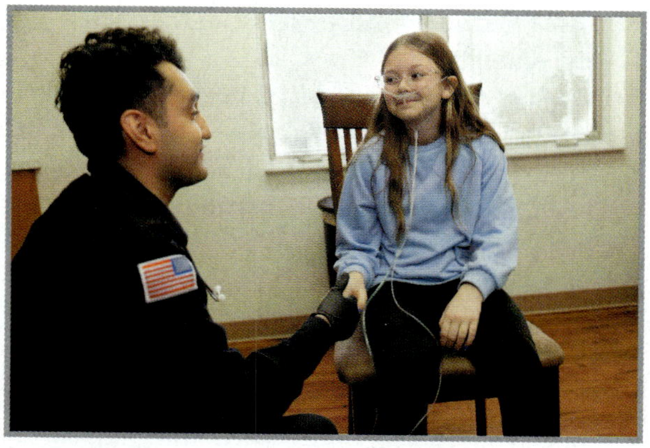

FIGURE 2-14 Approaching children and youth with special health care needs: Obtain a thorough history and identify developmentally appropriate approaches that work best with the child.

developmental level, not chronological age. To communicate, use language and techniques tailored to the child's cognitive level.

- Do not assume that the child with a physical disability has a mental impairment (**FIGURE 2-14**). Ask the caregiver about the child's level of function and interaction with others. To get at baseline functional level you might ask, "What would Johnny be doing right now if he was feeling well?"
- Display polite, professional behavior; acknowledge the caregivers' expertise; and take their concerns seriously. Families of chronically ill children usually have had extensive experience with the medical system. If most of their experiences have been good, they will very likely perceive the EMS clinician as an ally. However, if they have had bad experiences, they may feel a need to be highly vigilant in protecting their child and may be perceived as difficult or controlling.
- Keep in mind the amount of stress that the caregiver of a CYSHCN may be experiencing and be sympathetic. It is often helpful to acknowledge their stress about the care being provided.
- Ask the family/caregiver if they have an emergency information form or emergency protocols or action plans that provide important information about the patient.

Tips for the EMS Clinician

INFANT (0–12 MONTHS)

- Be diligent about keeping infants warm and dry to limit hypothermia.
- When assessing respiratory rate, count for a full 30 to 60 seconds.
- This is a particularly stressful time for parents adjusting to the eating, sleeping, and crying cycle; sometimes this is complicated by postpartum depression, which can be a risk factor for abuse.
- Persistent crying, irritability, or feeding difficulties can be a symptom of serious illness.
- Although infants sleep a lot, they should rouse easily; inability to rouse an infant should be considered an emergency.
- Parents are often the first to notice subtle changes. Take their concerns seriously, even if the initial assessment seems reassuring.
- Head control is limited until closer to 6 months of age, so when handling an infant, make sure to support the head and neck well.
- By 6 months of age, infants should make eye contact; lack of eye contact in a sick infant could be a sign of significant illness, depressed mental status, or delayed development.
- By 6 to 12 months, infants are at risk of experiencing foreign body aspiration and poisoning because of their exploration of the environment (eg, by crawling, using their hands) and placing objects into their mouths.
- Reduce separation anxiety by keeping the child and parent/caregiver together during an evaluation and involving the parent in the treatment if appropriate.
- Crawling and walking can increase exposure to physical dangers and injuries.

TODDLERS (12–36 MONTHS)

- Persistent crying or irritability can be a symptom of a serious illness.
- Because of a lack of molars, there is an increased risk of choking because children may not be able to grind up food before swallowing.
- Increased mobility increases exposure to physical dangers and injury.
- Distracting a child with a flashlight or toy may aid in physical examination.
- Allow a child to hold objects of importance to them (eg, blanket).
- Try to make the interaction as positive as possible; painful procedures make for lasting impressions.

PRESCHOOL CHILDREN (3–5 YEARS)

- The rapid increase in language means they understand much of what is said if simple terms are used.
- Respect the patient's modesty, and cover them up after the physical examination.
- The risk of foreign body airway obstruction continues to be high.
- Offer choices to the patient if appropriate (eg, "Should I listen to your front first or the back?").
- Do not waste time trying to use logic to convince preschoolers; they are concrete thinkers. Avoid using frightening or misleading comments.
- Appealing to their magical thinking may allow you to do more (eg, "This magic mist [nebulizer] will help you breathe better.").
- Communicate about procedures as close to doing them as possible.
- Respect modesty.

SCHOOL-AGED CHILDREN (6–12 YEARS)

- Provide simple explanations for illness and treatments.
- Ask the child about pain/symptoms first, then confirm with the parent.
- Be honest about painful procedures.
- If possible, provide a sense of control by giving choices.
- Respect modesty.
- Ask about school/sports/activities or interests to allow patients to warm up to you faster.

ADOLESCENTS (13–18 YEARS)

- Explain things as clearly and honestly as you would to an adult.
- Give choices when appropriate.
- Respect modesty.
- Be honest about procedures that will cause discomfort.
- Address concerns and fears about the lasting effects of their injuries.
- Adolescence includes hormonal surges, emotions, and peer pressure; there is an increased risk of substance abuse, self-endangerment, pregnancy, and dangerous sexual practices.

CHILDREN AND YOUTH WITH SPECIAL HEALTH CARE NEEDS

- Obtain information from the parent/caregiver.
- Ask the parent/caregiver what is "different" about the child that prompted the EMS call.
- Obtain a careful history from the parent/caregiver.
- Approach the child with respect and use techniques appropriate to their developmental level, not their age.
- Ask about the presence of a "go bag" and an emergency information form.

Summary

Understanding the developmental characteristics of each age group is essential for accurate assessment and treatment of the child in the prehospital environment. Good field care requires good communication with the child and family. The family may include a large number of people, all of whom become "patients." Children and youth with special health care needs pose additional challenges in assessment, but their caregivers can be a great asset in guiding field evaluation and management.

Every call experience offers the ability for an EMS clinician to learn something. With pediatric patients, the opportunities are greater than those with adults. Post-call self-evaluation and call critique can offer providers an opportunity to identify ways to improve for the next pediatric patient interaction.

CASE STUDY 3

You are called to a park where a 15-year-old was doing skateboard tricks and fell. He was not wearing a helmet and briefly lost consciousness. He now complains that his wrist hurts but wants to stay with his friends. A friend had called 9-1-1. He does not want to be examined, definitely does not want to go to the hospital, and starts to leave the scene as you approach him.

1. Is this teenager's reaction normal?
2. What techniques can help you adequately assess his injuries?

CASE STUDY ANSWERS

CASE STUDY 1

Even though the mother is crying, it is important to obtain additional history. Was the infant full-term? Did she have any problems with delivery or after birth? Has the infant had feeding problems or vomiting in the past? Any fever or diarrhea?

Infants in the first few months after birth have a limited range of behaviors, so anything out of the ordinary in the child's feeding, sleeping, or basic activity level raises concern about serious underlying illness or injury.

Reassuring the mother is important, but this infant may be critically ill and requires rapid assessment and transport. Although an infant's extremities may be mottled because of cold, mottling of the trunk is an extremely worrisome sign, reflecting poor perfusion. The possibility of **hypovolemic shock** is supported by the infant's cool extremities and history of vomiting.

Furthermore, although infants can develop abdominal distension because of crying and swallowing air, abdominal distension in association with vomiting and signs of shock (abnormal appearance and abnormal circulation to the skin) suggest serious pathology, such as an intestinal obstruction.

Move the infant quickly into the ambulance, explaining to the parent what you are doing and why. If local protocol permits, allow the parent to ride with you to the hospital. The infant should be transported and secured on the stretcher. It is never okay to allow a parent or caregiver to hold an infant on their lap while on the stretcher. Treatment of this infant includes administration of oxygen via a face mask and rapid transport to an emergency department. Prevention of heat loss by swaddling and applying a hat is important because **hypothermia** is a risk for a young infant. Consider vascular access en route, with a bolus of 20 mL/kg of crystalloid fluid.

The infant was found to have **malrotation with volvulus** and underwent emergency surgery, and did well.

CASE STUDY 2

Toddlers are often fearful of strangers, so enlisting the help of parents or caregivers makes patient assessment much easier. Allow the child to remain with the parent. Sit on the bed or crouch down to the child's eye level, and use a calm soothing voice. You can use distractions, such as a penlight, or ask about a stuffed animal on the bed to gain the child's attention and to evaluate interactivity. Ask the parent to remove the child's pajamas, and observe the work of breathing—including suprasternal, subcostal, or intercostal retractions—and respiratory rate.

Although your main concern is the child's respiratory status, you may have to perform other portions of the hands-on examination, such as touching or tickling the child's toes before you get to the chest. When listening to breath sounds, warm the stethoscope beforehand and explain what you are doing. If the child resists, you may be able to listen to a stuffed animal first, and allow the child to do the same, before resuming your examination.

Your assessment reveals the child's respiratory rate to be 32 breaths/min and heart rate 128 beats/min. You decide to give the child oxygen, but he refuses to keep the oxygen mask in place even with his parent's help, a response you recognize is typical of a toddler who is not seriously ill. For transport to the hospital, you secure the child on the stretcher, allowing his parent to accompany you in the ambulance, and direct blow-by oxygen in his direction.

At the emergency department, he is given nebulized epinephrine and oral dexamethasone for croup. The child is observed for 2 hours and then discharged home.

CASE STUDY 3

This teenager is asserting his independence but is not legally able to give consent or refuse care, unless he is emancipated. He may not realize the risks of occult injury. Show respect, be honest and nonjudgmental, and speak directly to him. Explain why it is important to check him for potentially serious injuries, and offer him the privacy of the ambulance to conduct the examination. If he still refuses care, attempt to contact his parents or caregivers or enlist the assistance of the police.

Suggested References

TEXTBOOKS

American Academy of Pediatrics, American College of Emergency Physicians. *APLS: The Pediatric Emergency Medicine Resource*. 5th ed. Jones & Bartlett Learning; 2012

Kliegman RM, St Geme 111 JW, Nelson WE, eds. *Nelson Textbook of Pediatrics*. 22st ed. Elsevier; 2025

Walls RM, Hockberger RS, Gausche-Hill M, Erickson TB, Wilcox S. *Rosen's Emergency Medicine: Concepts and Clinical Practice*. 10th ed. Elsevier; 2023

ARTICLE

Ghandour RM, Hirai AH, Kenney MK. Children and youth with special health care needs: a profile. *Pediatrics*. 2022;149 (Suppl 7):e2021056150D. doi:10.1542/peds.2021-056150D

OTHER RESOURCES

Code Green Campaign (first responder oriented mental health advocacy and education organization). 2025. www.codegreencampaign.org

Family Voices. FamilyVoices.org. 2025

Fire/EMS Helpline. 1–888–731-FIRE (3473)

CHAPTER 3

Respiratory Emergencies

Alexandra Cheetham, MD, MEd, FAAP
Tyler Molleur, MSN, RN, CEN, TCRN, CPEN, CTRN, CFRN, AEMT

LEARNING OBJECTIVES

1. **Differentiate among respiratory distress, respiratory failure, and respiratory arrest according to history, physical examination, and physiological monitoring.**
2. **Describe how to assess airway and breathing, including interpreting information from the Pediatric Assessment Triangle and the ABCDEs.**
3. **Interpret the physiologic information provided by pulse oximetry and capnometry, recognize situations in which each should be used, and recognize appropriate management responses to abnormal measurements.**
4. **Outline a general treatment strategy, going from the least to the most invasive, for children with respiratory compromise.**
5. **Contrast the key signs, symptoms, and management of upper airway obstruction versus lower airway obstruction.**
6. **Discuss possible complications of assisted ventilation and learn to anticipate the need to identify and correct these complications.**

Introduction

The most common chief complaints that emergency medical services (EMS) clinicians respond to are traumatic injury (28%), general illness (10%), and respiratory distress (9%). Of all conditions causing respiratory disease in children, asthma is the most common noninfectious cause. However, respiratory distress may also be associated with a myriad of other conditions, including viral illnesses, pneumonia, foreign bodies, and trauma. Good assessment and early intervention for pediatric respiratory problems can avert serious illness and preventable death and may shorten treatment time in the emergency department (ED).

Focusing on certain key physical signs and symptoms allows the EMS clinician to rapidly assess the effectiveness of gas exchange in the airways and lung alveoli. Using the Pediatric Assessment Triangle (PAT) is an important first step in determining the severity of disease, localizing the physiologic problem, and beginning treatment. Of the 3 aspects of the PAT, appearance and work of breathing are essential to the initial impression for a child in respiratory distress. Appearance reflects the overall state of ventilation and oxygenation. Increased work of breathing indicates either airway obstruction at some level or a problem in gas exchange at the alveolar level; it is often an early sign of hypoxia or hypercapnia. Fading respiratory effort is a sign of severe hypoxia or hypercapnia. Cyanosis of the skin or mucous membranes also indicates severe hypoxia and is part of the third aspect of the PAT: circulation to the skin.

After using the PAT to establish an initial impression, the primary assessment provides a more detailed assessment and includes assessing the work of breathing (this can be done in a nonthreatening manner by asking the parent or caregiver to lift the child's shirt or clothing), counting the respirations, performing hands-on chest auscultation, evaluating the heart rate, and obtaining pulse oximetry. This assessment not only provides a picture of respiratory function but also helps prioritize general and specific treatments, interventions, and timing of transport.

Respiratory Distress, Failure, and Arrest

Respiratory distress, failure, and arrest are 3 points on a continuum of physiologic response to different types of hypoxic stress. Using the PAT, respiratory distress is characterized by increased work of breathing and normal appearance. An abnormal appearance with increased work of breathing is consistent with respiratory failure/arrest. In addition, cyanosis may occur with respiratory failure/arrest. Causes of hypoxic stress are variable and include asthma, bronchiolitis, croup, pneumonia, and chest wall injury. Although these 3 points in the continuum (respiratory distress, failure, and arrest) have different clinical characteristics in theory, in reality they are part of a spectrum that is not black or white.

Respiratory distress is an abnormal physiological condition identified by increased work of breathing. Increased respiratory rate; supraclavicular, suprasternal, intercostal, or subcostal retractions; use of accessory muscles; and nasal flaring are signs that indicate increased work of breathing. These physical signs may be present alone or in combination and represent the patient's attempt to make up for decreased gas exchange in the lungs and airways and to maintain oxygenation and ventilation.

The child's appearance is relatively normal because oxygen delivery is still adequate.

Respiratory failure occurs when the infant or child exhausts their energy reserves and can no longer maintain oxygenation and ventilation. Respiratory failure may occur when chest wall muscles get tired after a long period of increased work of breathing (eg, a child with severe asthma who is very tight and has been working hard to breathe for several hours), when the insult is severe and progressive (eg, **fulminant pneumonia**), or when there is a failure of central respiratory drive (eg, a child with a severe closed-head injury). An abnormal appearance (lethargic, weak, fussy, poor feeding) or cyanosis in a child with increased work of breathing indicates respiratory failure. An abnormally low respiratory rate and decreased respiratory effort, usually with a decreasing heart rate, also indicate respiratory failure.

Respiratory failure must be treated immediately to restore good oxygenation and ventilation and to prevent respiratory arrest.

Signs of failure are a decreased level of consciousness, slow to agonal respirations, shallow respiratory depth, cyanosis, grunting, decreasing pulse oximetry, and bradycardia or inappropriate slowing of the heart rate.

Respiratory arrest means absence of effective breathing. If ventilation and oxygenation are not immediately supported, respiratory arrest rapidly progresses to full cardiopulmonary arrest. Most episodes of cardiac arrest in pediatric patients begin as respiratory arrest. Intervening at this point may prevent cardiac arrest.

Early intervention for children with respiratory distress may prevent progression to respiratory failure and arrest. If the child is experiencing respiratory failure, aggressive intervention will provide a far better chance of producing neurologically intact survivors

CASE STUDY 1

You are dispatched to the home of a 32-month-old boy who is having difficulty breathing. His mother says that for 2 days he has had a slight fever and has been "wheezing." He suddenly awoke tonight acutely short of breath and now is making a very loud noise each time he inhales. The child has no prior history of wheezing or respiratory illness.

The child is sitting on his mother's lap looking anxious but makes eye contact and cries when you approach. He makes loud, harsh noises with each inspiration. His color is pink, but he has marked supraclavicular and suprasternal retractions and nasal flaring. His respiratory rate is 38 breaths/min, and his heart rate is 160 beats/min. His blood pressure is not obtained. His skin is warm, and he has strong pulses and normal capillary refill time. He has good air movement with loud, harsh breath sounds heard on each inspiration.

1. How sick is this child?
2. Are this child's findings more likely to be caused by upper airway or lower airway obstruction, and how will you manage him in the field?

than treatment of respiratory arrest that progresses to cardiac arrest, which has an extremely low probability of survival.

Prearrival Preparation

Based on dispatch information and while en route to the scene, prepare mentally for management of respiratory distress and failure by reviewing the appropriate assessment techniques and treatment options for the child's age. This includes recalling an age-based approach to assessment, as outlined in Chapter 1; equipment needs; and the likely treatment and transport options. Also, anticipate the determinants of whether to stay on scene and treat or to manage the airway and transport immediately to the ED.

Scene Size-Up

Be sure the scene is safe and that there are no obvious illness or injury threats. Assess the environment for foreign body risks, medications, noxious gases, fumes, chemicals, or smoke. Document scene conditions if environmental factors may be contributing to anticipated respiratory problems. If indicated, make sure to wear personal protective equipment; question how many patients are in the home or facility; determine if additional resources are needed; and attempt to determine the mechanism of injury, nature of the illness, and need for spinal motion restriction.

General Assessment: The Pediatric Assessment Triangle

EVALUATING THE PRESENTING COMPLAINT

Find out the nature of the presenting complaint by asking several directed questions, as suggested in **TABLE 3–1**. After the primary assessment, in patients with mild distress, there is time to get a more complete SAMPLE history (SAMPLE standing for Signs & Symptoms, Allergies, Medications, Past medical history, Last oral intake, and Events leading to injury or illness) on scene as part of the focused history. If the child is in respiratory failure, do this later while en route to the ED.

TABLE 3–1 Key Questions About the Presenting Complaint

Key Question	Possible Medical Problem
Has your child ever had this kind of problem before?	Asthma, chronic lung disease
Is this the first time that your child has had trouble breathing?	Asthma, foreign body aspiration, bronchiolitis
Is your child taking any medications?	Asthma, chronic lung disease, congenital heart disease
Has your child had a fever?	Pneumonia, bronchiolitis, viral infections such as croup
Did your child suddenly start coughing/choking/gagging?	Foreign body aspiration or ingestion
Has your child had an injury to the chest?	Pulmonary contusion, pneumothorax
What primary care has your child received?	Allows differentiation between an acute condition (foreign body aspiration) vs an exacerbation of a chronic condition (asthma)

ASSESSMENT OF RESPIRATORY STATUS

Using the PAT

Begin the assessment with the PAT, as discussed in the chapter on patient assessment. Carefully evaluate appearance, work of breathing, and circulation to the skin. The PAT helps establish how sick the child is, an overall impression of the child, and the need for emergent intervention. **TABLE 1–2** in Chapter 1 lists physical features in the child to help make these clinical distinctions by simple observation and listening.

Appearance

Appearance reflects the adequacy of oxygenation and ventilation in a child with difficulty breathing. If the child is compensating effectively for the respiratory insult, the appearance is fairly normal, and the Tone, Interactiveness, Consolability, Look or gaze, and Speech or cry (TICLS) mnemonic (see **TABLE 1–1** in Chapter 1) shows an interactive child with good tone and color and with normal vocalizations who looks or gazes at someone. If the child is not compensating, the appearance is abnormal, and the child has abnormal findings in the TICLS mnemonic because the brain is impaired by hypoxia or hypercapnia. Abnormal appearance is a spectrum of clinical states, so that the severity of respiratory failure determines

ALS

Example 1: A 3-year-old child who has stridor and retractions, but is running around the room and has a normal appearance, requires general noninvasive treatment and transport. The child is compensating effectively and is only in respiratory distress.

Example 2: An 8-year-old child who is anxious and quiet, with wheezing and increased work of breathing, has an abnormal appearance and is probably hypoxic. The child is beginning to decompensate and is in early respiratory failure. In addition to general noninvasive treatment, this child requires immediate specific treatment on scene consisting of administration of a bronchodilator and oxygen, then rapid transport to an ED. The child should be monitored en route for response to the bronchodilator. End-tidal CO_2 monitoring by ALS providers would also be indicated for this patient.

Example 3: A 3-year-old child who has been working hard to breathe for hours and is now sleepy or poorly responsive has an abnormal appearance. The altered mental status is the result of severe hypoxia or hypercapnia, reflecting respiratory failure and impending respiratory arrest. These patients require immediate assisted ventilations with airway adjuncts, such as an oropharyngeal airway or a nasopharyngeal airway, using a bag-mask device on scene and possibly advanced airway procedures. This may include endotracheal intubation or insertion of a supraglottic airway.

how abnormal the child appears. Also, assessing appearance guides the urgency of basic life support (BLS) versus advanced life support (ALS) treatment. Even if ALS procedures are required, start with BLS procedures while preparing to implement ALS procedures based on local protocol.

Work of Breathing

To assess for adequate breathing, it is important to have the child appropriately exposed. Attempt to visualize the thorax in a nonthreatening manner while keeping the child warm. Look for signs of increased work of breathing, including the following:

1. Abnormal airway sounds (eg, snoring, stridor, wheezing, or grunting)
2. Retractions (suprasternal, supraclavicular, intercostal, subcostal)
3. Nasal flaring
4. Abnormal positioning (tripoding, "sniffing" position)
5. Head bobbing in infants

The significance of each of these findings is discussed in Chapter 1. These indicators of breathing effort help to identify the anatomical location of the problem (upper airway, lower airway, or lung alveoli), the severity of the physiological dysfunction (respiratory distress, failure, or arrest), and the urgency of need for treatment (immediate resuscitation, general treatment only on scene with specific treatment en route, general and specific treatment on scene). In addition to abnormal airway sounds (stridor, wheezing, and grunting), retractions and the use of accessory muscles may help localize the site of airway problems. Use of the accessory muscles of the neck and suprasternal and supraclavicular retractions occur more often with upper airway obstruction. Predominant subcostal and intercostal retractions and the use of abdominal muscles tend to localize an obstructive process to the lower airways. It is difficult to recognize some of these signs when the child is clothed; to best assess the patient, appropriately remove clothing to ascertain these other clinical signs.

Circulation to Skin

Finally, evaluate skin color. Cyanosis is an ominous sign, signaling profound hypoxia and the need for assisted ventilation. However, a child may have severe hypoxia without an obvious change in skin color. Pulse oximetry is very helpful; use it whenever available in a child with respiratory distress or respiratory failure.

Primary Assessment: The ABCDEs

After the PAT, perform the second portion of the primary assessment: the hands-on ABCDEs. There are 3 parts to the "B" or breathing evaluation:

1. Respiratory rate
2. Auscultation for air movement and abnormal breath sounds
3. Pulse oximetry

RESPIRATORY RATE

In the patient whose condition is not critical, determine the respiratory rate by sitting the child in the caregiver's lap and exposing the patient's chest. Count the rise and fall of the abdomen over 30 seconds, and then double that number. Normal respiratory rates vary in children of different ages (see Table 1–4 in Chapter 1). Always think about respiratory rates in the context of the PAT and the overall clinical assessment. Respiratory rate may be affected by level of activity, fever, anxiety, and metabolic state.

A respiratory rate of greater than 60 breaths/min is abnormal in a child of any age and should be a signal for careful evaluation for other signs of respiratory or circulatory problems. Even more dangerous is a rate that is too slow for age. A respiratory rate of less than 20 breaths/min in a sick child younger than 6 years of age, or a rate of less than 12 breaths/min in a sick child between 6 and 15 years of age, may be a sign of respiratory failure, and immediate intervention may be required.

AUSCULTATION FOR AIR MOVEMENT AND ABNORMAL BREATH SOUNDS

Assess air movement by placing the stethoscope and listening for the amount of air movement with each breath (**FIGURE 3–1**). Poor air movement may exist in children with respiratory problems for many reasons, as outlined in **TABLE 3–2**.

Assessing air movement, or the volume of air exchanged with each breath, allows clinical estimation of **tidal volume**. Tidal volume is one of 2 factors that determine minute ventilation (the volume of air exchanged per minute). **Minute ventilation** is the basis for gas exchange in the lungs.

$$\text{Minute Ventilation} = \text{Tidal Volume} \times \text{Respiratory Rate}$$

This equation shows the connection between tidal volume and respiratory rate. A child may not have enough gas exchange if tidal volume is low, even with a normal or fast respiratory rate. Also, a normal or increased tidal volume does not mean there is enough gas exchange if the respiratory rate is too slow.

While listening for air movement, also listen for abnormal breath sounds. Table 1–5 in Chapter 1 summarizes the types and causes of abnormal breath sounds. Stridor, which is usually inspiratory in nature (at least initially), is indicative of upper airway obstruction, whereas crackles and wheezes are associated with lower airway processes.

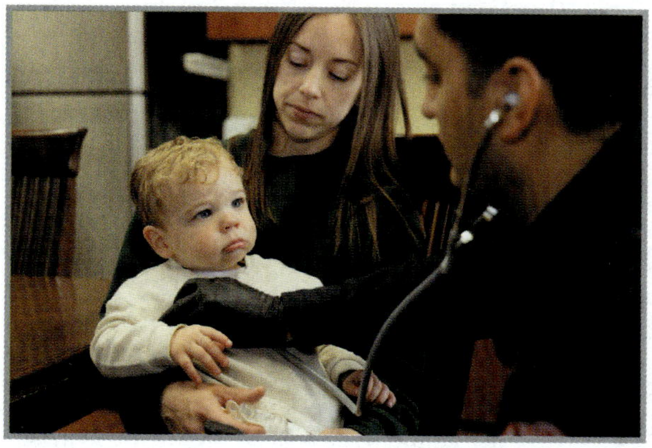

FIGURE 3–1 Assess air movement by placing the stethoscope and listening for the amount of movement with each breath (remember to use a small diaphragm and compare breath sounds side to side). In infants, if the chest is noisy, consider suctioning the nose and listening again.

TABLE 3–2 Causes of Poor Air Movement in Children

Functional Problem	Possible Causes
Obstruction of airway	Asthma, bronchiolitis, croup, foreign body
Restriction of chest wall movement	Chest wall injury, severe **scoliosis** or kyphosis
Chest wall muscle fatigue	Prolonged increased work of breathing, muscular dystrophy
Decreased central respiratory drive	Head injury, intoxication
Chest injury	Rib fractures, pulmonary contusion, pneumothorax

PULSE OXIMETRY

Pulse oximetry is a useful tool for detecting and measuring hypoxia. **FIGURE 3–2** illustrates possible sites for placement of the oximetry probe. **Procedure 9, Pulse Oximetry**, explains how to use a pulse oximeter. The pulse oximeter emits red light of 2 different wavelengths. These are absorbed differently by saturated and desaturated hemoglobin. The sensor on the pulse oximeter measures the transmission of the 2 wavelengths of red light, and a computer in the machine then determines the percentage of hemoglobin saturated with oxygen. When properly applied, *and if there is a good arterial tracing*, a reading of 95% or higher means normal blood oxygen saturation. *A value of 94% or less on room air is abnormal and is a signal to administer supplemental oxygen.* A reading of less than 90% in a patient on 100% oxygen usually indicates respiratory failure, unless the child has a chronic respiratory problem.

Patients with uncorrected cyanotic heart disease and some patients with chronic respiratory problems (eg, cystic fibrosis) have a low oxygen saturation at baseline. In this type of patient, obtain the baseline value from the caregiver and attempt to provide enough oxygen to get the child to their baseline pulse oximetry level. Providing more oxygen than is needed to achieve the baseline pulse oximetry level may actually suppress ventilation by reducing the child's hypoxic drive to breathe. In healthy children, hypercapnia or increased carbon dioxide pressure

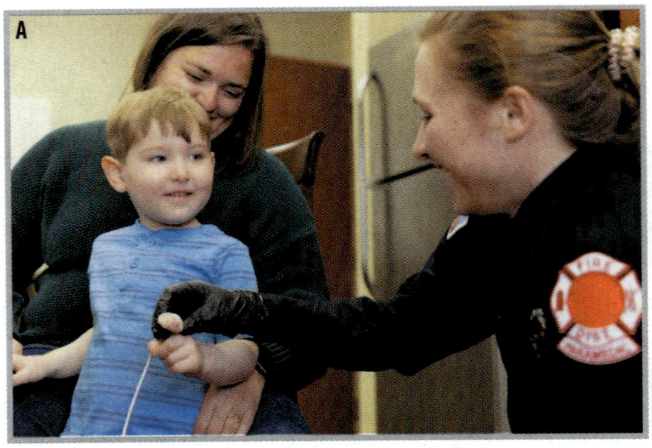

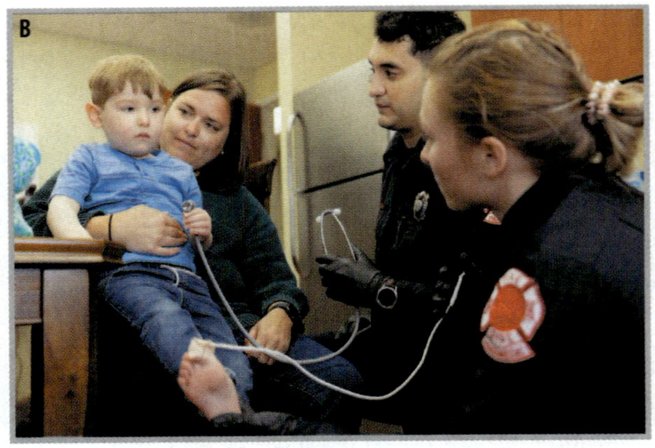

FIGURE 3–2 Possible sites for placement of the oximetry probe include the index finger **(A)** and the great toe **(B)**. Covering the probe after placement will help distract from its presence.

stimulates the drive to breathe, but in some children with chronic respiratory disease, hypercapnia is a constant state. In such cases, hypoxia becomes the stimulus to breathe. The preferred oxygen saturation rate is between 94% and 99%.

One must be careful not to overinterpret low oxygen saturation. Pulse oximetry is merely an adjunct to physical assessment. Falsely low readings are common with pulse oximetry. Movement by the child, cold extremities or a cold ambient temperature, and interference by light in the child's surroundings may cause inaccurate pulse oximetry readings. Check probe placement, the quality of the tracing, and the child's clinical state before treating. Conversely, inaccurate readings or the inability to obtain a reading may also occur in children in shock with poor perfusion. In these patients, it is important to administer oxygen even if they do not have respiratory distress and regardless of pulse oximeter readings to help optimize oxygen delivery during their shock state. It is also important not to underinterpret a normal pulse oximetry reading. *Sometimes, an apparently normal oxygen saturation (above 94%) may be present in a child with significant respiratory distress who is compensating by increased work of breathing.* Always use pulse oximetry in combination with physical assessment to ensure accurate interpretation of adequacy of breathing.

TIP

Remember, the pulse oximeter does not inform about the adequacy of ventilation. A patient who is receiving supplemental oxygen may have a normal pulse oximeter reading but not have adequate ventilation. **Capnometry**, which quantitatively measures exhaled carbon dioxide, monitors carbon dioxide levels and the adequacy of ventilation and provides a minute-by-minute picture of ventilatory status.

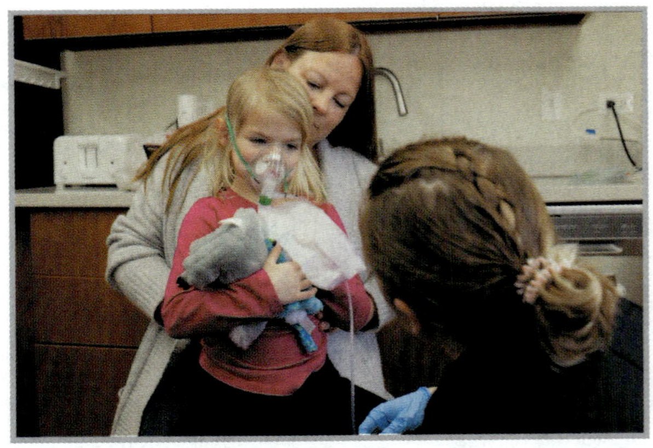

FIGURE 3–3 Always keep a child with respiratory distress in their position of comfort.

General Noninvasive Treatment

For every child in respiratory distress, begin general noninvasive treatment. *The general noninvasive treatment of every noncritical patient is the same—allow the patient to assume a position of comfort and supply oxygen, if tolerated* (**FIGURE 3–3**). This is the only treatment for patients in respiratory distress without upper or lower airway obstruction. If the child is in respiratory failure or arrest, perform assisted ventilation immediately with airway adjuncts and consider using advanced airways based on local protocols.

CAUTION

Be careful not to overinterpret low or normal oxygen saturation. Interpret oxygen saturation in the context of the patient's history and physical findings.

POSITIONING

A child in respiratory distress naturally moves into the position that provides the best air exchange,

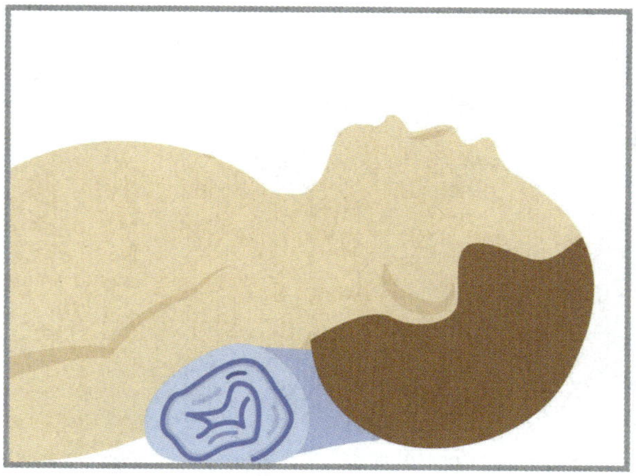

FIGURE 3–4 Sniffing position.

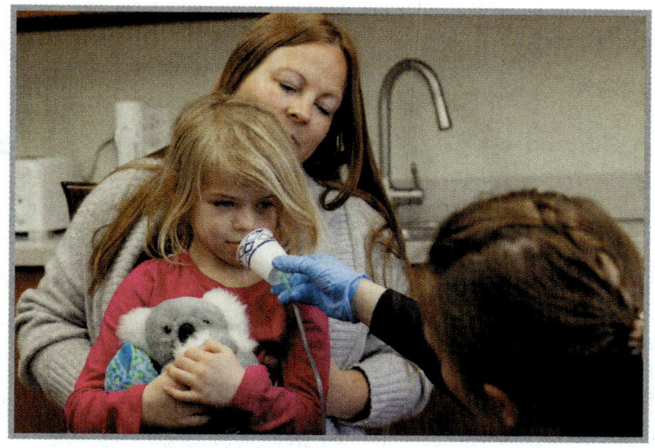

FIGURE 3–6 If the child resists application of a mask or nasal cannula, administer oxygen through a nonthreatening object, such as a cup.

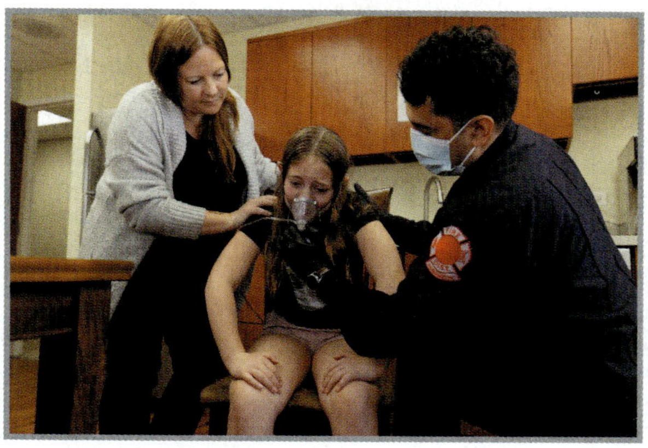

FIGURE 3–5 Tripod position.

called the position of comfort. For example, a child with severe upper airway obstruction may get into the sniffing position to straighten the airway and open the air passages (**FIGURE 3–4**). A child with severe lower airway obstruction may voluntarily take the tripod posture (sitting up and leaning forward on outstretched arms) to help accessory muscles (**FIGURE 3–5**). Infants and toddlers may be most comfortable in their caregiver's arms or lap. Do not move a child from their position of comfort, as this might worsen the respiratory distress. In the ambulance, keep the dyspneic child safely restrained in an upright position, unless the child requires assisted ventilations or has other physiological problems that require treatment in a supine position.

OXYGEN

Treatment with high-flow oxygen is usually safe. If the child has a chronic respiratory illness, be careful not to administer too much oxygen. The EMS clinician must weigh the possible benefits of giving oxygen against the risks of agitating the child and worsening the respiratory distress. This is a special concern in a child with an unstable airway. Infants with respiratory distress, cyanosis, or other signs of respiratory disease require high-flow 100% oxygen.

Because of concerns about oxygen toxicity in newborns, those without signs of hypoxia no longer require 100% oxygen, as explained in Chapter 12. For newborns in respiratory distress, start at 21% oxygen and titrate as needed to achieve an oxygen saturation of 94% or greater.

CAUTION

Do not move a child from their position of comfort.

Most children accept oxygen therapy, especially if the EMS clinician is creative in the approach. This often means getting the help of the caregiver. If a child resists the use of a mask or **nasal cannula**, ask the caregiver to give blow-by oxygen from the end of the oxygen tubing or from tubing inserted into a cup (**FIGURE 3–6**).

OXYGEN DELIVERY

Administer oxygen to any child with clinical signs of cardiopulmonary distress or failure or with a history suggesting possible abnormalities in gas exchange. The delivery method should provide the concentration of oxygen most appropriate for the child's condition, degree of cooperation, respiratory effort, and age.

For a step-by-step explanation of this procedure, see **Procedure 3, Oxygen Delivery.**

Summary of General and Initial Respiratory Assessment and General Noninvasive Treatment

The PAT is a good tool for determining the effectiveness of gas exchange, based on observation of appearance and work of breathing. If the PAT suggests respiratory distress, begin general noninvasive treatment with oxygen and keep the child in their position of comfort. The PAT also identifies the critically ill child in respiratory failure who requires immediate assisted ventilation. Obtaining the respiratory rate, listening for air movement, and determining oxygen saturation by pulse oximetry work in concert with the PAT. The primary assessment should allow an evaluation of severity and urgency for treatment and should establish whether specific treatment for upper or lower airway obstruction is indicated.

Specific Treatment for Respiratory Distress

After completing the primary assessment, consider specific treatment. The PAT and ABCDE assessment help determine whether the child has an upper or lower airway obstruction, lung disease, or disordered control of breathing (from such conditions as brain or nerve injury, poisoning, or sepsis). Snoring or stridor indicates upper airway obstruction; wheezing indicates lower airway obstruction. Separating true stridor from upper airway noise can sometimes be difficult because of nasal congestion. Breath sounds may also make it difficult to tell the difference between upper airway noise and true wheezing. Listen for breath sounds in the second or third intercostal space at the midaxillary line bilaterally (**FIGURE 3–7**). Consider the auscultation of breath sounds posteriorly between the scapula and spine bilaterally and lower lobes directly above the kidneys. At this location, it is easier to distinguish upper airway congestion from lower airway obstruction. When abnormal airway sounds are loudest with the stethoscope held near the child's nose rather than over the lungs, nasal congestion/obstruction is the likely cause.

The presence of abnormal breath sounds in a child with hypoxia and increased work of breathing suggests lung disease, such as pneumonia. Lastly, a child with hypoxia and *decreased* work of breathing may have respiratory failure resulting from airway obstruction or lung disease or disordered control of breathing caused by another insult to the brain or metabolic system.

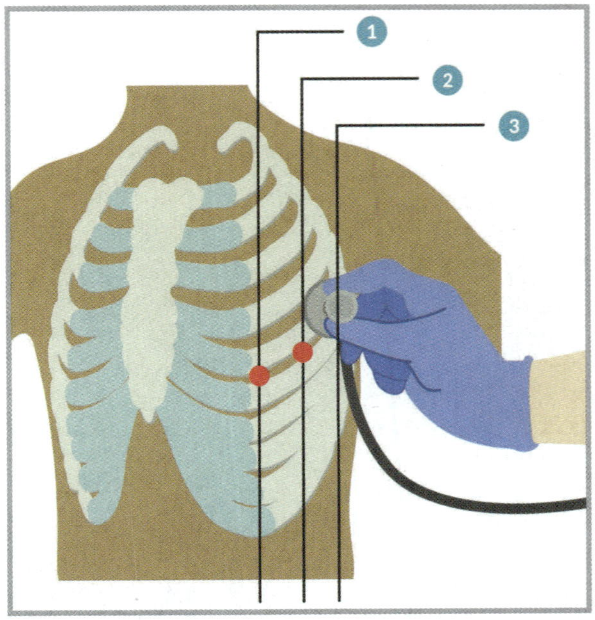

FIGURE 3–7 Listen for breath sounds. 1. Midclavicular line. 2. Anterior axillary. 3. Midaxillary line.

TIP

When abnormal airway sounds are loudest with the stethoscope held near the child's nose rather than over the lungs, nasal congestion/obstruction is the likely cause.

UPPER AIRWAY OBSTRUCTION

Proximal Airway Obstruction

In a patient with neurological impairment, loss of oropharyngeal muscle tone may cause upper airway obstruction and stridor because of the tongue and **mandible's** falling back and partially blocking the **pharynx**. This is a common problem in children during and after seizures. The head-tilt/chin-lift maneuver (**FIGURE 3–8**) or jaw-thrust maneuver (**FIGURE 3–9**) may relieve this **proximal** airway obstruction. When bag-mask ventilation is required, it may be helpful or even necessary to have 2 rescuers assist in airway management: one to hold the mask and perform jaw thrust, and the other to squeeze the bag (**FIGURE 3–10**). The use of airway adjuncts based on the level of consciousness may help with keeping the airway open, especially in larger children, children who are actively seizing, or children receiving ventilation (see **Procedure 5, Airway Adjuncts**).

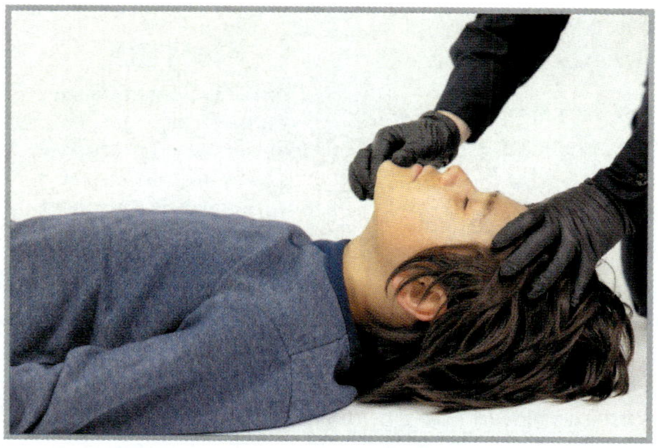

FIGURE 3-8 Use the head-tilt/chin-lift maneuver to place the child in a neutral position.

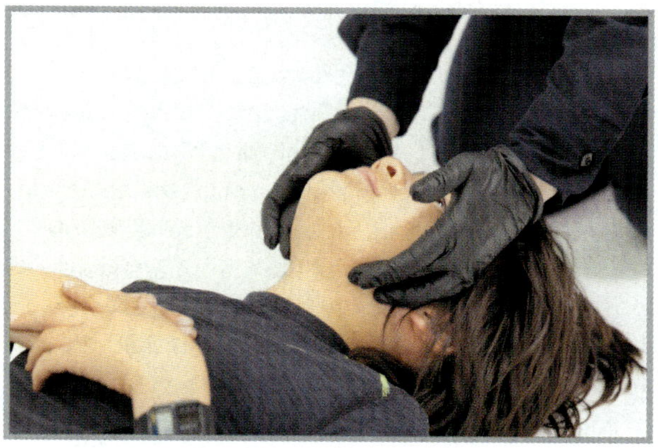

FIGURE 3-9 Use the jaw-thrust maneuver in a child with possible spinal injury.

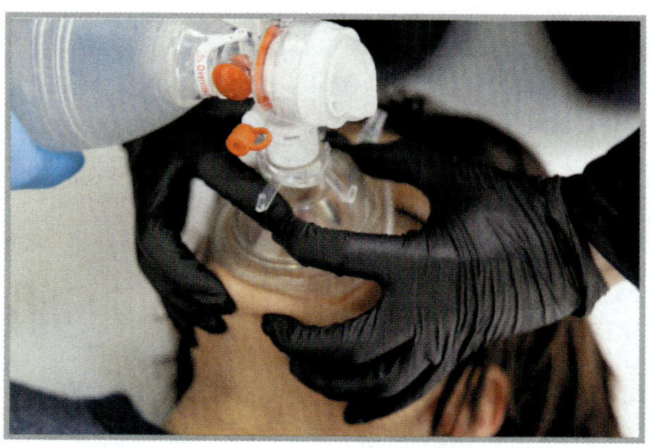

FIGURE 3-10 Two-rescuer technique for the jaw-thrust maneuver and positive-pressure ventilation.

Sometimes secretions, blood, or foreign bodies block the proximal upper airway. This is an important concern in the child with closed-head injury or seizures. Suctioning alone often relieves the upper airway obstruction caused by fluids or occluding objects in the mouth, pharynx, or nose.

Maintenance of an adequate airway may require placement of an oropharyngeal airway, a nasopharyngeal airway, an endotracheal tube, or other approved advanced airways. The role of endotracheal intubation in children in the prehospital setting has been brought into question by data demonstrating significant failure rates, induced hypoxia, airway injury, and endotracheal tube dislodgement. *Bag-mask ventilation is the key lifesaving technique that should be mastered by all EMS clinicians and provides adequate airway management for most pediatric patients.*

Alternative advanced airways, including supraglottic airways, can be considered in the early treatment of the child in respiratory failure or arrest. The particular type and brand are based on local emergency medical services (EMS) protocols.

Airway Obstruction Above the Thoracic Inlet

Upper airway obstruction beyond the proximal upper airway may result from a variety of causes. It is not necessary to make an exact diagnosis to provide appropriate care to children with upper airway obstruction. In most of these cases, simply allow the child to maintain their position of comfort and provide supplemental oxygen by the least invasive and least threatening means possible.

Causing the child to become more agitated or struggle may worsen the airway obstruction and precipitate the onset of a severe airway obstruction, leading to respiratory failure or respiratory arrest.

In an awake, alert child, upper airway obstruction and stridor are usually caused by croup, a viral disease with inflammation, edema, and narrowing of the larynx or trachea. Croup usually affects infants and toddlers. Most children with croup have experienced cold symptoms for a few days. The cold symptoms are followed by the development of a barking or "seal-like" cough, stridor, and various levels of respiratory distress. Patients usually have a low-grade fever, and symptoms are often worse at night. The severity of symptoms varies widely among patients, but the symptoms usually progress over days, rather than hours.

Treatment. In the prehospital setting, ensure the patient is in a position of comfort and provide supplemental oxygen. Nebulized saline may provide

> **TIP**
> Position of comfort, humidified oxygen, and avoidance of agitation are the best treatments for suspected croup.

ALS

Pharmacological Treatment of Croup. Nebulized epinephrine is a specific treatment for the upper airway inflammation associated with croup. Epinephrine is a potent α-and β-agonist and works through vasoconstriction to decrease the upper airway edema causing partial obstruction. If local EMS protocols permit, consider nebulized epinephrine therapy for children with stridor, increased work of breathing, poor air movement, blood oxygen saturation less than 94%, or altered appearance. Nebulized epinephrine is available in 2 formulations, and either is acceptable: racemic epinephrine and L-epinephrine.

Side effects of nebulized epinephrine include tachycardia, tremor, and vomiting. Children who receive nebulized epinephrine need a period of observation in the ED because of possible return of stridor after the medicine wears off. Very few children with croup require assisted ventilation in the prehospital setting. In the rare case of a child with croup and respiratory failure, begin bag-mask ventilation and reassess. A 2-person bag-mask ventilation technique may be necessary. Patients will also benefit from the administration of steroids, if available. The IM or IV route is likely to upset the child.

Dexamethasone 0.6 mg/kg up to a maximum of 16 mg can be given IV, IM, or orally.

Invasive Airway Management for Croup. Perform endotracheal intubation only in the unusual case of the child with respiratory failure who does not respond to bag-mask ventilation. Preparation for intubation includes choosing an endotracheal tube that is 1 or 2 sizes smaller than normal for age or length. Inflammation of the trachea at the subglottic level makes it difficult or impossible to use an endotracheal tube of normal size. Refer to local protocols when making the decision for drug-assisted intubation (formerly called rapid sequence intubation). Other advanced airways should also be considered based on local protocols and availability.

some comfort for the child. Having the caregiver assist by holding the nebulizer may be of benefit. If the child does not tolerate the treatment, transport in a position of comfort (**FIGURE 3–11**).

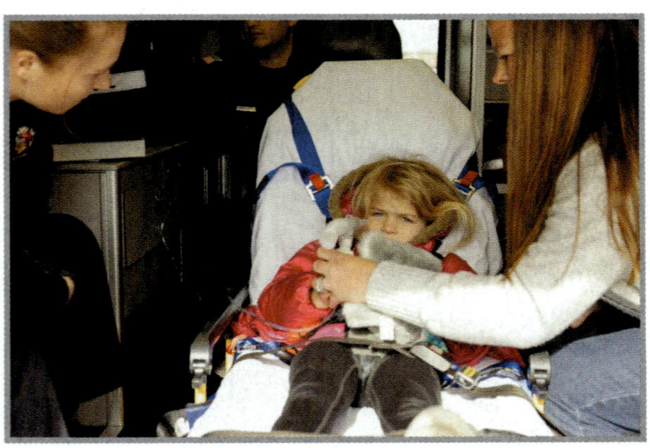

FIGURE 3–11 Ask the caregiver to assist in the administration of oxygen or nebulized saline.

Bacterial Upper Airway Infections

CAUTION

Stridor is often mistaken for wheezing. Stridor is an inspiratory sign of upper airway obstruction and may improve with an agent with vasoconstrictive properties, such as nebulized epinephrine.

Bacterial infections may also cause upper airway obstruction in children. Unlike viral croup, these infections tend to progress rapidly, with severe respiratory compromise developing over hours. The child with a bacterial upper airway infection usually is older than 12 months, appears ill or toxic, has fever, pain on swallowing, and may drool. Stridor may be present, but the child does not have the barking cough that is common with croup.

There are several possible causes of bacterial upper airway infections. **Epiglottitis**, inflammation of the **epiglottis**, is now extremely rare because of widespread vaccination of infants against the bacterium *Haemophilus influenzae* type B. A **retropharyngeal abscess** involves swelling of the retropharyngeal nodes that are located between the cervical vertebrae and esophagus. It usually occurs in children younger than 4 years and can mimic the presentation of epiglottitis. The child may have **torticollis**, or a stiff neck, and there may be swollen cervical lymph nodes. A **peritonsillar abscess** is a collection of pus adjacent to the tonsil. It tends to occur more often in adolescents and is often caused by group A streptococcus (so the child may be receiving antibiotics for a strep throat). The child complains of trouble speaking, is unable to open their mouth fully, and often drools. **Tracheitis** can occur in 2 forms. In the child without a tracheostomy, it can mimic the presentation of epiglottitis; in a child with a tracheostomy, it results in increased thick airway secretions.

Treatment. When a bacterial upper airway infection is suspected, provide only general noninvasive treatment with high-flow oxygen in a position of comfort. Avoid agitating the child by trying to place an intravenous line or attempting another maneuver, and quickly transport. If the child is in respiratory failure, initiate bag-mask ventilation and consider endotracheal intubation or a supraglottic airway.

Foreign Body Aspiration

Foreign body aspiration may cause mechanical obstruction anywhere in the airway, from the pharynx to the bronchus. A retained esophageal foreign

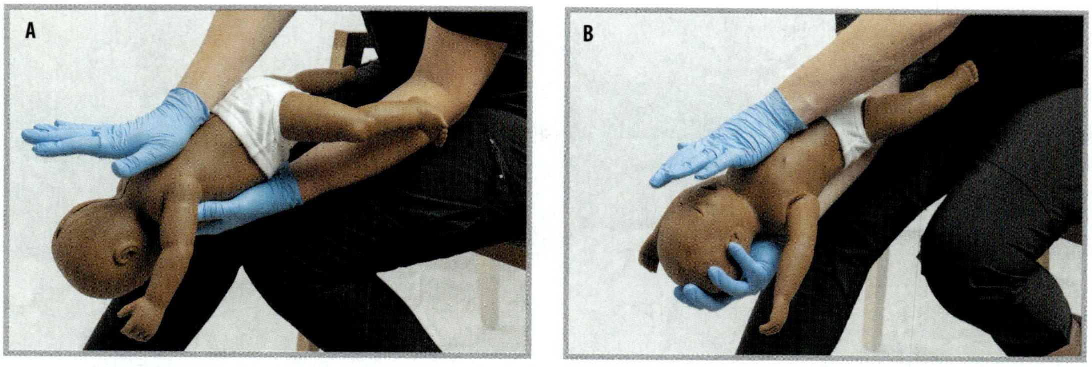

FIGURE 3–12 Foreign body airway maneuvers for a conscious infant. **A.** Use 5 back blows (slaps), followed by **B.** 5 chest thrusts in infants using the heel of your hand, with severe airway obstruction.

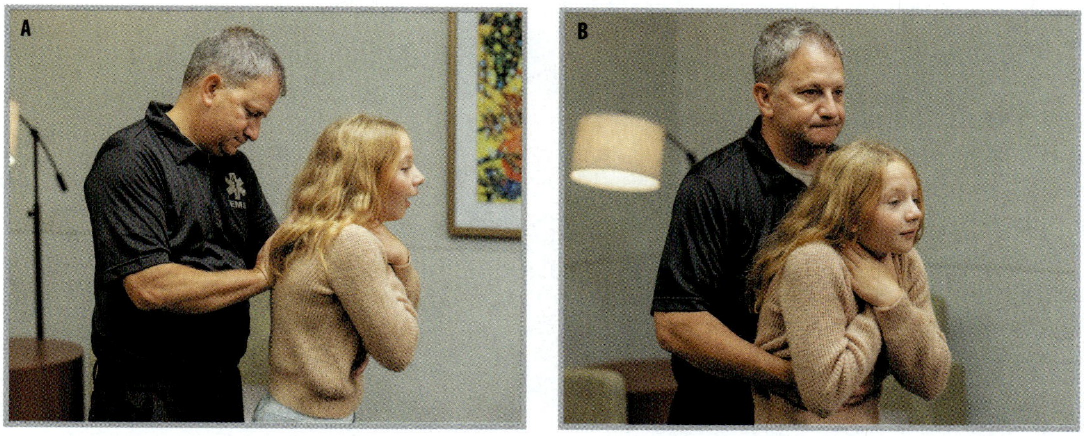

FIGURE 3–13 Foreign body airway maneuvers for a conscious child. **A.** Use 5 back blows followed by **B.** 5 abdominal thrusts to treat severe airway obstruction in the conscious child in the standing position.

body can also cause respiratory distress in an infant or a young child. This happens because the trachea is pliable and can be compressed by the adjacent distended **esophagus**. A typical history of foreign body aspiration includes the sudden onset of coughing, choking, gagging, and shortness of breath in a previously well child without a fever or other symptoms of upper respiratory tract infection. Older infants and toddlers, who explore their world by placing things in their mouths, are at highest risk.

Treatment. If the child can still cough, cry, or speak, the airway is only partially obstructed. Stridor or drooling may be present. Immediately transport these children, who are considered to have mild upper airway obstruction. Provide only general noninvasive treatment, avoid agitating the child, and keep the child in a position of comfort.

If the child has severe respiratory distress and is at risk of becoming worse during transport, be prepared to perform foreign body airway obstruction (FBAO) maneuvers for severe airway obstruction, as illustrated in **FIGURES 3–12** and **3–13**. **TABLE 3–3** summarizes these maneuvers. Consider these FBAO maneuvers if the child cannot cough, cry, or speak. *Never perform FBAO procedures if the child has mild airway obstruction (ie, can cough, cry, or speak).*

CASE STUDY 2

Your unit is dispatched to a child care center for a child in respiratory distress. On arrival, you and your partner find an 18-month-old girl who is very cyanotic and grasping her throat. The child care worker states that she believes the child choked on a grape. The child is making no audible noises and seems desperate for help.

1. What is the most important thing for you to do at this time?
2. If your initial steps failed, what would you do next?

TABLE 3–3 Foreign Body Airway Obstruction Maneuvers

Age	Technique
Infant (< 12 months)	Five back blows (slaps), followed by 5 chest thrusts using the heel of your hand on the sternum until unresponsive, then start CPR
Child (> 1 year)	Five back blows (slaps), followed by 5 abdominal thrusts until unresponsive, then start CPR

Abbreviation: CPR, cardiopulmonary resuscitation.

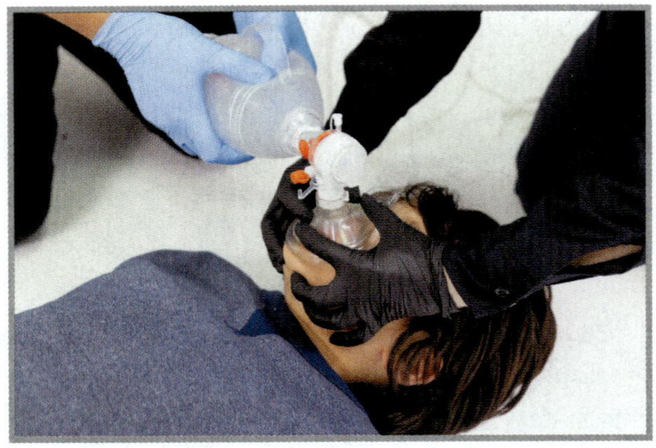

FIGURE 3–14 Two-person bag-mask ventilation technique.

Airway Obstruction and Foreign Body Removal

In the setting of severe airway obstruction, EMS clinicians can make the difference between life and death. Immediate removal of an airway foreign body can often be achieved using BLS procedures while the child is still conscious. Sometimes basic maneuvers are unsuccessful. In such cases, use of pediatric Magill forceps along with direct **laryngoscopy** may be the only option for removal. For a step-by-step explanation of this procedure, see **Procedure 6, Foreign Body Obstruction**.

Foreign Body Airway Obstruction Maneuvers. If the child has severe airway obstruction and BLS maneuvers fail to dislodge the foreign body to the mouth, where it can be easily removed, and the patient loses consciousness, begin cardiopulmonary resuscitation (CPR) with chest compressions, then open the airway. If not at the paramedic level, continue CPR and look for airway obstruction before delivering ventilations. Finger sweep FBAO only if the object is seen. *Do not* do a blind finger sweep. For advanced-level clinicians, if the foreign body can be seen at or above the level of the larynx, remove it using pediatric Magill forceps. If the child has severe airway obstruction and neither FBAO maneuvers nor direct laryngoscopy relieves the obstruction, attempt bag-mask ventilation, using the 2-person technique whenever possible (**FIGURE 3–14**). If bag-mask ventilation fails to achieve chest rise, consider endotracheal intubation, if in your scope of practice. Suction should be readily available when performing unconscious airway maneuvers.

Based on local protocols, cricothyrotomy might be considered for obstructions that cannot be removed.

Specific Treatment of Upper Airway Obstruction

When transporting any child with suspected mild upper airway obstruction, have airway equipment immediately available. Consider transporting the caregiver with any conscious child with airway obstruction, because this may keep the child calm. Also, the caregiver can help administer oxygen.

CAUTION

Never perform airway obstruction procedures if the child has only mild airway obstruction and can still cough, cry, or speak.

LOWER AIRWAY OBSTRUCTION

Bronchiolitis and asthma are the most common conditions causing lower airway obstruction in children. Foreign body aspiration is much less common and usually occurs in toddlers who have been otherwise well, and then suddenly start choking, coughing, or wheezing. *Wheezing is the clinical hallmark of lower airway obstruction of any cause.* Pneumonia can also cause lower airway disease, but usually without obstruction. A specific diagnosis of lower airway obstruction in the field is not necessary, and many times it is impossible to tell which of the 3 main conditions the child is experiencing: (1) bronchiolitis, (2) asthma, or (3) foreign body aspiration.

TIP

Attempt BLS maneuvers first in a child with suspected foreign body aspiration and a critical airway obstruction.

Asthma

Asthma is the most common chronic disease of childhood, affecting almost 5 million children in the United States. The ED admission rate for children with asthma younger than 5 years of age is more than twice the national average for all ages, and the mortality rate for children is rising. One-half of all pediatric asthma deaths occur in the out-of-hospital setting. The length of the final attack is less than 1 hour in many children, and less than 2 hours in one-half of children with asthma who die. Common reasons for an asthma attack include upper respiratory infection and exercise. Exposure to cold air, emotional stress, and passive exposure to smoke also may trigger attacks.

Asthma is a disease of small airway inflammation. The inflammatory reaction leads to bronchoconstriction, mucosal edema, and profuse secretions. These 3 factors in combination cause airflow obstruction and **ventilation-perfusion mismatch**. Clinically, children having an asthma attack show different degrees of tachypnea, tachycardia, increased work of breathing, and wheezing on exhalation; however, inspiratory wheezes can also be present. Pulse oximetry findings may be normal or low.

Carefully assess air movement by auscultation, both anteriorly and posteriorly; this helps to distinguish not only sounds, but also tidal volume. The person with asthma complaining of shortness of breath, but without wheezing on auscultation, may have too much airway obstruction to wheeze; this is also known as a silent chest (so little air is moving through the lungs that you cannot hear this abnormal lung sound). Aggressive bronchodilator treatment may improve airflow and increase audible wheezing. Beware of the following features of the primary assessment, which suggest severe bronchospasm and respiratory failure:

- Altered appearance
- Exhaustion
- Inability to recline
- Interrupted speech
- Severe retractions
- Decreased air movement or silent chest

In the focused history, several things suggest that a severe or potentially fatal attack may occur. These include the following:

- Prior intensive care unit admissions or intubation
- More than 3 ED visits in a year
- More than 2 hospital admissions in the past year
- Use of more than 1 metered-dose inhaler canister in the last month
- Use of bronchodilators more frequently than every 4 hours
- Progressive symptoms despite aggressive home therapy

Home therapy for asthma has several goals: preventing and controlling asthma symptoms, reducing the number and severity of attacks, and reversing existing airflow obstruction. Some children with a history of severe or frequent asthma attacks are taking daily medications (such as inhaled steroids), but most children receive treatment only during serious attacks. **TABLE 3-4** lists the medications frequently used in home asthma therapy for quick relief. It is important for the EMS clinician to recognize the difference between a daily medication for symptom maintenance (a "controller" medication) and a short-acting bronchodilator ("rescue" medication). The latter will be effective in treating acute symptoms, the former will not.

ALS

Asthma Treatment

Specific field treatment for wheezing includes either inhaled bronchodilators or intramuscular (IM) epinephrine. Some studies in adults have demonstrated a lower likelihood of admission and shorter ED length of stay for adult asthma patients with asthma who are treated with corticosteroids in the prehospital setting. Study results have been mixed in children. However, some prehospital protocols now include corticosteroid treatment as an option in pediatric patients with asthma. However, the full effect of prehospital corticosteroid treatment on patient outcome is not known. FIGURES 3-15, 3-16 and 3-17 illustrate administration of inhaled bronchodilators.

Treatment of Lower Airway Obstruction

For all children with lower airway obstruction, general noninvasive treatment is the first field action.

TABLE 3-4 Asthma: Common Home Therapy Quick-Relief Medications for Acute Asthma Attacks

Class of Medication	Medication	Mechanism of Action
β_2 agonists	Inhaled bronchodilators (albuterol [salbutamol]), levalbuterol	Relax bronchiole smooth muscle; prevent bronchospasm; rapid onset of action
Anticholinergics	Inhaled anticholinergics (ipratropium)	Relax bronchiole smooth muscle; decrease secretions; rapid onset of action
Anti-inflammatory medications	Oral corticosteroids (prednisone)	Block allergic response; reduce airway hyperresponsiveness; improve response to bronchodilators; delayed onset of action (2–12 hours)

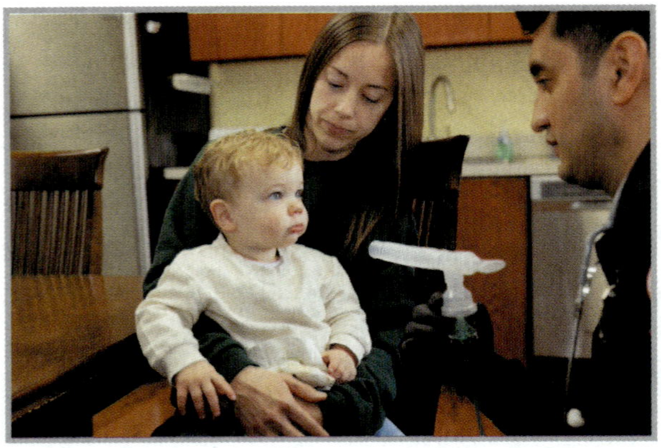

FIGURE 3–15 A nebulized bronchodilator can also be given without a mask using a blow-by technique.

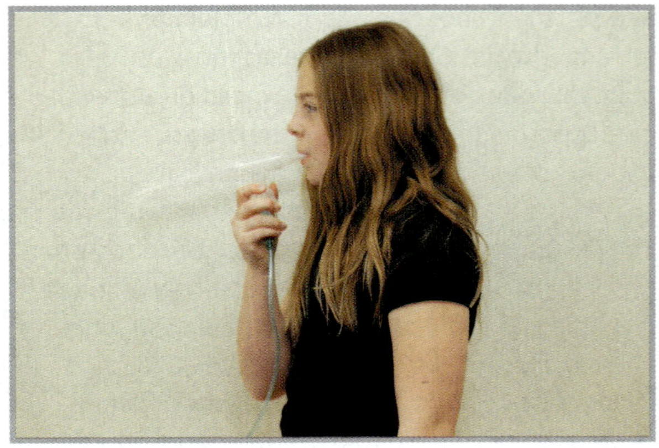

FIGURE 3–17 One method of delivering a bronchodilator is with an oxygen-powered nebulizer.

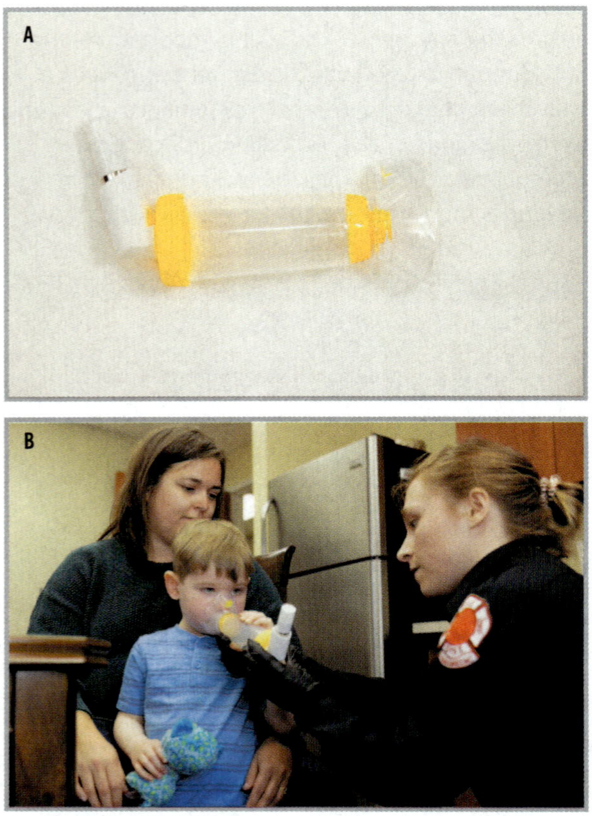

FIGURE 3–16 **A.** A metered-dose inhaler and spacer can be used with or without a mask. **B.** A metered-dose inhaler with spacer and mask can be used in children as young as 6 months.

Bronchodilators. Early bronchodilator therapy, on the scene and on the way to the ED, helps immediately open airways, relieve respiratory distress, and improve oxygen delivery in asthma. In patients whose condition is unstable or critical, continuous inhaled treatment with a β-agonist is the preferred approach, although IM epinephrine is acceptable in some patients who cannot cooperate with inhalation therapy, have severe respiratory distress, or have signs or symptoms consistent with anaphylaxis. For a step-by-step explanation of this **procedure,** see **Procedure 7, Bronchodilator Therapy,** and **Procedure 14, Intramuscular Injections.** An in-line bronchodilator used with continuous positive airway pressure (CPAP) can be used in older children based on local protocols.

Pharmacological Treatment of Wheezing. Albuterol (salbutamol) is the most commonly used inhaled bronchodilator. Because of its selective action on the bronchiole smooth muscles and its minimal effect on cardiac rate, the drug has a high margin of safety. In a child in critical condition with wheezing, treat with the highest dose and administer continuously. Unit dose vials of albuterol (salbutamol) premixed with saline are used by most prehospital systems. These vials provide 2.5 mg of albuterol (salbutamol) in a total volume of 3 mL. One vial is an acceptable initial dose for almost all children and adolescents. For patients in critical condition, the nebulizer may be refilled continuously, or 2 vials may be placed in the nebulizer initially and given immediately. Levalbuterol is an isomer of albuterol that has not been studied in the prehospital setting and has not been shown to offer any benefit over albuterol in the hospital setting.

Depending on local protocols, administer ipratropium with albuterol (salbutamol). Ipratropium is an anticholinergic agent that may provide additional bronchodilatation in addition to the β-agonist action of albuterol (salbutamol). Precautions include sensitivity to the effects of ipratropium or atropine. Adverse reactions include dry mouth, headache, cough, hoarseness, blurred vision, tachycardia, and occasionally flushing. Add it to a unit dose vial of albuterol (salbutamol) and administer together by nebulizer. Multiple doses of ipratropium provide added benefit in asthma exacerbations.

If a child cannot tolerate nebulized drug therapy or is moving air so poorly that the drug is not being inhaled, or in cases of possible anaphylaxis, administer IM epinephrine 1 mg/mL concentration (formerly known as 1:1000). Transport with cardiac monitoring if frequent nebulized treatments or IM epinephrine is necessary. **TABLE 3–5** summarizes the drugs and doses for field medication therapy.

In most cases of known asthma, begin a bronchodilator on scene before transport and then give additional doses en route, as indicated.

TABLE 3–5 Management of Wheezing: Bronchodilator Treatment

Medication	Dose
Albuterol (salbutamol)	Nebulized solution (1.25 mg/3 mL, 2.5 mg/3 mL, 5 mg/mL) Minimum dose: 2.5–5 mg every 20 minutes for 3 doses Repeat dose every 1–4 hours as needed; if not already prediluted, dilute in minimum of 2–3 mL saline for adequate nebulization May use continuously for patients in critical condition Metered dose Inhaler: 90 mcg per puff 4–8 puffs every 15–20 minutes for 3 doses
Ipratropium bromide inhalation solution	Nebulized solution (0.5 mg/2.5 mL) Children < 12 years: 0.25 mg nebulized every 20 minutes for 3 doses Children > 12 years: 0.5 mg nebulized every 20 minutes for 3 doses
Albuterol (salbutamol) metered-dose inhaler	90 µg per puff 4–8 puffs every 15–20 minutes for 3 doses
Epinephrine intramuscular injection (1 mg/mL)	Administer 0.01 mg/kg in critically ill patients with impending respiratory failure and no improvement despite use of inhaled bronchodilator (maximum dose, 0.3 mg); repeat every 5–15 minutes for a total of 3 doses
Magnesium sulfate	50 mg/kg IV over 20 minutes for patients in critical condition with impending respiratory failure and no improvement despite an inhaled bronchodilator (maximum dose, 2 g); monitor patients for hypotension or poor perfusion

Unit dose vials of 2.5 mg of albuterol (salbutamol) premixed with saline to a total volume of 3 mL may be used as an initial dose for children and adolescents of all ages. In critically ill patients, doses may be repeated continuously en route to the ED.

IM Injections. IM administration allows the medication to absorb slowly but steadily. The IM route may result in pain at the site (**FIGURE 3–18**). For a step-by-step explanation of this procedure, see **Procedure 14, Intramuscular Injections.**

IV Medications

Intravenous medication for a patient experiencing an asthma exacerbation can include corticosteroids. Two options are dexamethasone at 0.6 mg/kg IV, IM, or by mouth (maximum, 16 mg) or methylprednisolone at 1 to 2 mg/kg IV (maximum, 60 mg).

For patients not responsive to β-agonists with impending respiratory failure, ALS providers may consider the administration of magnesium sulfate at 50 mg/kg, with a maximum single dose of 2 g given over 20 minutes. Magnesium sulfate is an electrolyte and a smooth muscle relaxer. As a result, it provides relief from bronchoconstriction. A patient receiving magnesium sulfate should undergo continuous cardiac monitoring and frequent blood pressure assessments. One of the main side effects of magnesium is hypotension, which generally responds well to the administration of a fluid bolus.

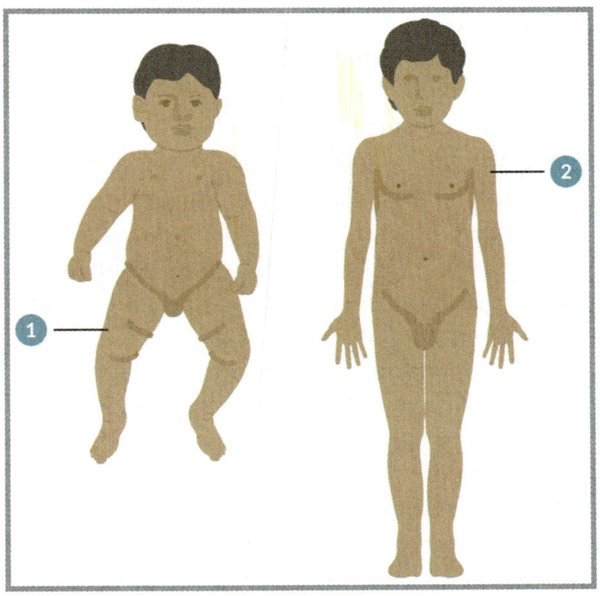

FIGURE 3–18 Common sites for IM injections. 1. Vastus lateralis. 2. Deltoid.

Assisted Ventilation. Because of the severe air trapping associated with bronchospasm, assisted ventilation may be associated with many complications and death. Positive-pressure ventilation requires very high inspiratory pressures and may result in pneumothorax or **pneumomediastinum**. Consider bag-mask ventilation and endotracheal intubation in a wheezing child only if the child is in respiratory failure and has failed to respond to high-flow oxygen and maximal bronchodilator therapy. While assisting ventilation in any patient with lower airway obstruction, slow rates (12–15 breaths/min in older children and adolescents, and a maximum rate of 20–30 breaths/min in infants) with long expiratory times are useful in minimizing barotrauma and complications.

TIP

When a child fails to respond to assisted ventilation with improvement in clinical status, quickly assess your equipment—from the oxygen tank to the patient—for mechanical failure.

Bronchiolitis

Bronchiolitis is a viral lower respiratory infection that usually affects infants and children younger than 2 years. Often caused by **respiratory syncytial virus (RSV)**, this infection is widespread in the winter months. The infection leads to destruction of the lining of the bronchioles, profuse secretions, and bronchoconstriction. Infants are particularly likely to develop bronchiolitis because of their small airway size, high resistance to airflow, and poor airway clearance. Airway edema and debris from sloughed cells and mucus are the primary mechanism in the pathophysiology of this infection.

Presenting complaints of bronchiolitis include upper respiratory infection symptoms, fever, cough, vomiting, poor feeding, poor sleep, and trouble breathing. Assessment shows variable degrees of increased work of breathing, tachypnea, diffuse wheezing, inspiratory crackles, tachycardia, and normal or low oxygen saturation.

Historic risk factors for respiratory failure in infants with suspected bronchiolitis include age younger than 2 months, history of prematurity, underlying lung disease, congenital heart disease, and immune deficiency. **TABLE 3–6** lists important clinical predictors of respiratory failure in children with suspected bronchiolitis. BLS treatment includes nasopharyngeal suctioning with a bulb syringe or a suction catheter attached to a suction canister (see **Procedure 4, Suctioning**). If the oxygen saturation is less than 94%, supply oxygen via nasal cannula or face mask.

TABLE 3–6 Predictors of Respiratory Failure in Suspected Bronchiolitis

Respiratory rate > 60 breaths/min with increased work of breathing
Heart rate > 200 beats/min or < 100 beats/min
Poor appearance (using PAT)
Blood oxygen saturation < 90% on supplemental oxygen

Abbreviation: PAT, Pediatric Assessment Triangle.

In the past, treatment of bronchiolitis included the use of bronchodilators, but studies have shown no benefit from their use in bronchiolitis. Once in the hospital, a high-flow nasal cannula (HFNC) circuit is often used to provide non-invasive respiratory support. High-flow nasal cannula therapy delivers a precisely controlled blend of air and oxygen, heated to body temperature and fully humidified, at high rates via a nasal cannula (higher than standard nasal cannula). High-flow nasal cannula works through multiple mechanisms: washing out carbon dioxide, generating a modest positive end-expiratory pressure (PEEP) to keep small airways open, reducing the work of breathing, ensuring stable delivery of oxygen, and enhancing patient comfort and mucus clearance through heating and humidification.

Foreign Body Aspiration

Children with lower airway obstruction caused by foreign body aspiration usually are only mildly ill. Unlike foreign bodies in the upper airway, it is rare to develop respiratory failure or severe airway obstruction from a small foreign body in the lower airway. Foreign body aspiration is most common in older infants and toddlers (**FIGURE 3–19**). Often, there is an abrupt onset of coughing or choking that may be followed by a period of relatively few symptoms. Tachypnea, increased work of breathing, and wheezing or decreased breath sounds, which are usually unilateral unless the foreign body is in the trachea, may develop rapidly or over a period of hours to days. The absence of a history of asthma or the symptoms of an upper respiratory infection in a child of the right age should suggest the possibility of foreign body aspiration. General noninvasive treatment, including allowing the child to assume a position of comfort and providing oxygen if tolerated, should be given to all patients. A trial of inhaled bronchodilators is

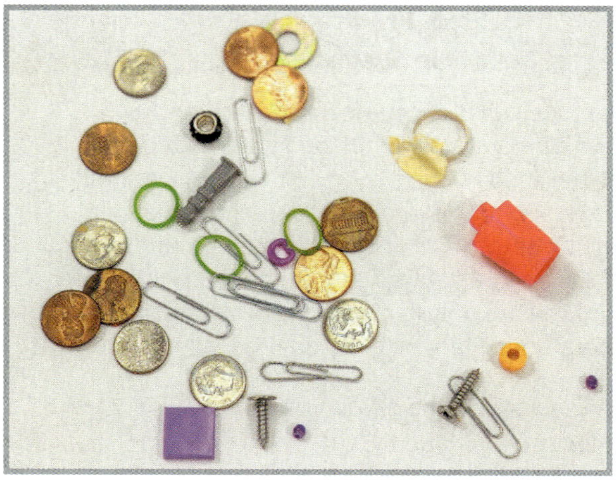

FIGURE 3–19 Examples of foreign bodies that can obstruct the airway.

reasonable if the diagnosis is unclear, but do not delay transport. Additional diagnostic tests may be done after arrival at the ED.

Lung Disease

In children, most lung disease is caused by pneumonia. Pneumonia may cause symptoms of lower airway disease and respiratory distress or failure in children. Almost all children with pneumonia have fever or a history of fever at some point in their illness. Most pneumonias in children are caused by viruses such as influenza. These children generally have symptoms that are less severe and of a more gradual onset than children with bacterial pneumonia.

Bacterial pneumonia in children occurs after aspiration or hematogenous seeding of bacteria into the lung. This is followed by an acute inflammatory reaction leading to the accumulation of fluid within the air spaces of the lung. At times, this may be accompanied by the development of a pleural effusion, or collection of fluid in the pleural space outside the lung parenchyma. Children with bacterial pneumonia usually have symptoms including fever; shaking; chills; tachypnea; and frequently nonspecific complaints such as lethargy or irritability, poor appetite, and occasionally chest pain. Cough may not develop until after a period of other, more nonspecific symptoms.

Physical findings may include fever, tachypnea, increased work of breathing, decreased breath sounds, and rales. Grunting respirations are relatively common in young children with any form of lung disease. Wheezes may be heard, especially with viral infections, but are not as common as rales or decreased breath sounds. In the absence of underlying illness, disability, or very young age, it is unusual for a child to abruptly develop respiratory failure caused by pneumonia. Respiratory distress is more likely.

Approach children with suspected pneumonia like any patient with symptoms of lower airway disease. Making the diagnosis is not as important as providing good supportive care. Provide general, noninvasive treatment to all patients. If the patient has wheezing, try bronchodilators. Patients with signs of respiratory failure may need assisted ventilation. Respiratory failure resulting from lung disease is more commonly seen in young infants, children with underlying neurologic or pulmonary disease, and children who have been ill for several days. There is no specific prehospital therapy for children with pneumonia.

Disordered Control of Breathing

Sometimes hypoxia or respiratory insufficiency is caused by problems in control of breathing. This category of respiratory disease includes that resulting from brain injury, spinal injury, poisoning, metabolic problems (eg, botulism, Guillain-Barré syndrome), postictal state, or sepsis. The hallmark of patients with disordered control of breathing is inadequate minute volume, from poor tidal volume or slow breathing rate. This can lead to hypoventilation, hypercarbia, and hypoxemia. Treatment includes opening the airway, ventilatory support with oxygen, bag-mask ventilation, and occasionally endotracheal intubation or other advanced airways.

Summary of Specific Treatment for Respiratory Distress

After identifying respiratory distress or failure and beginning general supportive measures, assess whether the anatomical level of the respiratory problem is in the upper or lower airway, using the PAT and the hands-on ABCDEs. Stridor is the hallmark of upper airway obstruction, wheezing is the hallmark of lower airway obstruction, grunting is the hallmark of lung disease, and inadequate minute volume and decreased work of breathing are the clinical markers for disordered control of breathing.

The most common cause of upper airway obstruction is croup. Specific treatment for croup includes nebulized epinephrine. Rarely, foreign bodies lodged at or above the vocal cords may be the cause of stridor in infants and toddlers. Frequent causes of lower

CASE STUDY 3

A caregiver calls 9-1-1 because a 4-month-old girl has had 3 days of cough, runny nose, and low-grade fever. The caregiver is concerned because the child seems to be working harder to breathe and is having a hard time taking feedings. On arrival, the child is found lying on the caregiver's lap. She appears sleepy and does not make eye contact or respond to examination. You note that her neck and belly muscles are pulling in. She has audible wheezing and deep subcostal and intercostal retractions. There is nasal flaring. Her skin is mottled. On a more detailed assessment, her respiratory rate is 70 breaths/min and heart rate is 170 beats/min. She has only fair air movement, and you hear high-pitched inspiratory and expiratory wheezes throughout. Pulse oximetry in room air is 78% with a pulse that corresponds to the patient's pulse on examination.

1. Is this child in respiratory distress or respiratory failure, and what is the level of airway obstruction?
2. What are the first steps in the treatment of this child?

airway obstruction are asthma and bronchiolitis. Bronchiolitis is a disease of children younger than age 2 years. Asthma is the most likely cause of wheezing in all children from infancy to adulthood. A nebulized bronchodilator, delivered continuously if necessary, is the specific treatment for asthma. Albuterol (salbutamol) and IM epinephrine have similar effectiveness as bronchodilators, and the anticholinergic ipratropium provides added benefit in patients with asthma. Start treatment on scene in patients with asthma.

Foreign body aspiration and pneumonia may present as lower airway problems, but there is no specific treatment for these conditions in the prehospital setting other than noninvasive measures for respiratory distress. Disordered control of breathing has many causes and often requires ventilatory support.

Management of Acute Respiratory Distress: Continuous Positive Airway Pressure

In children, severe respiratory distress may be challenging to manage. Escalating therapy may mitigate or delay the need for invasive interventions such as endotracheal intubation. Continuous positive airway pressure and noninvasive ventilation may provide a way to support and manage a child in acute respiratory distress and provide airway support. Continuous positive airway pressure attempts to open the peripheral airways in the lungs (**FIGURE 3–20**). Increased airway pressure may also support peripheral small airways during expiration.

Although the literature is not robust, there is evidence to suggest that CPAP may improve breathing in children with a variety of respiratory diseases, particularly bronchiolitis and asthma. The use of CPAP may allow for airway support and potential improvement in the child's status.

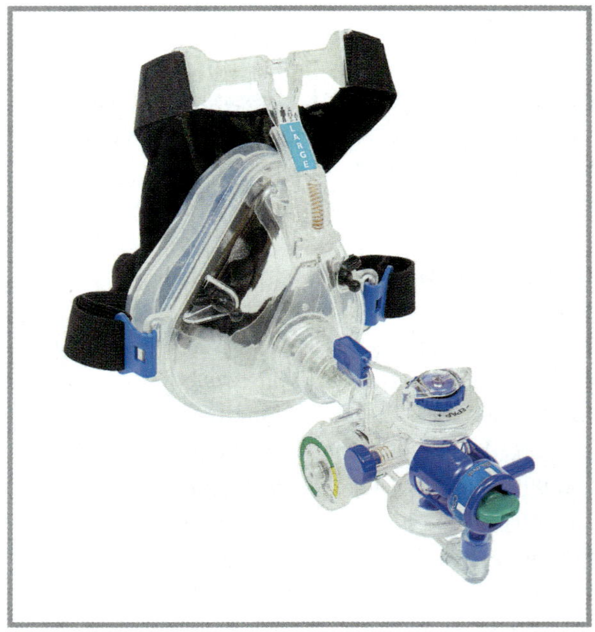

FIGURE 3–20 A disposable, single-use continuous positive airway pressure device.

Courtesy of Mercury Medical.

Management of Respiratory Failure

Regardless of the cause, initially treat every cooperative child in respiratory failure with general noninvasive measures. If upper or lower airway obstruction is present, attempt to provide specific treatment. However, if the child has an altered appearance or altered mental status and has signs of increased or decreased work of breathing (eg, flaring, grunting, gasping, apnea, or cyanosis), or if the child has a documented blood oxygen saturation of less than 90% on 100% oxygen via a nonrebreathing mask, the child is in respiratory failure or respiratory arrest. For this child, bypass general noninvasive treatment and consider immediately beginning assisted ventilation.

First, position the patient to maintain an open airway, with head-tilt/chin-lift or jaw thrust. Use a shoulder roll (sheet or towel) to help achieve a neutral airway position in infants and young children. A neutral airway position is achieved when the external auditory meatus (opening to the ear canal) and sternal notch are horizontally aligned. Then use suction. Suctioning is a basic technique to maintain an open airway. Children have tiny airways that are easily obstructed by secretions, vomitus, pus, blood, or foreign bodies. For a step-by-step explanation, see **Procedure 4, Suctioning.**

If the patient is unresponsive, use an airway adjunct. Adjuncts may immediately improve the child's spontaneous ventilation. In addition, they may allow more effective bag-mask ventilation and reduce gastric inflation. For a step-by-step explanation of this procedure, see **Procedure 5, Airway Adjuncts.**

Next, deliver assisted ventilation or positive-pressure ventilation using a bag-mask device. Bag-mask ventilation is usually the best method for providing oxygenation and ventilation during stabilization and transport. Use an age-appropriate rate of 30 breaths/min in infants and 20 breaths/min in older children. Saying the words, "squeeze, release, release" for children and "squeeze, release" for infants helps time the ventilations to avoid a rate that is too rapid. Ensure that there is good chest rise. Good bag-mask technique decreases the risk of gastric distention, a common complication leading to elevation of the **diaphragm**, decreased lung compliance, and increased risk of vomiting and aspiration of gastric contents. With severe lower airway obstruction, slower rates and longer expiratory times are indicated. Consider placing a nasogastric (NG) tube.

TIP

For an older child in respiratory failure who has increased work of breathing, ventilating at a rate of 20 breaths/min may assist the patient's respiratory effort.

Bag-Mask Ventilation

Bag-mask ventilation is one of the EMS clinician's most useful skills in pediatric prehospital care. Although the technique does not provide the definitive airway control that endotracheal intubation does, in most cases bag-mask ventilation is the best technique for providing oxygenation and ventilation during resuscitation and transport. For a step-by-step explanation of this procedure, see **Procedure 8, Bag-Mask Ventilation.**

CAUTION

Minimize gastric distention during bag-mask ventilation with good bagging technique.

TIP

If the child does not respond to bag-mask ventilation, or if there is a long transport time with a critically ill or injured child who has an unstable airway, consider endotracheal intubation.

ALS

Management With Endotracheal Intubation

The indications for endotracheal intubation in a child in the prehospital setting are limited and based on a careful and thorough assessment of risk versus benefit. Potential advantages of intubation include definitive airway control, decreased risk of aspiration, and ease of assisted ventilation. Potential complications include transient hypoxia and hypercapnia caused by prolonged intubation attempts; cardiac arrest as a result of prolonged hypoxia; unrecognized esophageal placement; elevation of intracranial pressure; aspiration of stomach contents; and injury to the teeth, mouth, tongue, palate, larynx, and soft tissues of the pharynx and neck.

Dislodgment of the tube from the trachea during patient movement or transport is common and may be catastrophic. If an intubated patient fails to respond with improved color, oxygen saturation, heart rate, and appearance, the DOPE mnemonic (dislodgments, obstruction, pneumothorax, equipment) may help to identify potential technical problems (TABLE 3–7). Most EMS systems require constant monitoring of proper placement of endotracheal tubes.

Continuous waveform capnometry (end–tidal CO_2) monitoring is the optimal method for monitoring patients with an advanced airway. Alternative advanced airways are also considerations for the treatment of patients needing ventilatory support; refer to local protocols and procedures.

CONTROVERSY

Avoid inserting a nasogastric or an orogastric tube unless ventilation is impaired by a distended stomach and there is no facial trauma.

Nasogastric and Orogastric Insertion

During positive-pressure ventilation, it is common to inflate the stomach and the lungs with air. Gastric inflation with air slows downward movement of the

TABLE 3-7 Troubleshooting the Endotracheal Tube: DOPE

	Problem	Assessment	Intervention
Dislodgments	Esophageal intubation	End-tidal carbon dioxide monitor or detector reads no or low carbon dioxide level or has poor waveform, or no color change Oxygen saturation < 90% Bradycardia Lack of chest rise with ventilation Auscultation of bubbling over the stomach	Extubate Bag-mask ventilation Reintubate
	Mainstem bronchus intubation	Asymmetric chest rise Asymmetric breath sounds	Pull tube back until breath sounds and chest rise are symmetric
	Accidental extubation	End-tidal carbon dioxide monitor/detector reads no or low carbon dioxide level, or has poor waveform, or no color change Oxygen saturation < 90% Bradycardia Lack of chest rise with ventilation Poor or absent air movement on auscultation	Bag-mask ventilation Reintubate
Obstruction	Tube blocked with blood, secretions, or kink	Decreased chest rise Decreased breath sounds bilaterally Oxygen saturation < 90% End-tidal carbon dioxide monitor/detector has abnormal waveform Increased resistance to bagging	Suction; if no improvement, extubate Bag-mask ventilation Reintubate
Pneumothorax	Tension pneumothorax, spontaneous or induced, compromises air exchange and may lead to decreased cardiac output	Asymmetric chest rise Asymmetric breath sounds Shock Oxygen saturation < 90% *Jugular venous distention *Tracheal deviation	Needle thoracostomy
Equipment	Big air leak around tube Activated pop-off valve on resuscitator Oxygen tubing disconnected Oxygen tank empty	Oxygen saturation < 90%	Check equipment, "patient-to-tank"

*Not easily assessed in young children.

diaphragm and decreases tidal volume, making ventilation more difficult and necessitating higher inspiratory pressures. In addition, inflation of the stomach with air increases the risk that the patient will vomit and aspirate. Gastric decompression with an NG or orogastric tube takes air from the stomach and helps positive-pressure ventilation.

However, use this technique only if there is difficulty ventilating the patient. Insertion may be painful and frightening to the child and family. For a step-by-step explanation of this procedure, see **Procedure 10, Orogastric and Nasogastric Tube Insertion.**

Endotracheal Intubation

Successful endotracheal intubation allows optimal oxygenation and ventilation, can provide a tube for medication delivery, and decreases the risk of aspiration and loss of airway control. A properly placed and secured endotracheal tube is a good tool for managing patients in critical condition, but the procedure can take a long time, and there can be frequent and serious complications. Every placement of an advanced airway must be confirmed for proper placement of the device. Exhaled carbon dioxide colorimetric devices or in-line capnometry or capnography

TABLE 3–8 Advantages and Disadvantages of Alternative Breathing Techniques

Technique	Advantages	Disadvantages
Supraglottic airway devices	Simple insertion Good airway seal Adapts to bag-mask equipment	Does not prevent aspiration
Gum elastic bougie	May facilitate endotracheal tube insertion	No equipment or data for infants and young children Prolonged attempts may worsen hypoxia
Laryngeal tube/subpharyngeal airway	Effective isolation of the airway Reduced risk of aspiration More reliable ventilation relative to bag-mask ventilation Does not require visualization of the glottis Less complicated to insert than esophageal-tracheal tube	Limited data published on the use of the laryngeal tube in children Potential for esophageal trauma
Drug-assisted intubation	Paralyzes child and eliminates muscle resistance Improves visualization Allows mild hyperventilation	Drugs remove spontaneous breathing Drugs may decrease blood pressure or respiratory rate Succinylcholine may cause high potassium
Cricothyrotomy	Provides tiny airway for lifesaving oxygenation or ventilation Bypasses obstruction	Technically difficult Bleeding Injury to other neck structures

should be used during the confirmation process. For a step-by-step explanation of this procedure, see **Procedure 11, Endotracheal Intubation**.

Alternative Breathing and Intubation Techniques

Advanced breathing techniques such as insertion of a supraglottic airway can be used as the primary airway management intervention, or in the case of failed endotracheal intubation, for pediatric respiratory failure or cardiac arrest. Rarely, standard bag-mask ventilation fails and endotracheal intubation is difficult or impossible. Examples of such patients are children with massive head trauma and airway edema or hematoma of the mouth or upper airway, or infants with significant congenital or acquired airway abnormalities who cannot be ventilated. In such dire circumstances, some EMS systems allow EMS clinicians to perform advanced breathing techniques, including use of a supraglottic airway. Additional adjuncts to assist in endotracheal intubation include the gum elastic bougie and **drug-assisted intubation**. Needle cricothyrotomy is another option, if necessary. None of these techniques has been well evaluated in children in the prehospital setting.

TABLE 3–8 summarizes the advantages and disadvantages of these alternative techniques. For a step-by step explanation of supraglottic airways (laryngeal mask airway, i-gel) and gum elastic bougie, see **Procedure 13, Supraglottic Airway Insertion and Pediatric Difficult Airway. Procedure 23, Needle Thoracostomy,** explains needle cricothyrotomy.

CONFIRMATION OF ENDOTRACHEAL TUBE PLACEMENT

Several products are currently available for confirming proper placement of the endotracheal tube. These include waveform end-tidal carbon dioxide monitors or capnometers, which reflect the blood carbon dioxide tension (**FIGURE 3–21**), and colorimetric end-tidal carbon dioxide detectors that give a qualitative reading.

The optimal method for tube confirmation in children in the prehospital setting is continuous waveform capnometry. Because the child's airway is so short, even slight movement of the endotracheal tube can lead to extubation or mainstem intubation. If capnometry shows no carbon dioxide, or if the colorimetric detector fails to change color with ventilation, these are indications that the endotracheal tube

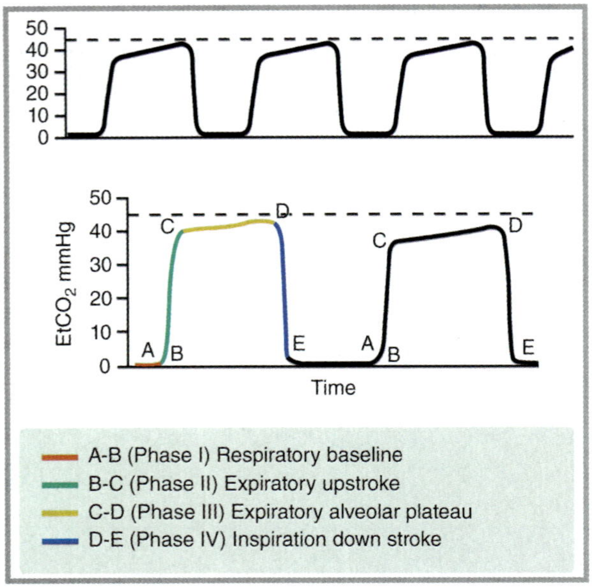

FIGURE 3-21 Normal end-tidal carbon dioxide waveform.

may not be in the trachea. In such cases, remove the endotracheal tube, perform bag-mask ventilation, and reintubate or attempt placement of a supraglottic device after 1 to 2 minutes of oxygenation and ventilation.

The only exception to this approach is the patient in full cardiopulmonary arrest, in whom pulmonary circulation may be too low to generate detectable expired carbon dioxide. In this case, if the capnometer shows a low or absent end-tidal carbon dioxide reading, or if the colorimetric device shows a tan color (low carbon dioxide), observe for chest rise, auscultate bilaterally for air movement, and attempt to visualize the tube passing through the vocal cords by direct laryngoscopy. If the endotracheal tube seems to be in the proper position, leave the tube in place.

> **TIP**
> The optimal method for tube confirmation in children in the prehospital setting is continuous waveform capnometry.

For a step-by-step explanation of these confirmation procedures, see **Procedure 12, Confirmation of Endotracheal Intubation and Use of End-Tidal Capnography**.

Summary of Management of Respiratory Failure

Respiratory failure or arrest can result from many different insults to the airway, mechanics of breathing, or gas exchange. Infection, trauma, and bronchospasm are important causes in children. Think respiratory failure when primary assessment reveals a child with altered appearance in the setting of significantly increased or decreased work of breathing. Bradycardia, poor air movement, and low oxygen saturation are key findings. In a child with respiratory failure or respiratory arrest, immediately begin assisted ventilation with a bag-mask device at an age-appropriate rate. Avoid gastric insufflation. Add specific treatment for airway obstruction, such as an inhaled bronchodilator, if indicated. Perform endotracheal intubation cautiously and be alert for the frequent DOPE complications in the intubated child whose condition suddenly worsens or who fails to respond. Always confirm proper placement of the endotracheal tube with continuous waveform capnometry or colorimetric carbon dioxide detection. In some EMS systems, advanced or alternative breathing techniques such as a supraglottic device are options in the child who cannot be ventilated by bag-mask ventilation or endotracheal intubation.

Primary Assessment: The Transport Decision—Stay or Go?

When a child has respiratory distress, begin general noninvasive treatment (position of comfort and oxygen) and consider specific treatment on scene. Never transport a child who is in respiratory failure without assisted ventilations. Also, never transport a child with a severely obstructed airway until after performing FBAO maneuvers. Immediate on-scene care to support breathing improves the outcomes in children with many respiratory emergencies. After opening the airway and providing assisted ventilation when necessary, or after simply providing general treatment, the EMS clinician must decide whether to stay on scene to assess further and treat specifically, or to go.

If the PAT and ABCDEs are normal and the child has no history of serious breathing problems, the child usually does not require urgent treatment or immediate transport. Take the time to obtain a focused history and physical examination and perform a detailed physical examination (trauma patient) on the scene if possible.

If the child has respiratory distress and signs of upper airway obstruction, transport is usually indicated after general noninvasive treatment. Consider specific treatment of suspected croup with a dose of nebulized epinephrine on the way to the ED, if available. *If the child has asthma and lower airway obstruction with wheezing, begin specific treatment with bronchodilators or IM epinephrine on scene, and continue bronchodilator treatment during transport to the closest medical facility.* Call in advance and let the ED know about the patient who is being transported to their facility.

For children in critical condition, consider endotracheal intubation or other advanced or alternative airways if the child is in respiratory failure and ventilation by bag-mask device is ineffective, or if an airway is difficult to maintain. However, endotracheal intubation increases scene time and delays the time to definitive care at the ED. A high rate of complications have been documented in prehospital studies of endotracheal intubation in children. Intubation skills tend to extinguish rapidly because they are used infrequently. Insertion of a different advanced airway (such as a supraglottic device) is a good alternative to endotracheal intubation in EMS systems where the protocol allows. In most cases, bag-mask ventilation is probably a better option.

Additional Assessment

If the child has minimal respiratory distress and there are no immediate safety concerns for the child or EMS clinician, consider obtaining the focused history and physical examination and performing a detailed physical examination (trauma patient) on scene. Use the SAMPLE mnemonic to find important features of the complete respiratory history. **TABLE 3–9** gives examples of a focused history in a child with a breathing problem.

Perform vigilant ongoing assessment of all children with respiratory distress or failure while on the way to the ED. Use the PAT to recall observational indicators of effective gas exchange, and watch respiratory rate, heart rate, and pulse oximetry. Be prepared to increase the level of respiratory support or to correct complications of therapy if the child's condition worsens or the child fails to respond.

TABLE 3–9 SAMPLE Components in a Child With Respiratory Distress

Component	Explanation
Signs and symptoms	Onset and nature of shortness of breath Presence of hoarseness, stridor, or wheezing Presence and quality of cough; chest pain
Allergies	Known allergies: food, medications, environmental Cigarette smoke exposure
Medications	Exact names and doses of ongoing drugs, including metered-dose inhalers and over-the-counter medications Recent use of steroids Timing and amount of last dose Timing and dose of analgesics and antipyretics
Past medical problems	History of asthma, chronic lung disease, or heart problems or prematurity Prior hospitalizations for breathing problems Prior intubations for breathing problems Immunizations
Last food or liquid	Timing of the child's last food or drink, including bottle or breastfeeding
Events leading to the injury or illness	Evidence of increased work of breathing Fever history Assessment by primary care physician

CASE STUDY ANSWERS

CASE STUDY 1

The child's general appearance is normal. He looks anxious, but makes eye contact and cries when you approach. The child's work of breathing is increased with marked supraclavicular and suprasternal retractions and nasal flaring. His color is pink. He has a normal circulatory status (pink with good perfusion).

This child is in respiratory distress, but does not seem to have progressed to respiratory failure. He is exhibiting many of the signs and symptoms of upper airway obstruction. His loud, harsh inspiratory breath sounds are consistent with stridor. This sound, along with the supraclavicular and suprasternal retractions, help localize the obstruction to the upper airway. He has increased work of breathing, but does not show any signs of hypoxia or hypercapnia (carbon dioxide retention). Upper airway obstruction and stridor in a young child after a few days of an upper respiratory infection are most consistent with croup, a swelling in the trachea below the area of the vocal cords caused by a viral infection. Other problems that may cause upper airway obstruction include foreign bodies, bacterial infections (eg, epiglottitis or retropharyngeal abscess), and airway edema caused by allergic reactions.

Regardless of the cause, the treatment of children with upper airway obstruction is similar and is based on the severity of the symptoms. Keep this patient in a position of comfort, administer oxygen for a pulse oximetry of < 94%, and transport to an ED for further care.

Nebulized medications (eg, epinephrine or racemic epinephrine) act as vasoconstrictors and decrease airway edema. These may be helpful en route to the ED. The child should be closely monitored because his upper airway obstruction may progress and respiratory failure may develop.

On arrival to the ED, the patient is given oral dexamethasone. At 1 hour, he requires an additional racemic epinephrine via a nebulizer. He is observed for another 2 hours and has a respiratory rate of 28 breaths/min and an oxygen saturation of 98% and no stridor at rest, so he is discharged home.

CASE STUDY 2

This is a choking child who needs BLS maneuvers first, such as 5 back blows followed by 5 abdominal thrusts, and, if unsuccessful, progression to ALS maneuvers by removing the FBAO using pediatric Magill forceps. This cannot be accomplished until the patient becomes unconscious. If the level of training prohibits the use of ALS skills, rapid transport to the ED while continuing chest compressions and ventilation or calling for an ALS intercept should be considered.

On arrival at the ED, an otolaryngologist removes the grape under direct visualization using a flexible bronchoscope, and the patient is admitted for observation.

CASE STUDY 3

According to the PAT, this child has an increased work of breathing, abnormal appearance, and poor circulation to the skin. She is in respiratory failure. Her wheezes and subcostal and intercostal retractions localize her airway obstruction to the lower airways. In the setting of the upper respiratory symptoms, fever, and progressive lower airway obstruction, the child probably has bronchiolitis. Open the child's airway, suction her nose, give high-flow oxygen, and begin bag-mask ventilation. Do not delay transport because the child is not likely to have an easily reversible condition. This is unlike the child with asthma, who will likely benefit from a dose of a bronchodilator begun on scene, before transport.

In the ED, the patient is placed on high-flow nasal cannula and admitted to the pediatric intensive care unit.

Suggested References

TEXTBOOKS

Gausche-Hill M. *Pediatric Airway Management for the Prehospital Professional*. Jones & Bartlett Learning; 2004

ARTICLES

Anders J, Brown K, Simpson J, Gausche-Hill M. Evidence and controversies in pediatric prehospital airway management. *Clin Pediatr Emerg Med*. 2014;15(1):28–37. https://www.sciencedirect.com/science/article/abs/pii/S1522840114000111

Bhende MS, Thompson AE. Evaluation of an end-tidal CO_2 detector during pediatric cardiopulmonary resuscitation. *Pediatrics*. 1995;95(3):395–399. PMID: 7862479 doi: 10.1542/peds.95.3.395

Brownstein D, Shugerman R, Cummings P, Rivara F, Copass M. Prehospital endotracheal intubation of children by paramedics. *Ann Emerg Med*. 1996;28(1):34–39. PMID: 8669736 doi:10.1016/S0196-0644(96)70136-1

Fishe JN, Garvan G, Bertrand A, et al. Early administration of steroids in the ambulance setting: an observational design trial (EASI-AS-ODT). *Acad Emerg Med*. 2024;31(1):49–60. PMID: 37786991 doi:10.1111/acem.14813

Gausche M, Lewis R, Stratton SJ, et al. Effect of out-of-hospital pediatric endotracheal intubation on survival and neurological outcome: a controlled clinical trial. *JAMA*. 2000;283(6):783–790. PMID: 10683058 doi: 10.1001/jama.283.6.783

Harris M, Lyng JW, Mandt M, et al. Prehospital pediatric respiratory distress and airway management interventions: an NAEMSP position statement and resource document. *Prehosp Emerg Care*. 2022;26(Supp 1):118–128. doi: 10.1080/10903127.2021.1994675

Jat KR, Mathew JL. Continuous positive airway pressure (CPAP) for acute bronchiolitis in children. *Cochrane Libr*. 2019;1(1):CD010473. PMID: 30701528 doi: 10.1002/14651858.CD010473.pub3

Joyner BL jr, Dewan M. Bavare A, et al. Part 6: Pediatric Basic Life Support: 2025 American Heart Association and American Academy of Pediatrics Guidelines for Cardiopulmonary Resuscitation and Emergency Cardiovascular Care. Pediatrics. 2025; doi: 10.1542/peds.2025-074350.

Kellner JD, Ohlsson A, Gadomski AM, Wang EEL. Efficacy of bronchodilator therapy in bronchiolitis—a meta-analysis. *Arch Pediatr Adolesc Med*. 1996;150(11):1166-1172. doi: 10.1001/archpedi.1996.02170360056009

Lasa JJ, Dhillon GS, Duff JP, et al. Pediatric Advanced Life Support: 2025 American Heart Association and American Academy of Pediatrics Guidelines for Cardiopulmonary Resuscitation and Emergency Cardiovascular Care. Pediatrics. 2025; doi: .10.1542/peds.2025-074351

Lerner EB, Dayan PS, Brown K, et al; Pediatric Emergency Care Applied Research Network (PECARN). Characteristics of the pediatric patients treated by the Pediatric Emergency Care Applied Research Network's affiliated EMS agencies. *Prehosp Emerg Care*. 2014;18(1):52–59. PMID: 24134593 doi: 10.3109/10903127.2013.836262

Lodeserto FJ, Lettich TM, Resaie SR. High-flow nasal cannula: Mechanisms of action and adult and pediatric indications. Cureus.2018.Nov26;10(11):e3639. Doi:10.7759/cureus.3639. PMID:30740281

Menon K, Sutcliffe T, Klassen TP. A randomized trial comparing the efficacy of epinephrine with salbutamol in the treatment of acute bronchiolitis. *J Pediatr*. 1995;126(6):1004–1007. PMID: 7776075 doi: 10.1016/S0022-3476(95)70234-2

Qureshi F, Pestian J, Davis P, Zaritsky A. Effect of nebulizedipratropium on hospitalization rates of children with asthma. *N Engl J Med*. 1998;339(15):1030–1035. doi: 10.1056/NEJM199810083391503

Ramgopal S, Naik VV, Komukai S, et al. The association of prehospital systemic corticosteroids with emergency department and in-hospital outcomes for patients with asthma exacerbations. *Acad Emerg Med*. 2024;31(7): 675–687. PMID: 38456349 doi: 10.1111/acem.14890

Riney L, Palmer S, Finlay E, et al. EMS administration of systemic corticosteroids to pediatric asthma patients: an analysis by severity and transport interval. *Prehosp Emerg Care*. 2023;27(7):900–907. PMID: 37428954 doi: 10.1080/10903127.2023.2234996

Sharieff GQ, Rodarte A, Wilton N, Bleyle D. The self-inflating bulb as an airway adjunct: is it reliable in children weighing less than 20 kilograms? *Acad Emerg Med*. 2003;10(4):303–308. PMID: 12670841 doi: 10.1197/aemj.10.4.303

Vitaliti G, Vitaliti MC, Finocchiaro MC, et al. Randomized comparison of helmet CPAP versus high-flow nasal cannula oxygen in pediatric respiratory distress. *Respir Care*. 2017;62(8):1036–1042. PMID: 28487415 doi: 10.4187/respcare.05384

Zar HJ, Ferkol TW. The global burden of respiratory disease—impact on child health. *Pediatr Pulmonol*. 2014;49(5):430–434. PMID: 24610581 doi: 10.1002/ppul.23030

ADDITIONAL RESOURCES

NASEMSO Medical Directors Council. National model EMS clinical guidelines. NAEMSO 2022. https://nasemso.org/content.aspx?page_id=22&club_id=157064&module_id=701974National Highway Traffic Safety Administration. National EMS scope of practice model 2019: including change notices 1.0 and 2.0. 2021. Report No. DOT HS 813 151. https://ldh.la.gov/assets/oph/ems/2021/210802 NationalScopeOfPractice.pdf

CHAPTER 4

Shock

Shea Duerring, MD, NRP, FAAP, FACEP, FAEMS
Kory Lane, MEd, NRP, FP-C, CCP-C, NCEE

LEARNING OBJECTIVES

1. **Describe how to assess circulation using the Pediatric Assessment Triangle (PAT), ABCDEs, and additional assessment.**
2. **Explain the relationship between shock and blood pressure.**
3. **Differentiate between compensated and hypotensive (decompensated) hypovolemic shock, and discuss appropriate management.**
4. **Distinguish the types of shock (hypovolemic, distributive, cardiogenic, and obstructive), and outline treatment.**
5. **Review septic shock, and discuss need for rapid recognition and therapy.**

Introduction

Emergencies involving shock, or inadequate perfusion, may be the result of hypovolemia, increased vascular permeability, cardiac failure, output obstruction, or a combination of any or all of these causes. **Hypovolemia** is the most common cause of inadequate perfusion in children. Hypovolemia is often precipitated by acute gastrointestinal losses or other illnesses, as well as by hemorrhage resulting from trauma or other causes of bleeding in children. Regardless of the type of emergency involving shock, early recognition and timely management can reduce the likelihood of serious morbidity or mortality.

Most perfusion problems in children arise from loss of intravascular fluid. The child's young, healthy cardiovascular system compensates for fluid loss by increasing the heart rate and reducing blood flow to nonessential anatomic areas through the mechanism of **peripheral vasoconstriction**, or "clamping down." Vasoconstriction limits blood flow to less essential peripheral sites, such as the skin, and preserves blood flow to the "core" organs, such as the brain, heart, lungs, and kidneys. The physiological process of restricting circulation to such areas as the skin and mucous membranes results in important physical signs of **hypoperfusion**. Children have a great ability to compensate for hypovolemia using these mechanisms and may maintain a normal blood pressure

CASE STUDY 1

A father calls 9-1-1 about a 6-month-old boy with a fever of 6 hours' duration. On your arrival, the child is listless. He will not interact and cries inconsolably when held. There are no abnormal airway sounds. Breathing is rapid without retractions or flaring. There is a purplish rash of the face, trunk, and legs. The brachial pulse is faint, the skin is warm to touch, and **capillary refill time (CRT)** is approximately 4 seconds. Respiratory rate is 60 breaths/min, and blood pressure is 50 mm Hg according to palpation. The cardiac monitor shows a heart rate of 190 beats/min.

1. What type of shock is present?
2. What differs in the management of this case versus treatment of pure hypovolemic or cardiogenic shock?

for age despite significant hypovolemia. Children can maintain a normal blood pressure even up to a loss of 30% of their blood volume; however, once they maximize these compensatory mechanisms, they can quickly decompensate. At that point, resuscitation efforts may be less successful. **Early recognition and treatment of shock is critical.**

Distributive shock is less common in children and is usually caused by **sepsis**. This type of shock primarily involves loss of vascular tone. Additionally, distributive shock can result from anaphylaxis, spinal cord injury, and toxin exposures.

Cardiogenic shock is unusual in pediatrics, except in children with **congenital heart disease**, **dysrhythmias**, or acquired **viral myocarditis**. Cardiogenic shock results from heart rates that are either too fast or too slow to support perfusion or from primary congestive heart failure. Regardless of the underlying cause, cardiac output is insufficient to meet perfusion requirements.

Obstructive shock is the rarest of all shock types in children. It is caused by **pericardial tamponade** or **tension pneumothorax**, secondary to injury to the chest. A third cause, pulmonary emboli, is extremely rare in children.

Identifying the type of shock can be difficult, especially when the **pathophysiology** is mixed. For example, bacterial toxins or ingested poisons may have adverse effects on **vascular tone** and **myocardial function**; sepsis may involve a volume deficit from third spacing (loss of plasma from the vascular space because of leaky blood vessels) and loss of vascular tone and **myocardial depression**. However, a careful history and physical assessment usually identify the cause of shock and drive appropriate management. Shock from any cause, if unrecognized or inadequately treated, may advance to cardiac arrest. After arrest has occurred, successful resuscitation is less likely.

Prearrival Preparation

Based on the dispatch information, prepare mentally for the assessment and management of a child with circulatory problems en route to the scene. Recall appropriate techniques for assessment; the role of vital signs; and the possible equipment, drug, and fluid requirements of the child, using length/weight-based tapes or tools. Consider when to stay and treat on scene and when to transport immediately.

Scene Size-Up

Be sure that the scene is safe. Evaluate the environment and document potentially important features, especially concerns regarding possible child maltreatment, or contagious infectious diseases, when personal protective equipment (PPE) is needed.

General Assessment: The Pediatric Assessment Triangle

EVALUATING THE PRESENTING COMPLAINT

On arrival, determine the child's presenting complaint. Key questions include the onset of illness, presence of fever, risk factors for sepsis, frequency and amount of fluid losses (vomiting and diarrhea), when the child last ate or drank, and history of possible congenital or cardiovascular problems. Ask if the child has been injured. In children with mild circulatory compromise who are not in shock, obtain a more complete SAMPLE history (with SAMPLE signifying signs & symptoms, allergies, medications, past medical history, last food or liquid, and events leading to the illness or injury) during the additional assessment.

ASSESSMENT OF CIRCULATION

Using the Pediatric Assessment Triangle

The Pediatric Assessment Triangle (PAT) is the first step in assessment of perfusion, as outlined in Chapter 1. The PAT evaluates 3 characteristics: (1) appearance, (2) work of breathing, and (3) circulation to skin. Knowing these characteristics helps to determine whether the child is sick or not sick, the type of physiological abnormality, and the urgency of need for treatment. Circulatory problems affect each of these characteristics in identifiable patterns.

Appearance

First, assess the child's appearance. A child with decreased core circulation caused by any shock type may have signs of poor brain perfusion and, therefore, altered mental status. The abnormality in the child's appearance will be variable, depending on the type of perfusion problem; the degree of circulatory insufficiency; and the presence of associated problems such as fever, head trauma, or intoxication.

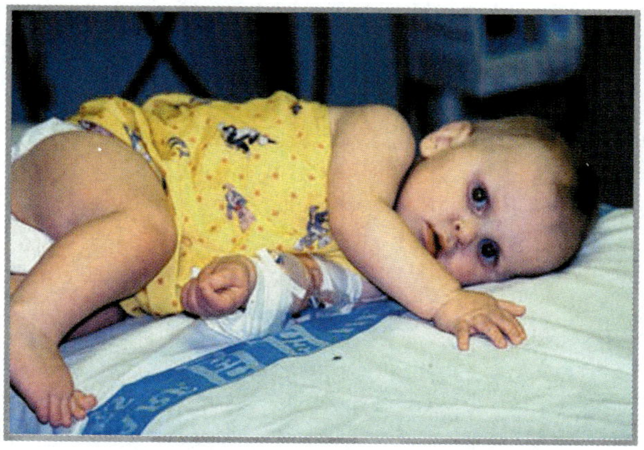

FIGURE 4-1 A child with decreased core circulation and too little blood and oxygen to the brain has an abnormal appearance. This dehydrated child has listlessness, poor motor activity, and decreased interactiveness.

Courtesy of Ron Dieckmann, MD.

Abnormalities in the appearance of a child with decreased core circulation include the following:

- Lethargy or listlessness
- Decreased motor activity
- Diminished interactiveness with caregivers, the EMS clinician, and the environment (**FIGURE 4-1**)
- Inconsolability
- Poor eye contact
- Weak cry

Sometimes the child in shock is restless and inconsolable. Appearance alone, however, is not an accurate sign of inadequate perfusion. An abnormal appearance may be caused by many things, such as poor oxygenation and ventilation, head trauma, hypothermia, drugs, or fever. Assessing appearance is a good way to tell if the child is ill, but not a good way to identify the physiological cause. Assessment tools other than the PAT, such as the hands-on ABCDE assessment, help determine the type of physiological problem and the presence or absence of abnormal perfusion.

Work of Breathing

Next, assess the work of breathing. If circulation to vital organs is decreased, the child's respiratory rate increases. **Effortless tachypnea**, sometimes known as silent tachypnea, is a fast respiratory rate without increased work of breathing. Effortless tachypnea is a common but nonspecific sign of shock. It reflects the child's attempt to blow off carbon dioxide and reduce the **metabolic acidosis** created by decreased perfusion to cells. Signs of increased work of breathing, such as abnormal positioning, retractions, flaring, or abnormal airway sounds (eg, grunting, stridor, or wheezing), are usually seen in the presence of a corresponding respiratory problem. These signs reflect poor gas exchange and **hypoxia**, typically from a primary lung problem. Although increased work of breathing is most commonly a function of respiratory disease, these signs may also occur with hypoxia from **pulmonary edema**; when cardiogenic shock results from **congestive heart failure**; or in anaphylaxis, when the respiratory system is a target organ.

Circulation to Skin

After assessing appearance and work of breathing, assess circulation by looking at skin color and checking capillary refill time (CRT). This is difficult to interpret if the environmental temperature is low, because **vasoconstriction**, as a reflexive effort to preserve heat, falsely alters skin findings, especially in infants. If possible, disrobe the child and look for mottling, pallor, and cyanosis, which reflect peripheral vasoconstriction or clamping down of nonessential skin perfusion to maintain essential core circulation. If a child has an abnormal appearance and abnormal skin signs in a warm ambient environment, the child may be in shock.

Primary Assessment: The ABCDEs

After the PAT, perform the hands-on ABCDE assessment (airway, breathing, circulation, disability, and exposure). After evaluating airway and breathing, as described in the previous chapters, assess circulation. There are 4 parts to the assessment of circulation: (1) heart rate (HR), (2) pulse quality, (3) skin temperature and capillary refill time (CRT), and (4) blood pressure.

HEART RATE

Tachycardia is the first sign of shock. Measure HR by feeling a pulse for 30 seconds, and then double the number. A normal HR is between 60 and 160 beats/min, depending on the child's age (see Chapter 2, Table 2-3, for a list of vital sign ranges in children). The brachial or radial areas are preferred sites at which to measure the pulse rate in infants and children, respectively. The carotid pulse is acceptable in older children and adolescents, but it is hard to locate in infants. If a pulse is difficult to feel, determine HR by listening to the heart sounds directly with a stethoscope placed on the medial side of the child's left nipple. However, be aware that the presence of a "normal" HR obtained by auscultation does

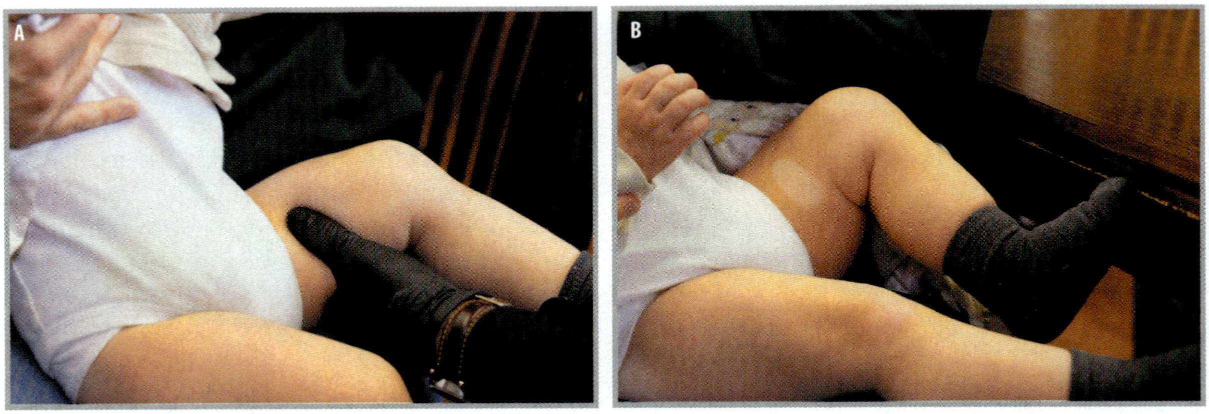

FIGURE 4–2 To determine CRT, first depress the skin (**A**), and then count the seconds before color returns (**B**). Capillary refill time should be less than 2 to 3 seconds in a child who is not cold.

not necessarily reflect adequate cardiac output and perfusion.

Interpreting HR may be difficult, as explained in Chapter 1. Ranges of normal HR change inversely with advancing age. Also, many conditions can increase HR, ranging from serious physiological problems to noxious stimuli that are rarely life threatening. Stimuli that can cause **tachycardia** include pain, fever, fear, cold, and anger. Interpret HR in the context of overall signs of perfusion, age, presence or absence of noxious stimuli, and observed trends. Although a single measurement of HR is usually of limited value in determining the degree of physiological derangement, a trend of mounting tachycardia, or a HR that is falling below the lower limits of normal, suggests a serious physiological problem. In addition, sustained tachycardia is a worrisome sign. Finally, be extremely vigilant when the child has **bradycardia**. Bradycardia in children is typically secondary to another cause and not a primary cardiac issue. Bradycardia may indicate hypoxia or an advanced state of shock.

PULSE QUALITY

Presence of a strong central pulse (carotid, femoral, or brachial in infants) with a strong peripheral pulse (**brachial**, **radial**, or **pedal** in children) suggests an adequate blood pressure. A strong central pulse with a weak peripheral pulse indicates a shock like state. If a brachial pulse is not palpable, the child is probably hypotensive and in hypotensive (decompensated) shock.

> **TIP**
>
> Tachycardia is often the first sign of shock in a pediatric patient.

SKIN TEMPERATURE AND CAPILLARY REFILL TIME (CRT)

The next part of the hands-on cardiovascular assessment involves evaluating skin signs. Check skin temperature for warmth at the hands, feet, thighs, or forearms. Cool hands and feet may be normal, but cool proximal extremities reflect poor perfusion and shunting of blood to the core. Determine CRT by pressing firmly on the skin. Capillary refill time should be less than 2 to 3 seconds in a child who is not cold (**FIGURE 4–2**). Again, inadequate core perfusion results in peripheral vasoconstriction, which manifests as cool skin and longer CRT. Although CRT is a good test of circulation in children, it must be interpreted in the context of overall signs of perfusion. The EMS clinician can become comfortable with the technique and interpretation of the key skin findings by practicing on every child.

BLOOD PRESSURE

A normal blood pressure does not rule out a shock like state because children are adept at compensating for shock. **Children in significant shock may have normal blood pressures until they decompensate.** However, consider taking a blood pressure. A high blood pressure value is not clinically significant in the field, unless the child has a history of hypertension, known renal disease, or acute head injury. However, a low blood pressure value is significant and means hypotensive (decompensated) shock. The challenges in the prehospital setting include knowing when to get a blood pressure reading, obtaining the blood pressure correctly, and interpreting it accurately.

Systolic blood pressure does not accurately reflect **intravascular volume** status until the acute volume loss is greater than 25% to 35% of normal circulating pediatric blood volume. This is because of the efficiency of compensation in a child, including vasoconstriction and an increase in HR. Therefore, a normal blood pressure does not mean the child has a normal blood volume or normal perfusion. A normal minimal systolic blood pressure in a child older than 1 year is greater than 70 + (2 × years of age). Proper equipment, technique, and patience are required to obtain an accurate blood pressure in an infant or a toddler. Because this can be a time-consuming process and may not contribute greatly to the clinical assessment of perfusion, especially in very young children, more time should be spent on assessing other signs of perfusion than on attempting to obtain a blood pressure measurement. Inadequate perfusion is better reflected in the other signs of perfusion described previously (skin color, HR, pulse quality, CRT, and skin temperature). In a child older than 3 years, make at least one blood pressure attempt. Use a cuff with a width two-thirds the length of the upper arm. Applying a cuff that is too large falsely decreases the blood pressure measurement.

CAUTION

A normal blood pressure does not rule out shock.

TIP

In children, one can use the combination of tachycardia, poor pulse quality, delayed CRT, and decreased mental status to diagnose shock, even with a normal blood pressure.

Additional Assessment

If the child is in stable condition after the primary assessment and does not require immediate treatment, and if there are no immediate safety concerns for the child or EMS clinician, conduct history taking and a physical examination and the detailed physical examination for a trauma patient on scene. Use the SAMPLE mnemonic (**TABLE 4–1**) to recall important features of the history in a child with inadequate perfusion. Use age-appropriate approaches to gain the child's trust and speak directly to him or her. Ask the caregiver to add to the child's history. Obtain the history from the caregiver if the child is too young to speak or is unable to cooperate.

After the history, perform a focused examination of the heart, peripheral circulation, and the abdomen. Then perform an anatomical examination of the entire body, as outlined in Chapter 1. If the child has a traumatic injury, also perform a detailed physical examination, searching for other injuries.

Perform an ongoing assessment of all children with perfusion problems while on the way to the emergency department (ED). The child's status may change during transport, so observe and document any physiological trends. Use the PAT to monitor effective perfusion, and watch respiratory rate, HR, blood pressure, and pulse oximetry. Keep a child who is in shock on a cardiac

TABLE 4–1 SAMPLE Components in a Child With Hypoperfusion Problems

Component	Features
Signs/Symptoms	Presence of vomiting or diarrhea Number of episodes of vomiting or diarrhea Vomiting blood or bile External hemorrhage Presence or absence of fever Rash Respiratory distress or shortness of breath (eg, in cardiogenic shock with congestive heart failure)
Allergies	Known allergies History of anaphylaxis
Medications	Exact names and dosages of ongoing medications Use of laxatives or antidiarrheal medications Chronic diuretic therapy Potential exposure to other medications or drugs Timing and doses of analgesic/antipyretics
Past medical problems	History of heart problems History of prematurity Prior hospitalizations for cardiovascular problems History of cancer, transplant, adrenal problems, or immunosuppressive medication
Last food or liquid	Timing of the child's last food or drink, including bottle or breast feedings
Events leading to the injury or illness	Travel Trauma Fever history Symptoms in family members Potential toxic exposure

monitor. Be prepared to increase the level of respiratory and cardiovascular support if the child's condition worsens or the child fails to respond to treatment.

Summary of Cardiovascular Assessment

The PAT provides a good first-line evaluation of perfusion: abnormal appearance, normal work of breathing, and poor circulation to skin suggest a perfusion problem. Pallor, mottling, and cyanosis all indicate poor peripheral perfusion. The circulatory portion of the hands-on ABCDEs consists of evaluating HR, pulse quality, skin temperature, CRT, and blood pressure. These physical features complement the PAT and help identify the type and severity of circulatory compromise. Vital signs can sometimes be misleading and must be correctly measured and interpreted for age. Trends in vital signs or persistence in abnormal vital signs, such as tachycardia, is a more accurate indicator of real physiological problems than mild vital sign abnormalities on primary assessment.

Using the Assessment to Identify Shock

Shock is inadequate perfusion at the tissue level, with insufficient oxygen delivery to maintain normal cellular function. Oxygenation and ventilation, HR, intravascular volume, myocardial function, and vascular stability are all determinants of effective systemic cardiovascular function. If any one of these factors is impaired by illness or injury, the body attempts to compensate and normalize perfusion through modification of other physiological components.

In a child, the physiological components at work are the same as those in an adult. However, there are some differences. The physiological compensatory mechanisms, such as vasoconstriction and tachycardia, are very efficient in a child. Vasoconstriction is so efficient that a line of demarcation can sometimes be seen on extremities, and mottling may be evident when circulation to the capillary beds has become stagnant. Sweating as a response to compensation, although common in an adult, does not always occur in a young child. Therefore, most children in shock have cool, dry skin versus pale, cool, diaphoretic skin. By adolescence, sweating as a response to compensation for shock is consistent. The last difference involves the child's energy reserves. A child does not have the amount of energy reserves that an adult has. The younger the child, the less the capacity for energy reserves. Infants in particular have high glucose needs with low energy stores. As a result, compensatory mechanisms, although efficient, cannot last as long as those of an adult. **Checking a blood glucose level is important in any child who is suspected of being in shock.**

Because of these differences, clinical signs of decreased perfusion include altered mental status, persistent tachycardia as a compensatory mechanism, and changes in skin color and temperature as a result of vasoconstriction. Do not expect sweating unless the child has increased work of breathing and is building up body heat. As long as vasoconstriction, increased HR, and increased myocardial contraction are supported by the child's reserves, systolic pressure is maintained and the child compensates. When the body's reserves begin to fail or are exhausted, perfusion to the vital organs, such as the brain, is compromised. Blood pressure falls, mental status is impaired, and organ systems fail.

There are 4 general classes of shock (hypovolemic, distributive, cardiogenic, and obstructive) (**TABLE 4–2**), reflecting impairment of the 3 major functional

CASE STUDY 2

9-1-1 receives a call about a lethargic 6-year-old girl. On your arrival, she is lying in bed and barely notices your entrance. There is no increased work of breathing, but you do notice that she is breathing fast. Her color is pale. Vital signs are as follows: heart rate, 160 beats/min; respiratory rate, 40 breaths/min; blood pressure, 70/40 mm Hg; Spo_2, 99% in room air. Her capillary refill time is 4 seconds. Her mother states that she has been vomiting and has had diarrhea for 3 days and cannot keep anything down.

1. Is this patient in shock?
2. If so, what type of shock is this?
3. What is the prehospital treatment?

TABLE 4-2 Summary of Different Types of Shock

Shock Type	Physiological Insult	Common Causes	Treatment
Hypovolemic	Volume loss	Hemorrhage Gastroenteritis (vomiting, diarrhea) Burns Prolonged poor fluid intake	Rapid transport Oxygen administration Intravenous fluid boluses Stop bleeding in trauma/hemorrhage
Distributive	Decreased vascular tone	Sepsis Anaphylaxis Drug overdose Spinal cord injury (neurogenic shock)	Rapid transport Oxygen administration Fluid administration Epinephrine for anaphylaxis Epinephrine or norepinephrine for septic shock
Cardiogenic	Heart failure	Congenital heart disease Cardiomyopathy Dysrhythmia Drug overdose	Rapid transport Oxygen administration Cautious crystalloid fluid administration, 10 mL/kg Consider a vasoactive agent, such as epinephrine, dopamine, or dobutamine For drug overdose, consider antidote therapy
Obstructive	Obstructed blood flow	Pericardial tamponade Pneumothorax	Rapid transport Oxygen administration Needle thoracostomy Fluid administration

components of circulation: (1) the blood volume (hypovolemic), (2) the vascular system (distributive), and (3) the heart (cardiogenic and obstructive). Studies of hypovolemia (the most common type of pediatric shock) have allowed researchers to describe the clinical signs that characterize the progression of shock from a compensated state (adequate systolic blood pressure) to an uncompensated state (hypotension). However, the clinical signs characterizing the progression of distributive, cardiogenic, or obstructive shock are not as well defined. This reflects the complex physiology of these other forms of shock.

Hypovolemic Shock

Hypovolemia (loss of fluid) is the most common cause of shock in children in the prehospital setting. Vomiting and diarrhea caused by gastroenteritis are the most common cause of hypovolemic shock. Bleeding from blunt injuries, such as falls or vehicle collisions with the child as a pedestrian, bicyclist, or passenger, is the most common cause of hemorrhagic hypovolemic shock.

The signs and symptoms of hypovolemic shock vary with the amount, duration, and timing of fluid loss. As intravascular volume is further compromised by ongoing fluid losses (such as profuse diarrhea or continued bleeding), the child may progress from compensated to decompensated shock.

COMPENSATED HYPOVOLEMIC SHOCK

Children who lose bodily fluids through minor blood loss or dehydration caused by gastroenteritis usually show no clinically significant effects on circulation. However, if fluid losses are more than about 5% of body weight, predictable adjustments occur in cardiovascular physiology. Sympathetic stimulation results in vasoconstriction and an increase in HR or tachycardia. As long as these processes maintain cardiac output to core organ systems, perfusion is maintained. This is **compensated shock**.

Vasoconstriction causes the following signs of abnormal circulation to the skin: delayed CRT, decreased pulse strength, poor skin color (pallor or mottling), and dry and cool or cold skin temperature. A cold environment or hypothermia may also cause vasoconstriction as a reflex to maintain body heat, which mimics poor perfusion. **Systolic blood pressure is normal in compensated shock.**

In the compensated stage of hypovolemic shock, appearance may be normal, or the child may appear slightly restless or less interactive. In a child with gastroenteritis, the appearance may be abnormal because of fever, which can alter appearance regardless of the circulatory status.

HYPOTENSIVE (DECOMPENSATED) HYPOVOLEMIC SHOCK

In **hypotensive shock**, perfusion is profoundly affected because compensatory mechanisms (increased HR and peripheral vasoconstriction) have failed to maintain sufficient circulation to core organs. The clinical signs are those of organ failure. Although a child in hypotensive shock may still be alert on the AVPU scale (see Chapter 1, Table 1–8), the appearance is abnormal on assessment because of inadequate brain perfusion. The child may be restless and agitated, sleepy, or poorly responsive. Hypotension, or low blood pressure for age, develops when there is about a 25% loss of intravascular volume (blood volume). Other late signs are effortless or silent tachypnea, extreme tachycardia, extreme pallor or presence of mottling, and cold skin temperature. If not reversed, hypotensive shock leads to cardiac failure, with bradycardia and respiratory failure, and then to cardiac arrest.

Although the course is less predictable, decreasing perfusion in children with distributive, cardiogenic, or obstructive shock results in progressive changes in appearance, skin signs, and work of breathing. For example, a child with cardiogenic shock may experience only tachycardia and diminished peripheral perfusion, and then progress to respiratory distress and lethargy as cardiac output worsens and congestive heart failure develops. In all shock types, hypotension is an ominous sign. More than one type of shock can occur concurrently in the same patient, as previously described.

Distributive Shock

In distributive shock, the child has decreased vascular muscle tone (peripheral vasodilation), impaired vascular integrity, or both in the presence of a normal circulating blood volume. This creates a relative hypovolemia, and can be thought of as operating with a "less than full" tank. This change in the capacity of the vascular system and relative hypovolemia lead to hypoperfusion to vital organs because of loss of vascular integrity. Patients with distributive shock may also have a component of hypovolemia. This is the case in a patient with sepsis, who in addition to loss of vascular tone has "capillary leak" caused by the effect of bacterial toxins—or, in the case of anaphylaxis, a capillary leak in the lungs or in the target tissues. In these situations, hypovolemia is the result of "third spacing" of fluid from the vascular space into the surrounding tissues.

The most common cause of distributive shock is sepsis. Identification of patients in early septic shock is challenging, especially in children in whom hypotension is usually a late finding. However, EMS clinicians should maintain a high index of suspicion in patients with fever, tachycardia, altered mental status, tachypnea, and signs of poor perfusion. Patients with known risk factors such as cancer and chronic immunodeficiency, including sickle cell disease, are at higher risk, but sepsis can develop in healthy children as well. Recognition is key, as early therapy can improve patients' outcomes.

Other causes of distributive shock include **anaphylaxis**, chemical intoxication with drugs that decrease vascular tone (eg, β-blockers, barbiturates), and spinal cord injury (above T6) with interruption of spinal sympathetic nerves to the muscle walls of peripheral arteries.

SPECIAL FEATURES IN ASSESSMENT OF DISTRIBUTIVE SHOCK

Signs of distributive shock reflect low peripheral vascular resistance (warm skin, bounding pulses, wide pulse pressure, changes in HR, hypotension) and decreased organ perfusion (abnormal appearance and behavior). These signs may vary with the specific cause, as noted in the descriptions of the 3 major types of shock. Although the progression of physical signs in distributive shock is not as predictable as that in hypovolemic shock, the late findings are indistinguishable from those of hypotensive shock resulting from any cause: abnormal appearance from poor brain perfusion and hypotension.

MAJOR TYPES OF DISTRIBUTIVE SHOCK

Sepsis

Sepsis occurs when any type of infection, usually bacterial or viral, overwhelms the body's defense system and sets in motion a systemic reaction called **systemic inflammatory response syndrome (SIRS)**.

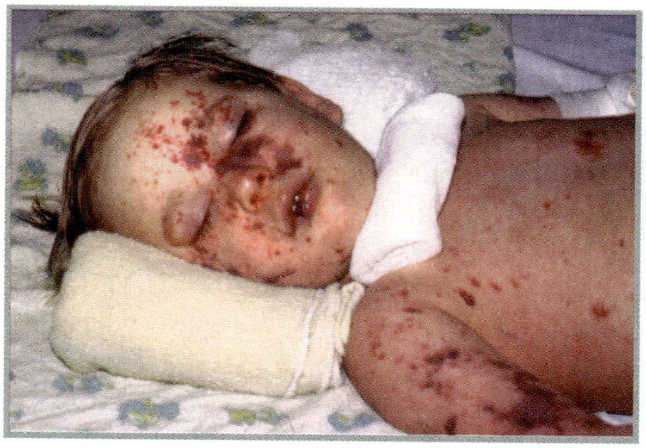

FIGURE 4–3 Purpura.

Courtesy of George Nankervis, MD

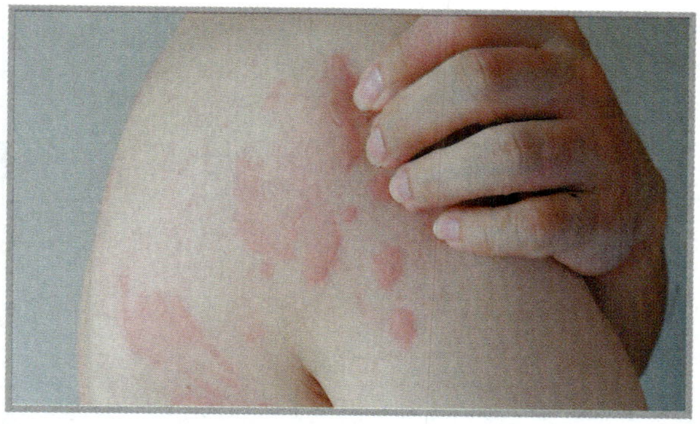

FIGURE 4–4 Hives suggest an allergic reaction and are usually present with anaphylaxis, the most extreme form of an allergic reaction.

wisely/Shutterstock.com

This leads to a generalized breakdown in core organ function, or multiple organ failure. Both can lead to death or serious long-term morbidity.

Distinctive signs of early septic shock are warm skin, tachycardia, and bounding pulses. A child with septic shock has an abnormal appearance that may include listlessness, lethargy, decreased interactiveness, restlessness, and poor consolability. Rash, fever, poor feeding, vomiting, diarrhea, and fussiness may also be present. This early phase may be brief, and patients with septic shock often exhibit signs of poor perfusion, similar to those with hypovolemic shock.

Ill children usually like to be held and cuddled. If a child with a fever does not want to be held but is more comfortable when left alone, the child may have **paradoxical irritability**. This may be a sign of meningitis, in which movement irritates the inflamed **meninges** (membranes covering the spinal cord and brain).

Sometimes, a child with septic shock has a **petechial rash** or **purpura** (nonblanching dark red or purple dots or splotches) (**FIGURE 4–3**). These skin lesions are the result of toxins that cause inflammation of the blood vessels and leakage of blood into the skin. Consider a child with shock in association with a rash and fever to have sepsis. The child may require aggressive volume resuscitation in the field, and EMS clinicians should use strict infection-control practices, including masks, to decrease their risk of infection.

Anaphylaxis

Anaphylaxis is a major allergic reaction that involves a generalized, multisystem response to an **antigen** (foreign protein). Anaphylaxis is defined as involvement of 2 body systems (ie, cutaneous, respiratory, gastrointestinal, or cardiovascular) in reaction to an antigen. Anaphylaxis can present with hives and vomiting, respiratory distress, or shock. The airways and cardiovascular system are important sites of this often life-threatening reaction. Common causes include insect stings by bees, wasps, or fire ants; peanuts; latex; or medication. A child in anaphylactic shock has hypoperfusion and possibly additional signs, such as stridor or wheezing, with increased work of breathing. The child also has an altered appearance with restlessness and agitation and sometimes a sense of impending doom. **Hives** (an itchy skin rash of raised wheals) (**FIGURE 4–4**) and angioedema (flushed, swollen skin) are also common. Signs and symptoms of anaphylactic shock depend on the target organ. This is why some victims of anaphylaxis experience vomiting, diarrhea, and hives, whereas others have angioedema, wheezing, and stridor. Prompt recognition with treatment of anaphylaxis is important in preventing mortality.

Shock Caused by Drug Intoxication

Numerous cardiovascular drugs can cause loss of vascular tone and hypoperfusion when ingested. **TABLE 4–3** lists common agents. The mechanism usually involves direct depressant effect on the cardiovascular system (slowing of the HR, decreased strength of contraction, and vasodilation).

Neurogenic Shock

Neurogenic shock is rare in children. It results from a mechanism of injury that involves the back, neck, or both and that interrupts nervous system pathways. There is a loss of sympathetic control by the autonomic nervous system. This is observed when the injury occurs at T6 or above. The result is vasodilation and impaired sympathetic stimulation of the heart.

TABLE 4–3 Drug Intoxications That May Cause Shock

Antihypertensives β-blockers Calcium antagonists Clonidine
Cyclic antidepressants
Iron
Opioids
Phenothiazines

The child has motor paralysis, hypotension, and bradycardia, with loss of the normal tachycardic response to actual or relative hypovolemia. With loss of the normal vascular reflex to maintain body heat, the body also loses heat to the environment.

TIP

If a trauma patient has a normal or slow HR and low blood pressure, think spinal cord injury and neurogenic shock.

Cardiogenic Shock

Cardiogenic shock is uncommon in children and is rarely diagnosed in the prehospital arena unless the child has a known cardiac history. In fact, the child's condition may be misdiagnosed as septic or hypovolemic shock, resulting in the administration of fluid boluses and **adrenergic agents**. The most likely cause is congenital heart disease, dysrhythmia, or cardiomyopathy resulting from myocarditis. **Myocarditis** is a disease of the heart muscle, usually caused by a virus. A **dysrhythmia**, such as **supraventricular tachycardia** or bradycardia (HR < 60 beats/min), may also cause cardiogenic shock. Overdose with a **cardiac medication**, such as a **calcium channel blocker** or β-blocker, is another possible etiology.

SPECIAL FEATURES IN ASSESSMENT OF CARDIOGENIC SHOCK

A history from the caregiver usually reveals that the child has had nonspecific symptoms, such as loss of appetite, poor feeding, lethargy, irritability, and inappropriate sweating over a period of days. The sweating is caused by the increased workload (work of breathing or work of the heart) and is an attempt to cool off the body. This is true of children with myocarditis and congenital heart disease. There is often a history of congenital heart disease or the presence of a midline chest scar from heart surgery (**FIGURE 4–5**). **TABLE 4–4** summarizes the common symptoms and signs of cardiogenic shock.

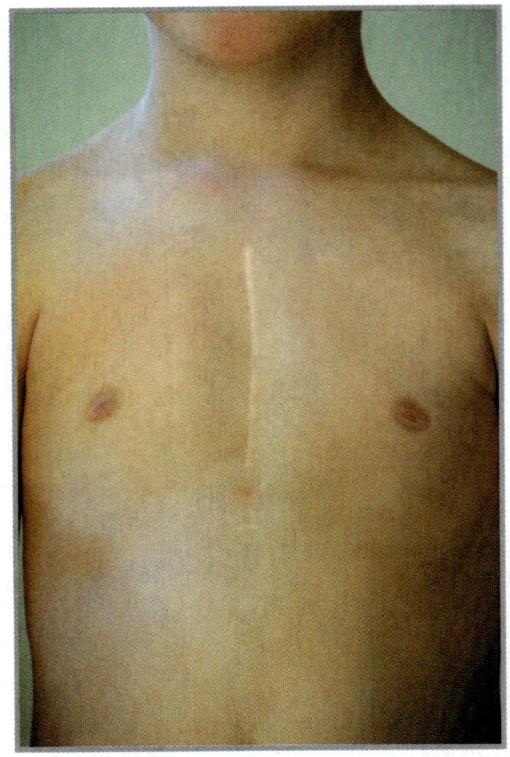

FIGURE 4–5 A midline sternal scar is an indicator of a cardiac history.

Perboge/iStockphoto.com

TIP

Cardiogenic shock can occur from HRs that are too fast or too slow.

Cardiogenic shock may develop from left heart failure, as impaired left heart function causes decreased core organ perfusion. On physical assessment, the child may appear abnormal—sluggish, irritable, or agitated—and the skin color mottled or cyanotic. The heart rate is rapid; blood pressure may be high (early), normal, or low (late). The skin is cool and the child may be **diaphoretic** (not dry as with hypovolemic shock), which is related to the increased workload. Pulmonary edema causes increased work of breathing and inspiratory crackles or wheezing. The increased workload may deplete energy stores, resulting in hypoglycemia. Checking blood glucose levels is recommended.

Increased right-sided cardiac pressures are also present in cardiogenic shock and result in liver

TABLE 4–4 Symptoms and Signs of Cardiogenic Shock

Possible Historical Findings in Cardiogenic Shock
Previous history of chest pain
Previous history of flulike symptoms associated with weakness and fatigue
Difficulty feeding because of fatigue and sweating during feeding in the breast- or bottle-fed infant
No history of fever
No history of volume loss (eg, diarrhea, vomiting, or blood loss)
Positive history of congenital heart disease
No history of asthma despite wheezing on examination
Persistent wheezing despite the administration of β-agonist (eg, **albuterol** [salbutamol])
History of cyanosis
Recent history of exercise intolerance
Possible Physical Findings
Tachypnea or grunting with clear lungs on examination
Unexplained dysrhythmias in the presence of a flulike illness
Tachycardia disproportionate to the degree of fever
Persistent or worsening tachycardia despite fluid administration
Heart murmur, friction rub, or gallop on examination
Presence of cyanosis that does not improve with the administration of oxygen
Crackles on lung examination
Peripheral edema or pitting edema
Hepatomegaly

enlargement (**hepatomegaly**). Hepatomegaly is an especially useful finding in infants and toddlers. Peripheral edema and **jugular venous distension** are rare in children. Cardiogenic shock can also occur because of HRs that are too fast or too slow. Because the origin of a heart rate–related problem is often congenital, assessment and treatment are discussed under congenital cardiac problems.

Obstructive Shock

Obstruction to either the right or left outflow tract from the heart results in obstructive shock. Pericardial tamponade and tension pneumothorax are 2 acute conditions that cause dramatic development of shock after blunt or penetrating injuries to the chest wall. **Hemopericardium** develops quickly after a gunshot or sharp object penetrates into a blood-filled heart chamber, usually the right ventricle. Blunt trauma to the chest at just the right time during the cardiac cycle can produce pressures great enough to rupture the tendons stabilizing the cardiac valves or rupture the tissue between the chambers of the heart. The hole in the wall of the heart provides a route for blood to escape into the space between the 2 pericardial membranes. Because the membranes do not stretch quickly, blood collects and collapses the right ventricle (tamponade). This interrupts venous return to the right heart and produces a profound drop in cardiac output.

Rarely, pericardial tamponade may develop after an infectious or inflammatory process in the chest. Cancer, chronic renal failure, or rheumatologic disease may cause pericardial fluid accumulation. This type of fluid accumulation is slow, and the membranes around the heart stretch. Therefore, obstructive shock caused by infectious or inflammatory processes rarely occurs.

Tension pneumothorax develops after a penetration into the pleural space. Sometimes blunt injury to the chest wall can also rupture alveoli, causing a pneumothorax, which may rapidly progress to a tension pneumothorax when vigorous ventilation with a bag-mask device occurs. Air and sometimes blood (hemothorax) collect between the 2 membranes of the pleura. When the pressure increases enough to cause a shift of the **mediastinum**, venous return to the right heart is impaired. This causes a drop in cardiac output and hypoperfusion.

In children or adolescents with cystic fibrosis, the lung may have blebs that rupture spontaneously, resulting in a pneumothorax, which can progress to a tension pneumothorax.

SPECIAL FEATURES IN ASSESSMENT OF OBSTRUCTIVE SHOCK

Penetrating injuries to the chest wall are often deceptive. The appearance of the wound may be benign and seem superficial. Consider all gunshot wounds or stab wounds to the chest as major penetrations into the heart or pleura. Other types of penetrations by sticks or sharp objects may also cause severe internal injury. Be especially vigilant when the penetration

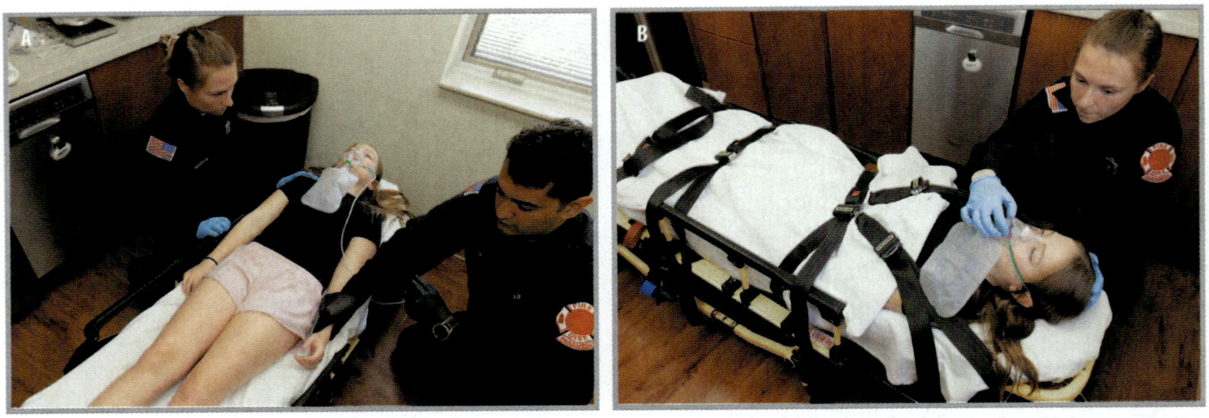

FIGURE 4–6 **A.** Treat suspected hypovolemic shock with high-flow oxygen and supine positioning. **B.** Keep the patient warm.

has an entry site in the area between the 2 nipples and the clavicles, because this is a high-risk location for cardiac injury. Blunt chest injury may also cause a pneumothorax that may progress to a tension pneumothorax. Suspect this condition in a child with a significant blunt mechanism of injury and signs of obstructive shock.

The cardinal features of obstructive shock are signs of decreased circulation in an injured child with increased jugular venous distension. The increased jugular pressures reflect the obstruction to venous return to the right ventricle. Sometimes, however, blood loss into the chest (hemothorax) or other related injuries may be associated with hemorrhage, so that jugular venous distension is not apparent. In the case of a tension pneumothorax, in addition to signs of obstructive shock, lung sounds are unequal or absent on the affected side, and ventilation is increasingly difficult. Because children have soft rib cages, they can experience significant underlying blunt chest injury in the absence of rib fractures and other outward signs. The presence of rib fractures in children indicates a significant amount of force to the chest wall.

General Noninvasive Treatment of Suspected Shock of All Types

Begin general noninvasive treatment of every child with suspected hypoperfusion after completing the PAT and initiating the hands-on ABCDEs. The general treatment is always the same: Allow the child to assume a position of comfort if the cause is medical (in the case of blunt trauma, spinal motion restriction should be considered [see Chapter 9]) and supply oxygen, as tolerated.

POSITIONING

Infants and toddlers may be most comfortable in their caregiver's arms or lap during assessment. If the primary assessment indicates that the child is physiologically unstable, place the child in a position of comfort that decreases their anxiety and activity. This is usually the supine position (**FIGURE 4–6**). Elevating the legs when the child is in the supine position or putting the child in a head-down position is not known to be effective. In a head-down position, the internal organs of the abdomen put pressure on the diaphragm, interfering with breathing; the resulting agitation increases oxygen demand and complicates treatment. In the supine position, alignment of the airway is aided by placing a towel under the shoulders and trunk of the child. This helps with ease of breathing. Keep the child warm, because children have a high surface-to-volume ratio and can lose body heat rapidly.

OXYGEN

Treat all children in shock with high-flow oxygen, regardless of the pulse oximetry value, to improve oxygen delivery. The EMS clinician must weigh the potential benefits of oxygen administration against the risk of agitating the child. Nasal cannulas are frequently better tolerated by children than oxygen face masks. "Blow-by" may be the only mechanism for delivering supplemental oxygen without upsetting the child and increasing the oxygen consumption.

> **TIP**
>
> Provide high-flow oxygen to all children in shock.

Specific Treatment of Hypovolemia

After the primary assessment and general supportive measures, provide additional specific treatment for shock. If the child has hypovolemic shock, consider starting early fluid resuscitation. A bolus of 20 mL/kg of crystalloid fluid such as normal saline (NS) or lactated Ringer (LR) solution is appropriate and may be repeated 2 times to replace intravascular volume. In trauma patients, always look carefully for bleeding sites and assume there may be internal bleeding. Apply direct pressure and/or tourniquets to stop external bleeding. Consider spinal motion restriction when appropriate, and splinting of injured extremities, as described in Chapter 7. Early administration of blood should be considered, if available, in the prehospital setting for patients with hypovolemia related to trauma.

ALS

If the child has severe fluid losses from vomiting or diarrhea, consider obtaining vascular access to administer fluids. If the child has hypotensive shock from illness, attempt an intravenous (IV) placement once in the field. Any further attempts should be made during transport to avoid a prolonged scene time. If the child is in extremis or is unconscious, consider an intraosseous (IO) needle insertion.

Intravenous Access

Intravenous access makes it easier to give medications and provides a way to give fluid therapy in patients with severe blood or fluid loss. Intravenous delivery is the reference standard for giving medication, because it permits rapid drug and fluid treatment and allows titration of important drugs. See Procedure 16, Intravenous Access.

IV Fluid Treatment of Compensated Hypovolemic Shock

If the child has mild to moderate volume losses as determined by HR, pulse quality, CRT, and skin temperature and has a normal blood pressure, they are in compensated shock. Make one attempt on scene to perform IV insertion and fluid administration. If unsuccessful, on the way to the hospital, obtain vascular access and administer IV crystalloid fluid in 20 mL/kg boluses to stabilize the patient. Although studies have shown improved outcomes in sepsis using LR, NS is still acceptable. Reassessment should be completed after each bolus, and the patient may require additional fluid boluses to correct the cardiopulmonary compromise.

IV Fluid Treatment of Hypotensive (Decompensated) Shock

If the child has hypotensive shock from illness, make one attempt on scene to establish vascular access. If the child is injured, delay all vascular access attempts until en route to the ED. Once access is established during transport, give 20-mL/kg boluses of IV crystalloid fluid as fast as possible. Consider IO needle insertion if vascular access cannot be obtained quickly and the child is unconscious. Repeat boluses (20 mL/kg up to 60 mL/kg) as needed to stabilize perfusion, based on ongoing reassessment of the PAT and vital signs. Using the "push-pull" method of fluid administration is an easy and precise way to administer IV fluids to a pediatric patient. This requires a 20-mL syringe and a 3-way stopcock attached to the end of the IV line. Twenty milliliters is drawn into the syringe, the stopcock is turned, and the fluid is given to the patient. The number of syringes given is equal to the patient's weight for a 20-mL/kg bolus. For older children, a pressure bag is an acceptable method for delivering larger volumes of fluid (see Procedure 26, Push-Pull Fluid Bolus).

IO Needle Insertion

Using an IO needle to give drugs or fluids is an excellent alternative to cannulating peripheral veins. The IO space is highly vascularized and functions as a noncollapsible vein. Needle insertion into this space is quick, simple, effective, and usually safe. Complications are infrequent and usually minor. See Procedure 17, Intraosseous Needle Insertion.

Treatment of Septic Shock

The mainstays of treatment are rapid administration of IV fluids and antibiotics. Timely fluid and antibiotic treatment has been shown to decrease mortality. An alert by EMS to the receiving ED has been shown to improve time to antibiotic treatment and fluid resuscitation; for a child in whom you suspect sepsis, rapid transport to the ED and alerting the ED that the patient may have sepsis can improve outcomes.

CAUTION

In a child with hypovolemic shock, crystalloid fluid boluses need to be given as fast as possible. Do not let the fluid just drip in.

Specific Treatment of Hypotensive (Decompensated) Distributive Shock

The primary difference between treatment of distributive and hypovolemic shock is the potential need for a vasoactive agent to improve vascular tone and heart muscle function when the child has distributive shock. Treat all shock conditions first with general noninvasive measures. Administer 100% high-flow

CASE STUDY 3

A 6-year-old boy at a birthday party is having trouble breathing, so 9-1-1 is called. On your arrival, the boy has swollen eyes but answers your questions about his name and age. He has increased work of breathing with audible wheezing. There are hives on his face and arms. The adult is not sure if he has a peanut allergy, and he may have eaten a birthday cake containing nuts. Vital signs are as follows: heart rate, 150 beats/min; respiratory rate, 50 breaths/min; blood pressure, 90/50 mm Hg; SpO_2, 90% in room air.

1. Is this child in shock?
2. What is the appropriate prehospital therapy?

oxygen, and put the poorly responsive child with shock in a supine position. Although LR is the preferred fluid for the treatment of sepsis, NS can also be used if LR is unavailable. After 3 fluid boluses, if the patient remains in decompensated shock, vasoactive therapy should be initiated. Epinephrine and norepinephrine are both acceptable vasoactive drugs in distributive shock; however, in children, epinephrine is generally considered to be the first-line vasoactive agent, and it can be administered in the field using a drip or by "push dose" epinephrine (0.1 mg/mL) administration.

ALS

Treatment of Distributive Shock

Attempt a vascular access on scene at least once. Deliver fluid boluses—20-mL/kg boluses up to 60 mL/kg—of a crystalloid solution on the way to the ED. The "push-pull" method or use of a pressure bag for fluid administration are rapid fluid delivery methods. If the child has lost protective airway reflexes or has refractory shock, support ventilation with a bag-mask device, endotracheal intubation, or a supraglottic airway.

If cardiopulmonary compromise (hypotension, markedly increased HR, and poor responsiveness) persists after volume therapy with up to 60 mL/kg of crystalloid fluid, early administration of a vasoactive agent (epinephrine or norepinephrine) should be considered. Epinephrine (0.1 mg/mL concentration) can be administered via drip at 0.1 to 1.0 µg/kg/min IV/IO for long transports, or by mixing 10 µg/mL ("push dose") epinephrine (0.1 mg/mL concentration) and administering 1 µg/kg (0.1 mL/kg) up to 10 µg/kg (1 mL/kg) IV/IO for shorter transport times, when mixing a drip is difficult and time consuming. Norepinephrine can be administered by drip at 0.05 to 2 µg/kg/min IV/IO. If epinephrine or norepinephrine is unavailable, use dopamine. Do not administer a vasoactive agent if you suspect untreated hypovolemia.

TREATMENT OF ANAPHYLAXIS

A child with anaphylaxis requires treatment with **epinephrine.** If respiratory symptoms are present, the administration of a β-agonist such as albuterol may be beneficial. If hives and angioedema are present, diphenhydramine may also be necessary (**FIGURE 4-7**). Unlike a simple allergic reaction, anaphylaxis has dangerous cardiovascular effects.

Epinephrine is the gold standard for treatment of anaphylaxis. It stimulates α- and β-adrenergic receptors, leading to 2 important effects: (1) constriction of the blood vessels to help counter the vasodilation and increased permeability of anaphylaxis (α effect), and (2) opening up the airways to help reverse the bronchospasm of anaphylaxis (β effect). For all children with anaphylaxis, administer epinephrine, 0.01 mg/kg (0.01 mL/kg) of a 1-g/mL concentration (maximum, 0.3 mg or 0.3 mL) intramuscularly (IM), or use an autoinjector of the correct dose (0.1, 0.15, or 0.3 mg). Intramuscular epinephrine should be given in the lateral thigh. For BLS providers, if the patient or parent has an epinephrine autoinjector, administer the

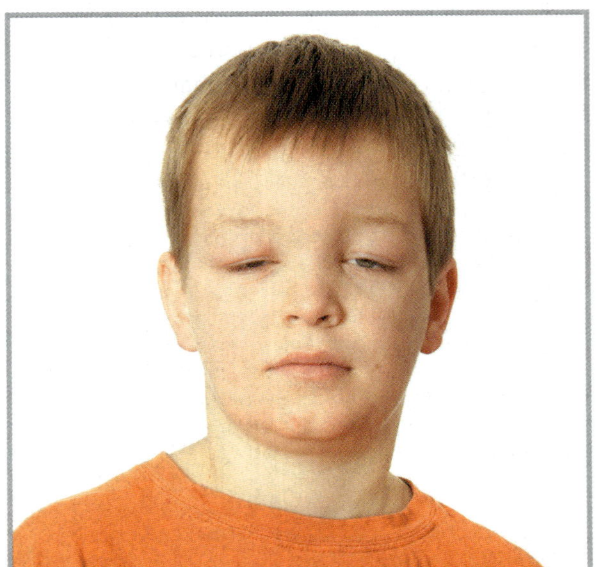

FIGURE 4-7 An allergic reaction, with edema of the eyes.

prescribed medication IM. Intranasal epinephrine is now available and approved for those patients 4 years and older who weigh 15 to <30 kg as a 1-mg nasal spray and for those >30 kg in a 2-mg spray. Epinephrine is a short-acting drug. If respiratory symptoms are present, administration of an inhaled β-agonist such as albuterol can be helpful. If hives or angioedema is present, diphenhydramine (1 mg/kg orally, IV, or IO; maximum, 50 mg) may also be necessary. Diphenhydramine works as a histamine blocker, specific for the histamine receptors that reside in the walls of the blood vessels and in the skin. Administration of this medication eases itching. The use of steroids such as methylprednisolone or dexamethasone is no longer recommended in the treatment of anaphylaxis in children.

Treatment of Cardiogenic Shock

If cardiogenic shock is suspected because of history or physical assessment findings, transport after general noninvasive treatment. On the way to the ED, consider vascular access. If the diagnosis of cardiogenic shock is uncertain, give a cautious fluid bolus of only 10 mL/kg of crystalloid fluid, and then reassess appearance, work of breathing, CRT, HR, and blood pressure. If there is no rhythm disturbance on the cardiac monitor (rate-related problems are discussed in Chapter 5) and the child remains poorly perfused after the initial fluid bolus, consider a vasoactive agent (epinephrine) after speaking to medical control, if the transport time is long. If epinephrine is unavailable, use dopamine or dobutamine. Start vasoactive agents at low doses, based on micrograms per kilogram, and then titrate to achieve acceptable perfusion (improved appearance and skin circulation and decreased HR and respiratory rate). If the child is known to be in congestive heart failure with cardiogenic shock, avoid fluid boluses and consider vasoactive therapy as front-line treatment if perfusion is severely compromised.

CAUTION

Do not withhold fluid from a child in cardiogenic shock; give it in boluses of 10 mL/kg and reassess.

The major difference in treatment of hypovolemic, distributive, and cardiogenic shock is the amount of fluid administration and consideration of a vasoactive agent.

ALS

Treatment of Obstructive Shock

The additional option for treatment of obstructive shock from a tension pneumothorax is needle thoracostomy to decrease air pressure, as explained in Procedure 23, Needle Thoracostomy.

This technique does not remove blood but relieves pressure in the pleural space. Rapid transport is an essential feature of field management of chest injury.

Primary Assessment: Transport Decision

After completing the primary assessment and beginning general treatment when appropriate, the EMS clinician must decide whether to go or stay on scene. Second, the EMS clinician must decide the destination based on the child's condition, local protocols, and distance to specialty hospitals. If the PAT and ABCDEs are normal and the child has no history of serious illness or injury mechanism, no anatomical abnormalities, and no pain, the child usually does not require urgent treatment or immediate transport. Take the time to get a history and perform a physical examination, and perform a detailed physical examination (trauma) on scene if possible. A child in this condition may be evaluated and managed at any hospital ED.

If the child has a serious mechanism of injury, a physiological or an anatomical abnormality, or severe pain, or if the scene is not safe, transport immediately. With such patients, conduct the additional assessment and attempt specific treatment on the way to the hospital, if possible. These children likely require transport to an ED with pediatric capabilities. An exception would be if their condition required stabilization to survive transport to the specialty center. In such instances, the child may need to be transported to the nearest hospital for stabilization and transfer.

The transport decision is sometimes difficult in a child with a suspected cardiovascular problem who needs vascular access. If the child is in compensated shock and has a palpable brachial pulse or normal blood pressure, protect the spine (if the child is injured), manage the airway and breathing, control hemorrhage, and transport immediately. Attempt vascular access for specific treatment on the way to the ED.

If the child is in hypotensive shock, the EMS clinician has several options, depending on the clinical condition of the child, local EMS system regulations, clinician comfort level, and the time to the nearest ED. If the child is injured, always transport immediately. If the child is ill with an abnormal appearance and hypotension, consider attempting a vascular access on scene, and then transporting without delay.

A final consideration in transport would be for children with preexisting or congenital conditions that are contributing to the shock state. In these instances, EMS clinicians should consider transport to the facility where the child normally receives care. This transport decision also reduces the chance of additional transfer for the child and family.

Summary of Shock States

There are 4 major classes of shock seen in children and adults: (1) hypovolemic, (2) distributive, (3) cardiogenic, and (4) obstructive. Hypovolemic shock is commonly the result of trauma and hemorrhage after injury. Vomiting and diarrhea leading to dehydration is the most common medical cause of hypovolemia. Distributive shock may result from sepsis, anaphylaxis, drug intoxication, or spinal injury. Always suspect sepsis in the infant or toddler who has a fever and an abnormal appearance. A petechial or purpuric skin rash is a red flag for sepsis. Cardiogenic shock caused by inadequate left ventricular contraction is rare in children and difficult to identify in the field, unless the child has a known congenital cardiac problem. Obstructive shock sometimes occurs in conjunction with significant chest wall injury. Clinical findings may reflect more than one type of shock pathophysiology. Treatment of all shock types includes general noninvasive interventions and then specific treatment based on clinical findings. Consider rapid fluid boluses in children who are hypotensive with an abnormal appearance.

CASE STUDY ANSWERS

CASE STUDY 1

This child has septic or distributive shock and is hypotensive. The rash is an ominous sign, and aggressive treatment is necessary to save the child's life. The appropriate first interventions are oxygen and assisted ventilation.

Attempt IV or IO access on scene once, and give a 20-mL/kg crystalloid fluid bolus as fast as possible, using the push-pull method or a pressure bag. Then, transport and deliver 20-mL/kg fluid boluses of crystalloid, to a maximum of 60 mL/kg, while en route as needed to correct perfusion. Reassess after each bolus. Consider giving a vasoactive agent (epinephrine or norepinephrine) if perfusion remains poor after administering 60 mL/kg of fluid and the transport time is long. Assisted ventilation or even endotracheal intubation may be necessary.

This case also requires universal precautions to protect the EMS clinician, because the child has a serious communicable disease. Direct specific questions about exposures and prophylactic treatment to your infection control personnel.

In the ED, the infant is given 2 additional fluid boluses and antibiotics. He is admitted to the pediatric intensive care unit and found to have meningococcemia, so the EMS clinicians are contacted about antibiotic prophylaxis.

CASE STUDY 2

This child is in hypotensive (decompensated) shock, because her blood pressure is low. The etiology is likely hypovolemia, related to the history of vomiting and diarrhea. Her lethargy can be caused by shock, but could also be caused by hypoglycemia. Prehospital treatment is to attempt IV or IO access on scene and give a 20-mL/kg normal crystalloid fluid bolus as fast as possible, using the push-pull method or a pressure bag. Begin transport and reassess. Give additional 20-mL/kg fluid boluses as needed to correct perfusion, to a maximum of 60 mL/kg, while en route to the ED. A bedside glucose level can also be obtained, and if it is low, 10% dextrose can be administered in addition to the IV fluids. In this case, the patient's glucose level is 50 mg/dL, and her weight is 20 kg, so 100 mL of 10% dextrose can be administered.

In the ED, she is more responsive, receives additional fluids, is able to take liquids on her own, and is discharged home.

CASE STUDY ANSWERS—cont'd

CASE STUDY 3

This is a case of anaphylaxis, and although this child is not in shock at this time, it could still develop. Anaphylaxis requires urgent IM administration of 0.01 mg/kg of epinephrine of the 1 mg/mL concentration. This child weighs 20 kg, so the dose is 0.2 mg (0.2 mL). This medication can be given by the patient's autoinjector, if available, at its prescribed dose. Administration of albuterol via a nebulizer may help his wheezing. Insertion of an IV line now can be useful to administer diphenhydramine. If the patient's blood pressure begins to drop (anaphylactic shock), a rapid infusion of a 20-mL/kg normal crystalloid fluid bolus is indicated. The patient may also need additional doses of epinephrine.

On arrival at the ED, the eye swelling and hives are improving, and he is no longer wheezing. Because he received IM epinephrine, he is observed for 2 hours and has no recurrence of symptoms. His parents and the patient are instructed on the use of injectable IM epinephrine, and given a prescription for this medication. The patient is told to avoid nuts and given a referral to see an allergist.

Suggested References

TEXTBOOKS

American Academy of Pediatrics and the American College of Emergency Physicians. *APLS: The Pediatric Emergency Medicine Resource.* 5th ed. Jones & Bartlett Learning; 2012

American College of Surgeons. *Advanced Trauma Life Support (ATLS) Student Course Manual,11*th ed. American College of Surgeons; 2025

Rogers JL. *Pathophysiology: The Biologic Basis for Disease in Adults and Children.* 9th ed. Elsevier; 2022:1727–1752

ARTICLES

Davis AL, Carcillo JA, Aneja RK, et al. American College of Critical Care Medicine clinical practice parameters for hemodynamic support of pediatric and neonatal septic shock. *Crit Care Med.* 2017;45(6):1061–1093. PMID: 28509730 doi: 10.1097/CCM.0000000000002425

Fuchs S, Terry M, Adelgais K, et al. Definitions and assessment approaches for emergency medical services for children. *Pediatrics.* 2016;138(6):e20161073. PMID: 27940682 doi: 10.1542/peds.2016-1073

Han YY, Carcillo JA, Dragotta MA, et al. Early reversal of pediatric-neonatal septic shock by community physicians is associated with improved outcome. *Pediatrics.* 2003;112(4):793–799. PMID: 14523168 doi: 10.1542/peds.112.4.793

Lasa JJ, Dhillon GS, Duff JP, et al. Part 8: Pediatric Advanced Life Support: 2025 American Heart Association and American Academy of Pediatrics Guidelines for Cardiopulmonary Resuscitation and Emergency Cardiovascular Care. Pediatrics. 2025; doi: 10.1542/peds.2025-074351.

Mhanna A, Beran A, Srour O, et al. Balanced crystalloids versus isotonic saline in pediatric sepsis: a comprehensive systematic review and meta-analysis. *Proc Bayl Univ Med Cent.* 2024;37(2):295–302. PMID: 38343480 doi: 10.1080/08998280.2024.2301904

Morris MC, Nadkarni VM. Pediatric cardiopulmonary-cerebral resuscitation: an overview and future directions. *Crit Care Clin.* 2003;19(3):337–364. PMID: 12848310 doi: 10.1016/S0749-0704(03)00003-4

Muraro A, Worm M, Alviani C, et al; European Academy of Allergy and Clinical Immunology, Food Allergy, Anaphylaxis Guidelines Group. EAACI guidelines: anaphylaxis (2021 update) *Allergy.* 2022;77(2):357–377. PMID: 34343358 doi: 10.1111/all.15032

Pflomm MJ (ed). Epinephrine 1mg nasal spray. *Med Lett Drugs Ther.* 2025:67(1727):71

Wang J, Lieberman JA, Wallace DV, Waserman S, Golden DBK. Anaphylaxis in practice: a guide to the 2023 practice parameter update. *J Allergy Clin Immunol Pract.* 2024;12(9):2325–2336. PMID: 38944199 doi: 10.1016/j.jaip.2024.06.036

Weiss SL, Peters MJ, Alhazzani W, et al. Surviving Sepsis Campaign International guidelines for the management of septic shock and sepsis-associated organ dysfunction in children. *Pediatr Crit Care Med.* 2020;21(2):e52–e106. PMID: 32032273 doi: 10.1097/PCC.0000000000002198

CHAPTER 5

Dysrhythmias and Resuscitation

Hoi See Tsao, MD, MPH
Evelyn F. Wilson, EdD, NRP, NCEE

LEARNING OBJECTIVES

1. **Describe how to assess circulation using the Pediatric Assessment Triangle (PAT), ABCDEs, and additional assessment.**
2. **Explain when to treat bradycardia and tachycardia, and discuss management.**
3. **Define indications for the use of the automated external defibrillator (AED) in pediatric patients.**
4. **List the links in the pediatric "chain of survival."**
5. **Order the steps in managing pediatric cardiac arrest caused by asystole, pulseless electrical activity (PEA), ventricular fibrillation (VF), and pulseless ventricular tachycardia (VT).**
6. **Describe the causes of primary cardiac arrest in the pediatric patient.**
7. **Discuss medical issues in children with congenital heart disease who may require the care of the emergency medical services (EMS) clinician.**

CASE STUDY 1

You have been dispatched for a 9-year-old child who is unconscious and not breathing. You arrive at a baseball field and find the child lying supine on the pitcher's mound. Teammates say he was hit in the chest by a baseball. The child is unresponsive, not breathing, and cyanotic, and he has no pulse. You begin cardiopulmonary resuscitation (CPR) while your partner attaches the AED.

1. How does management of VF or VT differ from treatment for **pulseless electrical activity (PEA)** or asystole?
2. Why should CPR be started as rapidly as possible and continued without interruptions?

Introduction

Cardiac arrest in pediatrics is uncommon in the prehospital setting. Survival to discharge from out-of-hospital cardiac arrest is 6% (3% for infants and 9% for children and adolescents). The primary cause of arrest in children is usually respiratory failure that deteriorates into cardiac arrest.

Although hypoxia leading to pulseless electrical activity (PEA) or asystole is the most common cause of pediatric arrest, a small percentage of patients may demonstrate **ventricular fibrillation (VF)** or **ventricular tachycardia (VT)**. Regardless of the type of cardiovascular emergency, early recognition and timely management are crucial to reduce serious morbidity or mortality.

Prearrival Preparation

Based on dispatch information, the EMS clinician needs to be prepared to assess, manage, and make transport decisions for a child exhibiting a symptomatic cardiac dysrhythmia, cardiac event, or cardiac arrest. Recall appropriate techniques for assessment; the role of vital signs; and the possible equipment, medications, fluid requirements, automated external defibrillator (AED), and electrical therapy a child may require. Consider when to stay and treat on scene and when to transport immediately.

Scene Size-Up

All EMS clinicians need to ensure that the scene is safe and note any significant findings that may be contributing factors to the situation. The EMS clinician must also assess the scene, as appropriate, for signs of child maltreatment.

General Assessment: The PAT

On arrival, if the child is unresponsive and not breathing, immediately check for a central pulse (brachial in an infant, carotid or femoral in a child). If there is no pulse, immediately start cardiopulmonary resuscitation (CPR). Attach an AED or defibrillator pads as soon as available. For an AED, follow prompts. For a defibrillator, follow the algorithm for VF/VT or asystole/PEA. If the child is responsive, proceed with the following.

EVALUATING THE PRESENTING COMPLAINT

Determine the child's presenting complaint. Gathering a complete history is a vital component in determining the cardiac event the patient may be experiencing. Attempt to gather a complete SAMPLE (**TABLE 5-1**) history during the primary assessment (with SAMPLE standing for Signs & Symptoms, Allergies, Medications, Past medical history, Last oral intake, and Events).

TABLE 5-1 SAMPLE Components in a Child With Cardiovascular Problems

Component	Features
Signs/symptoms	Presence of vomiting More cyanotic than usual Lower pulse oximeter reading Number of episodes of vomiting Presence or absence of fever Rash Respiratory distress or shortness of breath (eg, in cardiogenic shock with congestive heart failure)
Allergies	Known allergies and what reaction occurs History of anaphylaxis
Medications	Exact names and dosages of ongoing medications Chronic diuretic therapy Potential exposure to other medications or drugs Timing and doses of analgesics or antipyretics
Past medical problems	History of heart problems or heart surgery History of prematurity Prior hospitalizations for cardiovascular problems
Last food or liquid	Timing of the child's last food or drink, including bottle or breast feedings
Events leading to the injury or illness	Travel Trauma Fever history Symptoms in family members Potential toxic exposure

ASSESSMENT OF CIRCULATION

Using the PAT

The Pediatric Assessment Triangle (PAT) is the first step in assessment of circulation, as outlined in Chapter 1. The PAT evaluates 3 characteristics: (1) appearance, (2) work of breathing, and (3) circulation to skin. Knowing these characteristics helps to determine whether the child is sick or not sick, the type of physiological abnormality, and the urgency of treatment. Circulatory problems affect each of these characteristics in identifiable patterns.

Appearance

First, assess the child's appearance. A child with decreased core circulation caused by any cardiac compromise may have signs of poor brain perfusion. The abnormality in the child's appearance will be variable, depending on the type of perfusion problem and the degree of circulatory insufficiency. Abnormal features in the appearance of a child with decreased core circulation include the following:

- Lethargy or listlessness
- Decreased motor activity in infants, poor muscle tone
- Diminished interactiveness with caregivers, the EMS clinician, and the environment
- Inconsolability
- Poor eye contact
- Weak cry

Sometimes, the child with hemodynamic instability will be restless and inconsolable. *Appearance alone, however, is not a very accurate sign of circulatory problems*. Assessing appearance is a good way to tell if the child is ill, but not a good way to identify the physiological problem. Assessment tools other than the PAT, such as the hands-on ABCDE assessment (in which ABCDE stands for Airway, Breathing, Circulation, Disability [neurological status], and Exposure [skin/temperature]), will help determine the type of physiological problem and the presence or absence of abnormal perfusion.

Work of Breathing

Next, assess the work of breathing. If circulation to vital organs is decreased, the child's respiratory rate will increase. **Effortless tachypnea**, or a fast respiratory rate without increased work of breathing, is a common but nonspecific sign of hemodynamic instability. It reflects the child's attempt to blow off carbon dioxide and reduce the **metabolic acidosis** created by decreased perfusion to cells. Signs of increased work of breathing, such as abnormal positioning; retractions; nasal flaring; or abnormal airway sounds, such as grunting, stridor, or wheezing, may or may not be present in a child with a circulatory problem.

Circulation to Skin

After assessing the child's appearance and work of breathing, assess circulation by looking at skin color. This will be difficult to interpret if the environmental temperature is low, because **vasoconstriction**, as a reflexive effort to preserve heat, will falsely alter skin findings, especially in infants. Disrobe the child and look for mottling, pallor, and cyanosis, which reflect peripheral vasoconstriction or clamping down of nonessential skin perfusion to maintain essential core circulation. If a child has an abnormal appearance and abnormal skin signs in a warm ambient environment, the child may be hemodynamically unstable. Between your assessments, make sure to keep the child warm. Infants, especially neonates, are particularly susceptible to becoming unstable if they are hypothermic as a result of environmental conditions such as being unwrapped.

Primary Assessment: The ABCDEs

After the PAT, perform the hands-on ABCDE assessment. After evaluating the airway and breathing, as described in previous chapters, assess the circulation. There are 4 parts to the assessment of circulation:

1. Heart rate
2. Pulse quality
3. Skin temperature and capillary refill time
4. Blood pressure

HEART RATE

First, measure the heart rate by feeling the pulse for 30 seconds, and then double the number. A normal heart rate is between 60 and 160 beats/min, depending on the child's age, as noted in **TABLE 5–2**. In newborns, you can palpate the heart rate by holding the umbilical cord. The brachial area is the preferred site to measure heart rate in infants and children. The carotid pulse is acceptable in older children and adolescents, but it is hard to locate in infants. If a pulse is difficult to feel, determine heart rate by listening to the heart sounds directly with a stethoscope placed on the medial side of the child's left nipple. However, be aware that the presence of a "normal" heart rate by auscultation does not necessarily reflect adequate cardiac output and perfusion.

Interpreting the heart rate may be difficult, as explained in Chapter 1. Ranges of normal heart rates change inversely with advancing age. Also, many conditions can increase heart rate, ranging from serious physiological problems to noxious stimuli that are rarely life threatening. Certain common medications may also alter heart rate (high and low). Stimuli that can cause **tachycardia** include pain, fever, fear, and agitation. Interpret heart rate in the context of overall signs of perfusion, age, presence or absence of noxious stimuli, medications, and observed trends. Although a single measurement of heart rate is usually of limited value in determining the degree of physiological derangement, *a trend of mounting tachycardia, or a heart rate that is falling below the lower limits of normal, suggests a serious physiological problem*. In addition, sustained tachycardia is a worrisome sign. Finally, be extremely vigilant when the child has **bradycardia**, because this often indicates hypoxia or may be a sign of profound ischemia.

TABLE 5–2 Normal Heart Rate for Age

Age	Heart Rate (Beats/Min)
Infant (birth–12 months)	100–160
Toddler (1–3 years)	95–150
Preschooler (3–5 years)	80–140
School-aged child (6–12 years)	70–120
Adolescent (13–18 years)	60–100

PULSE QUALITY

The presence of a strong central pulse (carotid, femoral in children, **brachial** in infants) with a strong peripheral pulse (**radial**, in children) suggests a good blood pressure. A strong central pulse with a weak peripheral pulse indicates compensated shock. If a brachial pulse is not palpable, the child is probably hypotensive and is hemodynamically unstable.

> **CAUTION**
>
> **The carotid pulse is an acceptable site for measurement of the central pulse rate in older children and adolescents, but it is hard to locate in infants. In infants, the brachial pulse is easier to locate.**

SKIN TEMPERATURE AND CAPILLARY REFILL TIME

The next part of the hands-on cardiovascular assessment involves evaluating skin signs. Check skin temperature for warmth at the hands, feet, kneecaps, or forearms. Cool hands and feet may be normal, but cool proximal extremities reflect poor perfusion and shunting of blood to the core.

> **TIP**
>
> Practice CRT and pulse quality on every child. This will help you to become comfortable with the technique and interpret key findings accurately.

Capillary refill time (CRT) *should be less than 2 seconds in a child who is not cold.* Inadequate core perfusion results in peripheral vasoconstriction, which will manifest as cool skin and delayed CRT. Although CRT is a good test of circulation in children, it must be interpreted in the context of overall signs of perfusion. The EMS clinician can become comfortable with the technique and interpretation of the key skin findings by practicing on every child.

> **CAUTION**
>
> **CRT is a good test for circulation in children, but do not place heavy emphasis on this sign alone.**

BLOOD PRESSURE

Last, consider taking a blood pressure. A high blood pressure value in a child is not clinically significant in the field, unless the child has a history of hypertension, known renal disease, or acute head injury. However, a true low blood pressure value is significant for hemodynamic instability. The challenges in blood pressure measurement in children in the prehospital setting include knowing when to get a blood pressure reading, obtaining the blood pressure correctly, and interpreting it accurately.

A normal minimal systolic blood pressure in a child older than 1 year of age is determined with the following equation: greater than $70 + (2 \times \text{years of age})$. Proper equipment, technique, and patience are required to obtain an accurate blood pressure in an infant or a toddler. Because this can be a time-consuming process and may not contribute greatly to the clinical assessment of perfusion, in a child 3 years or younger, attempt a blood pressure measurement only once or skip it altogether. Inadequate perfusion will be better reflected in the other signs of perfusion described previously (heart rate, pulse quality, CRT, and skin temperature).

In a child older than 3 years of age, attempt to measure blood pressure at least once to provide a baseline for future assessments. Repeated vital signs provide trends that can yield useful information in determining the severity of the patient's condition. Use a cuff with a width that is two-thirds the length of the upper arm. Applying a cuff that is too large will falsely decrease the blood pressure measurement, and a cuff that is too small will falsely increase the measurement.

> **TIP**
>
> A normal minimal systolic blood pressure in a child older than 1 year of age is $70 + (2 \times \text{years of age})$. An infant should have a systolic blood pressure >70.

Additional Assessment

If the child is in stable condition after the primary assessment and does not require immediate treatment, and there are no immediate safety concerns for the child or EMS clinician, conduct the focused history and physical examination and the detailed physical examination on scene. Use the SAMPLE (**TABLE 5–1**) and OPQRST mnemonics (**TABLE 5–3**) to recall important features of the focused cardiovascular history. Use age-appropriate approaches to gain the child's trust and speak directly to them. Ask the caregiver to add to the child's history.

Obtain the history from the caregiver if the child is too young to speak or is unable to cooperate.

After obtaining the focused history, perform a focused examination of the heart, peripheral circulation, and abdomen. Then, perform an anatomical examination of the entire body, as outlined in Chapter 1. If the child has a traumatic injury, also conduct a detailed physical examination, searching for other injuries.

TABLE 5–3 The OPQRST of Pain

O—Onset **Key Question:** What were you doing when the pain/discomfort started?
P—Provocation/Palliation **Key Questions:** What makes the pain/discomfort better or worse? What have you tried to reduce the symptoms? Did it work? **Support Questions:** Has this ever happened before? If so, when?
Q—Quality **Key Question:** What does the pain feel like?
R—Region/Radiation **Key Question:** Can you point with one finger to the main area of pain/discomfort? **Support Questions:** Do you feel pain anywhere else? If so, can you show me or tell me where it is?
S—Severity **Key Question:** How bad is the pain or chief complaint on a scale of 1 to 10, with 1 being no pain and 10 being extreme pain? **Support Questions:** What is the worst pain you have ever experienced? How does this compare?
T—Time Frames **Key Question:** When did you first notice the symptoms? **Support Questions:** Have the symptoms been continuous? If not, has the feeling come and gone?

Perform an ongoing assessment of all children with cardiovascular problems while on the way to the emergency department (ED), observing for changes on the cardiorespiratory monitor. The child's status may change during transport, so observe and document any physiological trends. Use the PAT to monitor effective perfusion and watch the respiratory rate, heart rate, blood pressure, and pulse oximetry. Be prepared to increase the level of respiratory and cardiovascular support if the child's condition worsens or the child fails to respond to treatment.

Summary of Cardiovascular Assessment

The PAT provides a good first-line cardiovascular evaluation: abnormal appearance, abnormal work of breathing, and poor circulation to skin suggest a perfusion problem. Pallor, mottling, and cyanosis all indicate poor peripheral perfusion. The circulatory portion of the hands-on ABCDEs consists of evaluating heart rate, pulse quality, skin temperature, CRT, and blood pressure. These physical features complement the PAT and will help identify the type and severity of circulatory compromise. Vital signs can sometimes be misleading and must be correctly obtained and interpreted for age. Trends in vital signs, or persistence in abnormal vital signs, such as tachycardia, are more accurate indicators of real physiological problems than mild vital sign abnormalities on primary assessment.

Dysrhythmias

BRADYCARDIA

In children, bradycardia usually reflects hypoxia, rather than a primary cardiac problem. It is a pre-arrest rhythm, and the prognosis is ominous if left untreated. Immediate delivery of high-flow oxygen and **assisted ventilation** are essential. Untreated bradycardia can quickly cause cardiorespiratory compromise (altered mental status, signs of shock, hypotension) and ultimately death. In children with asthma or respiratory distress, bradycardia may indicate profound hypoxia. Pulse oximetry, when available, will help determine the degree of hypoxia in the field.

Congenital heart block is an extremely rare cause of bradycardia in infancy and early childhood. Drug overdose (eg, β-blockers, calcium channel blockers, digoxin, clonidine) is another possible cause of bradycardia. Bradycardia may also result from **vagal** stimulation during medical procedures or gastric tube placement. However, although bradycardia that develops during **laryngoscopy** or suctioning may be the result of vagal stimulation, hypoxia may be the true cause. If bradycardia does occur in this setting, stop the procedure, administer supplemental oxygen, and reassess the patient.

Bradycardia may also be a normal finding, especially in asymptomatic athletic adolescents. If bradycardia is an isolated finding, without signs of hemodynamic instability, in a well-perfused school-aged child or teenager, no treatment is necessary in the field.

ASSESSMENT OF THE CHILD WITH BRADYCARDIA

If the child has a heart rate below the normal range for age (see **TABLE 5–2**), evaluate carefully for signs of cardiopulmonary compromise. The PAT and ABCDEs, along with a brief history, will establish the likely cause, the severity of the problem, and the need for urgent treatment.

TREATMENT OF BRADYCARDIA

If the child is asymptomatic, consider no treatment, especially if the child is an adolescent, because slow heart rates are common in athletic teenagers. If the child has bradycardia and a primary assessment demonstrates oxygenation, ventilation, or cardiopulmonary compromise, provide 100% oxygen with bag-mask ventilation and begin transport. Attach cardiorespiratory monitor and monitor heart rate en route. Check the effectiveness of ventilation by observing for chest rise and an improvement in the PAT, heart rate, perfusion, pulse oximetry, and blood pressure.

ALS

Drug Therapy for Symptomatic Bradycardia. Oxygenation and ventilation are the primary treatments for bradycardia. If the heart rate does not rise in response to assisted ventilation, in most cases administer epinephrine as the first-line drug at a 0.1 mg/mL concentration—0.01 mg/kg or 0.1 mL/kg intravenous (IV) or intraosseous (IO)—every 3 to 5 minutes. If there is increased vagal tone (or poisoning by cholinergic drugs or agents, such as organophosphates) or a primary atrioventricular heart block, administer **atropine**, 0.02 mg/kg IV or IO (minimum dose 0.1 mg, maximum dose, 1 mg in a child, 2 mg in adolescents). When the child has a known reason for cholinergic-mediated bradycardia, such as congenital heart block, administer atropine and monitor the response; repeat once if indicated.

Before administering vasoactive agents, always assess for mechanical problems with oxygen delivery and ventilation. Check for disconnected oxygen tubing, poor mask seal, airway obstruction, inadequate chest rise, endotracheal tube blockage, or malposition. Other causes of bradycardia due to hypoxia or ischemia are pneumothorax, hypovolemia, cardiomyopathy, poisoning, or increased intracranial pressure.

When oxygenation, ventilation, and drug therapy for bradycardia fail, consider external electrical cardiac pacing of the heart.

Endotracheal Administration of Drugs. If neither IV nor IO access is available for giving drugs during resuscitation, the endotracheal route is an alternative for at least 4 pediatric drugs: lidocaine, epinephrine, atropine, and naloxone (recalled via the mnemonic LEAN). Although endotracheal drugs are not as effective as medications delivered by the IV or IO routes, endotracheal delivery is appropriate in the critically ill patient until IV or IO access is established. Use the technique for endotracheal drug delivery described in **Procedure 20, Endotracheal Tube Drug Instillation.**

When administering epinephrine through an endotracheal tube to a child who has no vascular or IO access, give epinephrine at the higher concentration of 1 mg/mL, and use the higher dose of 0.1 mg/kg (0.1 mL/kg). Note that this is the same total volume of epinephrine as the IV/IO dose, because the 10-fold dose has 10 times the concentration of 0.1 mg/mL. When administering atropine through an endotracheal tube, the dose is 2 to 3 times the IV/IO dose (0.04–0.06 mg/kg).

In rare situations, chest compressions for bradycardia are necessary. If the heart rate is below 60 beats/min and the child shows signs of cardiopulmonary compromise after oxygenation and assisted ventilation, begin chest compressions.

TACHYCARDIA

Tachycardia may be a nonspecific sign of fear, anxiety, pain, or fever and may not represent serious injury or illness. Tachycardia may also be a sign of a life-threatening problem, such as hypoxia, cardiac abnormality, or hypovolemia. Sinus tachycardia is the most common dysrhythmia in children, and treatment is generally limited to fluid administration, supplemental oxygen, pain medication, and transport to the ED.

CAUTION

Be extremely careful with IV/IO/endotracheal tube epinephrine, and check doses and concentration.

Assessment of the Child With Tachycardia

Tachycardia must be assessed in conjunction with the PAT and ABCDEs. Always ask about a history of congenital heart disease and check for midline chest scars from cardiac surgery.

There are 2 characteristics in the child's rhythm strip to measure and use as a basis for treatment, along with the perfusion assessment: (1) the heart rate per minute and (2) the width of the QRS complex. First, establish an accurate heart rate electronically from the rhythm strip. As in the assessment of bradycardia, interpret the heart rate according to knowledge of the normal range for age (see **TABLE 5–2**). Second, determine if there is cardiopulmonary compromise such as altered mental status, signs of shock, or hypotension. Third, establish the width of the QRS from the rhythm strip. If the QRS complex is less than or equal to 0.09 seconds (<2¼ standard boxes on the rhythm strip), consider the child to have a narrow complex tachycardia. If the width is greater than 0.09 seconds (>2¼ standard boxes on the rhythm strip), consider the child to have a wide complex tachycardia.

TABLE 5–4 distinguishes the features of a narrow complex sinus tachycardia from those of narrow complex supraventricular tachycardia (SVT) and wide complex VT.

Specific Treatment of Tachycardia

If the child is experiencing tachycardia, determine the appropriate treatment by establishing the perfusion status and by assessing the rhythm strip for heart rate and QRS duration.

TABLE 5-4 Features of ST, SVT, and VT

	History	Heart Rate	Variability	QRS Interval	Assessment	Possible Treatments
Sinus tachycardia	Fever Volume loss Hypoxia Pain Increased activity or exercise	< 220 beats/min (infant) < 180 beats/min (child)	Yes	Narrow ≤ 0.09 seconds	Hypovolemia Hypoxia Painful injury	Fluids Oxygen splinting Analgesia/sedation
Supraventricular tachycardia	Congenital heart disease Known SVT Nonspecific symptoms (eg, poor feeding, fussiness)	≥ 220 beats/min (often 240–300 beats/min) (infant) ≥ 180 beats/min (child)	No	Narrow ≤ 0.09 seconds	CHF or poor perfusion may be present	Vagal maneuvers (ice to face) Adenosine (stable) Synchronized cardioversion (unstable)
Ventricular tachycardia	Serious systemic illness Congenital heart disease Postoperative heart disease	> 150 beats/min	Yes	Wide > 0.09 seconds	CHF may be present	Synchronized cardioversion Defibrillation (VT without a pulse) Lidocaine Amiodarone

Abbreviations: CHF, congestive heart failure; ST, sinus tachycardia; SVT, supraventricular tachycardia; VT, ventricular tachycardia.

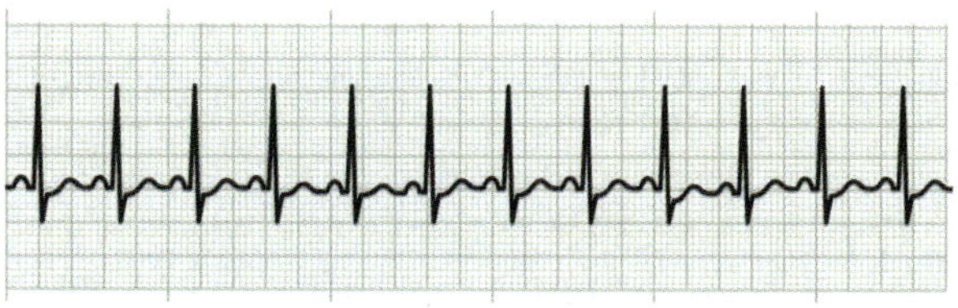

FIGURE 5-1 Electrocardiogram of sinus tachycardia.

Narrow Complex Tachycardia. If the child has a narrow QRS tachycardia (≤0.09 seconds), P waves are present, and the heart rate is variable and less than 220 beats/min in an infant, or less than 180 beats/min in a child, the cause is usually sinus tachycardia (**FIGURE 5-1**) due to noncardiac conditions (eg, hypoxia, hypovolemia, hyperthermia, hypoglycemia, metabolic abnormalities, toxins, fear, pain, or serious trauma to the chest). No specific cardiac medical management of the sinus tachycardia is needed. Instead, treat with fluids, oxygen, splinting, analgesia, or sedation as indicated by the associated condition. If there is no change in heart rate after treatment, consider other etiologies, such as SVT.

Specific Treatment of SVT. If the QRS is less than or equal to 0.09 seconds, P waves are absent or abnormal, and the heart rate is not variable and greater than or equal to 220 beats/min in an infant or greater than or equal to 180 beats/min in a child, consider SVT as the likely etiology. If the child has no previous history of SVT and is in stable condition, provide oxygen and transport to the ED. Delaying specific treatment for SVT until arrival at the hospital will permit the hospital staff to confirm SVT and to run a continuous electrocardiogram while actively managing the dysrhythmia. A patient with a confirmed diagnosis of SVT may need long-term treatment with cardiac medications.

ALS

If the patient has a prior history of SVT and is in stable condition, consider a vagal maneuver first. Ice to the face (if available) evokes the "diving reflex" and is an effective management tool for SVT in infants and toddlers. Place crushed ice in a plastic bag, glove, or washcloth and apply firmly over the mid-face (cheeks and bridge of nose) for approximately 15 seconds, until the rhythm changes or the patient's condition dictates immediate cessation of the procedure (FIGURE 5-2). Do not occlude the nose or mouth (to allow breathing), and provide constant reassurance to the parent and child. Avoid ocular pressure (pressure on the eyeballs) as a method of vagal stimulation in a child.

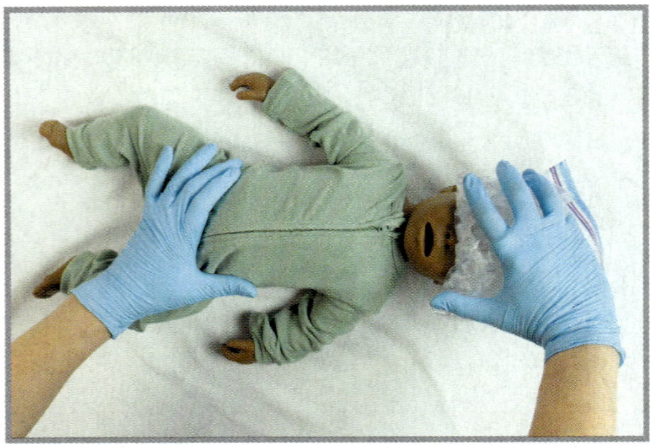

FIGURE 5–2 Placing a bag of ice on a child's face elicits the "diving reflex" and may convert supreventricular tachycardia to sinus rhythm.

ALS

If the patient with narrow complex tachycardia is in stable condition, and the heart rate does not convert to sinus rhythm after one attempt at vagal stimulation, administer adenosine at 0.1 mg/kg up to a maximum first dose of 6 mg rapid IV or IO push, and follow immediately with a 2- to 5-mL bolus of normal saline. Use an IV/IO access nearest to the heart and rapidly push adenosine followed by saline; a 3-way stopcock, if available, is a good tool to use when rapidly giving adenosine immediately followed by saline. Double the dose to 0.2 mg/kg if the rhythm does not convert after the first dose of adenosine (maximum second dose of12 mg). Be prepared to treat the untoward effects of adenosine; it is a very potent cardiac drug. If given properly, it is usually effective in the treatment of SVT. Brief runs of bradycardia or even several seconds of asystole commonly occur with adenosine administration. Sustained or fatal dysrhythmias (eg, asystole, VT, and VF) are rare, but possible. Caution should be used when administering adenosine in children who are already being treated with carbamazepine because it can result in prolonged heart block. Monitor the child closely, place defibrillator pads on the child prior to the administration of adenosine, and have a defibrillator and resuscitative drugs within reach.

If a child with suspected SVT has signs of cardiopulmonary compromise (abnormal mental status, signs of shock and hypotension), is in shock, or is unconscious, immediately administer synchronized electrical cardioversion at 0.5 to 1.0 J/kg as a starting electrical dose. If the initial shock is ineffective, double to 2 J/kg. If the child is in shock but still conscious and has vascular access, administer pain control and consider sedation, if needed, before delivering the electrical countershock. Do not delay electrical therapy for sedation. If electrical therapy fails to convert the child to sinus rhythm, consider using other antidysrhythmic drugs, such as amiodarone (5 mg/kg over 20–60 minutes) or procainamide (15 mg/kg over 20–60 minutes), as per local emergency medical services (EMS) system guidelines, or in discussion with online medical control.

TIP

The EMS clinician must be prepared to treat the adverse drug effects of all cardiac medications, even if the indication, dose, and route of delivery are correct.

Wide Complex Tachycardia. If the patient is conscious and has adequate perfusion, a heart rate of greater than 150 beats/min, and a QRS interval of greater than 0.09 seconds, they are probably in stable VT. Sinus tachycardia with a conduction abnormality (bundle branch block) may look like VT, but it usually occurs in a child with a history of heart disease or cardiac surgery.

CAUTION

Most tachycardia in children is a response to noncardiac stimuli (fever, fear, pain) and does not require dysrhythmia treatment.

Likewise, SVT with aberrant conduction can result in a wide complex rhythm. In such stable cases with wide complex tachycardias, provide oxygen and transport the patient to an appropriate ED, with close cardiac monitoring and equipment for defibrillation/cardioversion immediately available.

ALS

If the child has VT and is in stable condition, and the rhythm is monomorphic and regular, try a dose of adenosine first to determine if the rhythm is SVT with aberrant conduction. If the rhythm is VT, an antiarrhythmic can be used per EMS guidelines. If the child has VT and shows signs of poor perfusion, treat with synchronized electrical cardioversion (0.5 to 1 J/kg). If a second shock (2 J/kg) is unsuccessful, or if the tachycardia recurs quickly, consider antidysrhythmic drugs, such as amiodarone (5 mg/kg over 20–60 minutes) or procainamide (15 mg/kg over 30–60 minutes) per local EMS system guidelines. Do not administer amiodarone and procainamide together.

AUTOMATED EXTERNAL DEFIBRILLATOR

Cardiac arrest in children is usually the result of profound hypoxia or shock, which leads to **asystole**, or **pulseless electrical activity (PEA)**, the most frequent rhythms of pediatric cardiac arrest. Ventricular fibrillation, however, does occur in pediatrics. The typical VF case is a child out of the infant age group who has had a witnessed collapse. Etiologies for VF arrest in children include **myocarditis**, an infection of the heart muscle; long QT syndrome, a congenital cardiac conduction problem, and other inherited cardiac syndromes; **hypertrophic cardiomyopathy (HCM),** a hypertrophy of the ventricular septum and ventricles; and other cardiomyopathies. One other special circumstance for VF arrest is **commotio cordis**, which usually develops in a young athlete who is struck in the chest by a ball, stick, or other blunt object.

Perform rapid assessment for VF in all unresponsive children, begin CPR, apply the defibrillator or AED at the earliest opportunity and administer defibrillation if VF is present on the cardiac monitor or shock indicated by the AED. Be especially vigilant for VF when the child is older and has experienced a witnessed collapse. There is no demonstrated benefit to defibrillation of asystole, and this procedure will only delay the key interventions of chest compressions, ventilation, and oxygenation.

TIP

Treat pulseless ventricular tachycardia the same as ventricular fibrillation.

The AED (**FIGURE 5–3**) allows early recognition of VF and rapid defibrillation. The American Heart Association (AHA) guidelines recommend the use of an AED for treatment of VF in children of all ages, including infants. The AED has been shown to accurately identify VF and VT in young children and are also accurate in identifying pediatric rhythms that do not require defibrillation.

When used with a designated pediatric pad–cable system, these AEDs deliver an energy dose that is smaller than that delivered with adult pads. Use a pediatric AED or pediatric AED pads if available; however, an adult AED can be used on a child or an infant (one may consider putting pads anterior–posterior for an infant or anterolateral for a child as long as the pads are separated by 1-2 cm). For a pediatric arrest, use the AED as soon as possible.

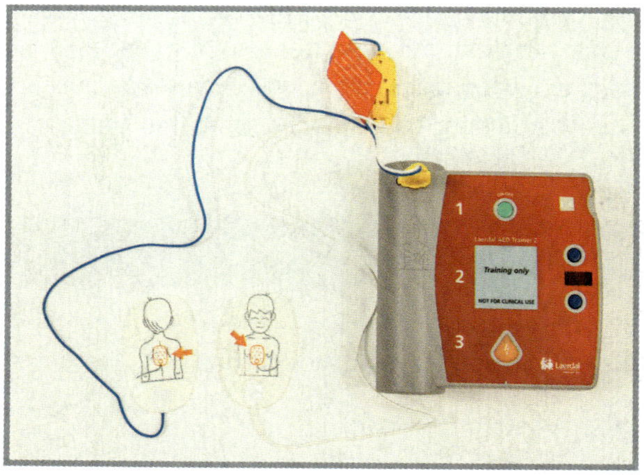

FIGURE 5–3 An AED.

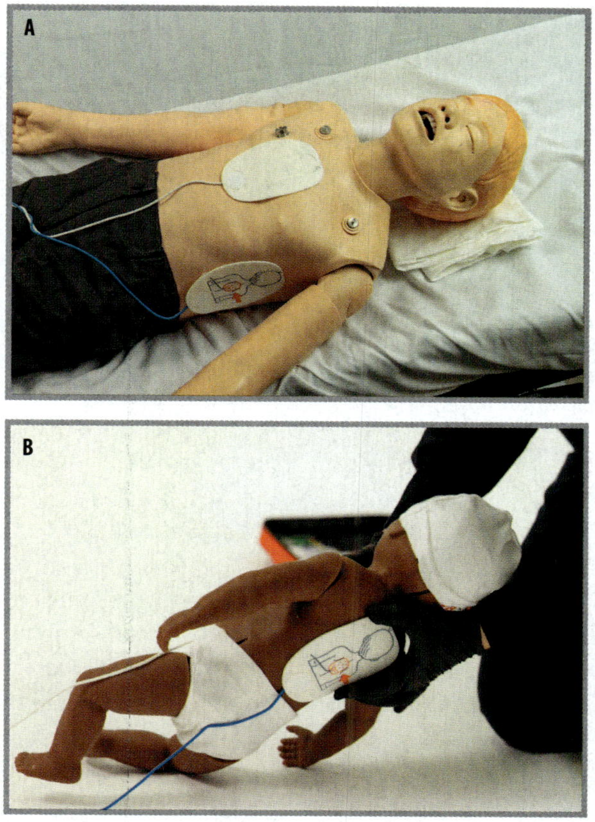

FIGURE 5–4 Using the AED on an unresponsive child in the **A.** anterolateral placement for a child and **B.** anterior–posterior position for an infant.

Studies show that even school-aged children with no experience or education in defibrillation can successfully operate an AED. **FIGURE 5–4** illustrates the use of an AED on a child and an infant.

TIP

AEDs can be used on anyone. Preferably use an AED with pediatric attenuator/cables for infants and children, but an adult AED can be used. For an unwitnessed cardiac arrest, begin CPR and use an AED as soon as it is available.

Summary of Dysrhythmias

Unlike adults, primary cardiac rhythm disturbances are rare in children. Bradycardia, a prearrest rhythm, almost always reflects profound hypoxia, and bag-mask ventilation should be initiated rapidly. Tachycardia is most commonly a sinus rhythm, but may represent SVT or VT. Although children can develop sinus tachycardia greater than 200 beats/min, perform a careful evaluation for hypovolemia

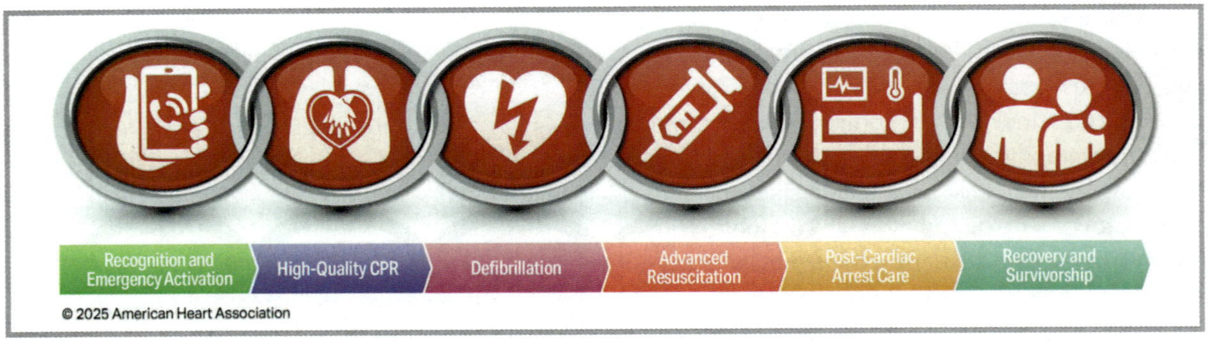

FIGURE 5–5 2025 American Heart Association cardiac arrest chain of survival. Reprinted with permission from American Heart Association. Highlights from the 2025 American Heart Association Guidelines for Cardiopulmonary Resuscitation and Emergency Cardiovascular Care. ©2025 American Heart Association, Inc. Accessed January 28, 2026. https://cpr.heart.org/-/media/CPR-Files/2025-documents-for-cpr-heart-edits-posting/Resuscitation-Science/252500_Hghlghts_2025ECCGuidelines.pdf?sc_lang=en

and hypoxia and other treatable causes, and then treat the identified causes.

Assume all rates over 220 beats/min in infants or over 180 beats/min in children and all wide complex (QRS $>$ 0.09 seconds) tachycardias are primary cardiac dysrhythmias. A patient in stable condition may need only general supportive care, regardless of cardiac rhythm. **Symptomatic ventricular dysrhythmias** may require drug therapy (with amiodarone or procainamide) and cardioversion or defibrillation. The AED is an important adjunct for EMS clinicians to use in unresponsive children with VF.

Cardiac Arrest

The emphasis for patients in cardiac arrest is based on early and excellent compressions. A single 6-link cardiac arrest chain of survival can be used for infants, children and adult (not newborns). The 6 links are recognition and emergency activation; high-quality CPR; defibrillation; advanced resuscitation; post-arrest cardiac care; and recovery and survivorship (**FIGURE 5–5**).

Survival from cardiac arrest depends on several factors, including time to CPR and the presenting rhythm. The shorter the "downtime" before basic life support (BLS) begins, the better the outcome. As in adults, pediatric EMS patients in VF are more likely to survive than are those in asystole, as long as there is early CPR and access to early defibrillation.

> **TIP**
> The only intervention associated with survival in pediatric asystolic cardiac arrest is time to onset of CPR.

CAUSES

In contrast to adults, pediatric cardiac arrest is almost always a secondary event, the result of profound hypoxia or shock. Cardiac arrest in children usually follows a primary respiratory arrest, often due to respiratory failure originating from common conditions such as pneumonia, bronchiolitis, or asthma. **Myocardial infarction** and **cardiac dysrhythmia**, frequent causes of cardiac arrest in adults, are extremely unusual in young children.

Children can experience arrest due to conditions such as HCM, which has a high incidence of sudden death and is the leading cause of cardiac death in both preadolescent and adolescent patients. Hypertrophic cardiomyopathy is a condition in which a child has profound hypertrophy of the ventricles and intraventricular septum, which causes an outflow obstruction. It also has effects on the coronary

> **CASE STUDY 2**
>
> You are volunteering as a health care professional at a local high school track meet when a 14-year-old boy collapses while running the 100-meter dash. You rush to his aid and find him apneic and pulseless. You immediately start CPR.
>
> 1. What should be the next step in your assessment/treatment of this child?
> 2. At what age is it appropriate to apply an AED to assess for VF in a child?

arteries, leading to a thickening of the lining of the artery, a narrowing in the vessel, and a decrease of flow to the myocardium.

Long QT syndrome is a congenital impairment of the electrophysiology of the heart that results in an increased risk of dysrhythmias, including bradycardia, torsade de pointes, and VF. Commotio cordis is another cause of cardiac arrest that occurs when a child is struck by a nonpenetrating object such as a baseball, hockey puck, or karate blow. The blow is most likely to be critical if it is over the center of the left ventricle. Because this results in VF and collapse, the presence of an AED is critical.

The highest incidence of cardiac arrest is in infancy, when **sudden unexpected infant death (SUID)**, infection, or child maltreatment precipitates respiratory failure. In toddlers and school-aged children, however, the causes of cardiac arrest change. In this older age group, the most likely causes are hemorrhagic shock and blunt trauma due to either vehicle-related injuries or falls.

ASSESSMENT IN CARDIAC ARREST

A child in cardiac arrest is unresponsive, apneic, and pulseless. The cardiac monitor will show a cardiac arrest rhythm: asystole, PEA, VT, or VF. Asystole is the most frequent rhythm; VF and VT are rare causes of cardiac arrest.

Asystole reflects profound hypoxia and ischemia. Pulseless electrical activity may represent a variety of ischemic, hypoxic, hypothermic, and traumatic insults. Some PEAs may arise from low-flow states with blood pressures too low to record in the prehospital setting. Ventricular fibrillation usually occurs in children older than 2 years due to a variety of conditions, including myocarditis, **congenital anomalies**, poisoning, electrocution, or hypoxia.

CHEST COMPRESSIONS

Chest compressions have become the focus of care in a patient in cardiac arrest. American Heart Association guidelines implemented the CAB (circulation–airway–breathing) sequence, which places emphasis on starting compressions more quickly and ensuring that compressions are the primary focus in a patient in cardiac arrest. Compression techniques differ for a child and an infant. For a child, 1 or 2 hands should be placed on the lower half of the sternum, the rate should be at least 100 to 120 per minute, and compression depth should be at least 2 inches (5 cm) with complete recoil (to ensure adequate preload). For an infant, as a single rescuer, the rescuer places either 2 thumbs (with hands encircling the infant's chest) or the heel of 1 hand at the nipple line and compresses at a rate of at least 100 to 120 per minute, with a depth of at least 1.5 inches (4 cm) with complete recoil. To ensure complete recoil, rescuers can visualize a sheet of paper passing between the rescuer's hand and the patient's chest between each compression. When performing 2-rescuer CPR in an infant, the 2 thumbs with hands encircling the chest technique is recommended. For the child and infant, when performing single-rescuer CPR, the ratio is 30:2 and changes to 15:2 when there are 2 rescuers. For children who have reached puberty and adolescents, use the adult compression depth of at least 5 cm (but no more than 6 cm) at a rate of 100 to 120 compressions per minute. Compression pauses for ventilation or switching compressors should be limited to no more than 10 seconds. For a step-by-step explanation of this procedure, see **FIGURE 5–6**.

Length-Based Drug Dosage

Treatment of infants and children in the prehospital setting is difficult because children of different ages require different sizes of equipment, different doses of medications, and different amounts of fluids. Length is a good index for drug dosing and equipment sizing during resuscitations (**FIGURE 5–7**). From a measured patient length, either a computerized resuscitation software program or a color-coded tape can provide correct doses and equipment sizes.

Computerized programs offer a wider range of drugs and additional safety features. For a step-by-step explanation of this procedure, see **Procedure 2, Length-Based Resuscitation Tapes**.

Presenting Cardiac Arrest Rhythm and Treatment

The top priorities in the care of a patient in cardiac arrest are circulation (emphasis on high-quality compressions), airway and breathing (bag-mask ventilation with an airway adjunct is adequate; consider endotracheal intubation or a supraglottic airway), and defibrillation (if indicated). The presenting cardiac rhythm is a major determinant of the treatment for cardiac arrest. When the child is pulseless and apneic, the treatment for asystole and PEA is the same.

BLS Health Care Professional Pediatric Cardiac Arrest Algorithm for the Single Rescuer—2025 Update

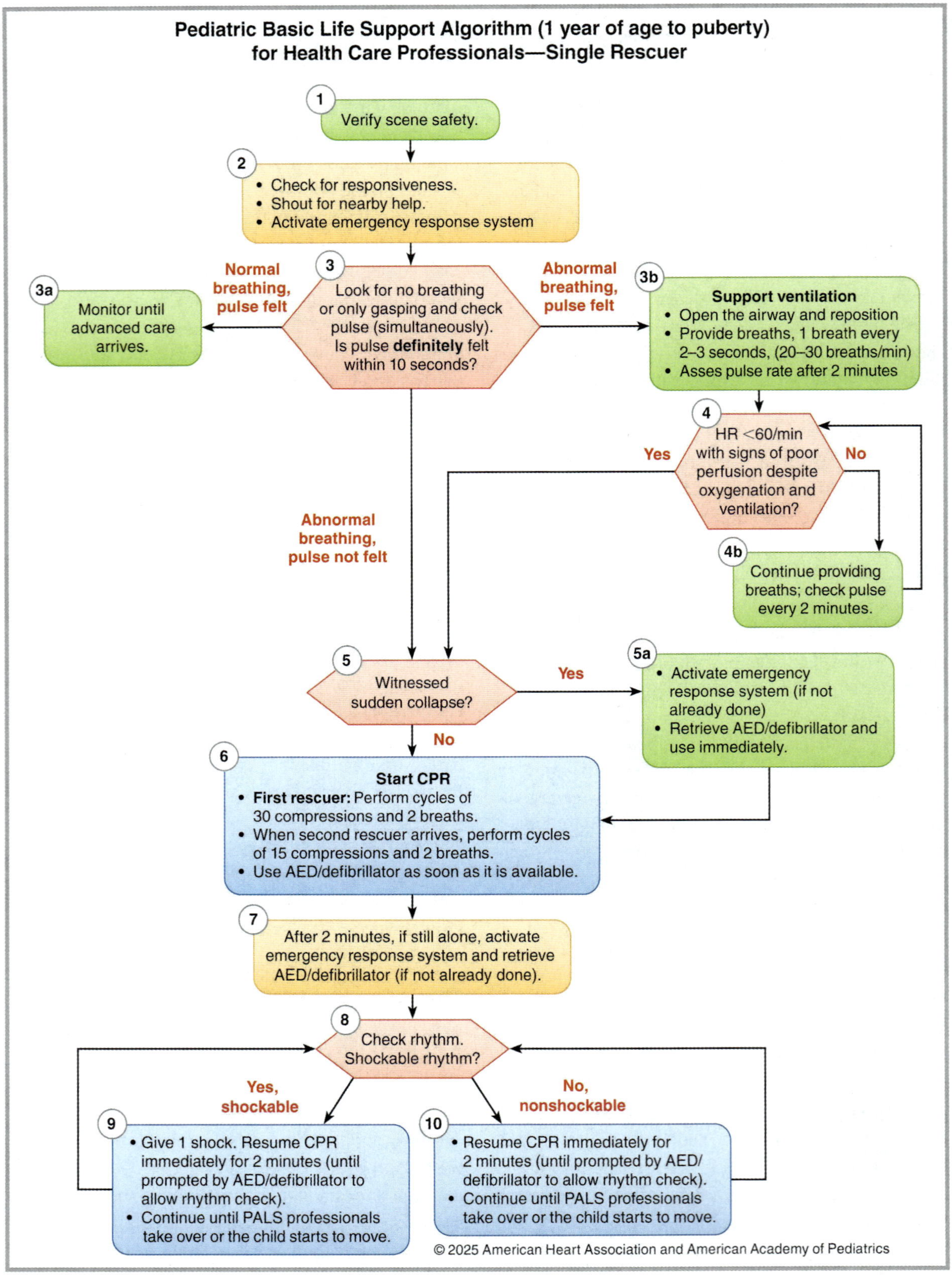

FIGURE 5–6 2025 AHA and AAP Guidelines criteria showing the pediatric BLS algorithm.

BLS Health Care Professional Pediatric Cardiac Arrest Algorithm for 2 or More Rescuers—2025 Update—Cont'd

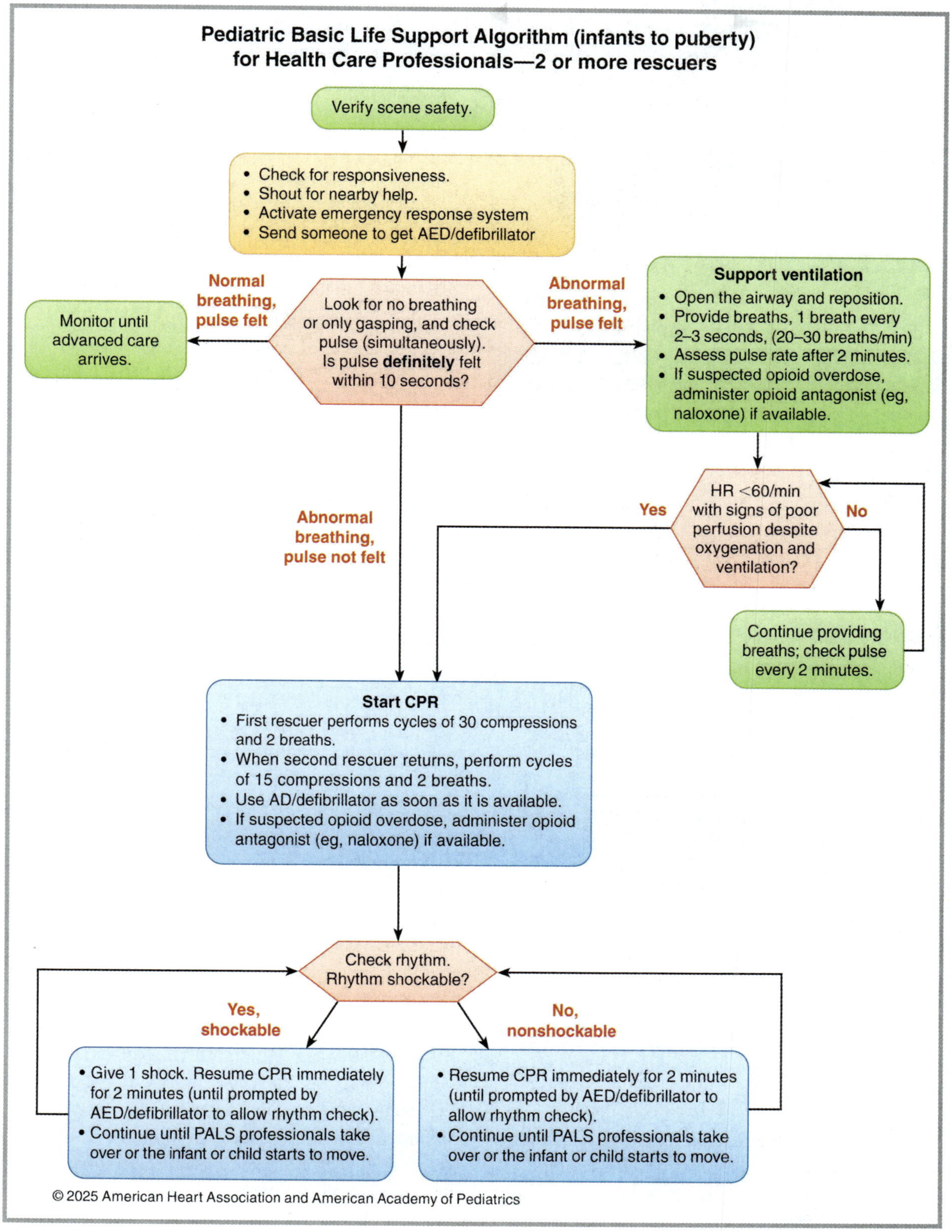

FIGURE 5-6 *(continued)*

Reproduced with permission from Lasa JJ, Dhillon GS, Duff JP, Hayes J, Kamath-Rayne BD, Levy A, Mahgoub M, Morgan RW, McCormick T, Roberts JS, Ross CE, Schexnayder SM, Sweberg T, Valdés SO, Topjian AA. Part 8: pediatric advanced life support: 2025 American Heart Association Guidelines for Cardiopulmonary Resuscitation and Emergency Cardiovascular Care. *Circulation*. 2025; 152(suppl 2):S479–S537. doi: 10.1161/CIR.0000000000001368

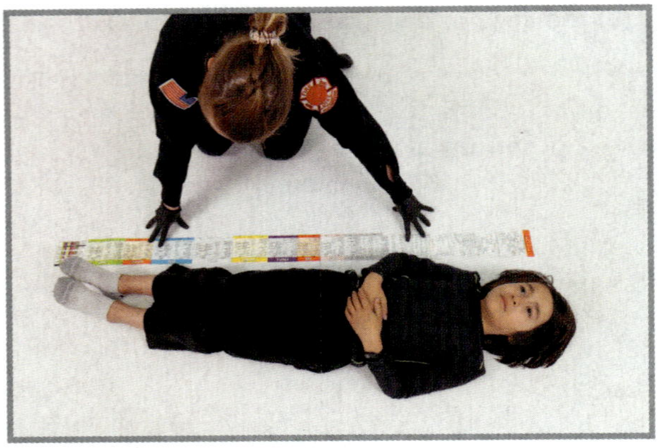

FIGURE 5-7 Resuscitation tape.

TABLE 5-5 Six Hs and Five Ts

Hypovolemia	Tension Pneumothorax
Hypoxia	Tamponade, cardiac
Hypoglycemia	Toxins
Hydrogen ion (acidosis)	Thrombosis (cardiac or pulmonary)
Hypokalemia/hyperkalemia	Trauma
Hypothermia	—

ALS

Asystole/PEA. Resuscitation efforts for nonshockable rhythms begin with high-quality CPR with an emphasis on chest compressions without interruption. Management of airway and breathing may be accomplished with assisted ventilation and an airway adjunct as the primary intervention as long as chest rise and compliance are noted. If the arrest is caused by respiratory failure, then an endotracheal tube or supraglottic airway becomes a priority. A cuffed endotracheal tube should be sized with the following equation: (age in years divided by 4) + 3.5.

Venous access can be accomplished IV or IO. All medications, fluids, and blood products administered IV can be administered IO.

Epinephrine is the drug of choice, administered at 0.01 mg/kg (0.1 mL/kg of 0.1 mg/mL concentration) IV/IO as soon as possible once asystole or PEA is recognized. High-quality BLS with adequate airway management is continued throughout the resuscitation, with pulse checks every 2 minutes and epinephrine administered every 3 to 5 minutes. Consider causes such as the 6 Hs and 5 Ts (**TABLE 5-5**).

Survival of pediatric cardiac arrest requires good BLS with high-quality compressions and ventilations (**FIGURE 5-8**). Intravenous or IO needle insertion and medication delivery are helpful, but are not primary determinants of survival. In addition, high-dose epinephrine has shown no increased survival when used in cardiac arrest. It may be considered in exceptional circumstances, such as a β-blocker overdose.

ALS

VF/Pulseless VT. VF/VT management should start with high-quality CPR while attaching the AED and identifying a shockable rhythm. The initial energy setting for the child should be at 2 J/kg, followed by 2 minutes of excellent CPR. During this time, IV access should be gained. Initial airway management should be maintained with a bag-mask device and an oropharyngeal airway as long as there is adequate chest rise and good compliance (an advanced airway may be considered further down the algorithm). When an airway is not maintainable with a bag-mask ventilation or the arrest is caused by a hypoxic event, an endotracheal tube or a supraglottic airway should be considered as soon as possible.

After 2 minutes of high-quality CPR, the patient is reassessed. If a pulse is not present, a shock is administered at 4 J/kg. The EMS clinician continues CPR, and the patient is given 0.01 mg/kg of epinephrine (0.1 mL/kg), at a 0.1 mg/mL concentration IV/IO, repeated every 3 to 5 minutes. Continued CPR is administered with pulse/rhythm checks every 2 minutes. Subsequent shocks are delivered at 4 J/kg, but can be increased to 10 J/kg, not to exceed the adult dose. Amiodarone may be administered for refractory VF/pulseless VT at 5 mg/kg, repeated up to 2 times to a total of 15 mg/kg. Lidocaine, 1 mg/kg as a loading dose with maintenance of 20 to 50 μg/kg/min by infusion, may also be given; repeat bolus if infusion is begun more than 15 minutes after the initial loading dose.

THE TRANSPORT DECISION: STAY OR GO

Deciding which pediatric patients in cardiac arrest require hospital transport is another important controversy. Of all children in out-of-hospital cardiac arrest, only 10% will survive. Predictors of survival include the type of presenting rhythm and early return of spontaneous circulation ($<$5 minutes) after BLS personnel arrive on scene. Survival of pulseless VT/VF is approximately 17%, versus about 4% for asystole. If children in cardiac arrest do not achieve return of spontaneous circulation (ROSC) with BLS and ALS care, the chance of survival is low. Regardless, initial treatment of a child in cardiac arrest should occur on scene in most cases. Patients who have ingested massive amounts of sedative-hypnotic drugs (eg, barbiturates) may have a greater chance of survival after prolonged resuscitation and deserve extended treatment before a decision to halt CPR.

In some cases, field resuscitation attempts can be stopped before transport if permitted by local EMS death-in-the-field policies. Although survival in unwitnessed out-of-hospital cardiac arrest is rare, EMS clinicians may be uncomfortable with discontinuing resuscitative efforts in children. When resuscitation is terminated, skillful communication with the child's caregivers is critical (**FIGURE 5-9**), as explained in Chapter 17. *Never leave a family member on scene*

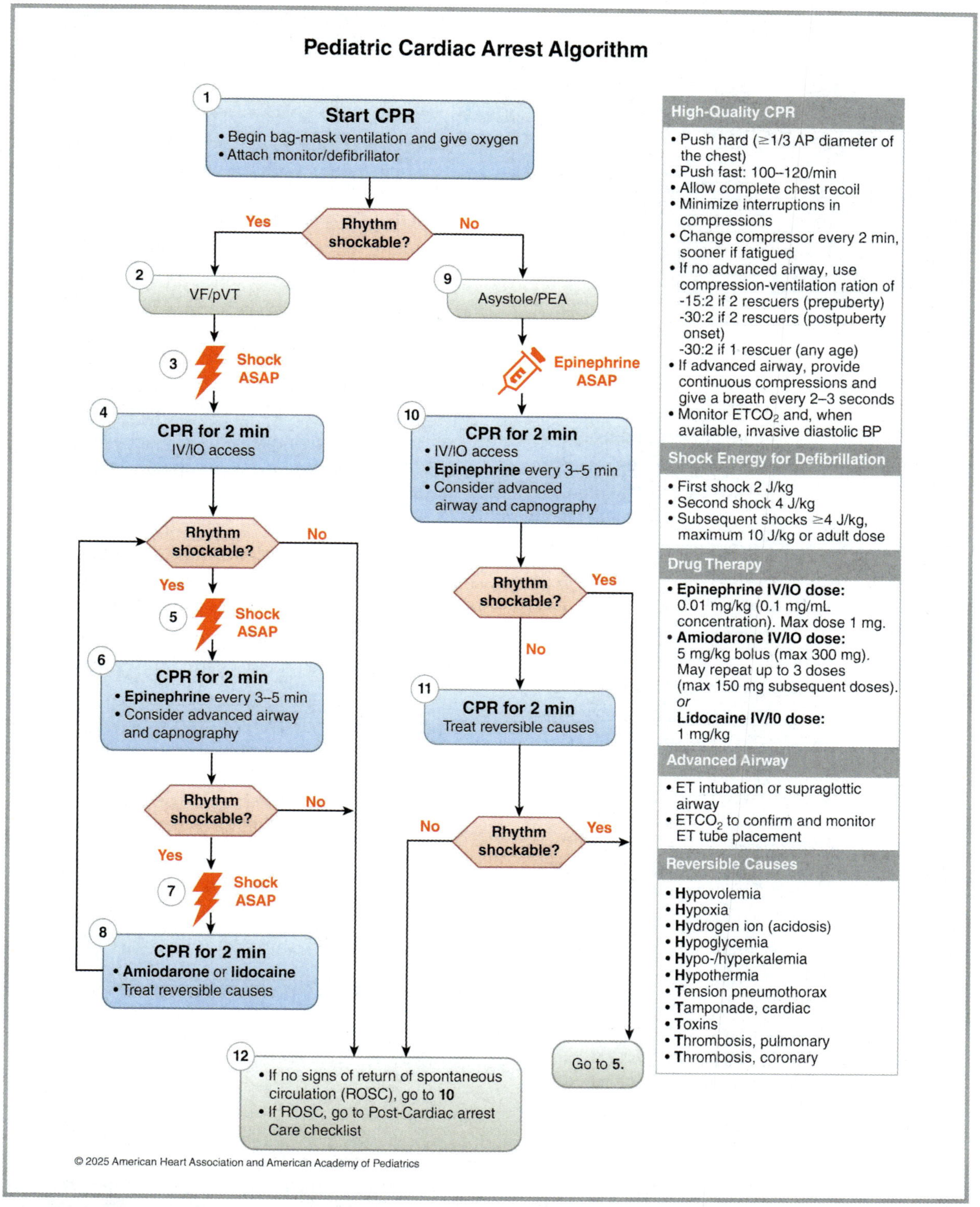

FIGURE 5–8 2025 American Heart Association and American Academy of Pediatrics guidelines criteria showing the pediatric cardiac arrest algorithm.

Reproduced with permission from Joyner BL, Dewan M, Bavare A, de Caen A, DiMaria K, Donofrio-Odmann J, Fosse G, Haskell S, Mahgoub M, Meckler G, Requist J, Schexnayder SM, Olech Smith M, Werho D, Raymond TT. Part 6: pediatric basic life support: 2025 American Heart Association and American Academy of Pediatrics Guidelines for Cardiopulmonary Resuscitation and Emergency Cardiovascular Care. *Circulation*. 2025;152(suppl2):S424–S447. doi: 10.1161/CIR.0000000000001370

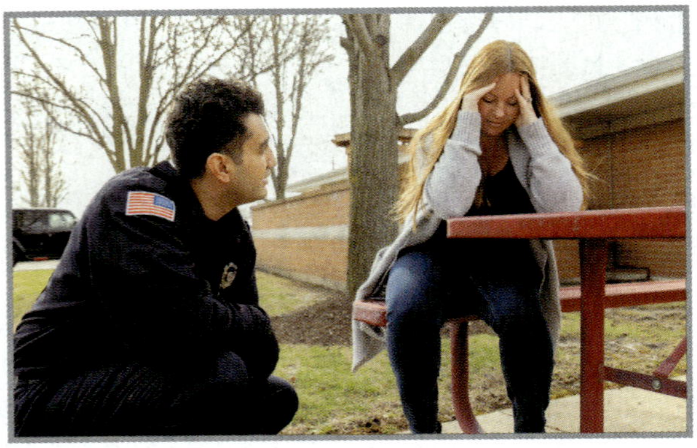

FIGURE 5–9 Skilled communication with the caregivers and family is imperative after the death of a child.

CAUTION
Never leave a family member on scene with a deceased child without appropriate supportive care.

with the deceased child without appropriate supportive personnel. A system to provide supportive care to the caregivers must be in place if EMS policy permits discontinuation of resuscitative efforts in the field. These services might be provided by social services personnel, pastoral care personnel, or grief counselors.

Cardiac arrest in children is associated with high provider stress. Critical incident stress debriefing may be helpful for EMS clinicians after such a tragedy.

TIP
Out-of-hospital cardiac arrest treatment requires good BLS skills.

Summary of Cardiac Arrest

Pediatric cardiac arrest is an uncommon event. Out-of-hospital arrest survival is low, and asystole is associated with the worst prognosis. Ventricular tachycardia or fibrillation usually occurs in older children and is associated with higher survival rates. Meticulous attention to chest compressions, airway, oxygenation, ventilation, and early defibrillation, when appropriate, will improve success. In all cases of pediatric cardiac arrest, grief counseling for the caregivers and critical incident stress debriefing for the EMS clinicians are extremely helpful.

Congenital Heart Disease

Children with congenital heart disease are at increased risk of experiencing the types of cardiovascular emergencies more commonly seen in the adult population, including dysrhythmias and congestive heart failure. These complications may present in infancy or as late as the teenage years. Advances in cardiovascular surgery have allowed the medical community to prolong the lives of children who, just decades ago, would have died in infancy. Many of these children are now living productive lives at home. EMS clinicians must be prepared to treat "adult problems" in this younger population.

The primary assessment and management of any child experiencing a cardiovascular emergency are the same: airway, breathing, and circulation. However, in any child with a possible cardiac pathology, include a "quick look" at the cardiac rhythm. These children may have treatable cardiac dysrhythmias.

Drowning

Drowning is suffocation after submersion in water. Drowning is the second leading cause of death due to unintentional injury in children younger than 9 years. Unfortunately, drowning is not limited to the summer months. In warmer climates, it occurs year-round, and in cooler climates it may occur as a result of submersion in lakes, buckets, hot tubs, and bathtubs (**FIGURE 5–10**).

PREVENTION

The best management of near-drowning is prevention. The installation of 4-sided locked fencing around swimming pools prevents up to 90% of childhood residential swimming pool drownings and

CASE STUDY 3

You are dispatched to the location of an unresponsive 2-year-old boy recently removed from a swimming pool. Estimated downtime is unknown, but the parents are on scene and state that the child had been missing for more than 30 minutes. The parents initiated CPR immediately. On arrival, you find the child to be cool, blue, apneic, and pulseless.

1. What is the most important intervention for this patient to improve his chances of survival?
2. Should the child be actively rewarmed?

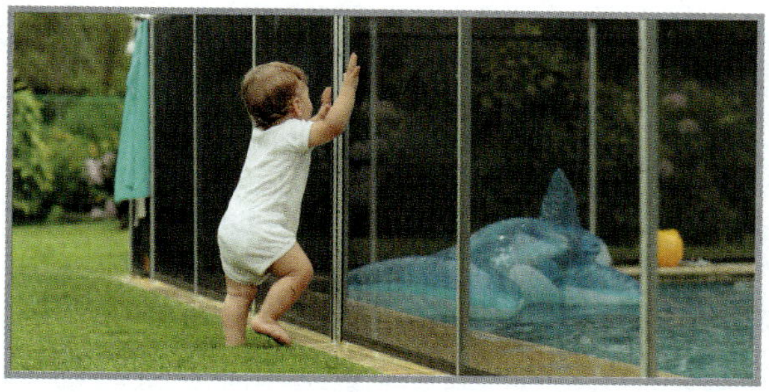

FIGURE 5–10 Drowning is the second leading cause of death due to unintentional injury among children aged 1–14 years. Installing four-sided isolation fencing around residential swimming pools is one of the most effective strategies to prevent childhood drowning.

Bricolage/Shuttershock.com

near-drownings. Eighty-five percent of boating-related drownings are preventable by wearing personal flotation devices. Other prevention methods include the following: wearing approved life jackets, providing swimming lessons for children, swimming where there are lifeguards, and close and active supervision of children in and around water.

TREATMENT

Early recognition of cardiac arrest and immediate CPR provided by bystanders have an important association with survival from severe submersion injuries. Advanced life support care has an unproven benefit.

If appropriately trained, provide in-water rescue breathing to an unresponsive child if it does not compromise the rescuer's safety.

Remove the patient from the water, if safe to do so, and quickly assess for responsiveness, breathing, and pulse. Because cardiac arrest in drowning is likely due to a severe hypoxemic mechanism, it is reasonable to initiate CPR with rescue breathing, then chest compressions by trained rescuers. It is also important to provide supplemental oxygen if available. On the other hand, lay rescuers can provide chest compressions, then rescue breaths. If they are unwilling, untrained, or unable to provide rescue breaths, provide chest compressions only until help arrives. Obtain an AED and wipe water from the child's chest before applying the pads. Protect the cervical spine if there is potential head or neck trauma. Perform chest compressions, airway management, oxygenation, and ventilation, and follow protocols for drug therapy and defibrillation/cardioversion depending on the presenting cardiac rhythm.

If the child has a pulse, open the airway and ensure appropriate oxygenation and ventilation, usually with a bag-mask device. Obtain IV or IO access and transport. Provide drug therapy, and rarely defibrillation/cardioversion, as indicated for shock or dysrhythmias.

CASE STUDY ANSWERS

CASE STUDY 1

This child could be experiencing VF/pulseless VT, PEA, or asystole. He is in cardiac arrest, and the appropriate first intervention is to provide excellent CPR and BLS care. Treatment for the patient will be based on the type of arrhythmia. It is likely that he suffered commotio cordis, which is ventricular fibrillation due to a blow to the chest.

The AED determined that the rhythm is VF, so delivering a shock is advised. After 1 shock, there is ROSC and the patient is transported to the hospital and admitted for observation.

CASE STUDY 2

This cardiac arrest appears to reflect a primary cardiac event. Begin 30 chest compressions to 2 ventilations and have 1 EMS clinician retrieve an AED. When the AED arrives, attach the pads and let it analyze the rhythm. If the AED indicates shock advised, deliver a shock and resume CPR for 2 minutes, then reanalyze the rhythm. If shockable, deliver a shock and resume CPR.

This child was in VF as a result of a previously undiagnosed disorder known as prolonged QT syndrome. Survivors of this disease often report a history of blackouts associated with exercise and stress. Other family members may also be affected by this disorder. A look back at the family history can uncover unexplained deaths of relatives at young ages.

The initial treatment for children in VF, as in adults, is rapid defibrillation. With the increasing availability of AEDs, many of these children will receive rapid recognition and defibrillation by bystanders.

The patient is transported to the hospital and admitted.

Continued

CASE STUDY ANSWERS—cont'd

CASE STUDY 3

After the child is removed from the water, begin CPR, starting with rescue breathing, then chest compressions, then provide bag-mask ventilation with 100% oxygen. Rushing to intubate this child, before providing effective bag-mask ventilation with 100% oxygen, may result in worsened hypoxia and hypercarbia. Most drownings cause airway spasm with little or no water entering the lungs, so bag-mask ventilations may be effective. The best anatomical location for palpating a pulse in a 2-year-old child is over the brachial artery, which is located just proximal to the elbow and medially to the biceps muscle.

Although there have been promising results in adult studies of hypothermia after cardiac arrest, pediatric studies have found no benefit. The hypothermic state may be protective of brain function, and rapid rewarming can introduce dysrhythmias. Therefore, remove wet clothing and provide rapid transport.

In the ED, the child is still in cardiac arrest, so receives continued CPR with 3 rounds of epinephrine and is intubated. Unfortunately, there is no ROSC, so the resuscitation is terminated after 20 minutes.

Suggested References

TEXTBOOKS

American Academy of Pediatrics. *Pediatric Education for Prehospital Professionals.* 4th ed revised. Fuchs S, McEvoy M, eds. Jones & Bartlett Learning; 2021

Horeczko T. Pediatric cardiac disorders. In: Walls RM, Hockberger RS, Gausche-Hill M, Erickson TM, eds. *Rosen's Emergency Medicine: Concepts and Clinical Practice.* 10th ed. Elsevier; 2023:2109–2131

ARTICLES

Del Rios M, Bartos JA, Panchal AR, Atkins DL, Cabanas JG, Cao D, Dainty KN, Dezfulian C, Donoghue AJ, Drennan IR, Elmer J, Hirsch KG, Idris AH, Joyner BL, Kamath-Rayne BD, Kleinman ME, Kurz MC, Lasa JJ, Lee HC, McBride ME, Raymond TT, Rittenberger, JC, Schexnayder SM, Szyld E, Topjian A, Wigginton JG, Previdi JK. Part 1: executive summary: 2025 American Heart Association Guidelines for Cardiopulmonary Resuscitation and Emergency Cardiovascular Care. *Circulation*. 2025;152(suppl): S284–S312. doi: 10.1161/CIR.0000000000001372

Fink EL, Prince DK, Kaltman JR, et al. Unchanged pediatric out-of-hospital cardiac arrest incidence and survival rates with regional variation in North America. *Resuscitation*. 2016;107:121–128.

Joyner BL, Dewan M, Bavare A, de Caen A, DiMaria K, Donofrio-Odmann J, Fosse G, Haskell S, Mahgoub M, Meckler G, Requist J, Schexnayder SM, Olech Smith M, Werho D, Raymond TT. Part 6: pediatric basic life support: 2025 American Heart Association and American Academy of Pediatrics Guidelines for Cardiopulmonary Resuscitation and Emergency Cardiovascular Care. Circulation. 2025;152(suppl2):S424–S447. doi: 10.1161/CIR.0000000000001370

Lasa JJ, Dhillon GS, Duff JP, et al. Part 8: Pediatric Advanced Life Support: 2025 American Heart Association and American Academy of Pediatrics Guidelines for Cardiopulmonary Resuscitation and Emergency Cardiovascular Care. Pediatrics. 2025; doi: 10.1542/peds.2025-074351.

McCallin TE, Dezfulian C, Bierens J, et al. 2024 American Heart Association and Academy of Pediatrics focused update on special circumstances: resuscitation following drowning: an update to the American Heart Association guidelines for cardiopulmonary resuscitation and emergency cardiovascular care. *Pediatrics*. 2024;154(6):e2024068444. PMID: 39530213 doi: 10.1542/peds.2024-068444

OTHER RESOURCES

Miyake CY. *Pediatric hypertrophic cardiomyopathy*. Accessed February 12, 2025. https://emedicine.medscape.com/article/189068-overview

Raghavan SS. Pediatric long QT syndrome. Accessed February 12, 2025. https://emedicine.medscape.com/article/891571-overview

Yabek SM. Commotio cordis. Accessed February 12, 2025. http://emedicine.medscape.com/article/902504-overview.

CHAPTER 6

Neurological Emergencies

Theresa Censoplano, MS, RN, NRP
Karen J. O'Connell, MD, MEd, FAAP

LEARNING OBJECTIVES

1. **Describe the major types of seizures, as well as the 2025 seizure classification and the management priorities for each.**
2. **Compare the advantages and disadvantages of various first-line and second-line medications and their routes of administration in status epilepticus.**
3. **Distinguish the common causes of altered mental status (AMS) in infants and children and outline management priorities.**
4. **Explain assessment of a child with AMS.**
5. **Discuss treatment of a child with AMS.**

Seizures

Seizures are caused by abnormal, sustained electrical discharges from a cluster of nerve cells in the brain. Seizures have varied presentations, depending on the location of the abnormal electrical activity in the brain and the age of the child. Seizures in the infant (0–12 months of age), whose central nervous system (CNS) is immature, can be very subtle, consisting only of abnormal gaze, focal motor activity, horizontal nystagmus, sustained muscle contractions, sucking motions, or "bicycling" (pedaling movements of the legs). In the older child, who has a more mature CNS, seizures are usually more obvious and typically manifest as repetitive muscular contractions (**tonic-clonic** activity) and/or unresponsiveness. Sustained or repetitive muscular contractions may be associated with upper-airway obstruction, resulting in poor air exchange, hypercarbia, and hypoxia. As a result, cyanosis is common.

NEW CLASSIFICATION OF SEIZURES

In 2025, the International League Against Epilepsy (ILAE) upgraded their classification of seizure types originally published in 2017. The 2017 classifications were based on presentation at onset and the 2025 revisions reflected implementation experience. The prior classification system, which had been used since 1981, did not reflect the inclusion of specific types of focal motor seizures and generalized seizures such as myoclonic-tonic-clonic or myoclonic-atonic. There was also no way to correctly categorize seizures with unknown onset. Obscure terminology was also used and could be confusing to those unfamiliar with the vocabulary. The expanded classification system, which reflects the signs and symptoms of seizure onset, is represented in **FIGURE 6–1**. The qualifiers for seizure onset are focal, generalized, or unknown. Focal seizures involve only one region of the brain, whereas generalized seizure onsets involve both hemispheres.

The next qualifier in focal seizures is level of consciousness or awareness. Focal seizures with awareness levels lend significance to how the seizure may influence the individual. The term "simple partial seizure and complex partial seizure" has now been replaced with the terms "focal aware seizure" and "focal impaired awareness seizure" (in which one is unaware of one's surroundings), respectively. Focal seizures affect only one hemisphere of the brain (and one part of the body), but may be nonconvulsive with only a loss of attention or eye blinking (absence or petit mal seizure). Focal seizures are classified according to whether consciousness is maintained. Focal seizures with no loss of consciousness are known as focal aware seizures; those associated with a loss of consciousness are known as focal impaired awareness seizures. Focal seizures are further subdivided according to the first sign or symptom, such as motor activity (can be **focal** and then either

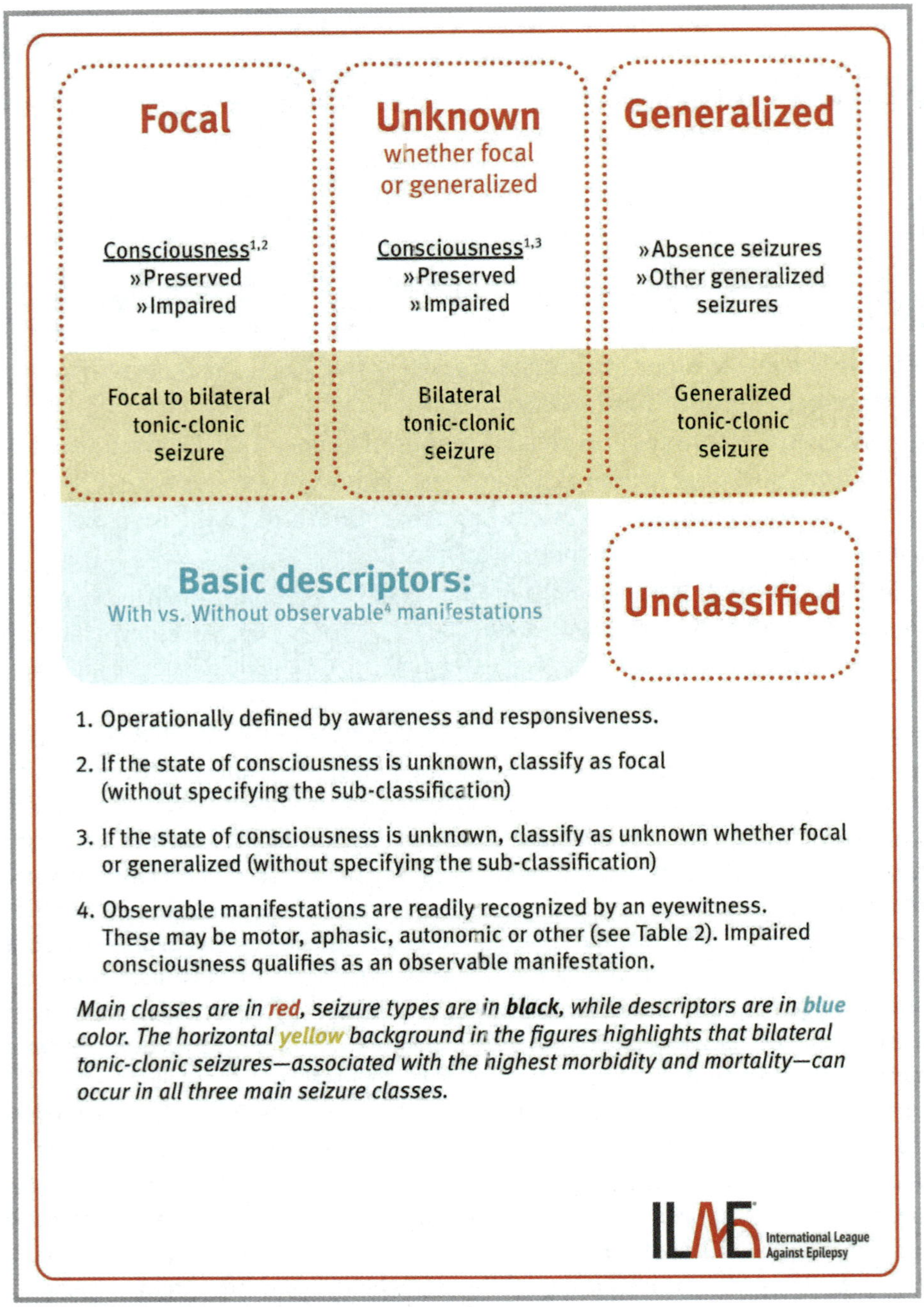

FIGURE 6–1 International League Against Epilepsy Basic 2025 Seizure Classification

generalize or spread to involve adjacent brain regions), sensory impairment (paresthesias, vertigo, visual or auditory symptoms), or autonomic changes (sweating, pupillary changes). Focal seizures can be further classified according to the presentation of motor symptoms. These seizures are divided into motor (with motor activity, such as tonic-clonic movements) and nonmotor (without motor activity, such as an absence seizure). During a focal impaired awareness seizure, the child may exhibit motor automatisms, such as chewing movements or bicycling movements of the legs.

Generalized seizures by definition include impaired awareness. Generalized seizures do not always involve abnormal muscle jerking, aka clonic activity, and are specifically categorized on the basis of motor features. Specific categories of generalized motor seizures include tonic-clonic, clonic, tonic, myoclonic, myotonic-tonic-clonic, myoclonic-atonic, atonic, and epileptic spasms.

CASE STUDY 1

You receive a call for a 2-year-old boy who was playing in the living room of his home when he began having a seizure, with jerking of his arms and legs that lasted for 10 to 15 minutes. On arrival at the scene, you find a child who has a decreased level of consciousness, responding only to painful stimuli. Lung sounds, work of breathing, and skin color are within normal limits. His respiratory rate is 12 breaths/min, his heart rate is 100 beats/min, his blood pressure is 90/58 mm Hg, and his oxygen saturation in room air is 92%. There are no focal neurological findings , nor is there any current seizure activity. The child's temperature is 38.6 °C (101.5 °F). His father tells you his son has had febrile seizures previously. He also says that because the seizure lasted so long, he gave his son rectal diazepam, as prescribed by his neurologist.

1. What other information would you want about this seizure and the child's medical history?
2. How should you treat this patient?
3. Should the child be transported?

Seizure onset is classified as unknown if the patient experiences an alteration in awareness or if the onset of the seizure is not witnessed. Such unknown whether focal or generalized seizures may later be grouped into focal or generalized categories when more information is obtained. It also may be impossible to determine the type of seizure at onset if information is lacking. To that end, the seizure may be characterized as unclassified.

There are also epilepsy syndromes, and affected infants and children may demonstrate a variety of seizure types. The term **epilepsy** refers to a chronic disorder that causes recurrent and unprovoked seizures over time, with or without a known underlying cause. Although caregivers of children with epilepsy may be very calm at the scene of a 911 call, those who are witnessing a seizure for the first time can be very frightened, may fear that the child is dying, and may have initiated cardiopulmonary resuscitation efforts. **Neonatal seizures** tend to be more subtle, because tonic-clonic activity may not occur during the first month of life. Deviated gaze or horizontal nystagmus and myoclonic seizures (a sudden, single muscle jerk) may be the only evidence of seizures in infants.

FEBRILE SEIZURES

The most frequent type of seizure in childhood is the febrile seizure. Approximately 5% of all children have at least 1 febrile seizure by 6 years of age, and more than one-half of these children never have another seizure. By definition, a **simple febrile seizure** is a generalized, tonic-clonic seizure of less than than 15 minutes' duration. It typically occurs in a febrile child who is between 6 months and 5 years of age and has no underlying neurological abnormalities, and it occurs only once in 24 hours. Simple febrile seizures do not cause brain injury, even if the child has more than one. Most simple febrile seizures stop spontaneously before the arrival of prehospital professionals. Risk factors for recurrence include age younger than 1 year at the time of the first febrile seizure, a family history of febrile seizure, or a seizure of complex nature.

Complex febrile seizures are those in which fever is present in an otherwise neurologically healthy child and which last longer than 15 minutes, are focal rather than generalized, and occur more than once in 24 hours. The presence of the additional findings changes the febrile seizure from simple to complex. This type of seizure has a higher association with serious illness. Most febrile seizures in children involve fevers of relatively benign etiology (otitis media, viral syndrome). Many febrile seizures occur with temperatures higher than 38.9 °C (102 °F), usually on the first day the child becomes febrile. Although there may be a brief postictal period, these children generally experience an improving level of consciousness and appear to be well. Children with fevers of more serious origins (meningitis) usually appear ill after the seizure resolves or may have associated symptoms (petechiae, neck stiffness). A child who has a seizure and a fever may not necessarily have had a febrile seizure and requires physician evaluation to exclude a serious disease such as meningitis, encephalitis, or sepsis. *A prehospital professional cannot make a diagnosis of a febrile seizure.*

CAUTION
A prehospital professional cannot make a diagnosis of a febrile seizure.

TIP

If the child begins to have another seizure, ensure airway, breathing, and circulation (the ABCs). If the seizure does not stop in 5 minutes, begin medication administration.

OTHER SEIZURE CAUSES

Although childhood seizures are frequently associated with fever, there are many other possible causes of seizures. These include trauma, especially head injury (accidental vs nonaccidental); metabolic derangements (hypoglycemia, hyperglycemia, hypocalcemia, hyponatremia, hypernatremia), neurological conditions (cerebral edema, brain tumor, intracranial hemorrhage, hemorrhagic or ischemic stroke), anoxic injury (cardiac arrest, carbon monoxide poisoning, profound shock, abuse, suffocation), poisoning (alcohol/drug of abuse, toxins), inborn errors of metabolism, epilepsy syndromes, and psychiatric causes (psychogenic nonepileptic seizures) There have been some cases of afebrile seizures attributed to COVID-19 , as well. **Afebrile seizures** are commonly seen in children with known epilepsy who have not received therapeutic doses of their anticonvulsant medication and experience breakthrough seizures. In addition, there is a sizeable group of children who have breakthrough seizures despite medication compliance; in this group, parents often call 911 when normal methods of controlling seizure activity are unsuccessful.

TIP

A seizure with a fever is not the same as a febrile seizure.

STATUS EPILEPTICUS

The classic definition of **status epilepticus** is either a series of 2 or more seizures without recovery of consciousness between the seizures, or a continuous seizure more than 20 minutes long. A newer "operational" definition of status epilepticus was developed in the late 1990s by a group of neurologists specializing in seizure management. On the basis of data indicating that most seizures stop spontaneously in less than 5 minutes, they redefined the term "status epilepticus" and set a threshold for initiating pharmacologic treatment as a seizure lasting longer than 5 minutes. Accordingly, any child who is actively seizing on the prehospital professional's arrival should be considered to be in status epilepticus, and the clinician should administer drug therapy to stop the seizure. Such patients inevitably have been seizing for at least 15 minutes, given the average response times in most emergency medical services (EMS) systems.

Status epilepticus may occur as the child's first seizure. The age of the child in status epilepticus helps identify the likely cause of the seizure. Children younger than 3 years tend to have acute, sometimes progressive causes of status epilepticus, such as hypoxia, infection, or toxic ingestion. Status epilepticus in children older than 3 years who tends to have chronic, static causes (eg, epilepsy, neurological disorder, an inborn metabolic disorder, or inadequate anticonvulsant treatment). Therefore, be especially vigilant in the care of infants and young children with status epilepticus, especially if they do not have a history of fever or epilepsy.

Status epilepticus is a medical emergency. Prompt treatment in the field is critical, because prolonged seizure activity is difficult to control pharmacologically. Stopping the seizure also facilitates airway management, support of oxygenation and ventilation, and transport. However, the risk of long-term neurological injury is most closely associated with the underlying cause and associated complications (hypercarbia, hypoxia). There are competing data on the impact of the duration of the seizure on neurological outcomes.

TIP

During status epilepticus, the risk of brain injury is most closely related to the cause of the seizure.

CONTROVERSY

When to treat a seizure is a matter of debate. Although many seizures stop spontaneously and do not need any treatment, some untreated children progress to the dangerous condition of status epilepticus. The best practical approach if the child is seizing on arrival is to treat them.

COMPLICATIONS

Seizures may cause hypoxia via airway obstruction, aspiration, or inadequate respiratory drive. Good prehospital management minimizes these complications. A second concern is brain injury caused by prolonged seizure activity in a child with a serious underlying condition, such as infection, overdose (including toxic exposures), hemorrhage, or congenital neurological problems. Children have fewer energy reserves than adults, and active seizure activity uses those reserves. Hypoglycemia can cause and/or prolong seizure activity.

Supporting airway and breathing, controlling seizure activity, diagnosing and subsequently treating hypoglycemia, and rapidly transporting the child to a facility with pediatric intensive care capability are the best strategies to minimize morbidity in this population of critically ill children.

TIP

Be especially vigilant in the care of infants and young children with status epilepticus if they do not have a history of fever or epilepsy.

Assessment and Treatment of the Actively Seizing Child

If a child is actively seizing when prehospital professionals arrive, there are several essential steps:

1. *Open the airway.*

   Managing the airway is the most important initial action (**TABLE 6–1**).

   Consider spinal motion restriction as part of airway management in a patient experiencing a posttraumatic seizure, although it is unlikely to be effective until the seizure activity has stopped. Padding under the child's head also helps protect against injury (**FIGURE 6–2**).

ALS

Positioning is the easiest method to maintain a clear airway in a young child. For an infant, toddler, or preschool-aged child, perform the chin lift or jaw thrust. If there are copious secretions, open the airway while placing the child in the lateral decubitus position (recovery position) (FIGURE 6–3). Suction secretions from the mouth, if possible. The insertion of a nasopharyngeal airway is the most useful tool after performing a chin lift or jaw thrust, because it provides an open airway around clenched teeth. Although an oropharyngeal airway can also be used, it is more difficult to insert if the teeth are clenched and may cause vomiting if the patient has a gag reflex.

Without the use of neuromuscular blockade agents, successful endotracheal intubation during a seizure is extremely difficult, and complication rates are high. *Do not attempt to intubate a seizing child.* If the airway cannot be maintained, attempt to stop the seizure through the administration of anticonvulsant medications. After the seizure is stopped, perform airway management as needed.

2. *Ensure adequate breathing.*

   Many seizures are associated with some degree of hypoventilation. Attempt to assist ventilation if the child has cyanosis or an oxygen saturation less than 90% on supplemental oxygen. Be

TABLE 6–1 Initial Airway Management in Seizing Children

Position the head to open the airway.
Clear the mouth with suction.
Consider the lateral decubitus position if the child is actively vomiting and suction is inadequate to control the airway.
Assess oxygenation and ventilation via bag-valve-mask device, continuous pulse oximetry, and end-tidal carbon dioxide monitoring, if available.
Give oxygen via nasal cannula/mask, as needed.
Consider a nasopharyngeal airway to relieve upper airway obstruction, especially if the teeth are clenched.

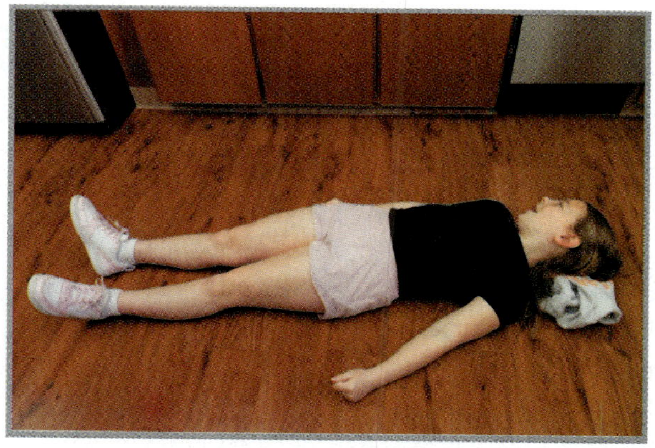

FIGURE 6–2 Padding under the child's head helps protect against injury.

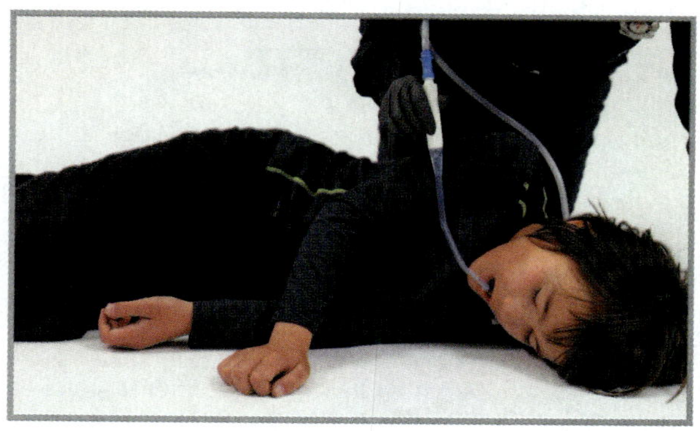

FIGURE 6–3 Position the head to open the airway, place the child in the lateral decubitus position, and clear the mouth of vomitus with suction.

CONTROVERSY

The best position in which to place the child during a seizure is controversial. A supine position may increase the risk of aspiration, but it allows easy airway and respiratory management. The lateral decubitus position provides some protection against aspiration but makes it more difficult to administer oxygen and assist breathing.

aware, however, that it is difficult to obtain an accurate pulse oximetry reading in a child who is having a seizure. Again, stopping the seizure is the key to successful ventilation. Opening the airway, coordinating ventilations with the patient's spontaneous respiratory effort, and expanding a rigid chest wall are technically difficult procedures to attempt during a generalized seizure. Often, the result of **assisted ventilation** is stomach inflation with air; therefore, advanced life support (ALS) clinicians should consider using a nasogastric tube to decompress the stomach if bag-mask ventilation visibly distends the abdomen. Importantly, ventilation effectiveness should be assessed via end-tidal carbon dioxide ($EtCO_2$) monitoring.

3. *Safeguard circulation.*
   Unless a child has seizures associated with sepsis or trauma, fluid resuscitation is generally not needed in the field or in transport. Signs of poor perfusion are most likely associated with prolonged seizure activity and related hypoxia. Once again, promptly treating the seizure would address these issues.
4. *Manage any disability.*
   Check the bedside glucose level and treat documented hypoglycemia, as described in **TABLE 6–2**.

ALS

Although most seizures stop before prehospital professionals arrive, the child who is still actively seizing should benefit from pharmacologic treatment. Consider options for anticonvulsant administration, in terms of medications approved by the EMS system and available routes of administration. The goal is to quickly stop the seizure while minimizing medication side effects. Research has shown that failure to adhere to treatment guidelines before transport was associated with admission to a higher level of care and longer hospitalizations. Guideline nonadherence often involves administering too many individual doses of underdosed first-line antiseizure medications. The longer status epilepticus continues, the higher the risk of requiring more aggressive interventions—hence the importance of administering adequate doses of antiepileptic medications.

Benzodiazepine drugs are excellent first-line anticonvulsants. Common drugs in this class are midazolam, lorazepam, and diazepam. TABLE 6–3 provides doses and routes of administration.

Although benzodiazepines all have the same mechanism of action, the time to peak effect and the duration of action vary with the specific agent used and its route of administration.

TABLE 6–2 Dextrose[a] Administration Guidelines During Seizures

Indications
▪ Infant or child with glucose level <60 mg/dL
▪ Newborn with glucose level <40 mg/dL
Treatment
▪ Newborn: babies: Dextrose 10% 2 mL/kg administered IV or IO
▪ Neonates, infants and children <2 years: Dextrose 10% 5 mL/kg administered IV or IO
▪ Children ≥2 years: Dextrose 10% 2 mL/kg or dextrose 10% 1 mL/kg administered IV or IO

[a]If the described forms of concentrated dextrose are not available, 5 mL/kg of dextrose 10% IV solution may be drawn up and given by syringe.
Abbreviations: IO, intraosseous; IV, intravenous.

ALS

Midazolam. Midazolam is another benzodiazepine that can be given to a patient without IV access and is a potent anticonvulsant, with a fast onset of action. Midazolam can be administered intramuscularly (IM) at a dose of 0.15 mg/kg. Because of its water solubility, midazolam is rapidly absorbed from the injection site and has excellent local tolerability. The pharmacodynamic effects of midazolam can be seen within minutes of its administration, and the seizure usually stops within 10 minutes. Although the onset of action of IM midazolam is delayed compared with that of intravenous (IV) diazepam, the overall time to cessation of seizure activity may be less considering the time and complexity of obtaining IV access in a seizing child. Midazolam can also be administered via IV and intraosseous (IO) routes (the dose is 0.1 mg/kg) and will work intranasally (IN). The IN dose is 0.2 mg/kg (maximum, 10 mg/dose), best administered via a nasal mucosal atomizer (FIGURE 6–4). The buccal route actually may be the best route for midazolam administration due to its rapid absorption, but it is not commonly used in the United States. Midazolam has been shown to be associated with minimal respiratory compromise in prehospital pediatric patients when administered via either IV or IM routes.

When administering any benzodiazepine by any route, watch closely for respiratory depression, a common side effect of this class of drugs, and be prepared to provide bag-valve-mask ventilatory support. Even in the case of apnea after benzodiazepine administration, a bag-valve-mask device usually suffices, because the respiratory-depressant effects of the drugs are transient. Endotracheal intubation is rarely necessary in such a case.

Lorazepam. Of the benzodiazepines, lorazepam (0.1 mg/kg; maximum, 4 mg/dose) probably has the best pharmacologic profile for seizure management. It has a rapid onset of action, can be administered IV

TABLE 6–3 Benzodiazepine Administration During Seizures

Generic Name	Initial Dose	Route	Pros	Cons
Diazepam	0.1–0.3 mg/kg	IV, IO	Rapid onset Inexpensive No refrigeration required	Sedating Respiratory depression Short duration of action for seizure control (15 minutes)
Diazepam	0.5 mg/kg	PR	Rapid onset No IV access required	Sedating Respiratory depression
Lorazepam	0.05–0.1 mg/kg	IV, IO	Rapid onset Long duration of action for seizure control (12–24 hours)	Must be stored away from heat and extreme temperature
Midazolam	0.1 mg/kg 0.15 mg/kg 0.2 mg/kg	IV/IO IM IN	Rapid onset	Medium duration of action for seizure control (30–120 minutes)

Abbreviations:IM, intramuscular; IN, intranasal; IO, intraosseous; IV, intravenous; PR, per rectum.

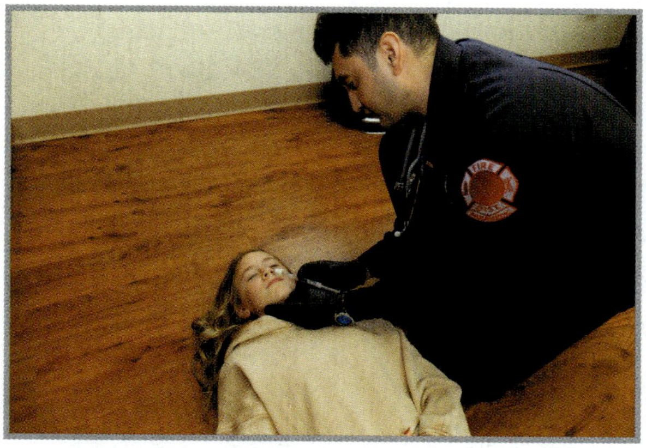

FIGURE 6–4 Administration of internasal midazolam.

or IO, and has a long half-life. Lorazepam is used to stop a seizure and can help to prevent further seizure activity for up to 8 hours, depending on the dose. There is little experience with prehospital rectal lorazepam administration in children, and doses are not well established. In general, this drug has not been widely used by prehospital professionals because of the manufacturer's recommendation regarding refrigeration (lorazepam may be stocked unrefrigerated on prehospital ALS units if it is replaced every 30 days).

Diazepam. Diazepam is a drug time-honored for treating status epilepticus. Intravenous or IO diazepam (0.15–0.2 mg/kg; maximum, 10 mg/dose) is an effective treatment for status epilepticus or prolonged seizures, but rapid IV administration may cause **respiratory depression**. Do not administer diazepam IM, because it is not well absorbed and is irritating to muscle tissue. Sublingual and IN administrations have been described, although there is little prehospital experience with these.

The task of cannulating a peripheral vein in a seizing child often slows down delivery of essential ALS drugs, especially in infants and toddlers. *The rectum is an effective alternative route for emergency diazepam administration*. Per rectum (PR) diazepam is effective, causes less respiratory depression, and is easy to administer. Use a higher dose than IV/IO of 0.2 to 0.5 mg/kg (maximum PR dose, 20 mg).

Rates of respiratory depression associated with PR diazepam are lower than those seen with IV diazepam; however, onset of action is longer, with time to clinical effect in the range of 5 minutes. For a step-by-step explanation of the rectal diazepam administration procedure, see **Procedure 21, Rectal Administration of Benzodiazepines**.

A common home medication is Diastat®, a form of rectal diazepam. Caregivers may have already administered Diastat to the child and then called for EMS assistance when the seizure did not stop. In this instance, administration of an additional IV, IO, or IM dose of a benzodiazepine may be necessary to stop the seizure.

Phenobarbital is preferred as the first-line drug in neonates at a dose of 40 mg/kg and is one of the second-line drugs for infants and children.

ALS

Intravenously administered diazepam begins to work quickly, but its anticonvulsant action is not long lasting. This may be a serious limitation in long field or transport times, so a second dose of IV diazepam (or another anticonvulsant medication, if available) may be necessary within 10 to 20 minutes. If the child is receiving phenobarbital or has received other benzodiazepines in the previous few hours, a second dosing of diazepam may not be necessary.

If a seizure does not stop after 2 doses of a benzodiazepine, further doses are unlikely to terminate the seizure. Consider a second-line drug if the local EMS system permits. Common choices for second-line anticonvulsants include phenytoin, fosphenytoin, levetiracetam, and phenobarbital, the dosing and administration of which are described in TABLE 6-4.

ALS

Fosphenytoin, a "prodrug" or metabolic precursor to phenytoin, is a second-line option when benzodiazepines have failed. In general, fosphenytoin is significantly preferred over phenytoin in children. Although fosphenytoin can be administered more quickly than phenytoin IV or IO and can also be given IM, it then takes about 15 minutes to metabolize to phenytoin, the active metabolite. *Hence, the total time it takes to achieve an effective drug level in the blood and brain to stop the seizure is approximately the same with phenytoin and fosphenytoin.* A disadvantage of fosphenytoin is that the drug is much more expensive than phenytoin.

Phenytoin is another second-line drug used in neonates, infants, and children. Phenytoin should be administered in normal saline only at a rate no faster than 1 mg/kg/min in children, to a maximum of 50 mg/min. The child should undergo cardiac monitoring and be watched carefully for bradycardia and hypotension, the most common serious complications of IV or IO phenytoin. Complications are caused by the diluent or mixing solution, propylene glycol.

Neither fosphenytoin nor phenytoin is indicated for seizures resulting from toxicologic ingestions or poisonings.

TIP

Always administer oxygen to a child who is having a seizure or who is postictal. For a seizure known to be drug induced, first-line anticonvulsants are benzodiazepines, followed by phenobarbital. There is no indication for use of fosphenytoin or phenytoin.

A subset of the pediatric population may be receiving complicated antiepileptic regimens because of complex epilepsy syndromes. As a result, some pediatric neurologists may have prescribed a sick seizure plan, which may be enacted in the prehospital setting.

CAUTION

When phenytoin comes in contact with glucose, it forms a gel that will occlude the IV line.

There is growing evidence to suggest the use of ketamine in the prehospital setting is a reasonable alternative to the guideline-supported second-line medications for pediatric seizures that are refractory to benzodiazepines. Most EMS systems may not have many of the second-line options available (eg, phenobarbital, phenytoin, levetiracetam). However, ketamine is common in most EMS drug formularies and does not result in the same respiratory depressive side effects as benzodiazepines when administered slowly or via infusion. Ketamine dosage for refractory seizures is 1 to 2 mg/kg IV or up to 3 mg/kg IM, which affords some benefit in children without IV access.

TRANSPORT

After providing airway and breathing support and administering a benzodiazepine, transport should be initiated. Some EMS regions allow administration of second-line anticonvulsant medications during transport. If reasonable, prehospital professionals should consider obtaining the patient history and performing the detailed physical examination on the way to the hospital.

TABLE 6-4 Second-Line Anticonvulsant Drug Administration

Generic Name	Initial Dose	Route	Rate of Infusion	Maximum Rate of Infusion
Fosphenytoin	20 mg/kg (PE)	IV, IO, IM	3 mg (PE)/kg/min	150 mg (PE)/min
Ketamine	1–2 mg/kg	IV, IO, IM	1 mg/kg/h	7 mg/kg/h[F]
Phenobarbital	20 mg/kg	IV, IO	1 mg/kg/min	50 mg/min
Phenytoin	20 mg/kg	IV, IO	1 mg/kg/min	50 mg/min

Abbreviations:IM, intramuscular; IO, intraosseous; IV, intravenous; PE, phenytoin equivalents.

During transport, ongoing patient assessments should be performed by using continuous cardiac monitoring, pulse oximetry, and $EtCO_2$ monitoring, if available. If a patient has not stopped seizing after administration of 2 doses of a benzodiazepine and a second-line drug (eg, fosphenytoin, phenytoin, phenobarbital), the risk of experiencing a prolonged seizure or refractory status epilepticus is high. Transport destination should be carefully considered, because this subset of children is likely to require intensive care.

Assessment of the Postictal Child

Usually, when the prehospital professionals arrive, the child's seizure is already over and the child is in a postictal state. This state is characterized by abnormal appearance with sleepiness, confusion, irritability, and decreased level of consciousness that may last from minutes to hours.

If the child is physiologically stable, it is reasonable to perform a complete assessment in the field, including history taking and physical examination, noting particular rashes or skin discoloration, as well as a detailed survey for patients who have experienced trauma. It is equally important to check blood glucose levels and to correct hypoglycemia, if present.

An example of a stable postictal patient is the child with a previous diagnosis of epilepsy who experiences a brief tonic-clonic seizure, or the child younger than 6 years with fever and a possible febrile seizure. Most children who have had a brief seizure show steady improvement in level of alertness, muscle tone, and interactivity within 15 to 30 minutes. Failure to reach normal mental status within a reasonable period after the seizure may reflect a more serious underlying problem and should trigger early transport with completion of the assessment en route to the hospital. **TABLE 6–5** lists some of the conditions that might lead to a prolonged postictal state and, in turn, to a need for urgent treatment in the emergency department (ED). If the child has had a seizure after head injury, provide spinal motion restriction, as discussed in Chapter 9.

If the postictal patient has a previous diagnosis of epilepsy, it is important to include in the history the name and dosage of anticonvulsant medications and when the last dose was given, as well as when the last blood levels were obtained and whether the levels were adequate. Equally important is determining the duration of the seizure and requesting a description of the motor activity, including where it started, how it progressed, and how long the child was unconscious. Some caregivers may even have video recordings of the seizure. This information helps determine the type of seizure (ie, focal, general, or unknown onset). The EMS clinicians should also inquire about head trauma (either preceding or following the seizure) and should consider the possibility of ingestion or overdose (either accidental or intentional), especially in toddlers and adolescents. Keep in mind that overdose of many nonprescription medications (eg, antihistamines) can cause seizures.

TABLE 6–5 Circumstances With a High Index of Suspicion In the Postictal Child

Posttraumatic seizure
Postingestion seizure
Seizure and sustained hypoxia (including postcardiac arrest)
Seizure in a neonate (<4 weeks of age)
First seizure in a child >6 years
More than 1 seizure
Seizure lasting longer than 5 minutes
Hypoglycemia

Summary of Seizures

Seizures are common in children, and frightened caregivers frequently call 911 to assist in managing this problem. Usually, the seizure has stopped before EMS clinicians' arrival, in which case the clinicians' tasks include only assessment of the postictal child and transport to the hospital with supportive care.

Sometimes the child is seizing on arrival and requires medical treatment. The treatment includes opening and clearing the airway, administering oxygen, and then administering a benzodiazepine medication, usually midazolam, lorazepam, or diazepam. Rectal diazepam stops most seizures in children. Effective alternatives are IV or IO lorazepam; IV, IO, IM, or IN midazolam; or IV or IO diazepam. The benzodiazepines often cause temporary respiratory depression, which may require assisted ventilation support without endotracheal intubation. If treatment with a benzodiazepine is unsuccessful, second-line drugs such as phenobarbital, phenytoin, and fosphenytoin (and even ketamine) are good options, according to local EMS protocols.

Altered Mental Status

Altered mental status (AMS) is an abnormal neurological state in which the child is less alert and interactive than their neurological status at baseline. The term AMS refers to a range of abnormal appearances, from irritability to total unresponsiveness. Sometimes the concern of the caretaker is vaguely expressed, and the complaint is simply that the child is "not acting right." Understanding normal developmental or age-related changes in behavior and listening carefully to the caregiver's opinion about alterations from an individual's normal state are key features in the assessment. A mnemonic lists many of the severe causes of AMS (**TABLE 6–6**): the 5 vowels in the alphabet (AEIOU), followed by tips (TIPPS). This mnemonic reflects the major causes of AMS, with infection being the most common.

TABLE 6–6 Possible Causes of Altered Mental Status: The AEIOU TIPPS Mnemonic

Alcohol
Epilepsy Endocrine disorders (eg, adrenal insufficiency; thyroid disease) Electrolyte abnormalities (eg, hyponatremia; hypernatremia; hypocalcemia; hypercalcemia)
Insulin (eg, diabetic ketoacidosis, hyperosmolar hyperglycemic state; hypoglycemia)
Overdose (eg, opiates)
Uremia Underdose (eg, missed doses of antiepileptic medications)
Trauma (eg, concussion, traumatic brain injury) Temperature (eg, hypothermia, hyperthermia)
Infection (eg, encephalitis, meningitis, sepsis) Intussusception
Psychogenic (eg, psychosis; psychogenic nonepileptic seizures; conversion disorder)
Poison
Shock Stroke (hemorrhagic vs ischemic) Space-occupying brain lesion

ASSESSMENT

EMS clinicians should use the Pediatric Assessment Triangle (PAT) and the disability component of the hands-on ABCDEs (airway, breathing, circulation, disability, exposure) to quickly assess the child's neurological status. These 2 parts of the primary assessment work in concert to evaluate both **cortical** and **brainstem functions**, as described in Chapter 1. There is a difference between abnormal appearance and AMS. Abnormal appearance is a more subtle measure of brain function and is evaluated via the TICLS mnemonic (tone, interactiveness, consolability, look/gaze, speech/cry). Altered mental status is a more severe signal of mental status alteration and is evaluated with the AVPU (alert-verbal-painful-unresponsive) scale. Although AMS is always associated with an abnormal appearance, some children with more subtle abnormalities in appearance would not have AMS according to the AVPU. For example, a child who is irritable or listless and has an abnormal appearance according to the PAT may be rated as alert on the AVPU scale of disability during the ABCDE hands-on evaluation.

Using the AVPU scale is a quick way to determine level of consciousness and to assess major changes in mental status during transport. A child with sepsis or intracranial hemorrhage, for example, has a serious degree of brain dysfunction and may score as verbal or lower on the AVPU.

Finally, EMS clinicians should observe the patient's **motor activity** and check the pupils. Assessment of motor activity includes watching for purposeful and symmetrical movement of extremities, **ataxia,** seizures, **posturing (decorticate** or **decerebrate**), or **flaccidity** (**hypotonia**). Pupils should be checked for size (small or large), equality, and response to light. Pupils may have abnormal size and/or reactivity in the presence of drugs, ongoing seizures, hypoxia, or neurological emergencies (eg, stroke, intracranial hypertension with impending cerebral herniation), as well as after cardiac arrest, among other factors. The presence of a deviated gaze is abnormal and should be noted and reported.

CASE STUDY 2

You respond to a call about an unresponsive child. The caregiver states that the 3-year-old boy could not be awakened from his nap. The child is sleeping on your arrival, with normal breath sounds and no evidence of retractions. He is pale. His respiratory rate is 24 breaths/min, the cardiac monitor shows a narrow complex with a rate of 160 beats/min, and his blood pressure is 68/46 mm Hg. His pupils are small and slow to constrict to light, and the child withdraws from painful stimuli. There is no sign of trauma. The caregiver states that the child has had a viral illness the past few days with vomiting and diarrhea.

1. What other assessment steps might be helpful in evaluating this child?
2. What are the immediate treatment priorities for this child?
3. What additional history may be helpful?

Look for a medical alert bracelet and ask about important medical history that may account for the child's AMS, such as diabetes or a seizure disorder.

TIP

There are many causes of AMS, but management must focus on the ABCs.

MANAGEMENT

Regardless of the cause of AMS, focus on the ABCs.

1. *Open the airway.*
   In the poorly responsive patient with compromised airway reflexes, suction the mouth to relieve potential obstruction from secretions or vomitus. If there is no **gag reflex** or if the patient is totally unresponsive, position the head and insert an oropharyngeal or nasopharyngeal airway. Consider spinal motion restriction if there is a suspicion of head or neck injury.
2. *Ensure adequate breathing.*
   Patients with AMS may have inadequate breathing, despite spontaneous respiratory effort, as indicated by inadequate respiratory rate or inadequate tidal volume. Administer high-flow oxygen via a nonrebreathing mask. Start assisted ventilation with 100% oxygen if the patient has cyanosis, has oxygen saturation less than 90% on high-flow oxygen via nonrebreathing mask, is breathing at a rate too slow for age, has shallow or irregular respiratory effort, or has a neurological examination finding that raises concern regarding impending cerebral herniation (eg, is unresponsive with a unilateral large, nonreactive pupil).

TIP

There is a difference between abnormal appearance and AMS. Abnormal appearance is a more subtle measure of brain function and is evaluated by using the TICLS mnemonic. Altered mental status is a more severe signal of mental status alteration and is evaluated by using the AVPU.

ALS

Consider endotracheal intubation to protect the airway and to avoid aspiration. Ventilate the patient with a suspected brain injury, but do not hyperventilate them unless the neurological examination results raise significant concern regarding impending cerebral herniation (see Chapter 3). Use $EtCO_2$ or waveform capnography to guide ventilations. Place the patient on a cardiac monitor and a pulse oximeter.

3. ***Safeguard circulation.***
   Establish vascular (or intraosseous) access. Always start isotonic fluids at a to-keep-open (TKO) rate, unless the child is in shock. Reassess the child's level of consciousness.

4. *Perform a bedside blood glucose test* (**FIGURE 6–5**).
   Obtain blood for **serum glucose** measurement and administer glucose to children with documented hypoglycemia. Hypoglycemia has been shown to worsen neurological outcomes in patients with documented brain injuries. If a bedside glucose test shows hypoglycemia (<40 mg/dL in a newborn, <60 mg/dL in a child), EMS clinicians should administer IV glucose, diluted as directed, or IM **glucagon** as outlined

in **TABLE 6–3**. **Oral glucose** may be administered to a child with diabetes and hypoglycemia who is conscious and able to follow commands appropriately.

5. *In the child with AMS and depressed respirations, consider naloxone administration.*
The naloxone dose is 0.1 mg/kg, with a usual maximum dose up to 2 mg. However, more is often required with synthetic opioid overdose. Naloxone may be administered by a variety of routes: IV, IM, IO, subcutaneous, IN, or endotracheally. Caution must be exercised when adminstering naloxone to a newborn with neonatal abstinence syndrome, because it may induce acute withdrawal symptoms and seizures. Instead of administering naloxone, consider supporting ventilations and transporting the newborn to the hospital. Causes of AMS, including pharmaceutical overdoses, should remain an important differential diagnosis in all pediatrics, regardless of age. Constricted pupils are a universal finding in pure opiate overdoses. This is not necessarily the case with synthetic narcotics, such as oxycodone.

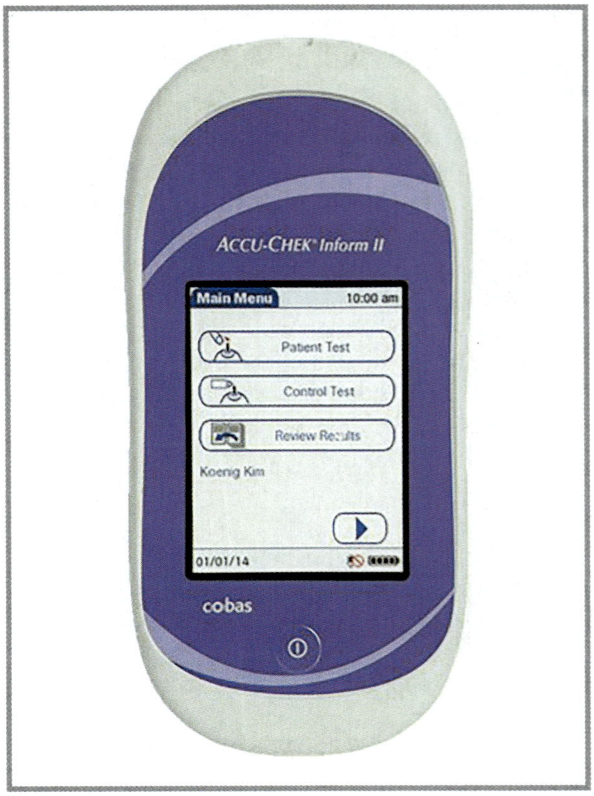

FIGURE 6–5 Perform a bedside blood glucose test.

Accu-Chek® Aviva used with permission of Roche Diagnostics.

CASE STUDY ANSWERS

CASE STUDY 1

It is important to determine if this child possibly experienced poisoning, head trauma, or other potential causes of seizures. In addition, the possibility of head trauma during the seizure should be determined. It may also be helpful to determine if this seizure was similar to previous seizures, when the last seizure occurred, and if the child has been taking his regular medication correctly.

All children with a history of seizure activity in the setting of fevers should be transported to the hospital, because it is impossible to diagnose a febrile seizure in the field. There are many causes of seizures, including serious infections (eg, meningitis, encephalitis, cerebral abscess, sepsis). This child also has a history of seizures, and there are factors, such as adequacy of current treatments, that require evaluation.

Continuous, careful monitoring during transport is especially important if drug therapy has been given, because administration of benzodiazepines, especially in combination with other seizure medications such as phenobarbital, can result in apnea or respiratory depression. Because this child is still not breathing adequately and his oxygen saturation is only 92%, airway maneuvers, 100% oxygen, and assisted ventilation are needed. If the child is still febrile, simple cooling methods, such as a cool towel to the forehead, may be useful. There is no need to apply ice packs to the body unless the child has heat stroke. Reassess the patient frequently, and be prepared for repeat seizures.

CASE STUDY ANSWERS—cont'd

At the hospital, the patient's anticonvulsant levels were determined to be subtherapeutic. Further investigation revealed a history of several days of nausea and vomiting resulting from a gastrointestinal illness. The patient was hydrated, received an intravenous dose of his anticonvulsant, and resumed his oral medications the following day when his nausea and vomiting resolved. He was discharged home the following day.

ALS

If multiple seizures occur or an additional seizure lasts longer than 5 minutes, consider treating with a benzodiazepine (rectal or IV diazepam; IV lorazepam; or IV, IN, or IM midazolam) and be prepared to manage airway and ventilation during transport. Although brief seizures do not require pharmacologic treatment, prompt treatment of seizures lasting longer than 5 minutes has the greatest success in terms of seizure cessation. Continuous, careful monitoring of airway and ventilation during transport is especially important if drug therapy has been given, because administration of benzodiazepines and phenobarbital can result in apnea or respiratory depression.

CASE STUDY 2

Oxygen saturation, temperature assessment, and blood glucose measurement can provide additional clues as to the cause of this child's AMS.

The possible etiology of the child's AMS is variable and includes head trauma, toxin ingestion, shock, sepsis, hypovolemia, hypoglycemia, or postictal period after a seizure. However, the initial treatment is the same regardless of cause: Open and manage the airway with positioning and administer 100% oxygen via nonrebreathing mask. If there is no trauma, place the patient in the sniffing position and use the jaw-thrust maneuver to maintain the airway. If respirations are shallow or irregular, or if oxygen saturation is less than 90% on supplemental oxygen, assist ventilation with an appropriately sized bag-mask device. Insert an oropharyngeal or nasopharyngeal airway as needed to maintain a patent airway.

ALS

Because the patient's blood pressure is low (calculated systolic blood pressure for a 3-year-old would be 76 [70 + (2 × age in years)], whereas the measured systolic blood pressure is 68), fluid boluses of 20 mL/kg should be administered. If the glucose level is less than 60 mg/dL, possibly due to vomiting and diarrhea, administer 25% dextrose (2 mL/kg) via IV bolus. If there is no IV access, administer glucagon IM. If bedside glucose level is within normal limits, consider other causes of AMS; the clinician may administer naloxone (0.1 mg/kg; maximum, 2 mg), if appropriate. Use a length-based resuscitation tape or computer software program, as described in Procedure 2, Length-Based Resuscitation Tapes, to determine drug doses.

Additional history questions to help determine the possible causes of the AMS may include whether the child has had fever or other symptoms besides the vomiting and diarrhea already reported; whether the child has been taking anything orally, especially fluids; whether urination has been adequate; if the child has any ongoing medical problems; whether there has been any possibility of trauma (especially head trauma) on the present day or in the recent past; and whether there is any possibility of drug or poison ingestion.

At the hospital, it was determined that the child was severely dehydrated and had multiple electrolyte abnormalities because of the vomiting and diarrhea. Intravenous fluids started in the field were continued, along with electrolyte replacement. Level of consciousness, blood pressure, and tachycardia all improved with fluid volume restoration. The child spent 24 hours in the pediatric intensive care unit and was discharged home 1 day later.

Suggested References

TEXTBOOKS

American Academy of Orthopaedic Surgeons. *Emergency Care and Transportation of the Sick and Injured.* 12th ed. Jones and Bartlett Learning; 2021

American Academy of Orthopaedic Surgeons. *Nancy Caroline's Emergency Care in the Streets.* 9th ed. Jones and Bartlett Learning; 2023

American Academy of Pediatrics; American College of Emergency Physicians. *APLS: The Pediatric Emergency Medicine Resource.* 5th ed. Jones and Bartlett Learning; 2012

Rogers JL, ed. *McCance & Heuther's Pathophysiology: The Biologic Basis for Disease in Adults and Children.* 9th ed. Mosby Elsevier; 2024

ARTICLES

Beniczky S, Trinka E, Wirrell E, Abdulla F, Al Baradie R, Alonso Vanegas M, et al. Updated classification of epileptic seizures: Position paper of the International League Against Epilepsy. Epilepsia. 2025;00:1–20. doi:10.1111/epi.1833

DiDomenico L, Garrity LC, Poisson KE, Broomall E. Enteral ketamine for status epilepticus in children with epilepsy. *Pediatr Neurol.* 2024;15841–48. doi:10.1016/j.pediatrneurol.2024.05.006

Geduld H, Hodkinson PW, Wallis LA. Validation of weight estimation by age and length based methods in the Western Cape, South Africa population. *Emerg Med J.* 2011;28(10):856–860. doi:10.1136/emj.2010.098640

Glauser T, Shinnar S, Gloss D, et al. Evidence-based guideline: treatment of convulsive status epilepticus in children and adults: report of the Guideline Committee of the American Epilepsy Society. *Epilepsy Curr.* 2016;16(1):48–61. doi:10.5698/1535-7597-16.1.48

Kuppermann N, Ghetti S, Schunk JE, et al; PECARN DKA FLUID Study Group. Clinical trial of fluid infusion rates for pediatric diabetic ketoacidosis. *N Engl J Med.* 2018;378(24):2275–2287. doi:10.1056/NEJMoa1716816

de Miguel Lavisier B, Molina Gutiérrez MÁ, Púa Torrejón RC, et al. Seizures in children with severe acute respiratory syndrome coronavirus 2 infection. *Pediatr Neurol.* 2024;157:151–156. doi:10.1016/j.pediatrneurol.2024.05.023

National Institutes of Health (U.S.); National Institute of Neurological Disorders and Stroke. (U.S.). Office of Communications and Public Liaison. *Febrile Seizures.* U.S. Department of Health and Human Services, Public Health Service, National Institutes of Health, 2012. Accessed April 18, 2025. https://www.ninds.nih.gov/health-information/disorders/febrile-seizures

Philpott NG, Dante SA, Philpott D, et al. Treatment guideline nonadherence pretransport associated with need for higher level of care in children transferred to a pediatric tertiary care center for status epilepticus. *Pediatr Emerg Care.* 2023;39(10):780–785. doi:10.1097/PEC.0000000000002952

Shah MI, Macias CG, Dayan PS, et al. An evidence-based guideline for pediatric prehospital seizure management using GRADE methodology. *Prehosp Emerg Care.* 2014; 18(suppl 1):15–24. doi:10.3109/10903127.2013.844874

Sorcher JL, Badaki-Makun O, Ngo TL. Unresponsive: a case of hyperglycemia and altered mental status. *Clin Pediatr Emerg Med.* 2019;20(4):100726. doi:10.1016/j.cpem.2019.100726

Vasquez A, Farias-Moeller R, Sánchez-Fernández I, et al; Pediatric Status Epilepticus Research Group (pSERG). Super-refractory status epilepticus in children: a retrospective cohort study. *Pediatr Crit Care Med.* 2021;22(12): e613–e625. doi:10.1097/PCC.0000000000002786

Vossler DG. Midazolam, ketamine, and propofol: while we slept, others worked on anesthetizing infusions for refractory status epilepticus. *Epilepsy Curr.* 2023;23(4):230–232 doi:10.1177/15357597231171240

Williams NC, Morgan LA, Friedman J, Siegler J. Ketamine efficacy for management of status epilepticus: considerations for prehospital clinicians. *Air Med J.* 2024;43(2): 84–89. doi:10.1016/j.amj.2023.09.011

CHAPTER 7

Infectious Diseases

Tabitha Cheng, MD
H. Joel Dishroon, PM, IC

LEARNING OBJECTIVES

1. **Discuss the association of fever and serious illness.**
2. **Describe the assessment and management of fever in children.**
3. **Identify common causes and symptoms of gastroenteritis in children.**
4. **Discuss the prehospital management of a pediatric patient with suspected gastroenteritis, including the prevention of disease transmission.**
5. **Explain the importance of recognizing and managing sepsis and meningitis in pediatric patients.**

Fever

Fever is a sign of infection or inflammation, rather than a disease itself. It is often misunderstood by parents. Most pediatric infections, whether viral or bacterial, are systemic and result in fevers. Children can experience high fevers (>40 °C/104 °F) as a result of minor illnesses, such as a cold, or more serious conditions such as pneumonia, meningitis, or sepsis. Temporal thermometers, commonly used by EMS clinicians, are accurate and less invasive than traditional thermometers and can be used to quickly measure temperature (**FIGURE 7-1**). Fever of any cause leads to an increase in the basal metabolic rate, which in turn raises respiratory rate, heart rate (tachycardia), cardiac output, and oxygen consumption. It also increases fluid and caloric needs; this can lead to volume depletion and hypoglycemia, especially because ill children often refuse food and fluids. In general, fevers are a common cause of concern for most parents, with many worrying that high temperatures may cause brain damage. However, there is no evidence to support this concern unless temperatures exceed 41.1 °C (106 °F). When fevers associated with infection do result in brain damage, it is typically the infection itself, not the fever, that causes damage. The focus for emergency medical services (EMS) clinicians should be the patient's history and presentation and assessment of the child's overall condition—level of consciousness, hydration status, and signs of serious infection—rather than the fever itself. Knowing the exact temperature is less important in field management because it rarely changes the treatment plan.

Important fever thresholds are as follows:

- A body temperature below 41.1 °C (106 °F) is generally not harmful.
- Temperatures at or above 41.1 °C (106 °F) could pose risks and warrant careful evaluation.

TIP

Fever less than 41.1 °C (106 °F) by itself does not cause brain damage.

ASSESSMENT

The primary assessment helps determine the severity of the child's illness and the urgency of the need for treatment. If the primary assessment result is normal, proceed with history taking and a focused physical examination. Ask about important signs and symptoms of infection, such as chills, **malaise**, poor feeding, **lethargy**, pulling of ears, vomiting, diarrhea, abdominal pain, presence of a rash or skin discoloration, stiff neck, headache, and irritability.

Ask about vaccination status and exposure to known communicable diseases of childhood. Many childhood illnesses begin with a fever before any other symptoms are present. Determine if the child has any significant medical history, because febrile children who may be immunodeficient (eg, patients

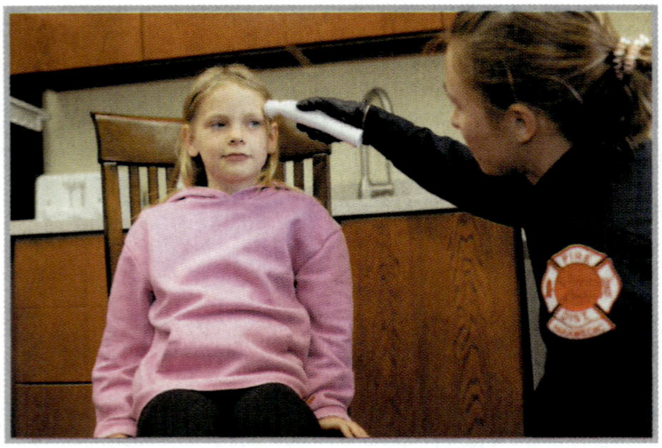

FIGURE 7-1 A temporal thermometer measures body temperature by being swiped across the skin of the forehead.

with **sickle cell disease**, cancer, or HIV, or who have undergone organ transplantation) are at higher risk of developing serious infection as the cause of fever.

Febrile respiratory infections are very common in children and are typically accompanied by tachycardia, tachypnea, nasal congestion, cough, and respiratory distress. Fever may make a child with a minor illness appear sicker than they really are, and parents often report a marked improvement in symptoms after administration of **antipyretics**, such as acetaminophen or ibuprofen. After the history, a physical examination should be performed to look for possible sources of infection.

Although the height of fever is not reflective of the degree of illness, certain findings suggest a serious underlying illness and must prompt rapid transport. These findings include a **bulging fontanelle** (if the child is $<$12 months of age, palpate with the child held upright or sitting up), photophobia (light sensitivity), nuchal rigidity (stiff neck), **paradoxical irritability** (an infant who is crankier when picked up and held than when left alone) (**FIGURE 7-2**), seizures, prolonged capillary refill time, or a petechial or purpuric rash (small red or purple spots, which could indicate a serious condition such as meningococcemia).

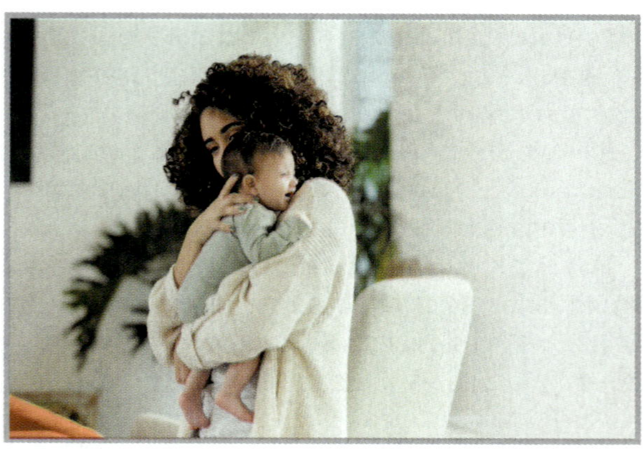

FIGURE 7-2 An infant experiencing paradoxical irritability.

Age and Fever

In addition to signs and symptoms, the child's age plays a critical role in fever assessment:

- Infants younger than 3 months:
  - Fever may be the only indication of serious infection. These infants often show nonspecific symptoms, such as
    - Fussiness
    - Poor feeding
    - Sleepiness
  - Infants younger than 3 weeks with a temperature of 38 °C (100.4 °F) or higher are considered to be at high risk and require immediate emergency department evaluation (blood, urine, and spinal fluid cultures, plus empiric **antibiotics**).
    - In the first days after birth, **jaundice** may be a sign of serious bacterial infection.
  - Infants aged 21 days to 2 months: Fever in these children requires a medical evaluation, including blood and urine cultures and evaluation of blood inflammatory markers, but they may be discharged with or without antibiotics if no abnormalities are found.
- Seizures and fever: A febrile seizure in any infant younger than 6 months warrants transport to a medical facility.

MANAGEMENT

Management of fever in a child with normal primary assessment findings involves the following steps:

1. *Prevent disease transmission to EMS clinicians.* Protect yourself by using standard precautions for infection control.
2. *Consider antipyretic administration* (in a child $\geq$6 months, if appropriate).
   For children older than 6 months, consider providing antipyretics if none has been administered in the past 4 hours.
   - Acetaminophen: Administer 15 mg/kg, orally or rectally (**FIGURE 7-3**).
   - Ibuprofen: Administer 10 mg/kg orally. Note that ibuprofen is not recommended for infants younger than 6 months or children with known kidney problems.

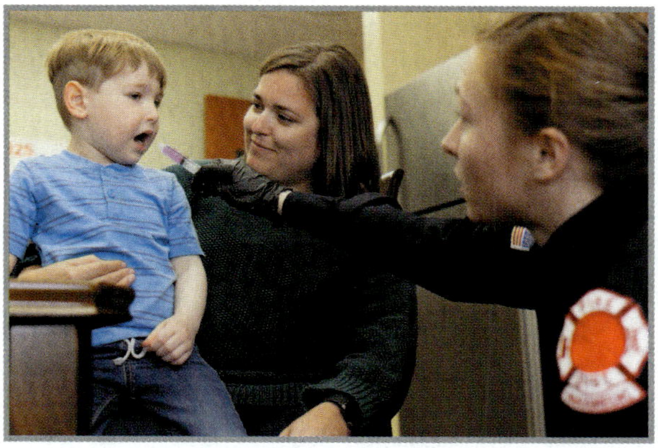

FIGURE 7–3 Administering antipyretics, such as acetaminophen, can help manage fever.

Considerations are as follows:

- Evaluate the child's level of consciousness and any history of recent vomiting before giving anything orally.
- Avoid aspirin owing to the risk of Reye syndrome in children with *Varicella* viral illnesses.

3. Provide cooling measures.
   Undress the child to help reduce fever but avoid causing hypothermia.
   Do not use ice, cold water, fans, or alcohol baths to cool the child, because these methods can be harmful or ineffective.
   Parent education: Inform caregivers that overbundling the child retains heat and may worsen the fever.
4. Reassure the caregiver that fever alone is not dangerous to the child.

CAUTION

Never use ice, cold water, fans, or alcohol baths to cool a feverish child.

Summary of Fever

Fever is typically a natural response to infection and is rarely dangerous on its own. However, prolonged fever increases the risk of dehydration. The age of the child and other associated signs and symptoms are important in determining probability of serious illness. Warning signs, such as a petechial or purpuric rash, stiff neck, light sensitivity, and/or altered mental status (AMS), are strong indicators of a potentially serious condition requiring emergent evaluation. In most febrile children, the primary actions for EMS clinicians involve simple cooling measures and transport if further evaluation is warranted.

Communicable Diseases

Many communicable diseases are common during childhood. Although most are viral in origin and are mild in terms of severity, infectious diseases on occasion cause significant compromise in the pediatric patient, resulting in the need for prehospital transport. Many childhood diseases have a respiratory component, a gastrointestinal (GI) component, or both. Respiratory diseases are addressed in Chapter 3. This section concentrates on the GI signs and symptoms of nausea, vomiting, and diarrhea, as well as sepsis and meningitis.

Nausea, Vomiting, and Diarrhea (Gastroenteritis)

Gastroenteritis, characterized by symptoms such as nausea, vomiting, and diarrhea, is an inflammation of the GI tract commonly seen in pediatric patients (**FIGURE 7–4**). Gastroenteritis can have numerous causes, including foodborne and waterborne illnesses, viruses, bacteria, antibiotic side effects, and parasites. Many of these are carried by pets. Viral agents are the most common culprits, with norovirus now being the most common cause of viral gastroenteritis in children in the United States. Regardless of the cause, gastroenteritis can lead to volume depletion, particularly in younger children. Be aware that the signs and symptoms often (but not always) associated with gastroenteritis—such as fever, abdominal pain, or vomiting—can also signal more

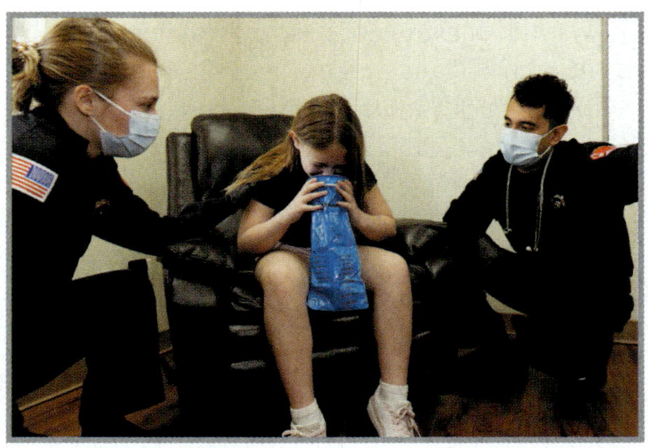

FIGURE 7–4 Gastroenteritis symptoms may include vomiting and nausea.

serious abdominal emergencies, such as appendicitis and bowel obstruction.

When assessing a pediatric patient, it is critical to identify the presence and sequence of symptoms such as nausea, vomiting, diarrhea, and fever. Some conditions are more common in certain age groups. For example, malrotation of the gut occurs in newborns, whereas pyloric stenosis presents with vomiting after feeding but without diarrhea or fever in young infants. In cases of food poisoning, such as *Salmonella* infection, symptoms typically begin with vomiting followed by diarrhea, and fever may appear hours after eating (usually 12–72 hours after ingestion). Although gastroenteritis is a common diagnosis, more serious causes of these symptoms must be excluded, and this determination cannot be made in the field.

ASSESSMENT

When evaluating a child with presumed gastroenteritis, focus primarily on assessing the child's hydration status.

The history should include questions about the following key aspects:

- Onset, sequence of events, and frequency of vomiting or diarrhea
- Relationship of symptoms to eating
- Amount of oral intake
- Number of wet diapers or frequency of urination in the past 8 hours
- Character of stool, including the presence of blood
- Last urination or wet diaper

The physical examination should focus on identifying signs of dehydration and include the following:

- Presence or absence of fever
- Level of consciousness
- Hydration status of mucous membranes (moist or dry)
- Presence or absence of tears
- Warmth of extremities and pulse quality
- Abdominal tenderness or distension

Always check a point-of-care glucose concentration in any child with a history of vomiting, diarrhea, and poor oral intake.

MANAGEMENT

Management of presumed gastroenteritis in the pediatric patient depends on the degree of dehydration. Additionally, prevention of disease transmission is a critical aspect of care.

1. *Prevent disease transmission.* Use standard precautions to reduce the risk of disease transmission, because gastroenteritis (whether bacterial, viral, or parasitic) is transmitted via the fecal-oral route. Even small amounts of pathogenic organisms can cause infection. Many organisms can survive on instruments and surfaces for hours, so hand hygiene and careful cleaning of equipment are essential.
2. *Provide supplemental fluids.*
   For the unstable pediatric patient, administer supplemental oxygen and manage the airway as needed.
   Provide advanced life support.
3. *Initiate fluid replacement for severe clinical dehydration:*
   If the child shows signs of severe dehydration (elevated heart rate, poor pulses, delayed capillary refill, cool extremities, abnormal skin color):
   - Establish vascular access, either intravenous or intraosseous.
   - Administer crystalloid fluid (20 mL/kg initial bolus).
   - Repeat the bolus to a total of 60 mL/kg until perfusion stabilizes.
4. *Treat hypoglycemia.*
5. *Reassess vital signs throughout treatment.*
6. *Transport the child.*

Transport decisions depend on the severity of dehydration and available resources.

A child with mild to moderate dehydration and ongoing vomiting or diarrhea may not need transport. Oral fluids can be provided if permitted by your EMS system.

For children showing signs of severe dehydration or shock, immediate fluid replacement before transport is critical.

Sepsis and Meningitis

Sepsis in children is a clinical syndrome characterized by **systemic inflammatory response syndrome (SIRS)** due to a suspected or confirmed infection. Systemic inflammatory response syndrome is defined by at least 2 of the following criteria (1 of which must be an abnormal temperature or white blood cell count):

1. Core temperature higher than 38.5 °C (101.3 °F) or less than 36 °C (96.8 °F)
2. Tachycardia with a heart rate more than 2 SDs above normal for age over a 0.5- to 4-hour period, or bradycardia (mean heart rate below 10th percentile for age) in infants younger than 1 year for 0.5 hours

3. Respiratory rate higher than 2 SDs above normal for age
4. **Leukocyte (white blood cell) count** elevated or depressed for age, or more than 10% immature neutrophils

Although EMS clinicians may not have access to all this information, the presence of fever, tachycardia, and/or tachypnea should raise suspicion regarding sepsis. Septic shock, which includes organ and cardiovascular dysfunction, is covered in Chapter 4.

Some children with sepsis also have **meningitis**, resulting from infection and inflammation of the meninges, the membranes that cover the brain and spinal cord. Other children experience sepsis or meningitis alone. Meningitis may be either viral (nonbacterial) or bacterial. Although aseptic meningitis may cause illness, it is rarely life threatening, whereas bacterial meningitis can progress rapidly, with the potential for death within hours to days. Symptoms, in addition to fever, may range from stiff neck and headache to signs of brainstem herniation.

Infants younger than 3 months are at highest risk of experiencing sepsis and bacterial meningitis, with causes varying according to age. The introduction of the *Haemophilus influenzae* type b (Hib) vaccine in the late 1980s significantly reduced the incidence of this illness. Bacterial sepsis and meningitis in the first month after birth are most commonly caused by bacteria acquired from the maternal vaginal area during delivery. These include *Escherichia coli*, group B *Streptococcus*, and *Listeria monocytogenes*.

For older infants and children, sepsis is more commonly acquired in the community, with bacterial causes including *Streptococcus pneumoniae* (common cause of ear infection, sinusitis, and pneumonia in children) and *Neisseria meningitidis* (meningococcus). **Meningococcal sepsis** or meningitis presents acutely with high fever, AMS, and a **petechial** or **purpuric rash**. This is a life-threatening emergency that requires rapid transport to the highest level of care available, because affected children can deteriorate rapidly and require aggressive life support. The pneumococcal vaccine, available throughout the United States, has reduced the incidence of childhood bacteremia and sepsis. Viral causes of meningitis, such as enteroviruses, are common, especially in the summer and fall.

Children with immunodeficiencies (eg, those who have cancer or have undergone organ transplantation) are also at higher risk of experiencing sepsis, particularly if they have indwelling central lines.

ASSESSMENT

In a child with presumed sepsis or meningitis who is physiologically unstable, limit the scene assessment and perform the focused history and physical examination during transport, if possible. The focused history should include the following:

- Known exposure to illness
- Perinatal history for infants younger than 1 month
- Onset and progression of symptoms
- Presence or absence of fever
- Associated symptoms and signs, such as irritability, vomiting, nuchal rigidity, and rash (petechiae or purpura)
- Immunization history

The physical examination should include assessment of the following:

- Fever
- Level of consciousness
- Adequacy of perfusion
- Nuchal rigidity
- Presence of a rash (petechiae or purpura)
- Photophobia

Owing to the hypermetabolic state in sepsis and meningitis, children can develop hypoglycemia and dehydration. Always check a point-of-care glucose concentration in any patient with presumed sepsis or meningitis.

MANAGEMENT

Management of pediatric sepsis or meningitis includes infection control and depends on the child's clinical presentation.

1. *Prevent disease transmission.*
   Use standard and respiratory precautions, including gowns, gloves, and masks, to avoid contact with patient secretions.
2. *Provide supplemental oxygen.*
   Unstable patients may need assisted ventilation or airway management.
3. *Establish vascular access.*
   Employ advanced life support.
4. *Initiate fluid replacement for inadequate perfusion.*
   For pediatric patients with inadequate perfusion, initiate crystalloid fluid replacement at 20 mL/kg as quickly as possible. Owing to

dehydration due to fever and the impact of bacterial toxins on blood vessels, repeat fluid boluses of 20 mL/kg up to 60 mL/kg of crystalloid fluid may be required to treat distributive shock and stabilize perfusion.

5. *Treat hypoglycemia.*
6. *Reassess vital signs frequently.*
   Use continuous cardiorespiratory monitoring and pulse oximetry, if available, and be prepared for deterioration during transport.
7. *Transport the child.*
   Transport these children by the highest level of service available to a facility equipped to manage critically ill children. Children with sepsis or meningitis generally require intensive care, so transport destination should be determined accordingly.

Suggested References

TEXTBOOKS

American Academy of Orthopaedic Surgeons. *Emergency Care and Transportation of the Sick and Injured.* 12th ed. Jones and Bartlett Learning; 2021

American Academy of Orthopaedic Surgeons. *Nancy Caroline's Emergency Care in the Streets.* 9th ed. Jones and Bartlett Learning; 2022

American Academy of Pediatrics; American College of Emergency Physicians. *APLS: The Pediatric Emergency Medicine Resource.* 5th ed. Jones and Bartlett Learning; 2012

Rogers JL, ed. *McCance & Huether's Pathophysiology: The Biologic Basis for Disease in Adults and Children.* 9th ed. Mosby Elsevier; 2022

Smith S; Advanced Life Support Group, eds. *Advanced Paediatric Life Support: The Practical Approach.* 7th ed. John Wiley & Sons Ltd; 2023. doi:10.1002/9781119716181

ARTICLES

Kuppermann N, Ghetti S, Schunk JE, et al; PECARN DKA FLUID Study Group. Clinical trial of fluid infusion rates for pediatric diabetic ketoacidosis. *N Engl J Med.* 2018;378(24):2275–2287. doi:10.1056/NEJMoa1716816

Pantell RH, Roberts KB, Adams WG, et al; Subcommittee on Febrile Infants. Evaluation and management of well-appearing febrile infants 8 to 60 days old. *Pediatrics.* 2021;148(2):e2021052228. doi:10.1542/peds.2021-052228

Shah MI, Macias CG, Dayan PS, et al. An evidence-based guideline for pediatric prehospital seizure management using GRADE methodology. *Prehosp Emerg Care.* 2014;18(sup1)(suppl 1):15–24. doi:10.3109/10903127.2013.844874

CHAPTER 8

Endocrine and Environmental Emergencies

Sean Davis, MSEd, CIC, NRP, FESI-2
Michael J. Stoner, MD, FAAP

LEARNING OBJECTIVES

1. **Outline the assessment and management of common endocrinological emergencies, including diabetes mellitus, congenital adrenal hyperplasia (CAH), cortisol deficiency, and panhypopituitarism.**
2. **Discuss the pathophysiology and management of hypoglycemia and hyperglycemia.**
3. **Outline the assessment and management of common environmental emergencies, including temperature emergencies, bites, and stings.**

ENDOCRINE DISORDERS

In children, common endocrine disorders include diabetes mellitus (DM), congenital adrenal hyperplasia (CAH), cortisol deficiency, and panhypopituitarism. Of these disorders, DM is the most common.

Diabetes Mellitus

Diabetes mellitus is a disorder associated with the hormone insulin. Insulin, produced by the pancreas, helps regulate blood glucose concentrations. Glucose is needed in the production of energy by the cells in the body. Without adequate amounts of insulin, cells cannot access circulating glucose and thus cannot create energy.

Diabetes mellitus is a disease of children and adults and comes in 2 major forms. Type 1 DM is a chronic immune-mediated destruction of the insulin-producing (β) cells. This leads to absolute insulin deficiency that requires treatment with insulin. Type 2 DM occurs when the cells are resistant to the insulin that is being produced.

Type 1 DM is more likely to develop in childhood. The exact underlying cause is unknown, but it is thought to be a combination of genetic and environmental causes.

There is an increasing prevalence of type 2 DM in childhood, and its etiology is linked to genetics and lifestyle. Affected children are usually adolescents (mid-puberty), often with associated obesity or poor activity levels. The child may be receiving oral hypoglycemic agents or may require insulin or other injectable medications.

TECHNOLOGY

Patients with DM have an inability to closely regulate their bodies' blood glucose concentrations intrinsically and require frequent extrinsic monitoring. Those with insulin dependence also require extraneous insulin to be administered. There are many devices on the market to perform this function.

Monitoring can be done from a simple glucometer, which requires a small sample of blood, usually from a fingertip that has been pricked with a lancet (**FIGURE 8–1**). Continuous glucose monitors are available that are inserted into the skin (approximately 1 cm) and reads the glucose concentration in the fluid around the tissue. These will provide an alert when the measurements are outside the set parameters. Newer models are Bluetooth enabled to connect to electronic devices such as a smart phone, not only alerting the user, but also tracking trends. Newer

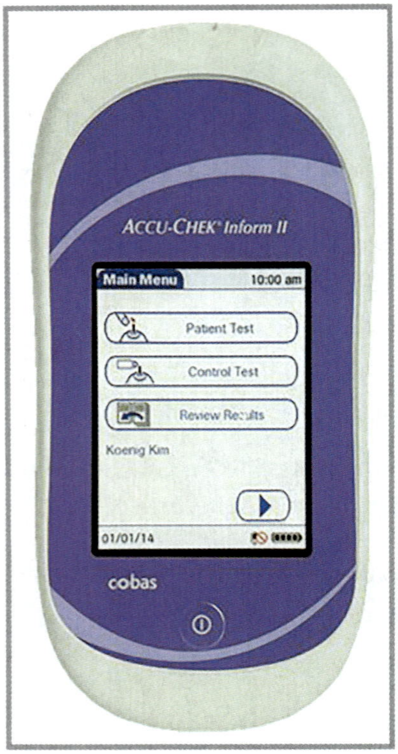

FIGURE 8–1 Perform a bedside blood glucose test using a glucometer.

ACCU-CHEK® is a trademark of Roche. © 2026 Roche

devices also have the ability to notify parents of children using these devices of significant changes in glucose concentrations.

Insulin delivery has also seen its share of progress, moving from a standard syringe used to administer insulin to the insulin pens now available. These allow the user to dial the exact amount of insulin needed. Taking it a step further, there are smart insulin pens that connect via Bluetooth to an application that can calculate and deliver the amount of insulin needed on the basis of current blood glucose concentrations and carbohydrates ingested. Finally, there is the insulin pump, which can be set to administer a continuous baseline infusion, bolus doses based on meals or elevated blood glucose concentrations, or a combination of these (**FIGURE 8–2**).

Technology has allowed us to put monitoring and delivery into a single device. There are insulin pumps that incorporate a continuous glucose monitoring system. The system will adjust the infusion of insulin according to the parameters entered and the current glucose concentration. This allows the user to experience fewer fluctuations of glucose and thus better controlled DM, which in turn leads to fewer complications.

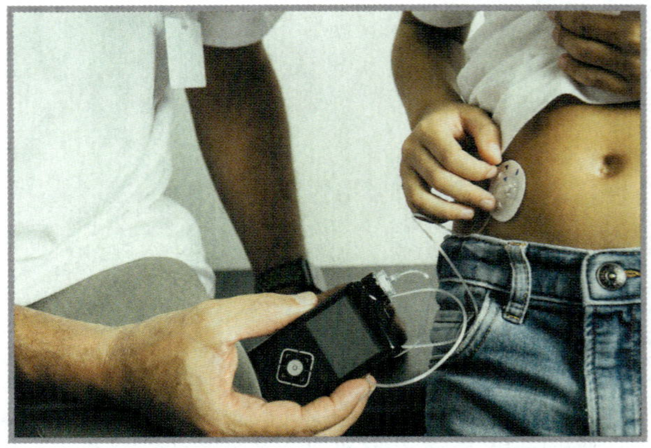

FIGURE 8–2 Insulin pumps administer a continuous baseline infusion, bolus doses based on meals or elevated blood glucose levels, or a combination of these.

Vadi Fuoco/iStockphoto.com

Technology is very helpful in day-to-day life but does have its pitfalls. Any of these devices can malfunction or become dislodged, interfering with either the monitoring of the glucose concentrations, the insulin delivery, or both. This can lead to episodes of hypoglycemia, hyperglycemia, or even diabetic ketoacidosis. Health care providers should not rely on the continuous glucose monitor as a sole source of information when determining acute treatment. Confirm readings with your glucometer when making treatment decisions. Also, if a patient is having an episode of hypoglycemia, be vigilant and assess for an insulin pump; if there is one, either remove it or shut it off so the patient does not continue to receive insulin in the face of hypoglycemia. This can be particularly important when the patient has a closed-loop system, in which an insulin pump is integrated with a continuous glucose monitor to automatically adjust basal insulin rates on the basis of blood glucose concentration. Administration of dextrose can result in increased insulin doses unless the insulin pump is turned off.

DIABETIC KETOACIDOSIS

Regardless of the type of DM, the onset of symptoms is relatively slow, over days (as in type 1 DM) to weeks (as in type 2 DM). Both types can present problems over time; the most emergent of these seen in the pediatric population is diabetic ketoacidosis (DKA).

Diabetic ketoacidosis results from the body's lacking insulin. Without insulin, the insulin-sensitive cells (muscle and fat) are unable to take up glucose from the blood, which leads to hyperglycemia. Glucagon and other hormones are also upregulated with the lack of insulin; this, in turn, stimulates breakdown of fats with conversion to free fatty acids and ketone bodies, which are acids, and leads to the syndrome of DKA. Signs of DKA can vary. If the blood glucose level exceeds the renal threshold for reabsorption, an osmotic diuresis is created. This results in frequent urination (**polyuria**) with corresponding loss of body water. The higher the blood glucose level, the higher amounts of body water are lost in the urine. Loss of body water causes dehydration, resulting in intense thirst (**polydipsia**), and fat breakdown leads to increased hunger (**polyphagia**). With the build of acids in the system, the body tries to compensate by blowing off carbon dioxide (inducing a respiratory alkalosis to compensate for the metabolic acidosis), resulting in the hallmark sign of **Kussmaul respirations**. These respirations are rapid and deep and have the odor of ketones or rotten fruit. Some early signs of DM and DKA include falling asleep in school, wetting the bed, having abnormal thirst, emitting the odor of ketones, and, in severe cases, experiencing altered mental status (AMS).

Emergency medical services (EMS) may be called for a child with AMS who has a history of abdominal pain, vomiting, and excessive thirst. The child is often severely dehydrated. In the presence of abdominal pain, nausea, and vomiting, sepsis may be suspected. If Kussmaul breathing is pronounced, this condition can also be confused with a respiratory emergency. The presence of a blood glucose level higher than 300 mg/dL, or hyperglycemia, may lead one to suspect the presence of DKA.

ASSESSMENT

Signs and symptoms of hyperglycemia can be hard to detect, especially because the onset is relatively slow. A key finding in hyperglycemia is dehydration. Depending on the blood glucose level, hypoperfusion may be evident, ranging from mild to severe. Tachycardia, rapid/deep respirations, and dry skin are all signs of volume depletion. In general, the higher the blood glucose level, the more extreme the dehydration.

MANAGEMENT

After general treatment measures are implemented, initiate intravenous (IV) access and administer isotonic fluid at 10 to 20 mL/kg over 30 to 60 minutes. Repeat boluses only if the child is hypotensive. If not hypotensive, keep IV fluids at 1 to 1.5 times maintenance rate. One serious complication of DKA is **cerebral edema,** with warning signs of headache and/ or a change in mental status. Monitor Glasgow Coma Scale (GCS) scores and reassess the patient frequently en route. If transport is prolonged, blood glucose monitoring should be done at least every hour.

HYPOGLYCEMIA

Hypoglycemia is defined as a serum glucose level of less than 40 mg/dL in a newborn or less than 60 mg/dL in a child. The most frequent scenario for out-of-hospital hypoglycemia is a child with known DM who uses too much insulin, exerts himself or herself excessively, delays a meal, or begins to vomit after taking insulin. Hypoglycemia may also occur in children with a history of almost any endocrine problem.

In nondiabetic infants, hypoglycemia may occur when the child has been working so hard that glycogen reserves become depleted (eg, when compensating for a cardiac defect or for an extreme respiratory rate). This is more common in infants and toddlers than in older children.

Hypoglycemia may also occur in children with sepsis. Check a point-of-care glucose level in any child who appears acutely ill, especially in the presence of abnormal appearance or AMS. Another cause of hypoglycemia in children is poor food intake in the face of an acute illness, such as gastroenteritis, especially in infants and toddlers with limited glycogen reserves.

ASSESSMENT

Signs and symptoms of hypoglycemia can be hard to detect, especially in younger infants who have mild hypoglycemia. The changing signs and symptoms are noted in **TABLE 8–1**. Tachycardia, tachypnea, sweating, agitation, and tremor all reflect increased catecholamine release as the body responds to inadequate sugar supplies to support cellular metabolism. When blood glucose is dangerously low, seizures, coma, and death can occur. It is important to note that hypoglycemia usually has a rapid onset, unlike hyperglycemia.

MANAGEMENT OF HYPOGLYCEMIA IN DIABETES MELLITUS

Children with type 1 (insulin-dependent) DM are often well aware of the signs and symptoms of hypoglycemia, on the basis of past experiences with

TABLE 8–1 Signs and Symptoms of Hypoglycemia

Mild	Hunger Irritability Weakness Agitation Tachypnea Tachycardia
Moderate	Anxiety Blurred vision Stomach ache Headache Dizziness Sweating Pallor Tremors Confusion
Severe	Seizure Coma

TABLE 8–2 Dextrose[a] Administration Guidelines During Seizures

Indications ▪ Infant or child with glucose level <60 mg/dL ▪ Newborn with glucose level <40 mg/dL
Treatment ▪ Newly born: give $D_{10}W$, 2 mL/kg IV or IO ▪ Neonate: give $D_{10}W$, 5 mL/kg IV or IO bolus ▪ Child <2 years old: give $D_{10}W$, 5 mL/kg IV or IO ▪ Child ≥2 years old: give $D_{25}W$, 2 mL/kg or $D_{50}W$, 1 mL/kg IV or IO bolus

[a]If described forms of concentrated dextrose are not available, 5 mL/kg of D_{10} IV solution may be drawn up and given by syringe.

insulin. If a patient with DM is at least physiologically stable and cooperative but has hypoglycemia according to blood glucose testing, allow them to attempt oral glucose replacement. Give 0.5 to 1.0 g/kg of sugar. There are 26 g of glucose in 8 oz (3 ¼ g/oz) of regular (not dietetic) soda, as well as in orange or apple juice. Milk may be an option, but it is usually not preferred because the protein and fat in the milk can slow absorption of the sugar.

Children taking oral hypoglycemic agents (type 2 DM) are also prone to hypoglycemia, although not as frequently as are children with type 1. When present in the child with type 2 DM, hypoglycemia can be more difficult to stabilize. Give the child oral glucose replacement if signs and symptoms of hypoglycemia occur and the child is physiologically stable and cooperative, or treat with IV **dextrose** or IV or intramuscular (IM) glucagon if the child has AMS.

TREATMENT OF HYPOGLYCEMIA

Treat hypoglycemia if the child has AMS and measured serum glucose of less than 40 mg/dL in a newborn or less than 60 mg/dL in a child older than 1 month, as outlined in **TABLE 8–2**. Children have different tolerances to hypoglycemia, so a child may be alert and cooperative with a blood glucose level between 40 and 50 mg/dL. A child in this condition can receive oral glucose, and an infant in this condition can breastfeed.

> **TIP**
> Signs and symptoms of hypoglycemia can be nonspecific.

For the physiologically unstable patient with hypoglycemia and AMS, IV or intraosseous (IO) dextrose should be administered immediately. Recheck the serum glucose level if scene time or transport is prolonged and repeat glucose doses as needed. Use 10% dextrose for infants, neonates, and those younger than 2 years. For those aged 2 years or older, 10% dextrose is still preferred in a peripheral IV, though 25% dextrose is also an option (see **TABLE 8–2**).

If there is no IV access, glucagon should be administered IO or IM (0.02–0.03 mg/kg, up to 1 mg). Repeat in 20 minutes as needed. Glucagon stimulates a transient increase of the blood glucose level if there are liver stores of glycogen (long chains of stored glucose molecules). It is important to note that the incidence of vomiting is increased in children when glucagon is administered. Take care to position the child to ensure airway patency within the first 15 to 20 minutes after administration.

Congenital Adrenal Hyperplasia

Congenital adrenal hyperplasia (CAH) is another endocrine disorder and involves the hormones of the adrenal glands. The adrenal glands help keep the body in balance by making the right amounts of **cortisol**, **aldosterone**, and **androgens**. Although there are many different types of CAH, the most common type (95%) results in a deficiency of cortisol and sometimes aldosterone. As a result, the body cannot appropriately adjust to illness or injury, resulting in fatigue, hypotension, hypoglycemia, or dehydration, and thus CAH may be severe and a threat to life.

Most children with this disorder carry emergency medication with them at all times. Usually, the medication is a steroid such as **hydrocortisone** or **dexamethasone**. Parents should be asked if they have given the stress dose steroid. If not, have them administer the medication if possible. If they have not given steroids, administer hydrocortisone (2 mg/kg) IV, IO, or IM per local protocol. Another dosing strategy recommended by the National Adrenal Disease Foundation is 25 mg of hydrocortisone for infants, 50 mg for school-aged children, and 100 mg for adolescents and young adults. Because the body is unable to adjust to stress, assessment and treatment include checking blood glucose level and administering dextrose as needed, monitoring blood pressure, and replacing fluids as necessary.

Cortisol Deficiency

This deficiency occurs when the adrenal glands do not produce enough cortisol. This may occur for a variety of reasons, including CAH, pituitary gland malfunction, failure of the adrenal gland itself, or long-term steroid use. When children are prescribed steroids for a period, the drugs must be withdrawn gradually to give the adrenal glands a chance to resume function. Normal management includes oral hydrocortisone or IM injections. In certain circumstances, the amount of hydrocortisone should be increased quickly. This is done by administering either oral or IM hydrocortisone.

In any case, when a child with cortisol deficiency becomes sick, many body systems are affected, including the ability to balance blood glucose and regulate body water. These children should always undergo a blood glucose check. Asking the parent or caregiver if the child's normal medication has been administered is appropriate. If the medication has not been administered, give hydrocortisone (2 mg/kg) IV, IO, or IM per local protocol, call the receiving facility, or follow the care plan (found with the rescue medication).

TIP

In a child with impaired adrenal gland function, administration of steroids (hydrocortisone) can be lifesaving.

Panhypopituitarism

This condition affects the pituitary gland, particularly the anterior pituitary, where thyroid-stimulating hormone, adrenocorticotropic hormone, growth hormone, and others are produced. As a result, many other glands of the child's endocrine system are also affected. Affected children are usually diagnosed in infancy, or they can develop the condition after removal of certain brain tumors. Parents or other caregivers generally are well educated in their child's condition. When a child suffering this condition becomes ill, hypoglycemia is common, and dehydration may also be present. These children also need hydrocortisone (2 mg/Kg) IV, IO, or IM.

TRANSPORT

With any child having an endocrine issue, transport is important. If the child is experiencing hyperglycemia, do not delay transport for administration of fluid. The child needs to be transported, so starting IV/IO access en route is appropriate.

However, if a low blood glucose level is present, treatment should be initiated immediately. After administering IV or IO dextrose or IM glucagon, reassess for a return to normal appearance and behavior. If the child with AMS does not return to normal in a few minutes after IV or IO administration or within 15 to 20 minutes after IM glucagon administration, transport immediately and conduct additional assessment on the way to the emergency department (ED). If the child returns to normal, consider doing additional assessment on scene. If the child has no history of DM or other endocrine problems and has either hyperglycemia or hypoglycemia, transport is indicated.

ADDITIONAL ASSESSMENT

Perform history taking when possible. Ask key questions, such as the following:

- How quickly did the symptoms progress?
- Does the patient have diabetes or any other known illness?

- If the patient has diabetes or another endocrine problem, has there been a recent change in medication or meals?
- Is the child receiving insulin, an oral hypoglycemia drug, or any other replacement medication?
- Is this the first episode? If not, how often does this happen?
- Is it possible that the child was exposed to drugs or alcohol?
- When was the last time the child had medication?
- How many caregivers are giving medications? Are they doubling up doses?

For newborns, ask the following questions:

- Has the mother received prenatal care?
- Did the mother have any medical problems with the pregnancy?
- Does the mother have diabetes or did she have gestational diabetes?
- What is the newborn being fed and how often?

After the history, a physical examination should be performed. It is important to continually reassess the patient's status. If the child has DM and received too much **insulin** and there are no physiological or anatomical abnormalities on reassessment, or if the child has another endocrine problem, consider contacting medical control. In some EMS systems, the child with type 1 DM who is not experiencing DKA may be left at the scene with management directed by the primary care physician in consultation with the caregiver. However, the circumstances with type 2 DM are somewhat different, because the oral drugs that are taken for this condition have a longer duration of action than does most insulin and the child may need ongoing administration of glucose to maintain appropriate blood glucose levels. *Patients with type 2 DM treated with oral agents who have experienced hypoglycemia should not be left on the scene.* If the child has an emergency medication that needs to be administered, or if the child has type 2 DM and is experiencing an episode of hypoglycemia, transport the child to the ED.

> **TIP**
>
> Do not leave patients on the scene if they have type 2 DM treated with oral agents and have experienced hypoglycemia.

Summary of Endocrine Disorders

Common endocrine disorders in children include diabetes mellitus, congenital adrenal hyperplasia, and cortisol deficiency. The caregiver may be the best judge of the child's condition, especially in the infant or toddler, in whom developmental assessment is more challenging. Appearance and the Alert, Verbal, Pain, Unresponsive (AVPU) scale work in concert to help assess the patient. Address the airway, breathing, and circulation (the ABCs) first and especially consider causes of dehydration, such as hyperglycemia, and reversible causes, such as hypoglycemia.

ENVIRONMENTAL EMERGENCIES

Common pediatric environmental emergencies include temperature-related problems, bites, and stings. Each of these emergencies can range from mild to severe. Match the intensity of the intervention to the severity of the illness or injury.

Heat-Related Emergencies

Heat-related emergencies involve 2 separate and distinct processes leading to 3 main heat-related emergencies:

- Heat cramps
- Heat exhaustion
- Heat stroke

Heat cramps and heat exhaustion are caused by a combination of fluid deficit and electrolyte imbalance. Heat stroke, however, is a result of a resetting of the heat-regulating mechanism in the hypothalamus of the brain, resulting in **hyperthermia**.

Heat cramps are a combination of electrolyte imbalance and dehydration in which the electrolyte imbalance precipitates muscle spasms, typically in the muscles of the long bones. Affected children complain of pain in their legs, arms, and sometimes abdomen. Because heat cramps usually occur during activity, the skin is warm and sweaty. Tachycardia may be present and may be caused by pain, high temperature, or dehydration. **Heat exhaustion** is a combination of electrolyte imbalance and dehydration in which the dehydration precipitates dizziness and/or syncope. Because a volume deficit is present, the skin is often pale, cool, and diaphoretic. Tachycardia and tachypnea are also common. Hypoglycemia is not common but should be assessed for and treated as necessary.

Heat stroke occurs when the body gains more heat than it loses, either through exertion or externally, and shows signs of multiorgan failure and central nervous system dysfunction. This is often with body temperatures higher than 40.6°C (105°F). As a result, the basal metabolic rate is greatly increased, and every body organ is affected. Because the enzymes within the organs and body systems are designed to work within a relatively narrow temperature range, organ failure occurs. Altered mental status, heart failure with pulmonary edema, kidney and liver failure, and profound hypotension are evident. Because of the increased metabolic rate, hypoglycemia is common. The skin is usually dry and red, tachycardia is extreme (usually > 150 beats/min), and tachypnea is present.

Heat-related emergencies, however, are rarely as clear cut as they are described. The child with heat exhaustion may have AMS, or the child with heat stroke may be sweating. Regardless of the type of heat-related emergency, it is very important that a heat-related emergency is recognized and treatment implemented. In the pediatric population, heat-related emergencies occur most commonly when young children are left in a closed car, or when older children who are not acclimated to heat participate in sports during periods of high environmental temperatures and do not hydrate adequately. Because of the difficulty of obtaining temperature readings in the field, the assessment of such patients often occurs without the benefit of an objective temperature measurement.

Physiologic considerations in infants and toddlers with heat-related emergencies include immature thermoregulatory systems, greater body surface area-to-mass ratio, and a reduced ability to dissipate heat (**TABLE 8–3**). These characteristics predispose infants and toddlers to experiencing heat-related emergencies, particularly heat stroke, much more quickly than older children.

ASSESSMENT

The history should include the following:

- Environmental temperature
- Duration of environmental exposure
- Activities and events before symptom development
- Preexisting medical conditions

TABLE 8–3 Typical Clinical Presentation of Heat-Related Emergencies

Clinical Presentation	Signs and Symptoms
Heat cramps	▪ Normal level of consciousness ▪ Slightly elevated body temperature ▪ Painful muscle spasms
Heat exhaustion	▪ Mild AMS ▪ Tachycardia, tachypnea, hypotension ▪ Core temperature 38–40°C (100.4–104°F) ▪ Fatigue ▪ Headache ▪ Diaphoresis
Heat stroke	▪ Severe AMS; confusion to coma ▪ Tachycardia, hypotension ▪ Core temperature > 40.6°C (105°F) ▪ Flushed, dry skin ▪ Nausea and vomiting

Abbreviation: AMS, altered mental status.

MANAGEMENT

The management of heat-related illness depends on the severity of symptoms, especially the patient's level of consciousness and cardiovascular status. Because the mechanism is different from fever caused by infections, use of antipyretics is not effective.

HEAT CRAMPS

- Ensure a cool environment.
- Remove excess clothing.
- Provide oral rehydration with an electrolyte-containing solution (preferable) or cool water.
- Establish vascular access with normal saline at a to-keep-open (TKO) rate.

HEAT EXHAUSTION

- Ensure a cool environment.
- Provide cool misting or light sponging with tepid water and allow moisture to evaporate.
- Fan the patient.

- Provide oral rehydration with an electrolyte-containing solution (preferable) or cool water.
- Establish vascular access and initiate fluid replacement with crystalloid fluid.

HEAT STROKE

- Ensure airway management, assist ventilations, and intubate if indicated.
- Establish vascular access and fluid replacement with crystalloid fluid at 20 mL/kg.
- Provide cool misting or light sponging with tepid water and allow moisture to evaporate.
- Use aggressive cooling measures: ice bags to axilla, groin, and neck; cold water immersion if immediate transport is delayed (**FIGURE 8–3**).
- Frequently remeasure core temperature.
- Treat hypoglycemia.
- Prevent shivering.
- Treat for shock.

> **TIP**
>
> Early recognition and frequent reassessment of a heat-related emergency are important, because the patient's temperature may continue to rise despite use of initial management techniques.

Summary of Heat-Related Emergencies

Rapid recognition of heat-related emergencies is essential to effective management. Reassess vital signs frequently to evaluate the patient's response to treatment. Aggressive cooling measures are required for heat stroke.

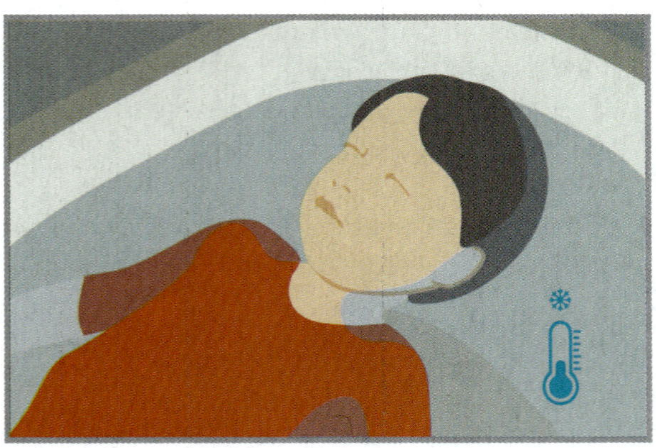

FIGURE 8–3 If immediate transport is delayed, use aggressive cooling measures, such as cold-water immersion.

Cold-Related Emergencies

Hypothermia is a core temperature of less than 35°C (95°F). Infants and toddlers are at especially high risk of experiencing hypothermia because of their greater body surface-area-to-mass ratio, decreased body fat, increased permeability of thin skin, and limited ability to shiver and produce heat. Extended exposure to a cold environment and immersion in cold water are the 2 most common causes of hypothermia in young children. Children with severe illness or injury may also develop hypothermia. Finally, infants and young children may experience hypothermia while being exposed for medical evaluation, especially in cold environments. The presence of hypothermia may precipitate or extend shock and complicate resuscitation, regardless of the underlying condition.

ASSESSMENT

History taking should include recent illness or injury and circumstances of exposure.

AIRWAY AND BREATHING

The physical examination should include special attention to airway and breathing. Because hypothermia leads to a slowing of metabolism, the child may hypoventilate, with slow or shallow respirations.

CIRCULATION

Bradycardia and hypotension may be present because of hypothermia itself or because of a concurrent hypoxic insult. Hypothermia may also lead to cardiac dysrhythmias or cardiac arrest, including pulseless electrical activity (PEA). Of note, it is one of the reversible causes of cardiac arrest. On examination, the skin is often pale and cool.

DISABILITY

Mental status may range from confusion to coma, depending on the degree of hypothermia. Again, hypoxia may be the underlying cause of AMS, especially in patients who have experienced submersion, so ensure the adequacy of oxygenation and ventilation. Depending on the circumstances, hypoglycemia may also be present.

CORE BODY TEMPERATURE

Obtain core body temperature, when possible, with a thermometer that registers less than 34 °C (94 °F).

Determine the degree of hypothermia according to the following classification:

- Mild: 35–36 °C (93–95 °F)
- Moderate: 30–34 °C (86–93 °F)
- Severe: less than 30 °C (< 86 °F)

Loss of the compensatory mechanism of shivering to generate heat is characteristic of moderate to severe hypothermia.

MANAGEMENT

Management of the patient with hypothermia depends on the core temperature.

1. *Support airway, breathing, and circulation as indicated.*
2. *Prevent heat loss.*
   It is crucial to prevent further heat loss. Remove wet clothing, dry the skin, and cover the patient after the examination is completed (**FIGURE 8–4**). Apply a hat or head wrap, because a high proportion of heat is lost through the head.
3. *Rewarm.*
   External, passive rewarming is appropriate for mild to moderate hypothermia. In the case of severe hypothermia, external rewarming may shunt cold blood to the core, leading to further complications. Core rewarming in the ED is the appropriate therapy for these patients.
   a. Mild hypothermia: apply warm blankets, increase ambient temperature of the ambulance; EMS clinicians should be uncomfortably warm.
   b. Moderate hypothermia: apply warm blankets, heat packs to axilla and groin.

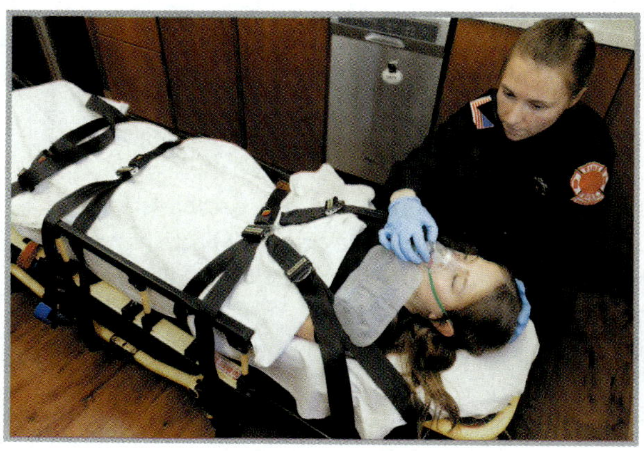

FIGURE 8–4 Cover patient after examination.

ALS

c. **Severe hypothermia: use cautious movement with gentle handling; use warmed, humidified oxygen; use warmed IV solution; treat hypoglycemia if present; provide rapid transport to a definitive care facility for core rewarming.**

Summary of Cold-Related Emergencies

Pediatric patients' physiological and developmental characteristics place them at risk of experiencing cold-related emergencies. Accurate assessment of the degree of hypothermia is essential to effective care of children in the prehospital environment.

TIP

Use caution when rewarming the pediatric patient with severe hypothermia in the prehospital environment, because cold acidic blood from the periphery could lead to further deterioration. Focus instead on preventing further heat loss and supporting airway, breathing, and circulation (the ABCs).

Bites and Stings

Bites and stings typically result in a puncture-type wound or laceration (**FIGURE 8–5**). Most of these injuries are minor. However, some stings, such as from a bumblebee or fire ant, may produce a severe

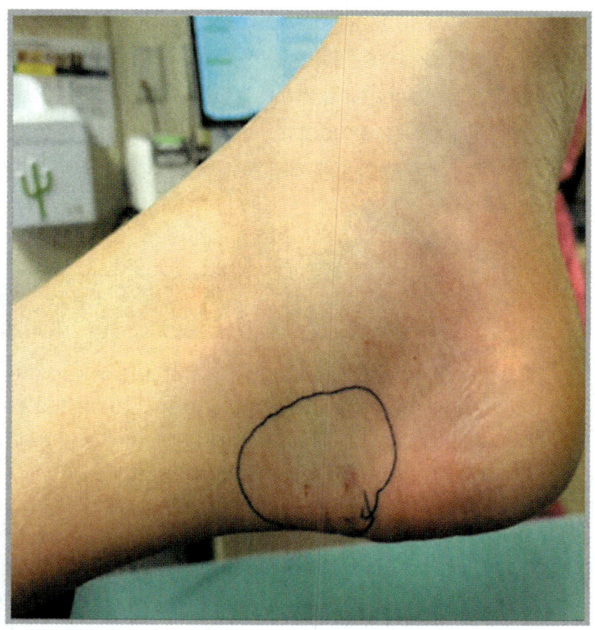

FIGURE 8–5 Snakebite resulting in puncture-type wound.

Courtesy of Justin Assioun, MD.

allergic or **anaphylactic reaction**. Some bites, such as from a rattlesnake, spider, or scorpion, can cause life-threatening **envenomation** or bleeding problems. Bites and stings may pose a greater risk to the pediatric patient because of their smaller body weight and higher metabolic rate.

ASSESSMENT

History taking should include the following:

- Time and type of bite or sting
- Activities since the injury
- Known allergies to bites or stings
- Immunization history

The physical examination should include special attention to the following:

- Be aware that clinical presentation varies depending on the type of bite, the presence or absence of envenomation, and the time since the bite occurred.
- Assess airway, breathing, and circulation; respiratory distress and **anaphylaxis** may be the initial signs of a bite envenomation.
- Inspect for type, anatomical location, and number of punctures or wounds.
- Assess for swelling, discoloration, and pain at or around the site.

MANAGEMENT: BITES

Management depends on the type of insect, snake, or animal involved in the envenomation.

General Management

- Support airway, breathing, and circulation; establish vascular access.
- Treat anaphylaxis if present (see Chapter 4).

Local Management

- Stop bleeding and perform wound care.
- If an envenomation is suspected, rinse area with water; for spider bites, consider cool compresses to the affected area to reduce swelling and pain. Neither cool compresses nor ice is recommended for snakebites.
- Minimize the activity level of the pediatric patient. Keep them in a supine position. Most venom is transported through the lymphatic system, and increased physical activity increases the rate of spread throughout the body.
- Immobilize an affected extremity at or below the level of the heart. It may be beneficial to keep the patient supine.
- Transport rapidly to evaluate for possible **antivenin** administration and for definitive care.
- Remove any clothing or jewelry on the affected area or limb.

MANAGEMENT: STINGS

General Management

- Support airway, breathing, and circulation; establish vascular access.
- Treat anaphylaxis if present (see Chapter 4).

Local Management

- Remove stinger if visible (swipe away with credit card).
- Apply cold compresses.
- Consider medications based on clinical presentation: epinephrine in the case of anaphylaxis; albuterol in the case of wheezing; diphenhydramine in the case of hives, itching, or swelling; analgesics as necessary.

CASE STUDY 1

A 6-year-old child was playing outside in the garden. The caregiver called 9-1-1 when the child started to have difficulty breathing. On arrival at the scene, the Pediatric Assessment Triangle reveals a pale, irritable child with audible wheezing and significant supraclavicular and subcostal retractions. Respiratory rate is 32 breaths/min, heart rate is 140 beats/min, and blood pressure is 90 mm Hg by palpation. During the physical examination, you note a red, swollen area on the side of the child's neck.

1. What are the possible causes of respiratory distress in this child?
2. What are the immediate management priorities?

Summary of Bites and Stings

Insect bites are common in children and may result in complications ranging from mild local reactions to life-threatening anaphylaxis. Other types of envenomation, such as snake bites or scorpion stings, are more specific to particular regions of the United States. Early recognition of the nature of the injury is important. Field treatment of anaphylaxis may be lifesaving. Prompt transport to a definitive care facility is crucial if antivenin treatment is needed.

> **TIP**
>
> Abnormal behavior may be the first clue that the pediatric patient has been bitten or stung. A thorough inspection of the patient's skin, particularly around the waist, distal extremities, axillae, and neck, may reveal the location of the bite or sting.

CASE STUDY ANSWERS

CASE STUDY 1

A previously healthy child playing outdoors with an acute onset of respiratory distress should be assessed for bites or stings and for exposure to possible environmental allergens or toxins, such as gardening-related chemicals. Also, it would be useful to determine if the child has a history of asthma or environmental allergies, including to bee stings. In this case, the presence of a swollen, reddened area suggests the possibility of an insect bite, most likely a hymenoptera (bee) sting, and the sudden onset of significant symptoms suggests anaphylaxis.

Supplemental oxygen and inhaled bronchodilators for wheezing should be provided. In addition, IM epinephrine should be administered because of the possibility of anaphylaxis.

At the hospital, the child was given additional antihistamines and oral steroids. She was observed for several hours and discharged home with a prescription for an epinephrine autoinjector. Education on use of the epinephrine autoinjector was provided to the family.

> **ALS**
>
> **If possible, establish vascular access and give IV diphenhydramine to help with symptoms. Watch for signs of shock and treat with IV fluids as appropriate. Even if the child shows marked improvement with these treatments, transport urgently because symptoms may recur as the medication effect wears off. Monitor carefully during transport.**

Suggested References

TEXTBOOKS

American Academy of Orthopaedic Surgeons. *Emergency Care and Transportation of the Sick and Injured.* 12th ed. Jones and Bartlett Learning; 2021

American Academy of Orthopaedic Surgeons. *Nancy Caroline's Emergency Care in the Streets.* 9th ed. Jones and Bartlett Learning; 2023

American Academy of Pediatrics and the American College of Emergency Physicians. *APLS: The Pediatric Emergency Medicine Resource.* 5th ed. Jones and Bartlett Learning; 2012

Rogers JL. *McCance & Brasher's Pathophysiology: The Biologic Basis for Disease in Adults and Children.* 9th ed. Mosby Elsevier; 2024

Smith S; Advanced Life Support Group, eds. *Advanced Paediatric Life Support: The Practical Approach.* 7th ed. John Wiley & Sons Ltd; 2023

ARTICLES

Arslanian S, Bacha F, Grey M, Marcus MD, White NH, Zeitler P. Evaluation and management of youth-onset type 2 diabetes: a position statement by the American Diabetes Association. *Diabetes Care.* 2018;41(12):2648–2668. PMID: 30425094 doi: 10.2337/dci18-0052

Epstein Y, Yanovich R. Heatstroke. *N Engl J Med.* 2019;380(25):2449–2459. PMID: 31216400 doi: 10.1056/NEJMra1810762

Libman I, Haynes A, Lyons S, et al. ISPAD clinical practice consensus guidelines 2022: definition, epidemiology, and classification of diabetes in children and adolescents. *Pediatr Diabetes*. 2022;23(8):1160–1174. PMID: 36537527 doi: 10.1111/pedi.13454

Wolfsdorf JI, Glaser N, Agus M, et al. ISPAD clinical practice consensus guidelines 2018: diabetic ketoacidosis and the hyperglycemic hyperosmolar state. *Pediatr Diabetes*. 2018;19(suppl 27):155–177. PMID: 29900641 doi: 10.1111/pedi.12701

CHAPTER 9

Trauma

Robert Sharkey, EMT-P, IC
Theresa A. Walls, MD, MPH, FAAP

LEARNING OBJECTIVES

1. **Explain the unique anatomical features of children that predispose them to injuries.**
2. **Sequence the primary assessment of the injured child.**
3. **Integrate the essential trauma interventions into the hands-on ABCDEs.**
4. **Assess sports concussions and return-to-play guidelines.**
5. **Distinguish different approaches in airway management of injured children.**
6. **Explain spinal motion restriction and the methods to achieve it.**
7. **Discuss assessment and treatment of pediatric burn patients.**

Introduction

One-half of the children transported by emergency medical services (EMS) have an acute injury. Fortunately, the most common injuries are minor, such as lacerations, minor or superficial burns, mild closed-head injuries, and extremity fractures. In minor trauma, the role of the EMS clinician is straightforward: Perform a scene size-up, assess for physiological or anatomical problems, and transport to the nearest appropriate emergency department (ED). Treatment may entail wound care, spinal motion restriction, splinting, and pain control when necessary.

Multisystem trauma, in contrast, provides the EMS clinician with a great challenge and demands a disciplined assessment and a child-specific approach to treatment. Most principles of adult trauma management can be effectively and safely applied to children. Important modifications in assessment are related to differences in mechanisms of injury, anatomy, and physiological responses. Modifications in treatment are related to differences in anatomy, equipment sizes, and emergency procedures.

Between infancy and adulthood, injuries are the most common cause of death. Intentional injuries, primarily nonaccidental trauma in infants and homicide and suicide in adolescents, are the leading mechanisms of traumatic death. Approximately 80% to 90% of pediatric trauma involves a blunt mechanism. This differs from the adult population, in which there is a higher incidence of penetrating injuries. Handgun injuries, however, are on the rise in children and are now the most common cause of penetrating injuries in adolescents.

Most injuries are preventable. Child restraint devices in automobiles, bicycle helmets, swimming pool fences, and window barriers have significantly reduced the incidence of blunt injuries and drowning. Stricter building codes have reduced the incidence of fires, although burns continue to be a leading cause of death in children younger than 14 years. Pediatric trauma challenges the EMS clinician to manage not just the injury and related physiological abnormalities, but also to treat the child's pain and communicate with and support the injured child and the affected family.

Pediatric emergencies are less frequent in the prehospital arena, which can lead to discomfort among EMS clinicians when treating these patients. This discomfort may stem from the inherent challenges of pediatric cases and the EMS clinician's perception of their own lack of preparedness. Additionally, incidents involving severe injury or death of a child can impose significant emotional strain on prehospital personnel. These situations often evoke fears and concerns that may be related to their own children's vulnerability, and may hinder their ability to maintain emotional detachment and affect their performance. However, education and experience in managing pediatric patients can enhance a EMS clinician's confidence, competence, and ability to remain composed in such high-stress situations. In the aftermath of particularly traumatic pediatric cases, critical incident

CASE STUDY 1

Your unit is dispatched to a call where a child has had a fall. You are greeted in the street by a neighbor who leads you to a 7-year-old boy who is lying face up on the grass next to a tall tree. The neighbor indicates that she observed the child fall about 20 feet out of the tree. No one has moved him. Your primary assessment reveals a child who is only responsive to painful stimuli. His breathing is shallow, with audible snoring sounds. His color is pale with slight cyanosis. The respiratory rate is 10 breaths/min, heart rate is 130 beats/min, and blood pressure is 76 mm Hg/palp. His skin is cool, the radial pulse is weak, and the capillary refill time is greater than 3 seconds. Pupils are equal and reactive. The oxygen saturation is 90%. The boy has a hematoma on the right side of his head. His right upper leg is swollen, with an obvious deformity of the right femur.

1. Based on the primary assessment and mechanism of injury, what are the child's most likely injuries?
2. Discuss the initial stabilization and prehospital management of this child.

stress management or employee assistance programs may offer valuable support to EMS clinicians, helping them cope with the emotional impact.

Fatal Injury Mechanisms

TABLE 9–1 summarizes the most frequent fatal mechanisms of injury in children and adolescents.

Unique Anatomical Features of Children: Effect on Injury Patterns

HEAD

Head injury is the most common serious traumatic injury in children. Even in multisystem trauma, the severity of **traumatic brain injury (TBI)** usually defines the patient's medical and functional outcome. Many of the essential interventions in managing pediatric trauma are directed at preserving brain function.

Until the child is 6 years old, the head is disproportionately large in relationship to overall body mass and surface area compared to adults. Because of this anatomical feature, in a fall or in an **acceleration-deceleration event**, such as a motor vehicle crash, the head functions like the heavy end of a lawn dart, becoming the lead point (**FIGURE 9–1**). Consequently, the head and brain of a child are more commonly injured in blunt trauma than they are in adults.

SPINAL COLUMN

As a group, children do not experience many vertebral fractures or dislocations. When vertebral fractures do occur, the event typically involves a high-energy mechanism (eg, motor vehicle crash or diving incident) with extreme **flexion** or extension or axial loading of the **spine**. Traumatic spinal cord injury, or disruption of the central nerve pathways, is also rare in children.

TABLE 9–1 Leading Mechanisms of Injury-Related Death

Age 0–4 Years	Age 5–9 Years	Age 10–14 Years	Age 15–19 Years
Suffocation	Vehicular trauma	Vehicular trauma	Firearm[a]
Drowning	Drowning	Firearm[a]	Vehicular trauma
Vehicular trauma	Firearm[a]	Suffocation[b]	Poisoning[b]
Firearm[a]	Fire/Burn	Drowning	Suffocation[b]
Fire/Burn	Suffocation[b]	Fire/Burn	Drowning

Data from 10 leading causes of injury deaths by age group, 2023, both sexes, all ages, all races. Centers for Disease Control and Prevention, Web-based Injury Statistics Query and Reporting System. Accessed February 8, 2026. https://wisqars.cdc.gov/pdfs/leading-causes-of-injury-deaths-by-age-group_2023_508.pdf

[a] Firearm deaths included homicides and suicides.

[b] Many suffocations and poisoning were suicides.

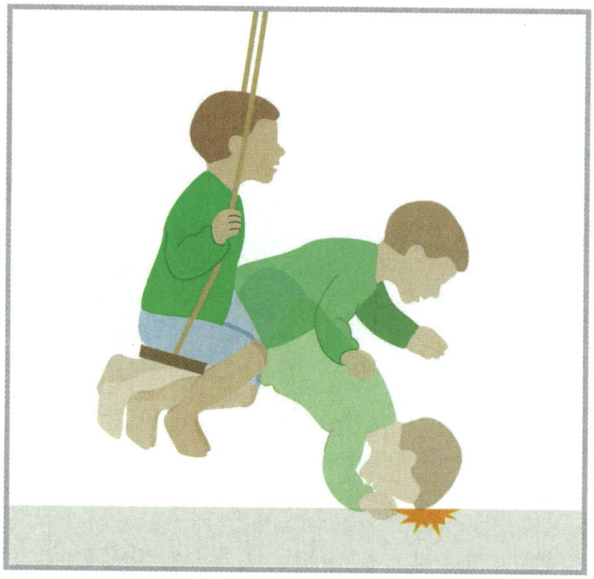

FIGURE 9–1 A disproportionately large head size in children explains their tendency to fall "head first," leading to a high rate of TBI.

The most common cervical spine injuries in children occur at the level of the high cervical spine. Weaker neck muscles and spinal ligaments, in conjunction with a "heavy" head, create greater vulnerability to acceleration-deceleration forces common in motor vehicle crashes and falls. In reality, most children with a high cervical injury are in cardiac arrest on the scene and die despite all medical interventions.

CAUTION

It is difficult to find a cervical collar that properly fits an infant or a toddler. When a properly sized collar is not available, use padding around the head and neck and stabilize the child's spine with padding to protect the spinal cord.

The most common lower spine injuries occur in the middle to lower **thoracic** spine. Mechanisms include direct blows, falls, or spinal **compression** during a motor vehicle crash from improper seat belt use. The use of booster seats in vehicles reduces these types of injuries by allowing proper fitting of the lap and shoulder belt.

TIP

Unintentional injuries are the No. 1 cause of death in all children aged 1 year through adolescence. However, since 2020, firearm-related injuries have surpassed motor vehicle crash injuries in those aged 1 to 19 years.

CHEST

The ribs of the child are more pliable and compressible than those of the adult because they are composed mainly of **cartilage**. For this reason, rib fractures and **flail chest** are uncommon in younger children, even with high-energy transfers. However, this bony compressibility in conjunction with a **chest wall** that is poorly protected by fat or muscle leads to direct transfer of energy to the lungs and heart on impact (**FIGURE 9–2**). Serious injuries of the thoracic organs can occur with or without external signs of injury, such as **abrasions**, bruises, or tenderness.

Pulmonary contusion, or bruising of the lung tissue itself, is the most common form of serious lung injury in children. You may suspect this condition in a child who sustains blunt chest trauma and has hypoxia or respiratory distress; however, pulmonary contusions may take time to fully develop and can only be diagnosed by radiography, which makes the distinction between pulmonary contusion and pneumothorax difficult in the field.

If a child has a blunt injury mechanism, there may be decreased breath sounds from a pulmonary contusion, so be careful about placing a needle in the pleural space, because a contusion is more likely than a tension pneumothorax. In contrast, a child with progressive hypoxia and respiratory distress after a penetrating injury probably does have a tension pneumothorax, and needle decompression is indicated.

Penetrating chest trauma may cause serious problems in oxygenation and ventilation. When the chest wall, back, or high abdomen is penetrated, look for a pneumothorax, a **tension**

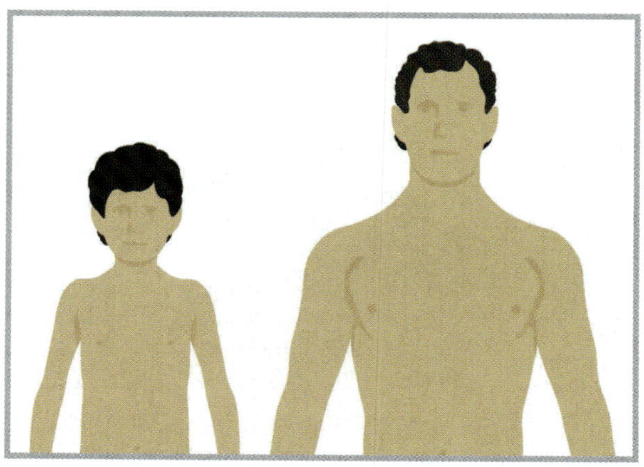

FIGURE 9–2 The child's chest wall is not well muscularized, so it lacks the soft tissue protection from injury that is present in adolescents and adults.

pneumothorax, and **sucking chest wounds**. These injuries are unusual in children but, if present, require specific and immediate lifesaving treatment in the field. **Needle decompression** may save the life of a child with a tension pneumothorax. The procedure is similar for a child and an adult, the major difference being the size of the catheter. The procedure is illustrated in **Procedure 23, Needle Thoracostomy**.

The diaphragm of a child can rise as high as the nipple line during full expiration. When there is blunt or penetrating trauma to the chest below the nipple line or below the scapula, internal injury may include both the chest and abdominal organs (**FIGURE 9–3**).

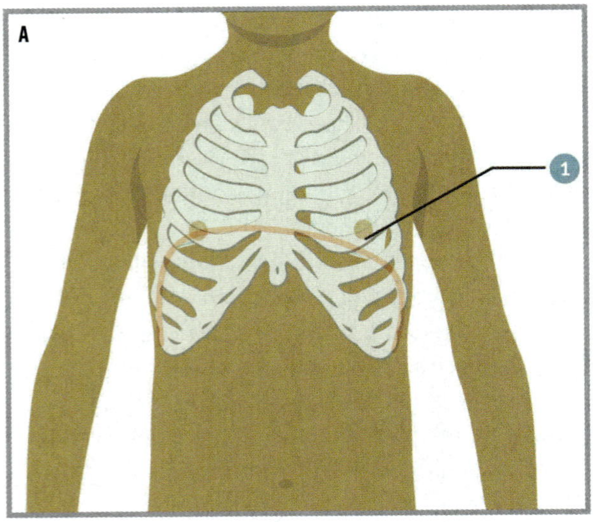

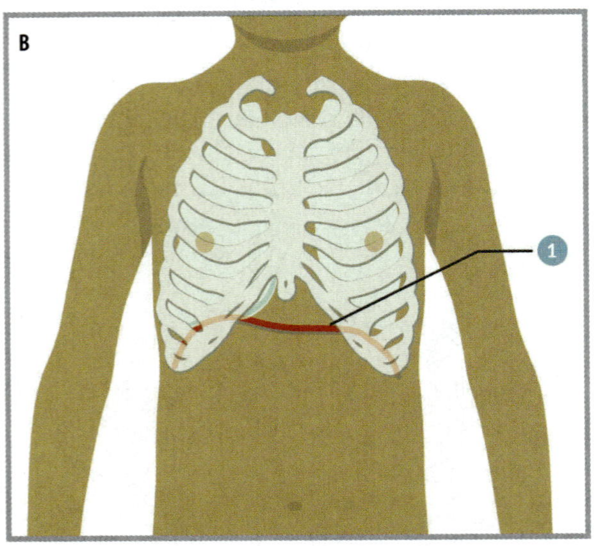

FIGURE 9–3 The diaphragm can rise as high as the nipple line during full expiration **(A)** and can flatten to the level of the lowest ribs during full inspiration. 1. Diaphragm. **(B)**. Therefore, injuries to the abdominal organs may occur after chest trauma. 1. Diaphragm.

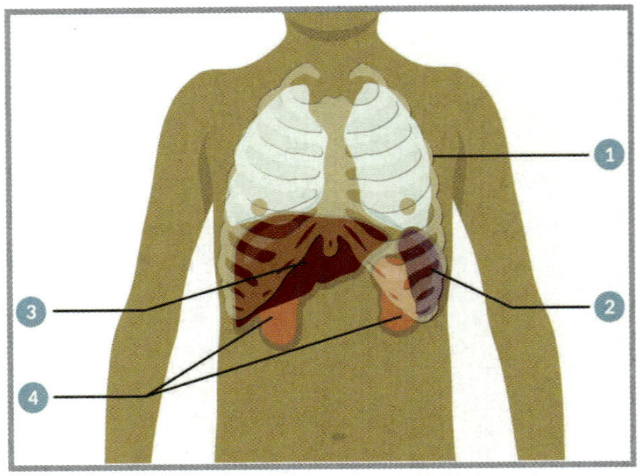

FIGURE 9–4 The solid organs of the upper abdominal cavity are disproportionately large and more exposed in children than in adults. They are poorly protected by the thin chest wall and undeveloped abdominal muscles. 1. Ribs, 2. Spleen, 3. Liver, 4. Kidneys.

ABDOMEN

The **abdomen** is often the site of serious blood loss in pediatric patients and is the most common site of injury causing shock. The solid organs of the upper abdominal cavity are the liver, **spleen**, and kidneys. These organs are disproportionately larger and more exposed than in adults and are poorly protected by the child's softer ribs and relatively undeveloped abdominal muscles (**FIGURE 9–4**). The liver is the largest abdominal organ, located in the right upper quadrant, and extends below the rib cage in infants, toddlers, and preschool-aged children. It is the most commonly injured abdominal organ in young children. The spleen, located in the left upper quadrant, is also commonly injured. Injuries to the hollow organs of the abdomen—the stomach, small bowel, and bladder—are less common than solid organ injuries. **Pelvic fractures** are uncommon in children, although they become more frequent in adolescents.

> **TIP**
>
> Because the child's chest wall is smaller, thinner, and less muscular than an adult's, lung sounds may be transmitted throughout the chest cavity, making it difficult to appreciate asymmetric breath sounds. Listening along the lateral sides of the chest wall under the axillae (armpits) may improve the ability to distinguish sound variability between the right and left lungs.

> **TIP**
>
> If there is penetration of the chest wall below the nipples, or below the scapula, anticipate abdominal injury as well as pneumothorax, including tension pneumothorax.

CAUTION

Remember that young children rely on their diaphragm to breathe, but also use abdominal muscles. Do not restrict the abdomen when protecting the patient's spine or restraining for transport.
Assume that every child with a serious trauma has a life-threatening abdominal injury. Many children with abdominal injury have no localizing signs and may not complain of pain. Fear, young age, or distracting injuries may hide signs and symptoms. When present, signs include progressive abdominal distension, rigidity, tenderness, abdominal wall contusions or abrasions, and hemodynamic instability.

TIP

The abdomen is the most frequent site of injury causing shock. Serial examinations greatly improve the accuracy of assessment of abdominal injury. In the injured child with multisystem blunt trauma, the EMS clinician should always have a high index of suspicion for intra-abdominal bleeding if shock presents.

EXTREMITIES

Compared with adults, children's bones are more flexible, and their muscles are not as well developed. They are especially vulnerable to fractures at the weak, cartilaginous growth plates near the ends of the bones (**FIGURE 9–5**). Fractures that disrupt the **periosteum** on only one side of the bone (often called **greenstick fractures**) are common, as are **buckle fractures** in which the pliant bone is compressed with **axial loading**. These fractures may be present in the absence of significant swelling, bruising, or deformity. *Suspect a fracture whenever there is point tenderness or limited range of motion, especially around a joint.*

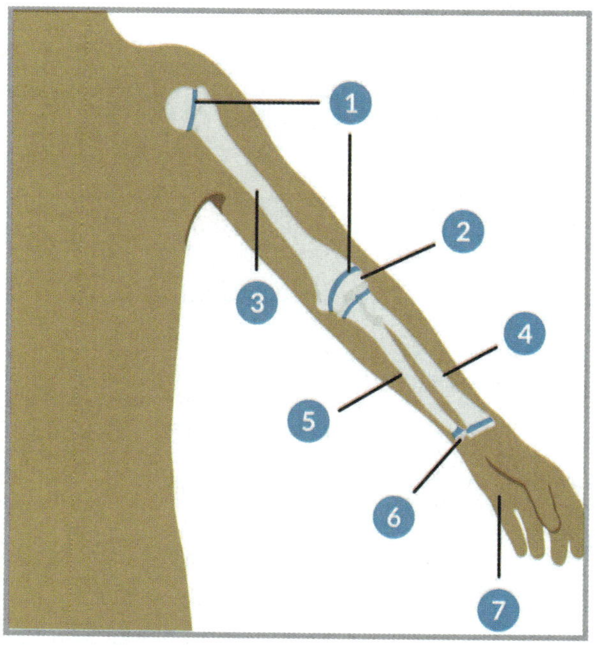

FIGURE 9–5 The physeal (growth) plates at the ends of children's bones are easily fractured. 1. Growth plates, 2. Elbow, 3. Humerus, 4. Radius, 5. Ulna, 6. Growth plate, 7. Hand.

CAUTION

Never overlook the possibility of solid organ injury when there has been blunt injury because fear, inability to speak, or distracting injuries may mask signs and symptoms.

ALS

Pain is frequently underestimated and undertreated in children. Consider analgesia for pain management in children with isolated extremity fractures. Morphine sulfate or fentanyl are the medications of choice for severe pain. Fentanyl can be given via the intranasal route with an atomizer (see Procedure 15, Intranasal Medication Administration). Repeat with half doses as needed for pain control. Fentanyl is faster acting than morphine and also has a shorter duration of action. Be extremely careful with morphine administration in children who have a serious injury mechanism or signs of compensated or decompensated shock. Morphine can drop the child's blood pressure and critical perfusion when it is administered to a hypovolemic patient. Always be alert for signs of respiratory depression, especially if multiple doses of an opioid are administered.

The most serious complications of extremity injuries are neurovascular problems and blood loss into the soft tissues at the fracture site. Blood loss may be severe in long-bone fractures (eg, fractures of the femur) or in pelvic fractures. Pain is the symptom usually associated with serious extremity injuries. It is important to check pulses after a splint is placed, which can also help with pain control.

TIP

Suspect an extremity fracture whenever findings include point tenderness or limited range of motion.

TIP

Injuries to the **physeal plate** or growth plate of a long bone can be permanently damaging to the limb.

SKIN

The skin provides temperature regulation. Children's skin is thinner and has a greater surface area in relation to their overall size and weight than the skin of adults. Because of this, heat transfer (loss or gain) from the skin can be rapid. Even without injuries that damage the skin, such as burns, injured children are at increased risk of experiencing hypothermia, which can in turn compromise core organ function. The signs and symptoms of hypothermia can mimic those of hypovolemia and shock. In infants, hypothermia may deplete vital glucose stores. To avoid hypothermia, especially in an infant or a toddler, prevent heat loss by ensuring that the child is dry and covered, and by limiting the time that the undressed child is exposed for assessment and procedures. Turn up the heat in the ambulance. For the temperature to be warm enough for an infant who is disrobed, it may be uncomfortably hot for an adult. In extremely hot environments, beware of hyperthermia.

Mechanism of Injury: Effect on Injury Patterns

The different mechanisms of injury in children in combination with their unique anatomical features lead to predictable patterns of injury. Head injury caused by blunt trauma is very common in children. Although there are many cases of minor closed-head injuries associated with play that do not have neurological consequences, high-energy impacts are often associated with traumatic brain injury (TBI). Because of a child's small size, high-energy blunt impacts can lead to **multisystem trauma**, including the head, chest, abdomen, and long bones.

TABLE 9–2 lists the common mechanisms of pediatric injury and the associated patterns of injury. **FIGURE 9–6** illustrates several typical injury sequences in children.

Assessment of the Injured Child

The initial steps in assessing the injured child follow the generic approach for all children outlined in Chapters 1 and 2. This includes prearrival mental preparation based on dispatch information and a scene size-up on arrival. Always use **universal precautions** or personal protective measures and equipment to prevent potentially harmful or infectious exposures to bodily fluids.

The on-scene trauma evaluation includes (1) general assessment using the Pediatric Assessment Triangle (PAT), (2) the primary assessment with the hands-on ABCDEs (Airway, Breathing, Circulation, Disability [neurological status], and Exposure [skin/temperature]), which has been modified for trauma to xABCDE, where x stands for exsanguination, then (3) additional assessment consisting of a focused history and physical examination and a detailed physical examination for trauma. A child with multisystem injuries needs a prioritized, efficient on-scene approach to assessment and

TABLE 9–2 Common Mechanisms and Associated Patterns of Pediatric Injury

Mechanism of Injury		Associated Patterns of Injury
Fall from a bicycle	Without helmet	Head and neck injuries, scalp and facial lacerations, upper-extremity fractures
	With helmet	Upper-extremity fractures
	Hitting handlebar	Internal abdominal injuries
Fall from a height	Low	Upper-extremity fractures
	Medium	Head and neck injuries, upper- and lower-extremity fractures
	High	Chest and abdominal injuries, head and neck injuries, upper- and lower-extremity fractures
Motor vehicle crash (child is passenger)	Unrestrained	Multiple traumas, head and neck injuries, scalp and facial lacerations
	Air bag	Head and neck, facial and eye injuries
	Restrained	Chest and abdominal injuries, cervical and lower-spine fractures
Motor vehicle crash (child is pedestrian)	Low speed	Lower-extremity fractures
	High speed	Chest and abdominal injuries, head and neck injuries, lower-extremity fractures

Reproduced with permission from American College of Surgeons, Committee on Trauma. *ATLS Advanced Trauma Life Support*. 10th ed. American College of Surgeons; 2018.

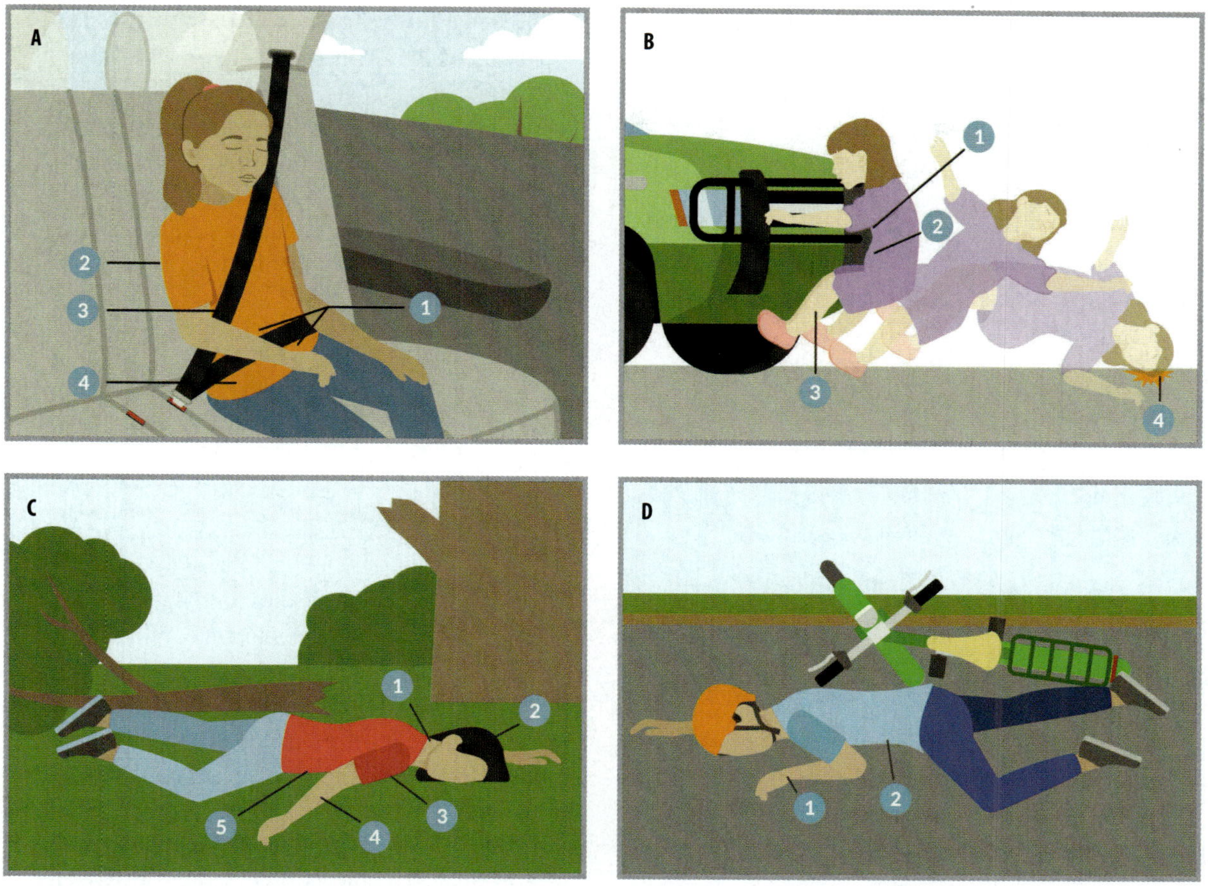

FIGURE 9–6 **A.** A restrained child in a motor vehicle crash may have a lap belt injury involving solid organs, bowel, and spine. 1. Solid organs, 2. Spine, 3. Seat belt, 4. Bowel. **B.** Children frequently sustain multisystem injuries involving the head, chest, abdomen, and long bones. 1. Chest, 2. Abdomen, 3. Leg, 4. Head. **C.** A fall from height frequently involves injuries to the head and neck, chest, abdomen, and the extremities. 1. Neck, 2. Head, 3. Chest, 4. Arm, 5. Abdomen. **D.** A fall over the handlebars of a bike may result in injuries to the abdomen and extremities. 1. Wrist, 2. Abdomen.

treatment and rapid transport to the appropriate regional trauma center. Typically, the EMS clinician gets no further than the primary assessment of a child with multisystem trauma, because the recognition and management of life-threatening physiological problems are the focus of field care. The anatomical problems identified in the additional assessment are generally not life-threatening and can be treated in the hospital when the child is physiologically stable.

The General Assessment

THE PAT

The PAT is the first part of the primary assessment of trauma patients as well as medical patients, and allows rapid determination of the type of physiological disturbance, severity of injury, and urgency of need for treatment.

APPEARANCE

Appearance reflects brain function, which may be abnormal in injured children because of **primary brain injury** (caused by direct trauma to the brain tissue itself) or **secondary brain injury** (caused by an indirect insult to the brain tissue by hypoxia or ischemia). The most likely causes of abnormal appearance in a pediatric trauma patient are closed-head injury; hypoxia; hemorrhage; and pain due to fractures, burns, and **soft-tissue injuries**.

Toxins may also cause an abnormal appearance or altered mental status, but are uncommon causes of poor responsiveness in the preschool- and school-aged trauma patient. However, toxins (most often recreational drugs) are an important contributor to trauma in the adolescent, who may have injuries caused by high-risk behaviors while "under the influence." **TABLE 9–3** lists common causes of abnormal appearance in injured children.

TABLE 9–3 Common Causes of Abnormal Appearance in Injured Children

Category of Injury	Examples
Primary brain injuries	Closed-head injury Cerebral edema Concussion Contusion Intracranial hematoma (subdural, epidural) Intracranial hemorrhage Penetrating brain injuries
Secondary brain injuries (ischemia and hypoxia)	Hemorrhage with hypoperfusion/shock due to Solid organ abdominal injury Hemothorax Pelvic fracture Hypoxia due to Aspiration of gastric contents Failure of central respiratory drive Pulmonary contusion Smoke inhalation Tension pneumothorax
Pain	Burns Fractures Soft-tissue injuries
Toxins	Alcohol Recreational drugs Carbon monoxide

TIP

There are many potential causes of abnormal appearance in a pediatric trauma patient, including closed-head injury; hypoxia; hemorrhage; and pain due to fractures, burns, and soft-tissue injuries.

WORK OF BREATHING

Work of breathing is increased by injuries that affect the airway, lungs, pleura, or chest wall. **TABLE 9–4** summarizes the injury-related causes of increased work of breathing in pediatric trauma patients. Effortless tachypnea, or a rapid respiratory rate in the absence of increased work of breathing, may be seen in a child with traumatic shock. This is a reflexive mechanism to compensate for **metabolic acidosis** (caused by **hypoperfusion**), by "blowing off" carbon dioxide.

TABLE 9–4 Injury-Related Causes of Increased Work of Breathing in Injured Children

Cause	Examples
Airway injuries	Hematomas or lacerations of the tongue, mouth, or neck
	Smoke and hot gas inhalation
	Penetrations into the upper airway
Chest injuries	Pulmonary contusion
	Sucking chest wound
	Tension pneumothorax/hemothorax
Abdominal injuries	Diaphragmatic injury
	Solid or hollow viscus injury with pain and "splinting"

Listen for abnormal airway sounds, such as stridor or change of speech, which may reflect tracheal injury or obstruction. Wheezing reflects lower airway irritation and bronchospasm. This may occur owing to inhalation of vaporized toxins. When children are victims of a structure fire, an inhalation injury should always be suspected.

Grunting, an infant's method of achieving positive end-expiratory pressure, indicates decreased gas exchange at the level of the alveoli and may be seen with pulmonary contusion. After listening, look for retractions and nasal flaring to further assess for hypoxia.

CIRCULATION TO SKIN

Circulation to skin reflects the blood flow to the skin and mucous membranes. Abnormal skin color and skin temperature in an injured child who is not in a cold environment suggests hypovolemia and poor perfusion. Hemorrhage due to abdominal solid organ injury is the most common cause of hypoperfusion and shock in pediatric trauma patients. The EMS clinician should consider direct pressure, packing, and the use of tourniquets in children with exsanguinating hemorrhage from an extremity to prevent blood loss. An isolated closed-head injury cannot account for signs of hypoperfusion or shock in children outside of infancy, because the closed space of the skull cannot accommodate a significant volume of blood. However, infants can lose large volumes of blood owing to intracranial bleeding, because the plates of the skull (sutures) are not yet fused, and the skull can expand under pressure.

FIGURE 9–7 and **FIGURE 9–8** show the PAT findings for the 2 most common patterns of major

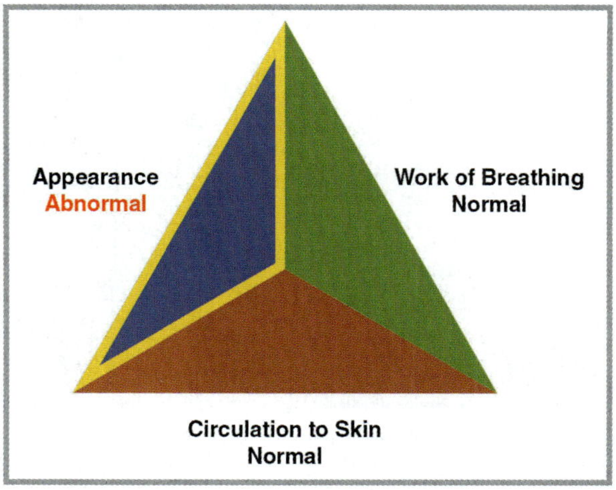

FIGURE 9–7 A patient with closed-head injury has an abnormal appearance, but normal work of breathing and normal circulation to skin.

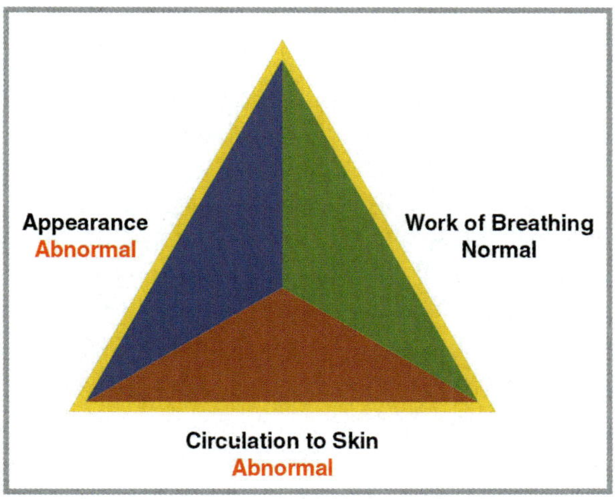

FIGURE 9–8 A patient with multisystem injury has an abnormal appearance, abnormal work of breathing, and abnormal circulation to skin.

pediatric trauma: closed-head injury and multisystem injury.

The Primary Assessment

HANDS-ON ABCDEs

The ABCDEs are the hands-on primary assessment. The trauma xABCDEs have a special focus on control of bleeding and spinal motion restriction. The pediatric assessment, including the PAT and ABCDEs, does not require any specialized equipment. Potentially life-threatening problems should be treated as they are identified in the ABCDE sequence. **TABLE 9–5** lists the key features of the pediatric trauma ABCDEs and interventions specific to the trauma patient.

TABLE 9–5 Pediatric Trauma xABCDEs

Element of Assessment	Special Interventions
exsanguination	Controlling bleeding; using pressure; packing; using tourniquets
Airway	Using jaw-thrust maneuver while maintaining cervical spinal motion restriction
	Suctioning airway of fluid or blood
	Considering airway adjunct
Breathing	Performing needle thoracostomy
	Applying dressing to sucking chest wound
Circulation	Controlling external hemorrhage
	Applying tourniquet
	Splinting fractured extremity
Disability	Managing elevated intracranial pressure (keeping head midline, keeping head of stretcher raised, using assisted ventilation to maintain normal CO_2 levels)
Exposure	Preventing heat loss

Exsanguination

Blood loss resulting from trauma is a preventable cause of death. Therefore, if you see bleeding, a critical first step is to apply pressure. If the wound is still bleeding, the wound can be packed and pressure reapplied. If the wound continues to bleed and is on an extremity, consider the use of a tourniquet (see **Procedure 25, Tourniquet Application**). If the wound is at a junctional location (axilla, groin, neck) or on the torso, wound packing and pressure are needed. If you have hemostatic gauze, that can be used for packing. Tranexamic acid (TXA) is an IV medication that stabilizes fibrin clots and blocks fibrinolysis, but it must be administered early after injury. According to local protocols, it can be given to children younger than 12 years in a dose of 15 mg/kg over 10 minutes and to those 12 years and older in a dose of 1 g over 10 minutes.

AIRWAY

After addressing exsanguination, airway maintenance is always a top priority. Trauma patients are at risk for airway obstruction from bleeding, **emesis**, edema, or foreign objects. Traumatic brain injury may cause loss of protective airway reflexes or impair central respiratory drive.

Consider spinal injury in a child with any of the following:

- Mechanism of injury involving high-velocity forces transmitted to the head or spine (eg, fall from a height, ejection from a motor vehicle, diving, axial loading)
- Altered mental status (AMS)
- Neck or spine pain/tenderness
- Inability to move the neck
- Neurological deficit (eg, acute weakness or loss of sensation after an injury)
- Deformity to the neck or spine

If the child has any of these findings, care should be taken to protect the spine to minimize risk of secondary injury. The current term for this practice is spinal motion restriction (SMR).

Spinal motion restriction may involve placing a cervical spine collar and/or securing the patient to a stretcher and taking care to minimize movement of the neck, especially when transferring the patient from scene to stretcher or into an ambulance. Use of a rigid backboard to immobilize the patient is now thought to cause potential harm. If a backboard or other rigid device is used to extricate a child or transfer them to a stretcher, the child should be removed from the rigid board as soon as possible, while maintaining spinal precautions. An injured child should be transported secured to a stretcher or in an appropriately sized car seat.

Although great care must be taken to prevent further injury in the unlikely event of an unstable spine injury, these concerns must not take precedence over appropriate management of the child's airway. ***An injured child is far more likely to die of untreated hypoxia or shock than of spinal trauma.***

Actions. If airway obstruction is present, use a jaw-thrust maneuver combined with manual SMR (**FIGURE 9–9**) to establish and maintain airway patency. Insert an oral **airway adjunct** if unable to maintain an open airway and the child has no gag reflex. Use suction to clear any fluid or a Magill forceps to remove foreign bodies from the mouth, nose, or upper airway. Be prepared to turn the child on their side and suction if they vomit, to prevent aspiration of stomach contents. Quickly but carefully logroll the patient while maintaining SMR if vomiting occurs.

CAUTION
Never let concern about spinal injury compromise appropriate management of the child's airway.

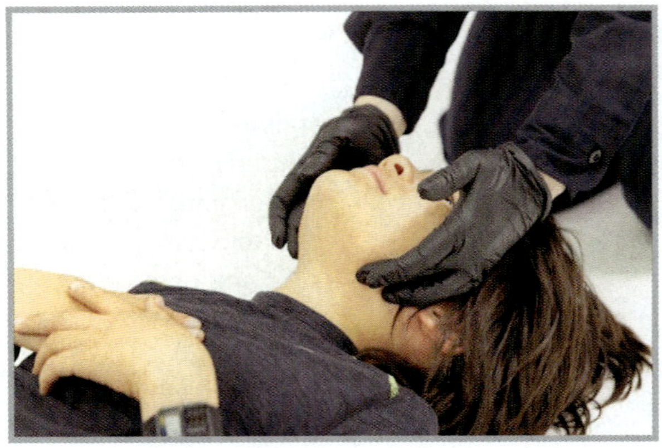

FIGURE 9–9 If airway obstruction is suspected in a child with possible spine injuries, use the modified jaw-thrust maneuver combined with manual spinal motion restriction.

The spinal column is made of 33 articulating bones—the vertebrae—and its structure changes significantly during childhood growth. The incidence and type of spinal injuries depend on the child's age and the mechanism of injury, and, in turn, are influenced by the child's developmental level and activity. Cervical spine trauma can lead to **quadriplegia**, the most devastating type of spinal injury. If cervical spine injury is suspected, an appropriately sized cervical collar should be applied. The use of a backboard should follow local trauma system protocols (**FIGURE 9–10**). Spinal cord injuries and lifelong paralysis may follow thoracic or lumbar trauma. For a step-by-step explanation of this procedure, see **Procedure 22, Spinal Motion Restriction**.

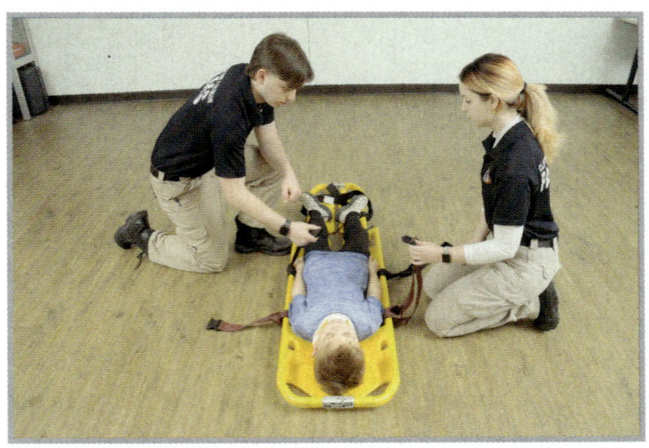

FIGURE 9–10 Spinal motion restriction may involve moving a nonambulatory child to a stretcher using a backboard or scoop stretcher to minimize motion of the spine.

BREATHING

Breathing is the second priority in the ABCDEs. Injuries to the airway, chest wall, lungs, or abdomen, as well as gastric distension caused by air swallowing, may compromise oxygenation and ventilation. Head and cervical spine injuries sometimes depress central respiratory drive mechanisms or diminish protective airway reflexes. Pulmonary aspiration of gastric contents is a common and potentially serious complication of head injuries that results in hypoxia and increased work of breathing.

Look for soft-tissue or penetrating injuries of the chest or back. Watch for the adequacy and symmetry of chest rise, and then listen with a stethoscope to assess air entry and equality of breath sounds. Feel the chest wall for **crepitus**, pain, or instability. Apply a pulse oximeter to assess for hypoxemia, because pallor and cyanosis can be late findings. A normal pulse oximetry reading does not, however, rule out respiratory distress. A child with profound tachypnea or increased work of breathing may need **assisted ventilation**, regardless of the reading on the oximeter, so they do not exhaust compensatory mechanisms.

Actions. If breathing is inadequate, position the child and assist ventilation. Lift the jaw into the mask; pushing the mask onto the face to make a seal may cause cervical spine flexion and exacerbate airway obstruction. The E-C clamp technique (**FIGURE 9–11**) helps with proper hand placement for a good mask-to-face seal. Consider inserting an airway adjunct to help maintain an open airway, although an oral airway is not tolerated by a child with an intact gag reflex.

Administer 100% oxygen by nonrebreathing mask or assisted ventilation. Use a properly fitted oxygen mask. Provide assisted ventilation with a bag-mask device if the child's respiratory effort is inadequate or if the child has deteriorating cardiopulmonary or mental status. Use the "squeeze-release-release" timing technique, because the tendency is to bag too fast. Allow a brief pause between each breath to minimize the chance of gastric distension. If the child has signs of increased intracranial pressure such as low heart rate, elevated blood pressure, and irregular respirations (**Cushing triad**), or signs of impending brainstem herniation, such as fixed and dilated pupils, unequal pupils, and/or **posturing**, use waveform or digital capnography to keep $EtCO_2$ between 35 and 45 mm Hg. Be extremely careful, because hyperventilation may decrease perfusion to the brain. In each breath, provide only enough tidal volume to achieve chest rise.

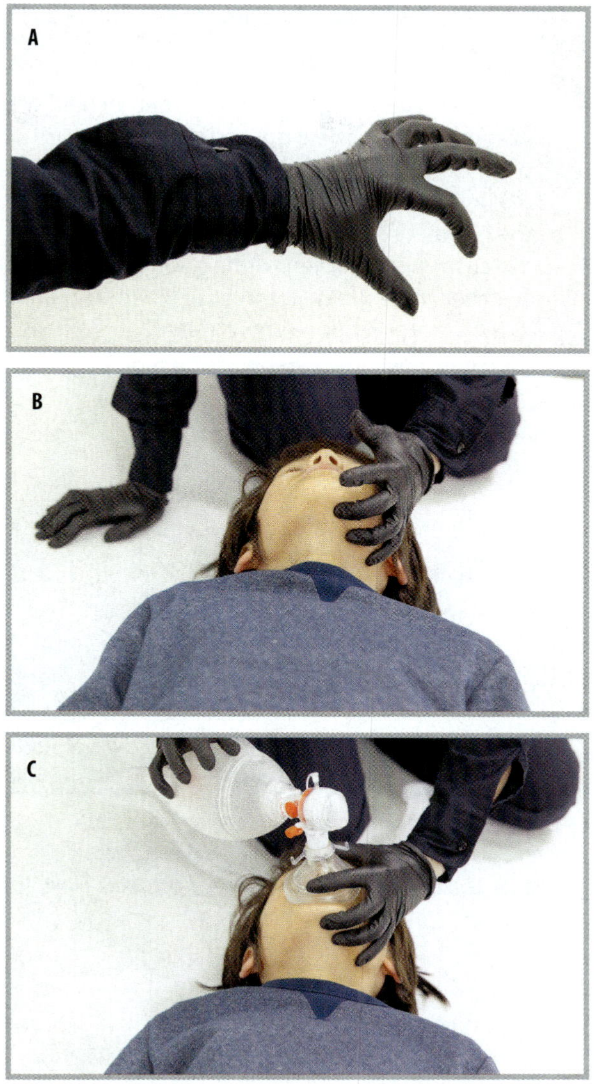

FIGURE 9–11 The E-C clamp technique facilitates proper hand placement for a good mask-to-face seal. **A.** Hand displaying the E-C shape. **B.** Fingers resting on the bony ridge of the jaw. **C.** Bag-mask ventilation in place.

Treating penetrating chest injuries, sucking chest wounds, impaled objects, and tension pneumothorax in children is the same as it is in adults. Cover sucking chest wounds with an **occlusive dressing**, such as petrolatum gauze, taped on 3 or 4 sides (depending on local protocol) (**FIGURE 9–12**) or a bandage/seal specially designed for sucking chest wounds. This technique allows trapped air to escape while helping to prevent the entrance of air and development of tension pneumothorax. Do not remove impaled objects. Instead, stabilize them in place.

CASE STUDY 2

You are dispatched to a local recreation field where a 6-year-old boy was struck in the head by a baseball bat that flew out of another player's hands while batting. The child has a large hematoma on his forehead and is crying in his coach's arms. The child did not lose consciousness, but is not making eye contact with you or his coach. Other than his altered appearance, the PAT is normal and the hands-on ABCDEs reveal normal vital signs and no other apparent injuries. The child becomes increasingly somnolent during your assessment and is difficult to arouse.

1. What is the greatest threat to life for this child?
2. What interventions are required?

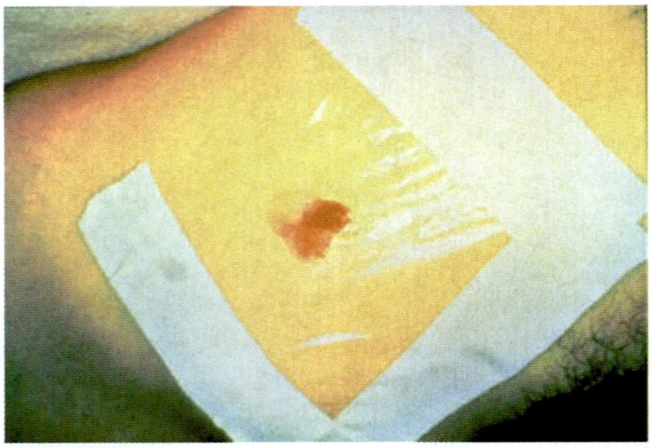

FIGURE 9–12 Management of a sucking chest wound. Cover sucking chest wounds with an occlusive dressing, such as a petrolatum gauze, taped on 3 or 4 sides. A defibrillator pad can also be used.

TIP

Pulmonary aspiration of gastric contents is a common and potentially serious complication of head injuries. Therefore, an orogastric tube should be inserted.

TIP

If a patient with penetrating chest trauma also has respiratory distress, hypoxia, and shock, perform needle decompression on the affected side to treat possible tension pneumothorax.

ALS

Management of Tension Pneumothorax. If a patient with penetrating chest trauma has increasing respiratory distress, hypoxia, and shock, perform needle decompression on the affected side to treat possible tension pneumothorax.

Needle decompression may also be necessary in the child with blunt chest injury if the child has serious blunt chest-wall injury and respiratory distress, especially if their condition worsens with assisted ventilation. In this situation, when there is a closed pneumothorax, positive-pressure ventilation quickly increases the air pressure in the pleural space, creating a dangerous level of "tension." Tension pneumothorax not only compromises ventilation of the affected lung, but also impairs venous return to the heart. This can lead to shock that is unresponsive to fluid resuscitation. Needle decompression of the tension pneumothorax improves oxygenation, ventilation, and perfusion. For a step-by-step explanation of this procedure, see **Procedure 23, Needle Thoracostomy.**

Management of Gastric Distension With a Nasogastric/Orogastric Tube. Assisted ventilation or prolonged crying can cause air swallowing and gastric distension. Nasogastric (NG) or orogastric (OG) tube placement may improve ventilation by decreasing the upward pressure on the diaphragm caused by the distended stomach and reducing the risk of vomiting. If possible, insert an OG tube after endotracheal intubation of a comatose patient because prior positive-pressure ventilation can cause gastric inflation. Contraindications for NG insertion include midfacial trauma and suspected basilar skull fracture (raccoon eyes, Battle sign, or suspected cerebrospinal fluid rhinorrhea or otorrhea) because of the risk of passing the tube through the disrupted cribriform plate into the cranial vault. In these cases, perform OG insertion. Weigh the benefits of gastric decompression against the possible complications of vomiting and aspiration during passage of the tube or after tube misplacement into the trachea. For a step-by-step explanation of this procedure, see **Procedure 10, Orogastric and Nasogastric Tube Insertion.**

CIRCULATION

Multisystem pediatric trauma more often involves respiratory failure than shock. Sometimes, however, shock develops because of external or internal bleeding, pneumothorax, spinal injury, or cardiac failure caused by cardiac contusion or **tamponade**. The combination of the PAT and the hands-on ABCDEs allows for ongoing perfusion evaluation. Measure heart rate continuously with a cardiac monitor or with frequent pulse checks. Tachycardia may be caused by pain, fear, cold, or anxiety, but a trend of rising heart rate suggests ongoing blood loss. Blood pressure measurement is not a good indicator of hypovolemia because a child can be in compensated shock with a normal blood pressure. When there is frank hypotension, assume the child is in hypotensive (decompensated) shock. If blood pressure is significantly higher than normal in a child with possible TBI, consider possible **intracranial hypertension/increased intracranial pressure**.

Because of the technical challenges of obtaining a reliable blood pressure, and because skin signs, capillary refill time, and pulse quality are good signs of perfusion, make only one attempt at measuring blood pressure in children older than 3 years. Make sure the blood pressure cuff size is correct, or the measurement will be inaccurate. In children younger than 3 years, taking the time on scene to obtain a blood pressure may be of limited value. Use other signs of perfusion such as mental status, pulse quality (peripheral vs central), capillary refill, and skin temperature.

Actions. Stop any visible external bleeding with direct pressure on the wound. Use sterile gauze or hemostatic gauze compresses, and use gloves and personal protective equipment. Splint any extremities with obvious deformity. Provide oxygen, and place the child in a supine position for transport. Consider tourniquet application if there is uncontrolled bleeding or massive hemorrhage of an extremity (see **Procedure 25, Tourniquet Application**).

Begin transport when the airway is properly secured, ventilation is adequate, and the child's spine is appropriately stabilized. In a poorly perfused, or hypotensive, patient, administer 20 mL/kg of isotonic fluid as rapidly as possible. Some EMS agencies now have prehospital blood transfusion protocols. Follow local protocols regarding the use of whole blood versus packed red blood cells.

> **TIP**
>
> Frequently reassess heart rate, preferably with an electronic monitor. Tachycardia may be a response to pain, fear, cold, or anxiety, but a trend of rising heart rate suggests ongoing blood loss.

> **TIP**
>
> Remember, the systolic blood pressure in a child aged 1 to 10 years should be greater than $70 + (2 \times \text{age in years})$. If not, the child is in hypotensive (decompensated) shock.

> **ALS**
>
> **Volume Resuscitation. If the child has signs of shock or significant ongoing blood loss, obtain vascular access and start volume resuscitation on the way to the ED. Look first for peripheral intravenous (IV) sites in the upper extremities. Attempt to secure 2 lines. Insert an intraosseous (IO) needle if IV access cannot be obtained immediately and the child has signs of hypotensive shock. Then administer 20 mL/kg of isotonic fluid as rapidly as possible.**

DISABILITY

Disability in the context of trauma care relates to TBI or spinal cord trauma. Injuries may be open or closed. Children may have primary or secondary brain injuries, or both.

Primary brain injury is the direct result of the traumatic insult and may include brain hemorrhage, **cerebral edema** (brain swelling), or **diffuse axonal injury**. Increased intracranial pressure may develop quickly after primary brain injury. Untreated, the downward spiral of increased intracranial pressure can lead to **brainstem herniation**, cardiopulmonary arrest, and **brain death**. By the time the EMS clinician reaches the scene, any damage that has occurred from the primary brain injury is complete.

Secondary brain injury results from central nervous system (CNS) hypoxia or ischemia and disorders of blood glucose. The EMS clinician has a key role in preventing secondary brain injury. Hypoxia may be the result of airway or chest injury, or of compromised central respiratory drive caused by the primary brain injury. Brain ischemia may result from hemorrhage, usually in the abdomen or chest. CNS cells cannot survive without sufficient blood glucose levels.

Ensuring adequate oxygenation, ventilation, and perfusion and normal blood glucose levels is key to preventing secondary brain injury.

A 9-1-1 call sometimes involves an infant with AMS, apnea, or seizures with no report of preceding trauma. Assessment of these infants may not reveal any findings suggestive of head trauma or TBI, despite the fact that they have sustained severe TBI. This is a typical scenario in **abusive head trauma**, where the infant is forcibly shaken by a caregiver, sometimes with impact of the baby's head against a fixed object. This mechanism involves severe acceleration-deceleration forces to the infant's brain and consequent diffuse axonal injury or intracranial hemorrhage. Abusive head trauma is discussed further in Chapter 13.

Assess the injured child's degree of neurological disability with the Alert, Verbal, Pain, Unresponsive (AVPU) scale (see Chapter 1, TABLE 1–8). Disability, as categorized in the AVPU scale, is not the same as "abnormal appearance" in the PAT. An injured child may have an abnormal appearance for many reasons other than brain or spinal cord injury, such as pain, fear, shock, hypoxia, or intoxication. Appearance may be quite abnormal in a child who is "alert" on the AVPU scale. Appearance is a more subtle indicator of overall physiological function in children than the AVPU. The AVPU scale is more helpful in categorizing children with severe neurological insults, including critical primary or secondary brain injuries.

Some EMS systems use the Pediatric Glasgow Coma Scale (PGCS) to assess neurological injury (**TABLE 9–6**). Neither the AVPU score nor the PGCS has been validated in young children. Although both systems attempt to objectively assess neurological function, the AVPU is less complex and easier to remember.

TABLE 9–6 Pediatric Glasgow Coma Scale

Score	Child	Infant
Eyes		
4	Opens eyes spontaneously	Opens eyes spontaneously
3	Opens eyes to speech	Opens eyes to speech
2	Opens eyes to pain	Opens eyes to pain
1	No response	No response
= Score (Eyes)		
Motor		
6	Obeys commands	Spontaneous movements
5	Localizes	Withdraws to touch
4	Withdraws	Withdraws to pain
3	Flexion	Flexion (**decorticate**)
2	Extension	Extension (**decerebrate**)
1	No response	No response
= Score (Motor)		
Verbal		
5	Oriented	Coos and babbles
4	Confused	Irritable cry
3	Inappropriate words	Cries to pain
2	Incomprehensible words	Moans to pain
1	No response	No response
= Score (Verbal)		
= Total Score (Eyes, Motor, Verbal). Scores will range from 3 to 15.		

Adapted with permission from James HE, Anas NG, Perkin RM. *Brain Insults in Infants and Children.* Grune & Stratton; 1985.

When using the PGCS, pay special attention to the motor component of the score, which has the highest value in predicting neurological outcome of TBI.

After evaluating the level of consciousness with the AVPU or the PGCS, note abnormal positioning (including posturing) and seizures, and check for pupil size, symmetry, and **reactivity**. Seizures are common with head injury in children. Beware of persistent horizontal nystagmus, which may indicate persistent seizure activity.

The pupils provide important information about brainstem function, and the pupillary examination helps determine the need for hyperventilation in patients who are at risk of experiencing brainstem herniation.

Concussion. Concussion, a mild form of TBI, occurs after a bump or blow to the head or as a result of a fall onto the head. These rotational and acceleration forces on the brain result in chemical changes and sometimes damage to the brain cells. Frequently sport related, loss of consciousness is seen in only 10% to 15% of concussed patients. Symptoms include headache, nausea or vomiting, double or blurry vision, confusion, dizziness, sensitivity to light (photophobia), sensitivity to noise (phonophobia), and concentration or memory problems. Although some of these may occur shortly after the injury, others may occur a few hours to days later. The child or adolescent may say that they do not feel well, but if the child appears dazed or stunned, is confused, answers questions slowly, moves clumsily, or cannot recall events before the injury, the child has suffered a concussion. If a child is involved in a sports activity, they should be removed from play. Recovery may require physical and cognitive rest and may take weeks to months. A second impact during the recovery phase may lead to rapid brain swelling and death. Patients who experience a concussion should be evaluated by a medical professional and should not return to play until they have been cleared to do so.

Actions. In pediatric trauma patients with AVPU values of P or U, provide assisted ventilation to maintain good oxygenation and adequate ventilation. Hypoxia is an important cause of secondary brain injury in these children with TBI. Hypoxia may be associated with increased intracranial pressure, a situation that may occur rapidly and sometimes deceptively in a child with a primary brain injury.

Children with TBI require oxygenation and ventilation, but the rate of ventilation is controversial. Although hyperventilation was widely recommended in the past as a way of rapidly decreasing intracranial pressure, extreme hyperventilation can cause decreased brain perfusion and secondary brain injury. Reserve hyperventilation for patients with TBI who have signs of increased intracranial pressure or signs of **impending brainstem herniation**, and use wave-form or digital capnography to keep $EtCO_2$ between 35 and 45 mm Hg.

Consider this intervention if the child has a severe neurological disability, as defined by a value of P or U on the AVPU scale; a score of less than 9 on the PGCS; or a fixed and **dilated** pupil, **asymmetrical** pupils, or posturing (decerebrate or decorticate).

TIP

A child with head trauma has impending brainstem herniation if the AVPU value is P or U; if the PGCS is less than 9; or there is a fixed dilated pupil, asymmetrical pupils, or posturing.

ALS

Management of Elevated Intracranial Pressure. If the child has AMS (not alert on AVPU or <15 on the PGCS), anticipate elevated intracranial pressure. The Cushing triad of bradycardia, elevated blood pressure, and irregular respirations occurs with elevated intracranial pressure. Take a graded approach to intracranial pressure management, always balancing risks and benefits of treatment.

- **Support the patient's head in a midline position to facilitate jugular venous return to the heart.**
- **If the patient is not in shock, elevate the head of the backboard or stretcher. Ensure adequate oxygenation and ventilation.**
- **Consider hyperventilation only in patients with signs of impending herniation syndrome. Use waveform or digital capnography to keep $EtCO_2$ above 35 mm Hg, preferably in a range from 35 to 45 mm Hg.**
- **If there is a head injury and hypovolemia, administer fluid to maintain brain perfusion. The injured brain hates ischemia.**
- **Mannitol or 3% hypertonic saline may be useful to acutely decrease intracranial pressure in a child with asymmetrical pupils or posturing, but it must be used with caution in a child with associated injuries who is at risk for hemorrhagic shock.**

EXPOSURE

Exposure is the last step in the primary assessment. Good exposure allows full assessment of the child's entire body, including the extremities. Quickly examine the back during the spinal stabilization procedure for soft-tissue or penetrating injuries. Assess circulation and neurological function **distal** to obvious or suspected extremity injuries. Although usually not life-threatening, complicated extremity injuries (eg, open fractures of the humerus or femur) may cause significant blood loss, vascular compromise, and pain. Remember to cover the patient after the examination to prevent heat loss and hypothermia.

CAUTION

Administration of mannitol can acutely decrease intracranial pressure through changes in CNS fluid distribution and diuresis. Do not administer mannitol to patients with hypovolemic shock.

Summary of Primary Assessment

The assessment of the injured child requires knowledge of anatomical and developmental differences that lead to pediatric-specific patterns of injury. The child's airway is small and easily obstructed, the lungs are vulnerable to contusion, and the solid organs and long bones are poorly protected. The EMS clinician's primary role in multisystem trauma is to ensure an open airway, assist ventilation, and minimize secondary brain injury. Treatment goals are to avoid hypoxia and hypotension. A brief time on scene and rapid transport to the ED are overriding priorities for all children who are physiologically unstable or have concerning mechanisms of injury. Vascular access and volume resuscitation are secondary tasks to be considered on the way to the hospital.

CAUTION

Mannitol is temperature sensitive. Do not store in temperatures lower than 7.22°C (45°F).

TIP

Use assisted ventilation to maintain oxygenation and to avoid carbon dioxide retention in pediatric trauma patients with AVPU scale values of P or U.

TIP

In the prehospital environment, endotracheal intubation is not always the optimal airway management tool.

Special Airway Considerations in Pediatric Trauma

Children with severe head injuries with neurological disability and impending herniation often require field interventions for the following reasons:

- To protect the airway and prevent aspiration
- To improve or control ventilation
- To improve or control oxygenation

Optimal airway management balances the potential risks of the procedure against the potential benefits to the patient. Although endotracheal intubation has long been considered the best method for airway management in a critically injured patient, the procedural risks are significant. These risks may include prolonged scene time, worsened hypoxia, vomiting and aspiration, elevation of intracranial pressure during laryngoscopy, or a misplaced tube. The decision to support ventilation using a bag-mask device versus an endotracheal tube or a supraglottic airway is complex and must take into consideration the following factors:

- Risk of increasing intracranial pressure (by increasing the child's combativeness or inducing gagging during the intubation procedure)
- Ability to access the airway
- Length of on-scene and transport times
- Personnel availability and experience
- Availability of a drug-assisted intubation protocol and training in its use

TABLE 9–7 lists the factors that the EMS clinician must consider to choose the optimal airway management approach for each patient.

ADVANCED AIRWAY MANAGEMENT OF THE PEDIATRIC TRAUMA PATIENT

If a severely injured child needs endotracheal intubation, the preferred path is orotracheal, with manual neutral stabilization of the cervical spine (see **Procedure 11, Endotracheal Intubation**).

Although blind nasotracheal intubation may cause less cervical spine motion in the adult than the orotracheal technique, the procedure is not applicable to children because of the anterior location of the **larynx** and the increased risk of **adenoidal** bleeding. *Do not attempt blind nasotracheal intubation in a child.*

Drug-assisted intubation (often called rapid sequence intubation) for pediatric endotracheal intubation, with sedatives and paralyzing drugs, is standard practice in many emergency departments and in a number of EMS regions. Its effectiveness, safety, and feasibility in the prehospital setting are controversial, and its use requires specialized training. See **Procedure 13, Supraglottic Airway Insertion and Pediatric Difficult Airway,** for a detailed explanation of this procedure.

TABLE 9–7 Factors Influencing Optimal Airway Management Decisions

Factors Favoring Basic Life Support (Bag-Mask Ventilation)
Combativeness, strong gag reflex
Presence of **trismus** (spasm of jaw muscles)
Short on-scene and transport times
Factors Favoring Advanced Life Support (Endotracheal Intubation/Supraglottic Airway)
Inability to ventilate with a bag-mask device
Unresponsive child
Absent gag reflex
Apnea, poor muscle tone
Long extrication or transport times
Limited personnel to assist during transport
Availability of a drug-assisted intubation protocol and training

CAUTION
Do not attempt blind nasotracheal intubation in children.

CONTROVERSY
The use of sedative and paralytic drugs to facilitate pediatric endotracheal intubation is standard practice in EDs and in a number of EMS regions. Its effectiveness and safety in the field are controversial, and its use requires specialized training.

The Primary Assessment

THE TRANSPORT DECISION: STAY OR GO?

After the primary assessment and initiation of life support, consider the timing for transport. *Immediately transport every pediatric trauma patient who has any abnormal physiological or anatomical findings/injury pattern mechanism of injury, or risk factors, or who in the EMS clinician's judgment requires immediate transport.* Trauma patients in stable condition who have apparently minor injuries may undergo further evaluation and treatment on scene. If the scene size-up suggests circumstances that could be dangerous to the child or EMS clinician, transport immediately. Potentially dangerous conditions that warrant immediate transport and completion of assessment in the ambulance include proximity to fire or hazardous materials, threatened violence, angry bystanders or caregivers, and suspected nonaccidental trauma.

Additional Assessment

The additional assessment consists of the focused history and physical examination and the detailed physical examination (trauma patient). This part of the assessment is directed at anatomical problems. Perform the focused history and physical examination and the detailed physical examination in the field only if the patient is physiologically stable and the conditions are safe. Otherwise, address these components of the assessment in the ambulance while on the way to the ED. In physiologically unstable patients, defer the additional assessment and perform it en route, if possible.

When obtaining the focused history, use the SAMPLE template (Signs & Symptoms, Allergies, Medications, Past medical problems, Last food or liquid, and Events leading to the injury), as outlined in Chapter 1. Focus only on points likely to affect primary trauma assessment and interventions. **TABLE 9–8** provides a SAMPLE template oriented to pediatric trauma patients.

The focused physical examination includes a careful look at the anatomy in the suspected areas of injury. This may involve a conscientious examination by exploration and palpation of the head and scalp in a child with a closed-head injury, observation and palpation of the back and axillae in a child with a penetrating chest injury, or inspection and palpation of the neck in a child with a strangulation injury.

The detailed physical examination (trauma) is head to toe in infants, toddlers, and toe to head in preschool-aged children, then a front-to-back complete physical examination of the patient is performed. This examination uses the traditional assessment tools of observation, palpation, and auscultation, as outlined in Chapter 1. While the child is on the way to the ED, perform ongoing reassessments, especially in patients with abnormal physiology. These include serial evaluations of the PAT, xABCDEs, pulse oximetry, vital signs (including heart rate and rhythm on the cardiac monitor), anatomical problems, and response to treatment. Be sure to monitor and treat pain, if possible. When the child arrives in the ED, diagnostic testing with blood tests and imaging studies may assist with continued assessment.

TABLE 9–8 SAMPLE History in Pediatric Trauma

Component	Explanation
Signs/symptoms	Time of event
	Nature of symptoms or pain
	Age-appropriate signs of distress
Allergies	Known drug reactions or other allergies
Medications	Long-term medications—timing and dose of last dose
	Timing and dose of **analgesic**/antipyretic medications
Past medical problems	Prior surgeries
	Immunizations
Last food or liquid	Time of the child's last food or drink, including bottle or breastfeeding
Events leading to the injury	Key events leading to the current incident
	Mechanism of injury
	Hazards at the scene

Summary of Additional Assessment

After the primary assessment, determine the timing of transport and the appropriate destination. Do an additional assessment, or an on-scene focused history and a physical examination and detailed physical examination, only in patients in stable condition in safe scene circumstances. All other patients require immediate transport with continuation of assessment on the way to the ED. Frequent reassessment is important in all injured patients. Transport severely injured pediatric patients to trauma centers rather than community hospitals when possible. Many state trauma programs have algorithms for directing patients, including children, to the appropriate level of care.

Spinal Motion Restriction and Splinting for Transport

Indications for SMR of children are the same as those for adults and are indicated for any child with a concerning mechanism of injury, signs of significant head injury, or multisystem trauma. When a cervical spine injury is suspected (discussed earlier), stabilize the neck using a properly sized pediatric extrication collar and/or a head immobilizer, when available. Otherwise, use properly secured towel rolls and tape. For a step-by-step description of this procedure, see **Procedure 22, Spinal Motion Restriction**.

Preschool-aged children may not be able to localize or communicate the presence of neck or back pain. Anatomical differences, specifically the large size of an infant's or a toddler's head, require modification of SMR procedures. For example, placing a thin (1-inch) layer of padding beneath a child's body from shoulders to hips before securing the child to the stretcher (**FIGURE 9–13**) helps to properly align the airway and the spinal column.

The spine does not stop at C-7, and SMR precautions should be used if a spinal injury is suspected. *Secure the patient against all axes of motion on the spine board or extrication device during extrication.* Near-vertical positioning may be necessary during extrication. Secure the patient against **lateral** movement by placing padding along the sides of the body to eliminate all space between the patient and the straps.

Avoid chin straps and other SMR aids that might impair ventilation. Leave room for chest expansion during breathing when tightening chest straps or flaps. Make sure cervical collars fit properly, or use manual spinal stabilization until the child can be secured to the stretcher if a properly sized collar is not available. Ensure that spinal stabilization equipment does not interfere with assessment and access to the patient. A child who does not have severe injuries, and in whom there is no concern regarding cervical spine or spinal injury, may not require SMR, according to local protocol.

Splinting deformed or painful extremities is also an important prehospital intervention. Splinting has several important functions: pain control, hemorrhage reduction, and preservation of neurovascular function. Unless the extremity shows signs of neurovascular compromise or the patient is experiencing severe pain, splint bones that may be fractured or dislocated in an "as is" position. Check pulses before and after splinting (**FIGURE 9–14**). An open femur fracture should be reduced by traction *only* if the traction can be maintained. This controls the bleeding at the fracture site and helps to control pain. Otherwise, unless circulation is compromised, leave bone exposed to avoid introducing further contamination by forcing fractured bone fragments back under the broken skin.

RESTRAINT OF CHILDREN DURING TRANSPORT

Make sure all persons riding in an ambulance are appropriately restrained. Secure children with possible spinal injury in a supine position on a stretcher. If the child has mild to moderate trauma without suggestion of spinal injury, use EMS system guidelines for age-appropriate restraint. All states have well-defined regulations regarding proper child restraint in a passenger vehicle. However, these regulations may not extend to ambulance transport. The appropriate use of a child restraint seat in an ambulance

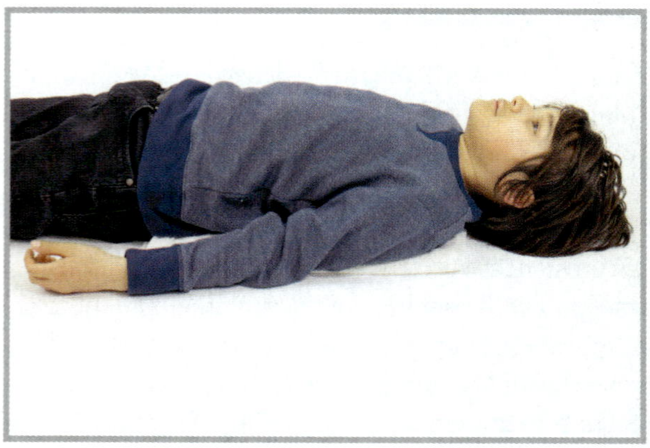

FIGURE 9–13 Keep the airway and spine in a neutral position by placing a layer of padding beneath the child's body from shoulders to hips before securing the child to the stretcher.

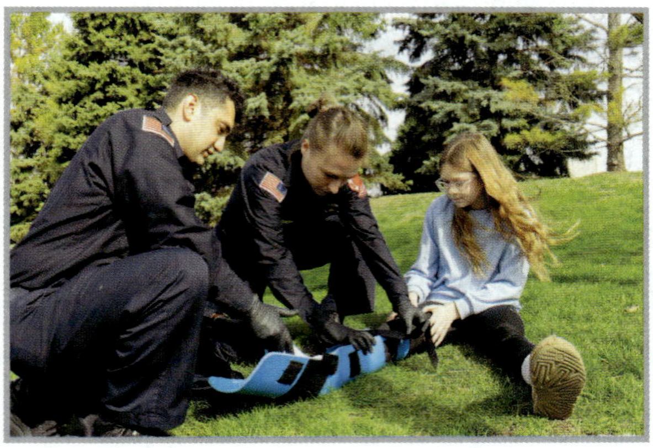

FIGURE 9–14 Splinting.

is controversial. When car seats are used for EMS transport, both the device and the method of securing the seat to the gurney must conform to industry standards and meet local requirements. If EMS local policy allows, have the child's caregiver remain within view or speaking distance of the child, as long as the caregiver's presence does not compromise the child's treatment or crew safety. Their presence is comforting for the conscious and **hemodynamically stable** child.

TIP

Although spinal injuries are not common in children, the high frequency of head injury means that SMR should be part of the care of most pediatric patients with a significant mechanism of blunt trauma.

TIP

The use of specially designed pediatric SMR devices is more efficient than on-scene modification of adult devices.

Pediatric Burn Patients

The assessment and management priorities for the burn patient are the same as those for any other trauma patient. Make sure the scene is safe before approaching the child. Always anticipate exposure to hazardous materials such as carbon monoxide or cyanide, and use protective measures. Get technical help, if needed, from authorities on hazardous materials.

ASSESSMENT

Assess the scene for risk factors for airway and breathing. Important considerations in patients with fire and smoke exposures include the following:

- Enclosed space
- Heavy smoke
- Fumes
- Steam
- Hot vapors
- Chemical hazards
- Explosions, with blunt or penetrating injury

Assess the patient for signs of smoke or particle inhalation and thermal burns of the airway. Provide 100% oxygen for suspected carbon monoxide poisoning in children with an abnormal appearance or AMS or in children exposed to fire or smoke in an enclosed space. Anticipate hidden injuries (especially abdominal) from a fall or a blast injury.

Make a quick estimation of the burned body surface area. A modified anatomical diagram of children of different ages gives an approximation of the burned body surface area, as shown in **FIGURE 9–15**. If such a diagram is not available, use the "rule of palms," which states that the patient's palm plus fingers equals 1% of body surface area (**FIGURE 9–16**). The percentage of burned body surface area is therefore roughly equal to the number of "patient palm plus fingers"–sized areas burned. Electronic apps that facilitate the calculation of percentage body surface area burned are available.

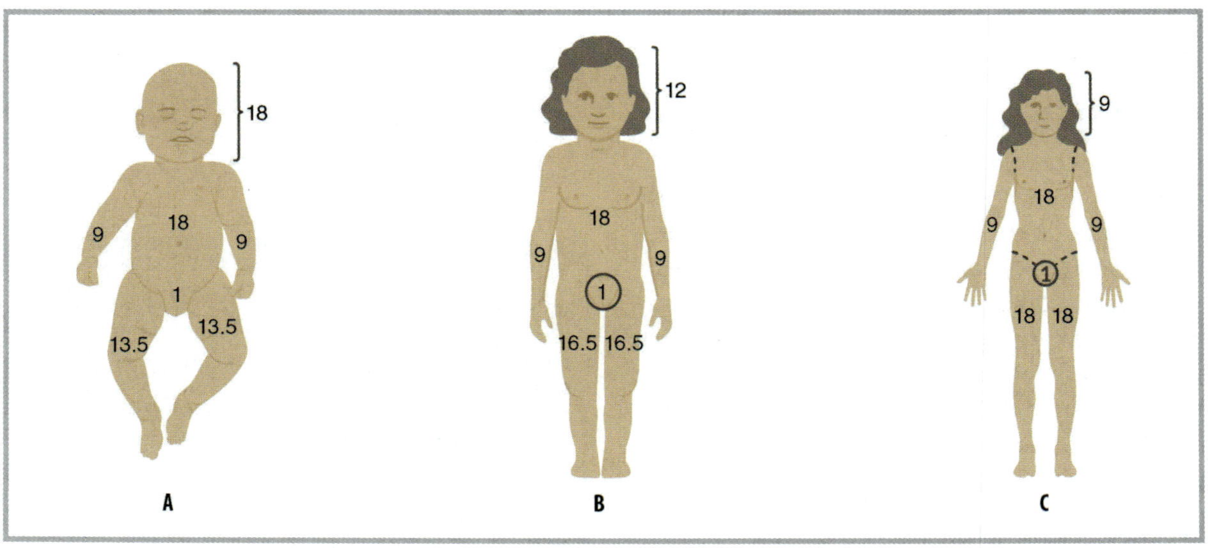

FIGURE 9–15 Modified anatomical diagrams of children of different ages give an approximation of involved body surface area for calculation of the extent of burn in **(A)** an infant, **(B)** a child, and **(C)** an adolescent.

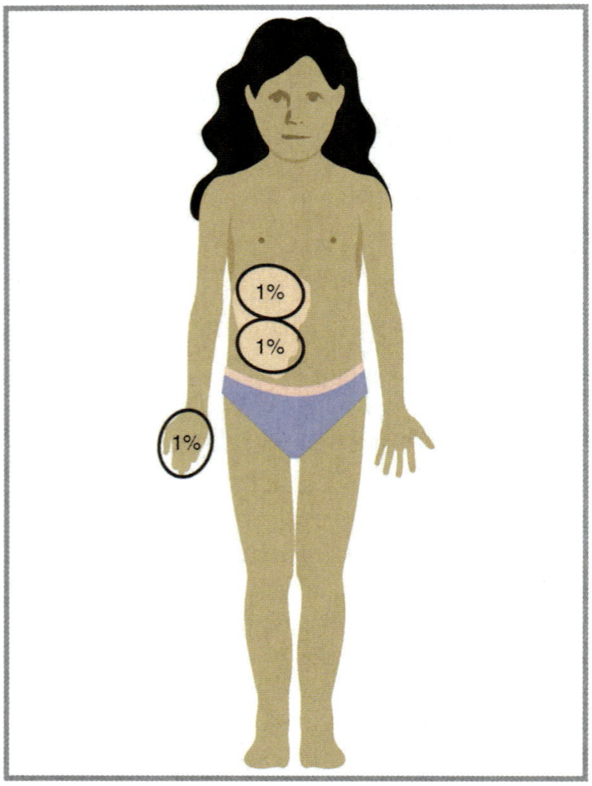

FIGURE 9-16 The palm plus fingers is approximately 1% of the body surface area.

Although most burns are unintentional, assess all burn patients for risk factors for nonaccidental injury. **Scald** and **contact burns** are common in children and are frequent findings in nonaccidental trauma, as explained in Chapter 13. A "pattern" burn (in which there is a clear demarcation of an object in the burned skin), "glove" or "stocking" distribution of a scald burn (**FIGURE 9-17**), or a history that is inconsistent with the injury raise suspicion of intentional injury.

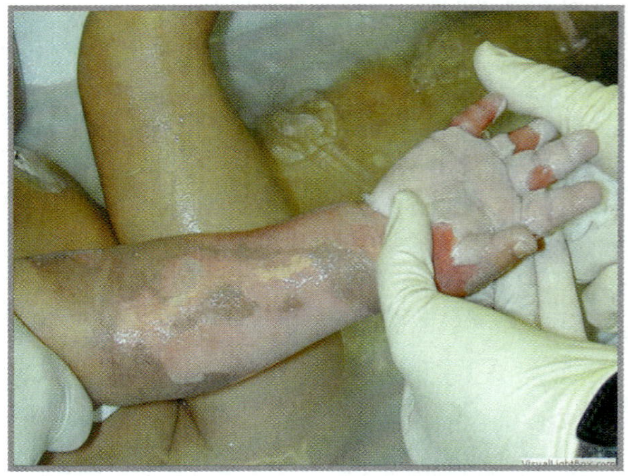

FIGURE 9-17 Consider intentional injury with a suspicious pattern of the burn, especially a "stocking" or "glove" distribution.

MANAGEMENT

Remove any burning clothes. Administer 100% oxygen to all patients with flame or blast burns. High-flow oxygen therapy is the only field treatment for suspected carbon monoxide poisoning. Because of the risk of hypothermia, do not flush or wet burned areas unless necessary to decontaminate or stop the burning process. Cover burned areas with clean dry sheets or burn **dressings**. Covering helps to reduce pain by minimizing exposure to air currents. *Do not apply ointments or creams to burn areas.*

Pain Management and Sedation. Fear and pain in children are frequently ignored or misinterpreted. Pain management is an important prehospital priority, especially in trauma and burn patients with long transport times. Infants and young children experience the same degree of pain as older children and adults; they just cannot express it in words.

Pain and anxiety are different things and require different treatments. Treat pain with an opioid analgesic drug, such as morphine or fentanyl when needed. Treat anxiety with a drug, such as a benzodiazepine (eg, diazepam or midazolam). For example, a child with continued pain after a burn needs morphine or fentanyl to control the principal problem, which is pain. Opioids, such as morphine or fentanyl, are pain killers, but they also provide some sedation. However, a child who is anxious or who has been intubated and is fighting the endotracheal tube needs a medication such as diazepam or midazolam because anxiety, not pain, is the problem.

CAUTION

Do not apply ointments or creams to burn areas.

ALS

Advanced Airway Management of the Pediatric Burn Patient. Consider early (before edema starts) endotracheal intubation in any patient exposed to a fire in an enclosed space with a suspected inhalation injury to the airway. Such patients may have abnormal airway sounds, abnormal positioning, and respiratory distress or failure. Singed or burned nasal hairs and carbonaceous sputum may also indicate airway injury. Smoke inhalation may cause bronchospasm. If wheezing is present, give a bronchodilator such as albuterol or administer intramuscular (IM) **epinephrine**.

Fluid Management of the Pediatric Burn Patient. Try to establish at least one IV line in patients with partial- or full-thickness burns greater than 5% of the body surface area, avoiding the burn site for IV insertion, if possible. Lactated Ringer is the initial resuscitation fluid of choice. If the burn is greater than 20% of the body surface area, administer fluids as follows: 5 years or younger, 125 mL/hour; 6 to 12 years of age, 250 mL/hour; and 13 years or older, 500 mL/hour. Only provide bolus fluids if the patient is hypotensive. If the burn is less than 20% of the body surface area, provide maintenance IV fluids. Fluid and heat are rapidly lost through disrupted skin, with the rate of loss proportionate to the percentage body surface area burned. Provide early analgesia and sedation, and titrate to effect. For longer transports, contact medical control to determine IV infusion rates.

Intravenous opioid analgesics are appropriate in hemodynamically stable trauma patients with burns or with isolated long-bone fractures or dislocations. If serious blood loss or bleeding is suspected, or if assessment suggests shock, avoid the use of opioids because of their tendency to contribute to hypotension. Compared with morphine, fentanyl may cause less hypotension.

Consider sedative drugs when transporting an awake, intubated child or a child who has received neuromuscular blocking agents (paralytics) to help with endotracheal intubation. Benzodiazepine drugs can also contribute to hypotension, so titrate the dose carefully.

TABLE 9–9 lists medications commonly used to treat pain or anxiety in a hemodynamically stable child after consultation with medical control, as per local EMS protocol.

TABLE 9–9 Advanced Life Support: Pharmacologic Management of Pain and Anxiety

Anxiety	
Diazepam	0.1 mg/kg IV (maximum 10 mg/dose)
Midazolam	0.05–0.1 mg/kg IV, IM, or IO; 0.2 mg/kg intranasal Maximum dose: 6 month-5 years: 6 mg >6 years: 10 mg
Pain	
Fentanyl	1 µg/kg/dose every 30-60 minutes IV, IO; 1-2 µg/kg intranasal
Morphine sulfate	*Neonates and infants* ≤6 *mo:* 0.05 mg/kg IM, IV, IO, or SQ
	Infants >6 months and children: 0.05–0.1 mg/kg IM, IV, IO, or SQ
	Adolescents: 3–4 mg IV or IO

Abbreviations: IM, intramuscular; IO, intraosseous; IV, intravenous; SQ, subcutaneous.

All IV sedatives and opioids cause respiratory depression. Administer via slow IV push over 3 to 5 minutes. Another option is to administer intranasal fentanyl. Give supplemental oxygen to all children receiving these medications. Place the child on a cardiac monitor and use pulse oximetry and waveform or digital capnography. Be ready to begin positive-pressure ventilation with a bag-mask device if the child develops respiratory depression. Naloxone (0.1 mg/kg/dose to a maximum single dose of 2 mg IV/IO/intranasal/endotracheal tube) may temporarily reverse respiratory depression caused by opioid administration. Keep in mind that use of naloxone also negates any analgesic effect and prevents further positive effects of opioids until the naloxone has been metabolized by the child's body.

CAUTION

Avoid opioids in multiple-trauma patients whose condition is unstable because these drugs may contribute to hypotension.

Treat circulatory compromise with IV fluid boluses of 20 mL/kg.

TIP

Pain and anxiety are different things and require different treatments.

Transport Decisions. The American Burn Association criteria for transfer to a burn center include the following: partial-thickness burns of more than 10% body surface area; burns involving the face, hands, feet, genitals, perineum, and major joints; and full-thickness burns. If there is a burn center in close proximity that can handle pediatric burns, transport to this location would be ideal. If there is no facility available, transport the child to the hospital based on local protocol. If needed, the child can then be transferred to a burn center.

Summary of Burns

Burns are common pediatric injuries but usually are small and require only first aid. Burns involving the airway, burns covering more than 5% of body surface area, or full-thickness burns require important field interventions, including possible airway protection, fluid administration and pain control. Burns from fires in enclosed spaces raise the possibility of carbon monoxide and cyanide poisoning. Pain is a universal feature of burns, and analgesia is usually a primary intervention.

CASE STUDY 3

You are dispatched to a child who has been run over by a vehicle. On arrival, you notice a full-sized sport utility vehicle parked in the middle of the road and a 6-year-old girl, conscious and alert, lying on the ground. She has no abnormal airway sounds or increased work of breathing, and her skin is pale. According to bystanders, the child was walking behind the car when her dad backed up. The patient is cool and clammy to the touch. The respiratory rate is 40 breaths/min, the heart rate is 146 beats/min, and you are unable to obtain a blood pressure. Lung sounds are decreased in lower fields. While exposing the child, you notice a tire track impression across the abdomen and sternum area. Pulse oximetry is 87% on room air.

1. What critical injuries do you suspect?
2. What are your treatment and transport priorities?

CASE STUDY ANSWERS

CASE STUDY 1

This patient requires immediate treatment and transport. The patient has sustained multisystem trauma to the head and lower extremities, and the primary assessment confirms respiratory failure and shock. Snoring respirations are likely caused by airway obstruction from soft tissues or blood. Positioning the airway and suctioning may alleviate the problem. Perform rapid SMR.

The patient is hypoxic with a slow respiratory rate due to his altered level of consciousness.

Perform a jaw thrust and provide oxygen at 100% by positive-pressure ventilation. Consider supraglottic airway or endotracheal intubation if the oxygenation does not improve with less-invasive airway management.

Stabilize the femur with a splint. Start IVs en route to the hospital and initiate fluid resuscitation. Transport rapidly to a trauma center with pediatric expertise.

At the hospital, the child is found to have a subdural hematoma and femur fracture and is admitted to the hospital.

CASE STUDY 2

This child appears to have an isolated head injury and TBI. The child's rapid deterioration suggests an expanding intracranial hematoma, which may be life-threatening. Provide SMR, and be prepared for vomiting. Administer 100% oxygen. Rapidly transport.

Establish an IV line en route for the administration of medications and leave at a keep-vein-open rate. Consider use of an OG tube to relieve gastric distension from crying and to limit the possibility of aspiration.

Transport to a facility with pediatric neurosurgical capability; if such care is not available in your community, consider rendezvous with an air ambulance service. This is a surgical emergency, and immediate access to operative care may make the difference between the life and death of this child.

The patient is found to have an epidural hematoma and is taken to the operating room for evacuation.

CASE STUDY ANSWERS—cont'd

CASE STUDY 3

The injuries to this child are life-threatening and she appears to be in shock. Transport immediately after spinal stabilization and provision of 100% oxygen. Consider the use of a pelvic binder or sheet.

Do not prolong scene time with IV attempts. Give fluid resuscitation during transport. Provide blood if indicated by local protocol.

This child is at risk of having sustained massive internal injury, including abdominal solid organ hemorrhage (liver, spleen, and kidneys); viscus rupture of the stomach, small bowel, and large bowel; and pelvic fracture. The source of bleeding is not relevant to field care, but the recognition and treatment of hypotensive (decompensated) shock are critical.

Transport to the highest level of trauma care available in your community, based on local trauma triage protocol. This child requires rapid radiological assessment of the extent of injury and possibly early operative intervention.

In the ED, she is given IV fluids and is intubated. She is found to have a splenic laceration, rib fractures, and a pulmonary contusion, and is admitted to the pediatric intensive care unit.

Although there have been promising results in adult studies of hypothermia after cardiac arrest, pediatric studies have found no benefit. The hypothermic state may be protective of brain function, and rapid rewarming can introduce dysrhythmias. Therefore, remove wet clothing and provide rapid transport.

In the ED, the child is still in cardiac arrest, so receives continued CPR with 3 rounds of epinephrine and is intubated. Unfortunately, there is no return of spontaneous circulation, so the resuscitation is terminated after 20 minutes.

Suggested References

TEXTBOOKS

Alson RL, Han K, Campbell JK. *International Trauma Life Support for Emergency Care Providers.* 9th ed. Pearson; 2019

American Academy of Pediatrics and the American College of Emergency Physicians. *APLS: The Pediatric Emergency Medicine Resource.* 5th ed. Jones and Bartlett Learning; 2012

American College of Surgeons, Committee on Trauma. *ATLS Advanced Traumas Life Support.* 11th ed. American College of Surgeons; 2025

Bledsoe B, Porter R, Cherry R. *Essentials of Paramedic Care.* 2nd ed. Prentice Hall; 2011

National Association of Emergency Medical Technicians. *PHTLS: Prehospital Trauma Life Support.* 10th ed. Jones and Bartlett Learning; 2024

ARTICLES

Adelgais KM, Brown K. Pediatric prehospital pain management: impact of advocacy and research. *Clin Pediatr Emerg Med.* 2014;15(1):49–58. doi:10.1016/j.cpem.2014.01.005

Atabaki SM. Prehospital evaluation and management of traumatic brain injury in children. *Clin Pediatr Emerg Med.* 2006;7(2):94–104. doi:10.1016/j.cpem.2006.03.003

Fischer PE, Perina DG, Delbridge TR, et al. Spinal motion restriction in the trauma patient–a joint position statement. *Prehosp Emerg Care.* 2018;22(6):659–661. doi:10.1016/j.cpem.2006.03.003

Goldstick JE, Cunningham RM. Current causes of death in children and adolescents in the United States. *N Engl J Med.* 2022;386(20):1955–1956. doi:10.1056/NEJMc2201761

Kochanek PM, Tasker RC, Carney N, et al. Guidelines for the managemnet of pediatrics sever traumatic brain injury, Third edition: Update of the Brain Trauma Foundation guidelines. *Pediatr Crit Care Med.* 2019;20:S1-82. doi:10.1097/PCC.0000000000001735

Leonard JC, Browne LR, Ahmad FA, et al. Cervical spine injury risk factors in children with blunt trauma. *Pediatrics.* 2019;144(1):e20183221. doi:10.1542/peds.2018-3221

Lerner EB, Dayan PS, Brown K, et al; Pediatric Emergency Care Applied Research Network (PECARN). Characteristics of the pediatric patients treated by the Pediatric Emergency Care Applied Research Network's affiliated EMS agencies. *Prehosp Emerg Care.* 2014;18(1):52–59. doi:10.3109/10903127.2013.836262

Sadow KB, Teach SJ. Prehospital intravenous fluid therapy in the pediatric trauma patient. *Clin Pediatr Emerg Med.* 2001;2(1):23–27. doi:10.1016/S1522-8401(01)90022-9

Shah MI. Prehospital management of pediatric trauma. *Clin Pediatr Emerg Med.* 2010;11(1):10–17. doi:10.1016/j.cpem.2009.12.003

Stansfield R, Morris D, Jesulola E. The use of transexamic acid (TXA) for the management of hemorrhage in trauma patients in the prehospital environment: literature review and descriptive analysis of principal themes. *Shock*. 2020;53(3):277–283. doi:10.1097/SHK.0000000000001389

OTHER RESOURCES

American College of Surgeons. National Guidelines for the Field Triage of Injured Patients. Accessed April 8, 2025. https://www.facs.org/quality-programs/trauma/systems/field-triage-guidelines/

Centers for Disease Control and Prevention. Heads up. Concussion basics. Accessed April 8, 2025. https://www.cdc.gov/heads-up/index.html

Centers for Disease Control and Prevention. Leading causes of death, 2023 United States. Accessed February 8, 2026. https://wisqars.cdc.gov/creat-table

Centers for Disease Control and Prevention. National Center for Injury Prevention and Control. WISQARS. Web-based Injury Statistics Query and Reporting System. Accessed April 8, 2025. https://wisqars.cdc.gov

CHAPTER 10

Toxicology

Elizabeth Blizzard, BA, NRP, FP-C, CCP-C
Ann Dietrich, MD, FAAP, FACEP

LEARNING OBJECTIVES

1. **Identify the age groups at risk of experiencing toxic exposures and the substance and management issues unique to each group.**
2. **Describe the physical assessment of the child with a suspected toxic exposure.**
3. **Explain the risks and benefits of different forms of gastrointestinal decontamination.**
4. **Discuss the use of antidotes in a child with a toxic exposure.**
5. **Identify situations where phone, online, or direct contact with the regional poison center might influence the assessment and treatment of toxic exposures.**

Introduction

A toxic exposure is something causing harmful effects including illness, injury, or death by various routes of exposure (eg, an ingestion, inhalation, injection, topical application to eyes or skin). Children experience such exposures for a myriad of reasons, including unintentional ingestions of poisons, environmental exposures, and deliberate intoxications. An example of an unintentional exposure is a toddler who ingests a caregiver's medication. An environmental exposure might be a child who inhales carbon monoxide during a house fire, or a child with a systemic reaction to skin contact with an insecticide or other chemical. Intentional intoxications include recreational drug or alcohol exposures and attempted suicides.

Age-Related Differences in Toxic Exposures

Toxic exposures are a common pediatric prehospital complaint. Although children younger than 6 years account for almost 40% of the total exposures for all age groups, according to 2023 data from America's Poison Centers, the percentage of fatalities in this age group remains low at 1.9% (**TABLE 10–1**). Although the number of reported exposures for the adolescent population (13–19 years) is relatively low at 8.6%, the mortality rate is much higher at 4.5% of fatalities, and it is usually caused by intentional exposure. Most toxic exposures in infants and children younger than 6 years are nontoxic or minimally toxic. The toddler is a fearless, curious individual who explores the world by placing objects in their mouth (**FIGURE 10–1**). Because toddler ingestions are unintentional, and most nonfood items ingested are not very palatable, poisonings in this age group often involve small volumes of a single substance. The most common ingestions in young children include cleaning substances, analgesics, cosmetics and personal care products, dietary supplements/herbals/homeopathic medications, and foreign bodies/toys. The great majority of toddlers are initially asymptomatic; however, toddlers may experience significant symptoms without a known history or witnessed ingestion, particularly of cannabis and opioids. Providers should consider this possibility and survey the scene to better understand possible causes. In addition, it is important to keep

TABLE 10–1 Toxicological Cases 2023: America's Poison Centers Toxic Exposure Surveillance System

Total reported cases	2,080,659
Patients <3 years of age	583,922 (28.4%)
Patients <6 years of age	828,669 (39.8%)
Total patients <20 years of age	1,158,039 (55.6%)

Data from Gummin DD, Mowry JB, Beuhler MC, et al. 2023 Annual Report of the National Poison Data System (NPDS) from American's Poison Centers: 41st Annual Report. *Clin Toxicol.* 2024;62(12): 793–1027. doi:10.1080/15563650.2024.2412423

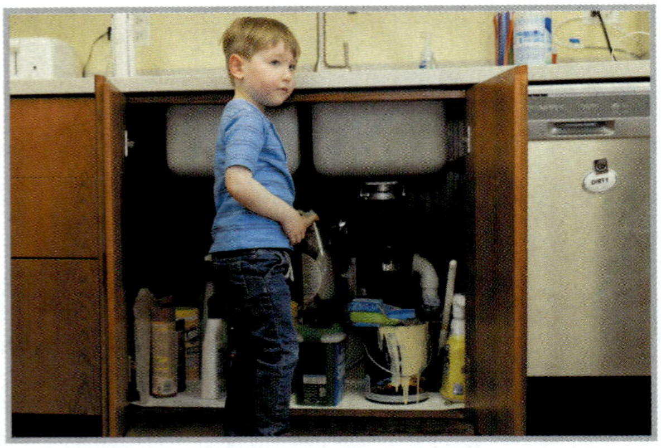

FIGURE 10–1 Toddlers are "oral explorers"; they will try to taste or swallow almost any substance.

in mind that the initially asymptomatic child may have dangerously high levels of a toxin in their body that may not become apparent until much later. In the absence of any apparent life threats, obtaining a thorough history before making a transportation disposition is absolutely imperative. In this age group, analgesics, stimulants and street drugs, and fumes/gas/vapors caused the most fatalities.

Button (disk) batteries usually pass through the digestive tract without a problem, but can get stuck in the esophagus or anywhere else in the body. If there is suspicion that a child has ingested a battery (or one is stuck in the nose, ear, or elsewhere), attempt to find out exactly what kind of battery it is and bring the child to the emergency department (ED). Providers should also consider this possibility when "coin" ingestion is reported, as the 2 are easily confused. More than one-third of patients with disk batteries lodged in the esophagus are initially asymptomatic. Symptoms develop when the battery begins to erode and damages surrounding tissues. Most batteries pass through the gastrointestinal tract in 1 to 4 days, but a lodged battery can cause esophageal or tracheal injury or life-threatening hemorrhage. The risk is highest with 20-mm batteries, which are larger and more likely to become lodged, while batteries smaller than 12 mm pose a lower risk. Co-ingestion of a magnet with the battery also increases the risk of serious injury. If a battery ingestion is known or suspected, oral administration of 10 mL of honey for patients older than 12 months may prevent esophageal damage. Children aged 6 to 12 years are less likely to ingest nonfood articles or nonprescribed medications. Although most exposures continue to be unintentional in this age group, intentional exposure begins to play a role, particularly among the middle school–aged group.

Among adolescents (13–19 years), toxic exposures are usually intentional, most often as a suicide attempt, but sometimes a result of recreational misuse. Intentional exposures lead to more ED visits and hospital admissions than unintentional exposures. In suicide attempts, adolescents usually ingest 2 or more substances, often in large quantities. Recreational misuse often involves alcohol in addition to another recreational drug. The number of fatalities in this age group is increasing. Statistics represent an underestimation of the true incidence, because statistics only include those cases reported to the poison center database. Adolescents may also experiment with creative ways to get high that involve substances they can access easily. Huffing usually involves common household products, such as markers, glue, aerosol air freshener or hair spray, spray paint, correction fluid, gasoline, and other products. These substances are inexpensive, easy to find in many homes, and do not seem suspicious to parents. Botanical substances such as salvia and jimson weed (hallucinogens) are also easy to grow or obtain. The internet may provide access to a wide variety of illegal drugs that were previously more difficult for teens to obtain. One example is "bath salts," a group of synthetic cathinones that mimic the symptoms of

CASE STUDY 1

A mother calls 9-1-1 because her 3-year-old toddler is drooling and having trouble breathing. On arrival at the home, you find a young boy coughing. He has no abnormal airway sounds, no flaring, and no retractions. His skin is pink. The respiratory rate is 32 breaths/min, the pulse oximetry finding is 98%, and the heart rate is 120 beats/min. His lungs are clear. On further assessment, you note that the child has a brightly colored laundry packet in his hand that has been bitten into. His mother states that she was doing the laundry when she received a telephone call and left her son briefly.

1. What are key aspects of the scene size-up?
2. Outline transport and management priorities.

methamphetamine and can cause agitation, tachycardia, violent behavior, and hallucinations; luckily, they are now illegal to sell. "K2" or "spice" is synthetic marijuana; symptoms include mood elevation and altered perception, but it can also cause tachycardia, palpitations, elevated blood pressure, and nausea. Another popular synthetic drug is "ecstasy" or "Molly." This is 3,4 methylenedioxymethamphetamine (MDMA), and it has stimulant and hallucinogenic properties. It causes an elated mood, euphoria, and increased energy, but it also causes tachycardia and hypertension. Because this drug can affect the body's ability to regulate temperature, it can lead to hyperthermia, resulting in dehydration; heart, kidney, and liver failure; and seizures. Providers need to be aware of new trends in drug use, and are often the first people to alert a health department or an ED after treating a patient.

It is important to keep in mind crew member safety, because some substances may result in an unintentional exposure for providers. Providers need to use personal protective equipment (PPE)—specifically gloves to avoid skin contact—whenever the use of substances such as organophosphates or hydrogen sulfide is suspected.

With the legalization of marijuana in some states, children may be at higher risk of exposure to these substances/products. In particular, marijuana is found in edibles that may be packaged to look like children's snacks or candy. In children, marijuana can cause significant respiratory depression. An increasing number of children also have been exposed to fentanyl.

Another problem continues to be the exposure of young children to the chemicals used in methamphetamine laboratories and the use of methamphetamines. Crew safety in these situations is critical because of explosion and fire hazards. Methamphetamine can cause delusional and violent behavior in a teenage patient. Restraints may be necessary if approved by local medical protocol.

Exposures that do not fit the usual pattern of pediatric poisoning should be carefully examined for the possibility of child maltreatment. Examples include large exposures or multisubstance ingestions, or repeated ingestions in children younger than 6 years. An unusual form of abuse involves deliberate intoxication of infants or young children, a condition called **factitious disorder imposed on another (FDIA)** (formerly called Munchausen syndrome by proxy). This is a mental health condition in which a caregiver fabricates or induces physical or psychological symptoms in another person, typically a child or dependent adult, to gain attention, sympathy, or medical care. In these cases, the caregiver frequently possesses more than average medical information and is trying to induce a state of illness in the child in an attempt to bring attention to themself. Children with such exposures may be especially difficult to identify because the intoxication is secretive and often long-term. It is important to alert child protective services and the receiving ED as required by local laws and regulations, as well as departmental policy.

COMMON SUBSTANCES RESPONSIBLE FOR SERIOUS POISONINGS IN CHILDREN

Most poisonings occur in the home. **TABLE 10–2** lists common substances responsible for poisonings according to age.

Summary of Age-Related Differences in Toxic Exposures

Most toxic exposures in children are minor and involve household products. The most common patient is the toddler who unintentionally ingests a single agent in small quantity and is asymptomatic. The second most common patient is the adolescent who uses recreational drugs or who is making a suicide attempt or gesture. Adolescent exposures often consist of more than 1 drug and often involve large quantities. Common serious exposures in young children involve analgesics, whereas those in adolescents involve analgesics, alcohol, and recreational

TABLE 10–2 Top 10 Substances Involved in Toxic Exposures

Children (<5 years of age)	Adults >20 years of age
Cleaning substances (household)	Analgesics[a]
Analgesics[a]	Cardiovascular drugs
Cosmetics/personal care products	Antidepressants
Foreign bodies/toys/miscellaneous	Sedatives/hypnotics/antipsychotics
Dietary supplements/herbals/homeopathic	Cleaning products (household)

[a]Analgesics include aspirin, acetaminophen, ibuprofen, and opioid analgesics such as methadone, fentanyl, and morphine.

drugs. An unusual form of intoxication in young children involves a condition called factitious disorder imposed on another, a complex form of deliberate poisoning or abuse of a child by a caregiver.

TIP

Most patients with toxic exposures are toddlers or preschool-aged children. There is usually only one poison involved, the exposure is usually small and unintentional, and the child is asymptomatic.

Prearrival Preparation and Scene Size-Up

Sometimes, at the time of dispatch, the toxin has already been identified by the caregiver, the poison center, or another health care professional. In such cases, immediately contact medical control or the poison center, depending on local emergency medical services (EMS) protocol. They can help clarify the toxicity of the agent and priorities in assessment and treatment. In other cases, in which the dispatch involves a toddler or an adolescent with a sudden change in behavior, consider a toxic exposure. Poison center resources can be substantial and provide great insight into the appropriate treatment needed for the ingested substance.

On arrival, first perform the scene size-up. Note if there are potentially hazardous toxins in the area or on the patient's clothes or skin. Assess the scene for methamphetamine that might pose a risk to the crew. If it is present, determine whether immediate patient decontamination is safe to perform. The poison center or other public health agency may assist in defining risk and the need to mobilize other personnel (eg, hazardous materials team). Pay close attention to scene safety when dealing with adolescents with sudden behavioral changes, because some common substances of abuse can lead to paranoia and sudden violent actions.

If there is a possible toxin or hazardous material, secure the scene and minimize the risk of toxic exposures to the EMS crew through the skin, eyes, or lungs by use of PPE. Use all your senses to gather information at the scene. Pay particular attention to your initial impression of smell on the scene. Some dangerous toxins quickly overwhelm the sense of smell, rendering it useless after just a few sniffs (olfactory fatigue). Other toxins have an odor only at low levels, such as hydrogen sulfide. The rotten egg odor given off by this chemical overwhelms the sense of smell, and one cannot smell it at high toxic levels. Other key smells include bitter almonds (cyanide) and garlic (organophosphates, arsenic). Pay attention to confined spaces, and remember that some toxic gases are heavier than air and may affect children first or may only be in low-lying areas, such as cesspools or ditches.

Any poisoning call with multiple patients reporting the same symptoms raises concern about environmental toxins, and providers should be cautious when entering the scene. Be aware of the possibility of a mass exposure to a toxic substance, because of either unintentional or deliberate action (eg, bioterrorism). If a disaster or mass-casualty event is suspected, implement disaster response preparedness (see Chapter 16).

TIP

Bring bottles, containers, plastic bags, suspicious substances, plants, or syringes to the ED.

TIP

Ask caregivers to look around (eg, in purses, under the child's bed) to help determine what could have been ingested.

TIP

The adolescent who makes a suicide attempt or gesture must be transported to the ED for medical and psychological assessment, even if the child refuses. This is essential even if the injury or immediate medical risk is assessed as trivial.

Next, look over the surrounding area. Bring any bottles, containers, or plastic bags containing possible toxins and samples of ingested plants or syringes to the ED along with the patient (**FIGURE 10–2**). If the caregiver refuses to let a poisoned child be transported to the hospital, ask medical control to talk to the caregiver over the telephone or radio. If this strategy does not work, then request assistance from law enforcement personnel.

CAUTION

Never forget about toxic hazards on scene. Watch out for absorbable toxins and protect the skin and eyes by using gloves and other personal protective equipment.

Role of the Poison Center

Every state in the United States is covered by a designated regional poison control center. The telephone number within the state is usually toll-free. For ease of access, there is also a national toll-free

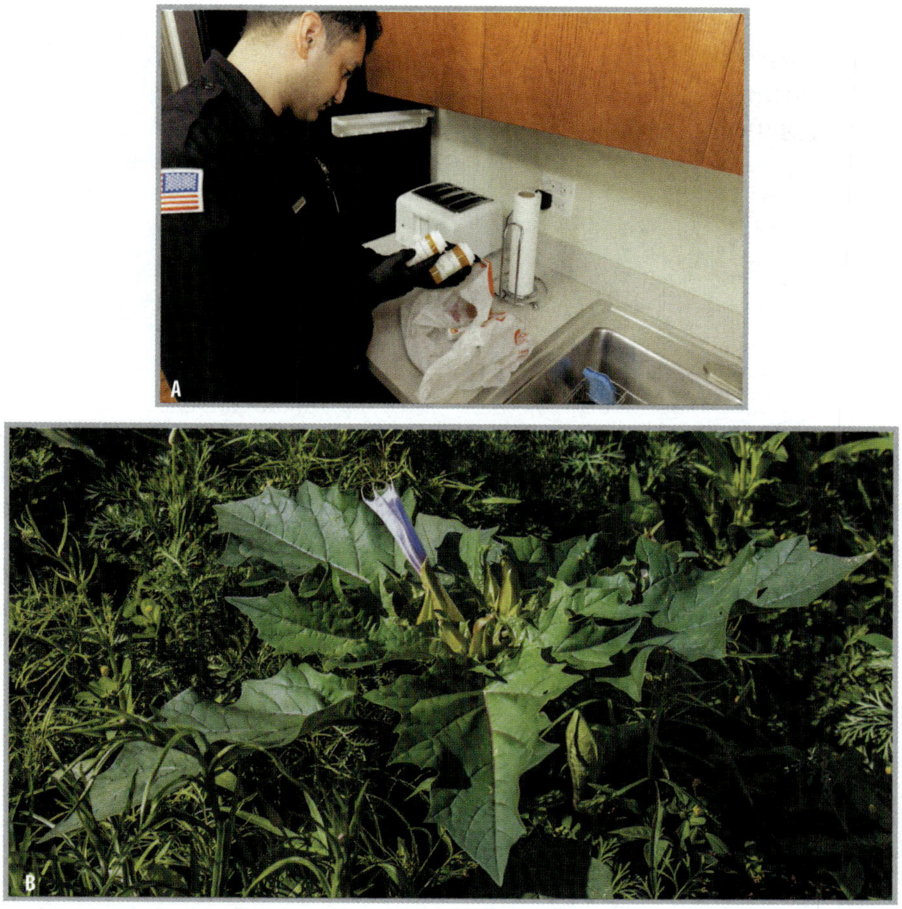

FIGURE 10–2 Bring any bottles or plant samples to the ED. **A.** Bottles and containers. **B.** The poisonous plant jimson weed.

number (1-800-222-1222) that is available 24 hours a day, 7 days a week. At the other end of the telephone are specialists who can provide information about the potential toxicity of a substance or adverse effects and can recommend home or hospital management. Caregivers often call the poison center for advice before, or while awaiting, the arrival of the EMS clinician. The poison center can also be accessed online at poisonhelp.org.

TIP

The poison center has a key role in individual and community prevention and treatment of toxic exposures. Save the nationwide toll-free number (1-800-222-1222) in the phone you use for work and consider posting it in the ambulance.

The regional poison center can also be a valuable resource to the EMS clinician when managing children with a toxic exposure. Local EMS system protocol should define the circumstances when contact with the poison center must be made by medical control and when EMS clinicians can make the call directly.

TIP

Poison centers have the capability to follow up with continuing reassessment by telephone.

Assessment of the Child With a Possible Toxic Exposure

GENERAL ASSESSMENT

After the rapid scene size-up and environmental evaluation for toxins, assess the child. Use age-appropriate techniques to approach the patient, as outlined in Chapters 1 and 2, and conduct a general assessment (pediatric assessment triangle [PAT]), a primary assessment, and then an additional assessment when appropriate. If the child's condition is unstable, treat the physiological abnormalities detected in the general (PAT) and primary assessments, and then transport. En route, do a reassessment and additional assessments, if possible.

A detailed history is the best tool for overall assessment of risk and for determining the urgency of need

TABLE 10–3 "TART" Chart

Toxin	Amount	Route	Time
Name of substance type (pill, capsule, liquid, seed, root, flower, suppository, patch)	Milligrams or other amount if known; include approximate number of pills or seeds, amount of liquid, and so forth (note if any spilled on floor or clothes) Note any vomitus Take with you if possible	By mouth, snorted, smoked, injected, rectal, skin, eyes, nose, and so forth	Approximate time of first exposure or ingestion Include duration and whether in confined space, if applicable Last known time patient was acting normally

for treatment in pediatric poisoning. It is usually more accurate than a physical evaluation in determining the specific type of toxic exposure. In the first few minutes, the important questions are as follows: (1) the identity of the agent, (2) the route of exposure (ingestion, inhalation, injection, topical), (3) the time since the exposure occurred, and (4) the amount of the agent involved in the exposure; if unknown, assume the worst-case scenario. Using the acronym TART can help one remember: T = Toxin, A = Amount, R = Route, T = Time. See **TABLE 10–3**.

SPECIAL CONSIDERATIONS IN THE PRIMARY ASSESSMENT

After the PAT, perform the hands-on ABCDEs (Airway, Breathing, Circulation, Disability [neurological status], and Exposure [skin/temperature]) to complete the primary assessment, and then immediately treat any physiological abnormalities. Special elements of the physical assessment that may help identify the type of poison include breath odor, vital signs, pupillary size, skin temperature, and skin condition (eg, color, sweating). An odor of bitter almonds may be caused by cyanide, a sweet smell by ethylene glycol, or garlic odor by organophosphates. Also, look for stains, powders, and burns on the skin or clothes. Use assessment information to match the patient's signs and symptoms with possible toxidromes, identifiable clinical patterns of single-agent intoxications. **TABLE 10–4** outlines the signs and symptoms of important toxidromes in pediatrics.

AIRWAY

Clear, maintain, and control the airway in a child with a suspected toxic exposure who has altered mental status (AMS). This may happen in a child exposed to a **sedative** or **hypnotic drug**, such as a benzodiazepine or a barbiturate. Beware of the child who has ingested a **caustic** agent, such as **lye**. This child may have severe burns of the esophagus and experience drooling, **dysphagia**, and signs of upper airway obstruction. Have a suction unit on hand; if using it becomes necessary, do so gently to avoid making the child vomit.

TABLE 10–4 Common Toxidromes

Toxidrome	Agents	Signs and Symptoms
Anticholinergics	Antihistamines, cyclic antidepressants	Identified according to the mnemonic "Hot as a hare, red as a beet" (hot, dry skin; hyperthermia), "blind as a bat" (dilated pupils), "mad as a hatter" (delirium, hallucinations); similar to sympathomimetic toxidrome but differentiated by dry skin
Cholinergics	Organophosphates	DUMBELS: diarrhea/diaphoresis, urination, miosis (constricted pupils), bradycardia/bronchoconstriction, emesis, lacrimation, salivation SLUDGEM: salivation, lacrimation, urination, defecation, gastrointestinal upset, emesis, muscle weakness
Nicotinic	Nicotine	MTWTFSS (days of week): mydriasis, tachycardia, weakness, tremors, fasciculations, seizures, somnolence
Opioids	Morphine, fentanyl, methadone	Hypoventilation, bradycardia, hypotension, miosis, apnea
Sympathomimetics	Cocaine, amphetamines, other stimulants	Tachycardia, hypertension, hyperthermia, mydriasis (dilated pupils), diaphoresis (sweating); similar to anticholinergic toxidrome, but differentiated by diaphoresis (wet skin)

BREATHING

Give 100% supplemental oxygen by a nonrebreathing mask if there is AMS, respiratory distress, or a history of exposure to a toxic substance known to cause breathing problems. One example of this type of toxic exposure is **hydrocarbon** inhalation. Obtain pulse oximetry, but be aware that the reading is not accurate for some toxic exposures, notably carbon monoxide or cyanide poisoning. Sedative or hypnotic drugs, opioids, and gamma hydroxybutyrate may decrease the respiratory rate, whereas **sympathomimetic agents** (cocaine, amphetamines), **phencyclidine (PCP)**, and aspirin may increase the respiratory rate.

Close monitoring of the airway is essential to evaluate the adequacy of breathing so that intervention with a bag-mask device with supplemental oxygen can be started without delay if necessary. End-tidal capnography is helpful to monitor respiratory status.

CIRCULATION

If the child has eaten or swallowed a possible cardiac toxin, place the child on a cardiac monitor to watch for dysrhythmias. Such drugs as β-blockers, digoxin, or calcium channel blockers may decrease the heart rate, whereas sympathomimetic agents and anticholinergic agents (**scopolamine**, antihistamines, and jimson weed) may increase the heart rate. Skin can be warm and dry because of such drugs as older antihistamines and anticholinergics, whereas the skin may be hot and sweaty because of sympathomimetics, organophosphates, aspirin, and PCP.

DISABILITY

Altered mental state is a common effect of many different chemical exposures. Recreational drug use with sedatives or hypnotics depresses the central nervous system (CNS). Sympathomimetic drugs may stimulate the CNS and cause excitement, agitation, paranoia, or hallucinations. Cyclic antidepressants may cause seizures or coma. In a comatose or unresponsive patient, always consider the other common causes of AMS, such as a head injury, seizure, or hypoglycemia (which may accompany alcohol or β-blocker ingestion). Check the bedside glucose level in any patient with AMS, even if toxins are suspected, and treat as needed. **TABLE 10–5** outlines the signs and symptoms of specific agents in pediatric patients.

TABLE 10–5 Specific Agents

Agent	Alternate Names	Signs and Symptoms
Ecstasy	3,4-methylenedioxymethamphetamine, mephedrone (MDMA), and/or methylenedioxypyrovalerone, "Molly"	Euphoria, increased energy, intense visual perceptions Complications: hyperthermia, hypertension, tachycardia, seizures, dehydration, myocardial infarction, intracerebral hemorrhage
γ-hydroxybutyrate γ-butyrolactone	GHB, "date rape drug" GBL (GHB precursor)	Initially drowsiness, dizziness, and disorientation; high doses result in bradycardia, hypoventilation, and apnea
Rohypnol	Flunitrazepam, "roachies," "roofies"	Drowsiness, sedation, amnesia, blackout
Second-generation (atypical) antipsychotics	Olanzapine (Zyprexa™), risperidone (Risperdal™), aripiprazole (Abilify™), ziprasidone (Geodon™), quetiapine (Seroquel™)	Drowsiness, QT prolongation, stomach pain; can also cause neuroleptic malignant syndrome (NMS), a rare, but life-threatening, idiosyncratic reaction to these antipsychotics/neuroleptic medications that is characterized by fever, muscular rigidity, hypertonicity, altered mental status, and autonomic dysfunction; NMS often occurs shortly after the initiation of neuroleptic treatment or after dose increases
Selective serotonin reuptake inhibitors (SSRIs)	Sertraline (Zoloft™), fluoxetine (Prozac™), paroxetine (Paxil™), fluvoxamine (Luvox™)	Restlessness, hallucinations, shivering, diaphoresis, nausea, diarrhea, headache; these medications can also cause serotonin syndrome, which is characterized by agitated delirium, high fever, elevated blood pressure, tachycardia, and diaphoresis, can occur within minutes of exposure to the precipitating agent, and can deteriorate to shock and muscle rigidity.
Synthetic cannabinoids	Spice, "synthetic marijuana," K2, fake weed	Elevated mood, relaxation, altered perception Complications: agitation, hallucinations, severe paranoia, seizures, vomiting, tachycardia, hypertension, myocardial ischemia
Synthetic cathinones	"Bath salts"	Tachycardia, hypertension, euphoria, paranoia, agitation, hallucinations, violent behavior, sweating, nausea, vomiting, dizziness, panic attacks

EXPOSURE

Undress the child and look for evidence of toxic exposure to the eyes and skin. Many substances, such as hydrocarbons, irritate the eyes. Other toxic substances, such as **hydrochloric acid**, are caustic to skin. **Organophosphate insecticides** can be inhaled and also enter through the skin and can cause a severe **cholinergic crisis** with diaphoresis (sweating), diarrhea, urination, **miosis** (small pupils), bradycardia, bronchoconstriction, emesis, tearing, and **salivation**. The mnemonic DUMBELS (Diarrhea/Diaphoresis, Urination, Miosis, Bradycardia/Bronchoconstriction, Emesis, Lacrimation, Salivation) helps identify signs of cholinergic drug intoxication. In some systems, the mnemonic SLUDGEM is used: Salivation, Lacrimation, Urination, Defecation, Gastrointestinal pain, Emesis, and Muscle twitching (seizures or coma). These signs, coupled with agitation and respiratory distress, signal a severe possible environmental exposure, as discussed in Chapter 16.

INITIAL MANAGEMENT OF TOXIC EXPOSURES

After the primary assessment, determine the need for treatment and transport of the poisoned child by combining the physical assessment with a risk assessment. The physical assessment is a way to determine the child's physiological stability and the overall urgency of need for treatment and transport. The risk assessment evaluates the probability of serious toxicity (early and delayed) from the exposure. *Perform the risk assessment with knowledge of the identity of the drug involved, time since ingestion or exposure, and amount of poison involved. The child's weight should also be considered* (see **TABLE 10–6**). The poison center can provide much of this information.

Common toxic agents, such as aspirin, acetaminophen, or iron, have predictable physiological effects that are determined by how much of the drug was taken, time since exposure, and amount of drug per kilogram of body weight. By collecting information and evidence at the scene, the EMS clinician serves an important role in later ED testing and treatment. Be sure to ask about *all* medications (prescription and over the counter), preparations, and other substances to which the child may have been exposed. Caregivers may not realize that some topical preparations (eg, liniments or wart treatments) contain salicylate and can contribute to the same or similar potential salicylate toxicity as that when a child ingests aspirin or some common herbal preparations and oils, many of which also contain salicylates.

Sometimes, the EMS clinician's risk assessment determines that a child has had a potentially lethal exposure, although the child is physiologically stable. Indeed, in a small child, 1 ingested pill or teaspoon of some common medications can kill. **TABLE 10–7** lists potentially dangerous agents that may be fatal to a toddler after a tiny toxic exposure (eg, one pill).

Iron poisoning is one of the leading causes of fatal poisonings in young children. Tasty chewable children's vitamins have, on average, 17 mg of iron, and the tempting new chewable gummy prenatal vitamins have 27 mg each. A young child can easily mistake either of these for candy and eat excessive amounts. Consider that seriously toxic doses begin at 60 mg/kg of iron (20 mg/kg of elemental iron), and as the ingestion climbs toward 120 mg/kg and higher, the poisoning can easily be lethal without prompt treatment. Gather all bottles, and when pills are missing, assume that the child has eaten them until proven otherwise.

TABLE 10–6 Risk Assessment

Assess the chances of serious toxicity from these 5 pieces of information:
1. The agent involved and its lethality, usually identified through consultation with medical control or the poison center
2. Amount of the toxin, dosage form or strength, pills or liquid (in milligrams when possible)
3. Child's weight
4. Route of exposure
5. Time since the exposure or last time patient was acting normally

CONTROVERSY

If the child is in stable condition and has a history of a single, small ingestion of a low-risk agent, some EMS systems allow nontransport in consultation with medical control. Although this approach may be medically sound, it eliminates an opportunity for ED assessment of psychosocial risk factors.

TIP

In suspected toxic exposures, perform risk assessment to determine the probability of serious toxicity.

TIP

Nicotine in any form (eg, gum, patch, lozenge, e-cigarettes) can be toxic if ingested. Signs and symptoms include vomiting, sweating, drowsiness/tiredness, shaking, confusion, seizures, and death.

CASE STUDY 2

You respond to a call for a 3-year-old who just ingested all of her mother's prenatal iron gummies (approximately 30). On your arrival, the child is active and running around the room, but complaining that her "tummy hurts." She has no increased work of breathing, and her skin is pink. Her respiratory rate is 22 breaths/min, heart rate is 110 beats/min, and blood pressure is 90/60 mm Hg. Her physical examination reveals no abnormalities. The mother hands you the empty bottle of fruit-flavored chewable prenatal gummy vitamins. Reading the label, you learn that each vitamin contains 27 mg of iron.

1. Do you need to transport this child to the hospital?
2. Should you give the child activated charcoal?

TABLE 10–7 Potentially Lethal Toddler Ingestions in 1 or 2 doses

Medicine	Lethal Dose
Calcium antagonists	40 mg/kg
Camphor	One to two teaspoons of oil
Chloroquine	One 500-mg tablet
Clonidine	One 0.3-mg tablet
Glyburide	Two 5-mg tablets
Imipramine	One 150-mg tablet
Lindane (lice removal—not available in the United States)	Two teaspoons (10 mL) of 1% lotion
Diphenoxylate/atropine (Lomotil™ Rx strength)	Two 2.5-mg tablets
Methadone	5 mg/kg
Nicotine (liquid) (eg, vaping liquids)	One teaspoon (5 mL) (13 mg/kg)
Oil of wintergreen (methyl salicylate)	One teaspoon (5 mL) (200 mg/kg)
Phenothiazines	20 mg/kg
Propranolol	One or two 160-mg tablets
Quinidine	50 mg/kg
Theophylline	One 500-mg tablet
Tricyclic antidepressants (eg, amitriptyline)	15 mg/kg
Toxic alcohols (eg, methanol, ethylene glycol)	0.3 mL/kg
Verapamil	One or two 240-mg tablets (50 mg/kg)

THE TRANSPORT DECISION: STAY OR GO?

After the primary assessment, initial treatment, and risk assessment, consider whether to transport immediately, performing additional assessment and treatment on the way to the ED, or stay on the scene. If the results of the physical assessment and the risk assessment reveal an asymptomatic child and the ingestion of a small amount of a single low-risk agent, consider nontransport after appropriate consultation with medical oversight or the poison center. This is controversial, however, because some EMS systems consider hospital transport necessary in all toxic exposure cases. Other systems allow the poison center to manage minor ingestions exclusively over the telephone. Always follow the advice of your local medical control.

If the physical assessment indicates that the child has any physiological abnormality, or if the risk assessment indicates that the toxic exposure is potentially harmful, transport and perform additional assessment on the way to the ED, if possible. The onset of symptoms varies with the substance involved. A child without symptoms on arrival of the EMS clinician may still have ingested a lethal dose of a substance. For example, ingestions of acetaminophen, a common household over-the-counter medicine, may be extremely dangerous but cause no early symptoms. History from the scene is critical to the management in the ED.

In serious poisonings, the patient may benefit from in-hospital therapies such as dialysis or specific antidotes, so ideally the patient should be transported where this therapy is available.

TIP

Most preadolescent pediatric poisonings do not require any treatment in the field; however, EMS does carry some antidotes that can be given en route, if necessary.

ADDITIONAL ASSESSMENT

If the child has no physical abnormalities and is asymptomatic, and if the risk assessment indicates no serious toxicity, perform a complete assessment on

TABLE 10–8 The Pediatric SAMPLE for Toxic Exposures

Component	Explanation
Signs and symptoms	Time of suspected exposure Behavior changes in child Emesis and content of vomitus
Allergies	Known drug reactions or other allergies
Medications	Identity of suspected toxin Amount of toxin exposure (count pills or measure volume) Pill or chemical containers on scene Exact names and doses of prescribed medications
Past medical problems	Previous illnesses or injuries
Last food or liquid	Timing of the child's last food or drink Type and time of home treatment
Events leading to the exposure	Key events leading to the exposure Type of exposure (inhaled, injected, ingested, or absorbed through the skin) Poison center contact

scene. Additional assessment includes the focused history and physical examination and the detailed physical examination (for trauma). Sometimes, it is more appropriate to perform this additional assessment on the way to the ED. **TABLE 10–8** lists important aspects of patient history in a suspected toxic exposure, presented in the standard SAMPLE format. During the primary assessment and the risk assessment, the EMS clinician will have already obtained some of the SAMPLE history.

Summary of Assessment of the Child With a Possible Toxic Exposure

Every child with a toxic exposure needs a careful physical assessment and risk assessment. The physical assessment includes all of the features of the standard assessment, with an emphasis on the history, which is usually the most important part of the toxicologic evaluation. Preparation begins on the way to the scene with dispatch information about the age of the patient, the type and potential toxicity of exposure, and the need for PPE. Preparation then continues with the scene size-up and environmental assessment. If multiple patients are involved, consider disaster plan activation to ensure that adequate resources are available to respond.

After the physical assessment, the risk assessment helps determine if there might be serious toxicity based on the type of toxin involved, the amount of the toxin, the weight of the child, the route of exposure, and the time since the exposure. The risk assessment elicits important information about expected physiological effects, the need for treatment, and the timing of transport. The poison center often plays a key role in helping to decide about treatment and transport.

Toxicologic Management

The EMS clinician has 3 options for toxicologic management of serious or potentially lethal exposures: (1) decontamination to reduce local or systemic exposure to the toxin, including absorption and distribution, (2) enhancement of natural elimination or increasing the speed of removal of the toxin, or (3) antidote administration to reverse the actions of the poison directly. In most cases, documenting a thorough history, evaluating the risk assessment, and appropriate transport supporting the ABCs (airway, breathing, circulation) are the best treatment.

DECONTAMINATION

After the treatment and transport decision, consider decontamination. There are several ways to decontaminate, depending on the toxin and the type of exposure.

Skin

If there is a chance that the poison could have been **absorbed** through the skin, remove the child's clothing. The EMS clinician must protect their own skin and eyes by using gloves and protective gear. Flood the skin with large amounts of warm water for 15 to 20 minutes (if time allows and no apparent life threats take priority), and then wash it well with mild soap and water, avoiding harsh scrubbing.

Eyes

Immediately wash out the eyes if there has been direct eye contact (**FIGURE 10–3**). **Alkali** burns with caustic agents, such as lye, are the most dangerous. Flush the eyes for 20 minutes using normal saline or water. Attach intravenous (IV) tubing to the bag of normal

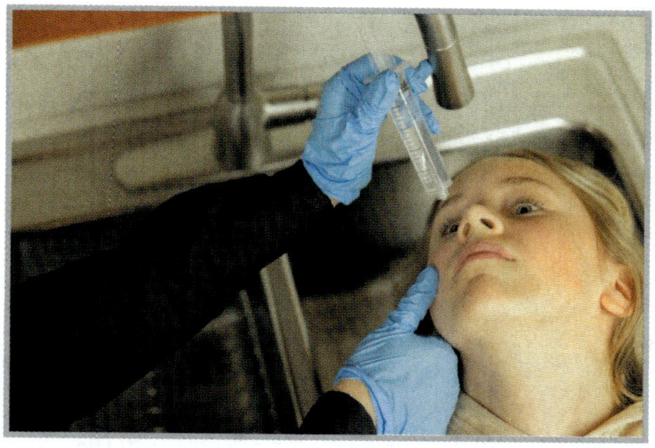

FIGURE 10–3 Immediately wash out the eyes if there has been direct eye contact.

TABLE 10–9 Toxins Poorly Adsorbed by Activated Charcoal: "PHAILS"

Pesticides, potassium
Hydrocarbons
Acid, alkali, alcohol
Iron
Lithium
Solvents

saline and flush the eye with the end of the IV tubing. If this is not possible, hold the patient's head under the sink and pour water into the eye from a pitcher or cup. When the eyes are the main area of exposure, continue flushing during transport if possible.

Gastrointestinal Decontamination

Before any **gastrointestinal (GI) decontamination**, contact medical control or the poison center, depending on EMS protocol. In some cases, it may be beneficial to dilute mild **acid** or alkali ingestions by asking the alert patient to drink an 8-oz glass of milk or water. Dilution is contraindicated when there is absent gag reflex, airway compromise, diminished level of consciousness, or ingestion of a hydrocarbon corrosive or caustics (strong alkalis and acids).

> **TIP**
>
> **Ipecac**, an old-time remedy for ingestions, is no longer manufactured in the United States, but may have been given in the home by the caregiver. Make note of this and the time it was given. The vomiting induced by ipecac does not remove significant amounts of ingested toxins from the stomach and may cause prolonged emesis, delaying the administration of activated charcoal.

Activated Charcoal. Most high-risk ingestions in toddlers and preschool children do not require any prehospital treatment. Use activated charcoal only when recommended by medical control or the poison center, based on local protocols. In cases in which GI decontamination is necessary, consider using activated charcoal. Activated charcoal is made from burned wood products. The surfaces are "activated" by steam or chemical treatment, so the material can irreversibly **adsorb** ingested toxins in the stomach and small bowel, reducing bloodstream absorption of the toxins if given quickly after exposure. Charcoal itself is not absorbed from the GI tract, nor is it metabolized. Activated charcoal has no odor or taste, but has a granular consistency that makes many children unwilling to drink it. Charcoal administration is messy, even with a cooperative child. In a child with altered or deteriorating mental status, aspiration of charcoal can lead to serious pulmonary consequences. Limited data are available on the use of activated charcoal in the prehospital setting, and the risks of prolonged scene time must be weighed against the potential benefits of rapid transport and early ED management, including making intubation more difficult. Some agents are not adsorbed by activated charcoal, as noted in **TABLE 10–9**.

Administration of Activated Charcoal. The activated charcoal dose is 10 times the mass of the ingested substance. However, because the actual amount of ingested material is usually not known, use 1 to 2 g/kg of the child's body weight. Activated charcoal begins working immediately, and it is most effective when given within 1 hour of ingestion (**FIGURE 10–4**).

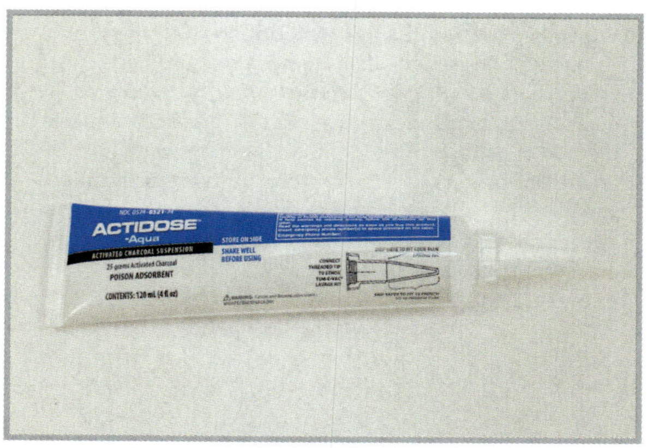

FIGURE 10–4 Activated charcoal is a treatment option for potentially serious ingestions of bindable toxins.

TABLE 10–10 Activated Charcoal: Guidelines for Use

Product Information	A highly adsorbent, tasteless material made from wood pulp
Indication	To limit amount of drug absorbed by the body in most toxic ingestions (ie, intestinal decontamination) Repeated doses may enhance the elimination process
Technique	If advised, mix 1–2 g/kg patient weight with water to form a **slurry**; if the quantity of ingested substance is known, give 10 times the ingested dose of the toxin by weight (maximum dose, 100 g) Administer orally (or by nasogastric tube in rare situations) Consider adding a flavoring agent to make the slurry more acceptable
Contraindications	Loss of gag reflex Altered mental status Unwillingness to take the drug voluntarily **Corrosive**/caustic substance ingestion Drugs not adsorbed by charcoal
Adverse effects	**Constipation** or intestinal **bezoar** (large foreign-body mass in gut) Pulmonary aspiration Diarrhea and dehydration may occur in children younger than 1 year who are given a combined **cathartic** (eg, sorbitol) and activated charcoal

Never force a child to take activated charcoal, because this may lead to aspiration and pulmonary complications. If local EMS policy allows, consider adding a flavoring agent (eg, cola, juice, milk) to make the mixture more acceptable to drink, then transport the child. Some formulations of activated charcoal also contain sorbitol. **Do not use charcoal and sorbitol formulations in children** because of the risk of causing electrolyte abnormalities and dehydration due to diarrhea. **TABLE 10–10** summarizes activated charcoal and guidelines for its use.

ALS

The child must be in stable condition and cooperative to receive activated charcoal. Because young children or adolescents may not want to drink the activated charcoal, some EMS systems use a nasogastric tube as an alternative method of delivery if the ingestion is potentially serious or lethal. Delivery of activated charcoal by nasogastric tube can be dangerous and must be reserved for highly unusual circumstances in which the transport time is long and risk assessment indicates severe toxicity.

TIP

The biggest problem with field use of activated charcoal is the difficulty in getting children to take it.

CONTROVERSY

The value of activated charcoal for prehospital treatment of ingestions is unproven. Although the treatment has a possible advantage of early binding of toxins in the gut, there are potential complications, such as aspiration and bowel obstruction.

ENHANCEMENT OF ELIMINATION

Sorbitol is a cathartic medication that is mixed with many commercial activated charcoal preparations. Cathartics have been promoted to clear the bound toxin from the gut and help speed up elimination. The effectiveness of cathartics has not been proved, and sorbitol is not an approved drug in most EMS systems. EMS clinicians may think they are giving pure activated charcoal when the preparation actually is a mixture of activated charcoal and sorbitol. Sorbitol may cause nausea, vomiting, abdominal discomfort, diarrhea, and electrolyte disturbances in young children. *Therefore, never use a cathartic in children in the prehospital setting unless recommended by the poison center.*

ANTIDOTES

Antidotes are medications that reverse or treat the adverse effects of toxic ingestions. EMS clinicians carry several antidotes (**TABLE 10–11**) that may be life-saving for poisoned patients. Use these medications

TABLE 10–11 Commonly Available Prehospital Antidotes

Poison	Antidote
Carbon monoxide	Oxygen
Cyanide	Hydroxocobalamin or nitrites and sodium thiosulfate
Organophosphate	Atropine/pralidoxime (2-PAM)
Tricyclic antidepressants, salicylates	Sodium bicarbonate
Opioids	Naloxone
β-blockers	Glucagon
Calcium channel blockers	Calcium
Benzodiazepine	Flumazenil
Oral hypoglycemics	Glucose, glucagon

with knowledge of the type of ingestion or exposure, patient's clinical status, and possible adverse effects associated with the antidote, and as advised by the medical director and local protocols.

Naloxone is an antidote used frequently in adult patients with suspected opioid overdose. It can have a therapeutic and diagnostic effect in selected pediatric patients. If the child has signs of an opioid ingestion or overdose (respiratory depression, bradycardia, coma, small pupils), administer 0.1 mg/kg. Although the maximum dose has been 2 mg, a higher dose is often needed for a fentanyl overdose. Although IV is the preferred route, it can be given intramuscularly (IM), intraosseously, intranasally, endotracheally, or via nebulizer. In fact, the packaged nasal spray is available only in a 4-mg dose. The child may then awaken slightly or fully, but the main goal of naloxone treatment is improvement in vital signs, especially respiration. The duration of action of naloxone is 20 to 60 minutes, so repeat doses may be necessary if a longer-acting opioid (eg, methadone, fentanyl) is involved. When administering naloxone, as with adults, give the lowest effective dose and administer slowly. In adolescents with a chronic substance abuse disorder to opioids, administering naloxone too rapidly may induce undesired acute withdrawal symptoms. Have suction on hand in case vomiting occurs. To prevent danger to the EMS crew, it is also important to prepare for the possibility that the patient will awaken violently.

Although flumazenil is an effective benzodiazepine antagonist, do not use this antidote routinely for patients with AMS of unknown cause. One of the most common causes of AMS in children is the postictal state after a seizure. If flumazenil is given and the child has further seizures, benzodiazepines are not effective. Also, flumazenil may precipitate seizures if administered to a patient who is receiving long-term therapeutic doses of a benzodiazepine.

Sodium bicarbonate helps reverse the adverse cardiac effects seen with cyclic antidepressant overdoses, including conduction abnormalities. It alkalinizes the blood to reverse the sodium channel blockade caused by the drugs. The dose is 1 to 2 mEq/kg IV, administered slowly. It can also be used for salicylate poisoning.

Glucagon, a drug familiar to EMS clinicians because of its role in the treatment of hypoglycemia, can help improve the low heart rate caused by an overdose of calcium channel blockers. Although there are no good pediatric studies, the suggested dosage of glucagon is 0.05 mg/kg followed by 0.07 mg/kg/h (maximum, 5 mg/h) given IV. Note that this is higher than the usual dose of glucagon administered for hypoglycemia.

Calcium channel blockers are a frequently prescribed medication for hypertension in adults. Pediatric ingestions may result in severe toxicity that is similar to a β-blocker overdose, including bradycardia and hypotension. There also can be secondary respiratory and neurological effects (respiratory depression, decreased level of consciousness). Intravenous fluids are the first line of therapy, and calcium can be beneficial. Administer either IV calcium chloride 10% (20 mg/kg = 0.2 mL/kg) or IV calcium gluconate 10% (60 mg/kg = 0.6 mL/kg) slowly. Calcium gluconate is recommended by peripheral IV in children. The patient needs to be on a cardiac monitor during administration of these drugs and during transport. Vasoactive agents such as epinephrine are also beneficial for hypotension after a calcium channel blocker overdose.

Organophosphates

The mnemonics DUMBELS and SLUDGEM (see **TABLE 10–4**) summarize the clinical hallmarks of organophosphate poisoning toxidrome. Treatment involves several steps:

1. Ensure your personal protection (use protective gloves and other protective clothing to prevent exposure).

2. Remove contaminated clothes and place them in a bag.
3. Perform the primary assessment, and ensure adequate oxygenation and ventilation.
4. Decontaminate the patient (flush the skin with large amounts of water; wash the skin, hair, and under the nails well with soap and water).
5. Flush exposed eyes with large amounts of warm water or saline.
6. If the child has symptoms of severe poisoning, consider treatment with the antidote atropine. The drug helps reverse the muscarinic organophosphate effects (salivation, bronchorrhea, bronchospasm, bradycardia, respiratory depression, seizures, coma). The initial pediatric dose is 0.05 mg/kg IV (a higher-than-usual atropine dose). Repeat doses until the airway is dry and the child has adequate perfusion. Also consider administration of pralidoxime (2-PAM), if available. This drug restores the enzyme that is deactivated by organophosphate poisons, reversing toxicity. It is only effective for certain organophosphates and within a limited period of time. The use of benzodiazepines to control seizures is also indicated.

With the advent of possible chemical terrorism incidents, much attention has been paid to the side effects of organophosphates, which are the same as those for such nerve agents as sarin gas. Because some EMS agencies have distributed MARK 1 or MARK 2 kits to their providers for management of chemical terrorism, it is important to realize that the medication doses in these autoinjector kits are for adults. However, in severe, life-threatening pediatric cases, administer the contents of these kits to children 3 years or older by IM injection. Keep in mind that the likelihood of responding to a child involved in an event of weapons of mass destruction is far lower than the likelihood of responding on a sunny afternoon to a child poisoned by one of the many household and commercial pesticide preparations containing organophosphates.

Summary of Toxicologic Management

Most children with toxic exposures do not require treatment of any kind in the field. Consider nontransport after consultation with medical control or the poison center only if the child is asymptomatic and has ingested a small amount of a single low-risk substance, and there are no red flags for child neglect or maltreatment. In other circumstances, when physical assessment and risk assessment together show physiological instability or possible toxicity, treatment is indicated. After managing the ABCDEs, consider toxicologic management by decontamination or, in special situations, administering an antidote. Perform skin and eye decontamination when indicated. Attempt GI decontamination for serious or potentially fatal ingestions according to local protocol. Activated charcoal is a useful binding agent for many types of toxic ingestions, but it can be safely administered only to a cooperative child. Sorbitol is contraindicated in children. Several antidotes carried by EMS clinicians may be diagnostic, therapeutic, and even lifesaving. More advanced antidote therapies are best administered in the ED or hospital setting. Remember to educate the family or caregiver about poisoning prevention if circumstances allow, as discussed in Chapter 19.

Medicolegal Issues

There are several scenarios in which medicolegal issues play an important role in the management of toxicologic emergencies in children. If the caregiver refuses therapy and transport to the hospital, ask medical control to talk to them over the telephone. If this strategy does not work, then request assistance from law enforcement personnel.

An adolescent who makes any suicide attempt or gesture must be transported to the ED. An individual who has attempted suicide is legally incompetent to make treatment decisions and cannot refuse transport. In some cases, law enforcement must become involved in scene management. Place the patient in temporary protective custody and transport them to the hospital (see Chapter 17).

Legal problems can also arise with an adolescent due to emancipated minor laws, allowing them to **consent for care** as well as the illegal use of alcohol or recreational drugs. If an adolescent has taken a potentially toxic dose of medication, or has life-threatening complications of drug use or overdose, treat according to the emergency exception rule (the doctrine of implied consent), as explained in Chapter 17. Leave the legal issues of alcohol or drug use to law enforcement officials.

CASE STUDY 3

You respond to a call about a seizing girl at a park. On arrival, you find a group of high-school students surrounding a girl who is lying on the ground having a tonic-clonic seizure. She is unresponsive and cyanotic. Her heart rate is 90 beats/min and respiratory rate is 6 breaths/min, and you are unable to obtain a blood pressure.

The students tell you she is 16 years old and that they were partying after a football game, smoking some "spice" and drinking beer. The patient was happy and dancing 1 minute, then she became agitated and started to seize. The students deny any head trauma. She has been seizing for 10 minutes.

1. What are your initial treatment management priorities?
2. Can you treat and transport this patient without parental consent?

CASE STUDY ANSWERS

CASE STUDY 1

Scene size-up should include ensuring your safety with gloves and other PPE as needed. Note if there has been skin or eye involvement in addition to ingestion. If present, remove the child's clothes and undertake skin and eye decontamination.

The emergence of brightly colored laundry pods has resulted in numerous pediatric ingestions. The toddler will usually bite into the pod and swallow the liquid. The main issue is the components of these pods. They often contain a detergent and surfactant, but some contain alkaline substances.

The most likely symptoms from these ingestions are vomiting, coughing, and drowsiness, but if an alkali is present, mouth burns, drooling, and airway compromise can occur.

Rapidly transport this child to the hospital, frequently reassessing his airway. Bring the bitten pod, as well as an intact one, to the ED. Allow the child to sit upright in a position of comfort. Administer blow-by oxygen because a face mask will likely not be tolerated. Contact with medical control or poison control (1-800-222-1222) can provide information on potential complications to anticipate in transport, such as airway edema, stridor, or wheezing. Do not give anything by mouth, including charcoal or fluids, because of the risk of vomiting.

The child is taken to the operating room by otolaryngology clinicians (ear, nose, and throat) and found to have mild burns of his esophagus.

CASE STUDY 2

Although this child appears well, this is a potentially dangerous ingestion. Iron is one of the most common fatal ingestions in children. There are 4 phases to an iron ingestion. The initial phase begins with the ingestion and lasts 6 hours. Common signs and symptoms in mild ingestion include nausea and vomiting. Stage 2 (at 6–12 hours) is the quiet phase, during which the child appears well. It is not until stage 3 (12–24 hours after ingestion) that the child begins to show signs of toxicity, including GI hemorrhage, hypotension, AMS, and renal and hepatic failure. Stage 4 is the postrecovery phase, during which GI strictures can still occur. Because the extent of toxicity cannot be predicted from early symptoms, a cautious approach is warranted. Transport any child who has ingested iron-containing pills to the hospital for further evaluation unless the poison center has been contacted and has determined that this is a nontoxic ingestion based on the nature and number of pills taken. This child requires transport to the hospital. Bring any pill bottles to the ED to ensure proper identification and risk assessment. Because iron is not absorbed by activated charcoal, do not attempt GI decontamination.

In the ED, laboratory samples are drawn and fluids given. Treatment with deferoxamine is started to chelate the iron, and the patient is admitted.

Continued

CASE STUDY ANSWERS—cont'd

CASE STUDY 3

The first priority is to establish an effective airway and begin bag-mask ventilation with 100% oxygen, because respiratory failure is present. Based on local protocols, you can provide medications such as intranasal or IV midazolam or rectal diazepam. In addition, naloxone may be given.

Some questions to ask the patient's friends include a SAMPLE history:

- Signs and symptoms: Did anyone see her before she started to seize? Was she acting normally?
- Allergies: Any known drug reactions or other allergies?
- Medications: Does she take any medications (both prescription and nonprescription, such as herbs/vitamins)? Was she drinking any alcohol? Does she use illicit drugs? Did anyone see other drugs being passed around?
- Past medical problems: Does she have any medical problems?
- Last food or liquid: When was the last time anyone saw her with something to eat or drink?
- Events: What was she doing before she began to seize?

Because they admit to smoking "spice," the real question is whether there were any other drugs in the mixture besides synthetic marijuana. The key finding of a seizure can be caused by this drug, but also consider hypoglycemia due to alcohol ingestion. Once the seizure has stopped, reassess vital signs and transport to the hospital with bag-mask ventilation and IV fluids.

Even without the girl's assent or her parents' consent, you are legally bound to treat and transport this patient because she has a life-threatening condition.

In the ED, she is intubated and admitted to the pediatric intensive care unit.

Suggested References

TEXTBOOKS

American Academy of Pediatrics and the American College of Emergency Physicians. *APLS: The Pediatric Emergency Medicine Resource*. 5th ed. Jones and Bartlett Learning; 2012

Dieckmann R. Toxic exposures. In: Seidel J, Henderson D, eds. *Prehospital Care of Pediatric Emergencies*. 2nd ed. Jones and Bartlett Learning; 1997:122–129

Olson KR, Smollin CG, Anderson IB, et al, eds. *Poisoning & Drug Overdose*. 8th ed. McGraw Hill; 2022

Tenenbein M, Macias CG, Sharieff GQ, Yamamoto LG, Schafermeyer RW, eds. *Strange and Schafermeyer's Pediatric Emergency Medicine*. 5th ed. McGraw Hill; 2019

ARTICLES

Bar-Oz B, Levichek Z, Koren G. Medications that can be fatal for a toddler with one tablet or teaspoonful: a 2004 update. *Paediatr Drugs*. 2004;6(2):123–126. doi:10.2165/00148581-200406020-00005

Bonney AG, Mazor S, Goldman RD. Laundry detergent capsules and pediatric poisoning. *Can Fam Physician*. 2013;59(12):1295–1296, e535–e537. PMID: 24336541

Graudis A, Lee HM, Druda D. Calcium channel antagonist and beta-blocker overdose: antidotes and adjunct therapies. *Br J Clin Pharmacol*. 2015;81(3):453–461. doi:10.1111/bcp.12763

Gummin DD, Mowry JB, Beuhler MC, et al. 2023 Annual Report of the National Poison Data System (NPDS) from American's Poison Centers: 41st Annual Report. *Clin Toxicol*. 2024;62(12):793–1027. doi:10.1080/15563650.2024.2412423

Kim JW, Baum CR. Liquid nicotine toxicity. *Pediatr Emerg Care*. 2015;31(7):517–521. doi:10.1097/PEC.0000000000000486

Lowry JA, Leeder JS. Over-the-counter medications: update on cough and cold preparations. *Pediatr Rev*. 2015;36(7):286–298. doi:10.1542/pir.36.7.286

Liebelt EL, Shannon MW. Small doses, big problems: a selected review of highly toxic common medications. *Pediatr Emerg Care*. 1993;9(5):292–297. PMID:8247936

Osterhoudt KC. The toxic toddler: drugs that can kill in small doses. *Contemp Pediatr*. 2000;3:73.

Stromberg PE, Burt MH, Rose SR, Cumpston KL, Emswiler MP, Wills BK. Airway compromise in children exposed to single-use laundry detergent pods: a poison center observational case series. *Am J Emerg Med*. 2015;33(3):349–351 doi:10.1016/j.ajem.2014.11.044

Velez LI, Shepherd JG, Goto CS. Approach to the child with occult toxic exposure. *UpToDate*. Wolters Kluwer. Accessed November 18, 2024. https://www.uptodate.com/contents/approach-to-the-child-with-occult-toxic-exposure

Wang GS, Hall K, Vigil D, Banerji S, Monte A, VanDyke M. Marijuana and acute health care contacts in Colorado. *Prev Med*. 2017;104:24–30. doi:10.1016/j.ypmed.2017.03.022

OTHER RESOURCES

National Institute on Drug Abuse. Drugs A to Z. Accessed May 10, 2025. https://www.drugabuse.gov/reserach-topics/drugs-a-to-z.

Poisoning statistics, 2023, national data. Poison Control. Accessed November 18, 2024. https://www.poison.org/poison-statistics-national

Swallowed a button battery? Battery in the nose or ear? Poison Control. Accessed April 15, 2025. https://www.poison.org/battery

CHAPTER 11

Behavioral Emergencies

Dawn Poetter, Oregon Paramedic
Archana Reddy Bongurala, MD, FAAP

LEARNING OBJECTIVES

1. **Describe neurodevelopmental and psychiatric conditions in children and adolescents that may present with behavioral emergencies, including autism spectrum disorder (ASD), attention-deficit/hyperactivity disorder (ADHD), behavior or conduct disorders, anxiety, and depression.**
2. **Discuss the management of behavioral emergencies in children.**
3. **Explain suicidal ideation and proper evaluation of suicidal patients.**
4. **Review management of common suicidal intentional ingestions.**
5. **Discuss de-escalation methods for agitated patients.**
6. **Provide information on chemical restraint.**
7. **Review issues that may arise during patient restraint.**

Introduction

Behavioral emergencies in children and adolescents are a significant public health issue, resulting in numerous emergency department (ED) visits and prehospital patient encounters. From 2018 to 2021, more than 11% of all pediatric prehospital incidents involved behavioral emergencies. Pediatric behavioral emergencies increased by 60% from 2007 to 2016, and there was a 300% rise in suicide/self-harm presentations during the same period. The frequency of these encounters creates considerable pressure on prehospital clinicians and EMS systems (**FIGURE 11-1**).

Behavioral health emergencies may present alone, as part of, or together with other special health care needs. The most common disorders diagnosed in childhood include attention-deficit/hyperactivity disorder (ADHD), behavior disorders (including oppositional defiant disorder [ODD] and conduct disorder), anxiety, and depression. One in 6 US children between 2 and 8 years of age have been diagnosed with a mental, behavioral, or developmental disorder (the latter includes autism spectrum disorder [ASD]). Behavior issues are more common in those 6 to 11 years old, while diagnoses of anxiety and depression increase with age. Often, those with ASD and ADHD are included as a subset of children with special health care needs.

There are many barriers to effective treatment, including limited resources for inpatient and outpatient treatment of mental health problems and a shortage of mental health care providers. Additionally, identifying and treating behavioral health emergencies is challenging because they may present at nearly any age, from toddlerhood to adolescence, and can occur in a variety of settings, including the school and home environment. Onset may occur gradually or suddenly.

Examples of behavioral emergencies in children include suicidal behavior such as self-harm or intentional ingestions, depression with suicidal ideation, and ODD with aggressive behavior. Behavioral emergencies may also present in children without a previous formal diagnosis. Prehospital clinicians should be aware of behaviors that need to be brought to the attention of the ED at handoff to facilitate care by mental health experts.

Common Pediatric Psychiatric and Behavioral Conditions

To fully understand the types of behavioral emergencies faced by prehospital providers, it is important to define and describe common pediatric psychiatric

CASE STUDY 1

You are called to the scene of a 6-year-old boy who was stung by a bee while playing outside at a summer barbecue. On your arrival, the child's mother states that the boy began crying and pointing at his arm. The mother noted a welt with surrounding redness, along with swelling of the child's lips. She also states that her son has been inconsolable since the sting. The mother reports her son has no allergies and a history of mild asthma, with use of an albuterol inhaler as needed. She also reports that her son has been diagnosed with ASD. As a result, he can be very difficult to calm when upset and becomes very anxious around medical providers.

Your assessment reveals an agitated child seated near his mother, crying and kicking his legs. He appears anxious. His actual work of breathing is difficult to determine because of his crying; his skin is pink. You note swelling of his lips and around the eyes and urticaria on his neck and arms. The child is pulling away and will not make eye contact with prehospital providers; however, you are now able to hear expiratory wheezes between cries. The child is uncooperative with your examination, and you are unable to obtain vital signs, but respirations appear to be fast and the hives are spreading. The mother sent another family member to retrieve the child's favorite blanket and stuffed animal.

1. What are the key principles in assessing this child?
2. Describe treatment and transport approaches.

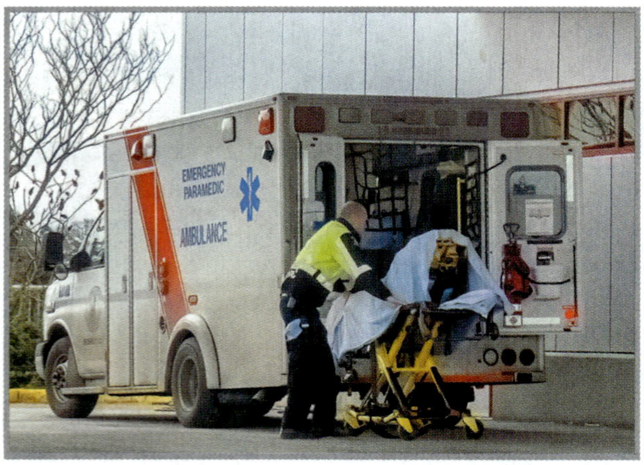

FIGURE 11-1 Behavioral health emergencies in children and adolescents are a significant public health issue, resulting in numerous emergency department visits and prehospital patient encounters.

Marvin Samuel Tolentino Pineda/iStockphoto.com

TABLE 11-1 Missed Developmental Milestones in Autism Spectrum Disorder

Age	Clinical Manifestations
6 months	Few or no big smiles or other engaging expressions Limited or no eye contact
9 months	Little or no back-and-forth sharing of sounds, smiles, or other facial expressions
12 months	Little or no babbling Little or no back-and-forth gestures such as pointing, showing, reaching, or waving Little or no response to name
16 months	Very few or no words
24 months	Very few or no meaningful 2-word phrases (not including imitating or repeating)

conditions, including ASD, ADHD, ODD, depression, bipolar disorder, and schizophrenia.

AUTISM SPECTRUM DISORDER

Of the aforementioned conditions, ASD presents at the earliest age. ASD is defined in the *Diagnostic and Statistical Manual of Mental Disorders, Fifth Edition* (*DSM-5*), as a neurodevelopmental disorder characterized by 2 primary features: (1) persistent deficits in social communication or interaction with others and (2) repetitive and restrictive patterns of behavior or actions. Because this is a spectrum disorder, the outward signs of a child with autism can range from mild to severe. Most children on the autism spectrum have sensory sensitivities including hypersensitivity to environmental stimuli such as light, sound, and touch or hyposensitivity to painful stimuli such as a broken bone. These symptoms typically present early in development, sometimes as young as 6 months (see **TABLE 11-1**). As such, according to the American Academy of Pediatrics, all children should be screened at 18 and 24 months of age so that early diagnosis and therapeutic interventions can be provided. Unfortunately, most children are not diagnosed until after 4 years of age. Recent research and innovations such as technology-assisted eye-movement tracking have facilitated earlier diagnosis and improved our understanding of ASD. According to the Centers for Disease Control and Prevention, autism affects an estimated 1 in 36 children in the United States today. It is 4 times more common in boys than in girls and affects all races, ethnicities, and socioeconomic groups. There has been a significant increase in the diagnosis of this disorder in recent years.

Treatment of children with ASD often involves a multidisciplinary team consisting of psychiatrists, pediatricians, behavioral therapists, psychologists, teachers, and social workers, along with many others (**FIGURE 11–2**). For some patients with significant agitation or severe and frequent behavioral outbursts, medications, such as α-2 adrenergic agonists (eg, guanfacine [Intuniv®, Tenex®] and clonidine [Catapres®]), stimulants (eg, methylphenidate [Ritalin®, Concerta®]), or selective serotonin reuptake inhibitors (SSRIs) (eg, fluoxetine) (Prozac®) may be prescribed. Rarely, atypical antipsychotics such as risperidone are required if initial pharmacotherapy fails.

Prehospital providers may be called to care for an individual with autism who is experiencing a medical, traumatic, or behavioral emergency, and the approach taken to scene size-up, history taking, assessment, intervention, and transport will require special attention to ensure the best outcome for the child and family. Patients who have communication difficulties commonly communicate pain and other symptoms with behavioral outbursts, including self-injurious behavior. A sudden change in behavior in a child who is nonverbal or has limited communication abilities warrants a thorough physical evaluation.

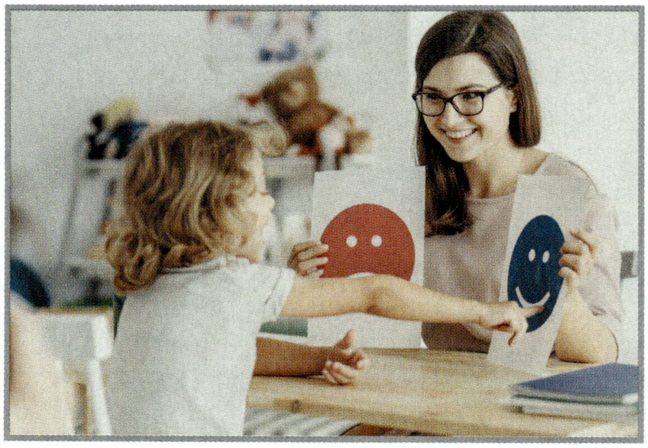

FIGURE 11–2 Visual supports, such as emotion cards, are commonly used by behavioral therapists, psychologists, educators, and health care providers to help children with autism spectrum disorder identify and communicate feelings.

KatarzynaBialasiewicz/iStockphoto.com

> **TIP**
>
> *Do not* assume that a behavioral emergency has a behavioral cause. Children with ASD or other communication difficulties may communicate their pain or distress with behavioral outbursts.

Children with ASD are at risk of wandering or running away from help, drowning, or experiencing other accidental injuries. They also have difficulty understanding and communicating when stress levels are increased, such as in an emergency, and may be frightened or scared by strangers or medical providers. As a result, they may exhibit aggression, agitation, or outbursts that may make it difficult for prehospital providers to care for them. In such situations, children with ASD who may typically communicate with minimal difficulty may suddenly become nonverbal, repeat words or movements, or take increased time to respond to questions or requests. Adjustments can be made when responding to, caring for, and transporting a child with known ASD. For example, avoiding lights and sirens, loud noises, and quick sudden movements, when possible, can help alleviate some of the sensory sensitivities that can heighten during an emergency in a child with ASD.

Additionally, it is often helpful to have a discussion with the parent or caregiver regarding calming or de-escalation techniques that have worked in the past. Although many children with ASD have presentations similar to those of other children, as with any pediatric patient, prehospital providers will need to rely on information provided by family members or other caregivers to ascertain what may be normal or baseline for a child. Caregiver participation is also necessary in helping to keep the patient calm and cooperative during an assessment. Keep instructions simple, explain what you are going to be doing to the child before you do it, have family available as a resource, and minimize portions of the examination that may be overstimulating. It is also best to limit the number of prehospital providers involved in the assessment—preferably just you and your partner—to help reduce anxiety in the child with ASD, unless additional assistance is needed on scene. It is helpful to work slowly, avoid sudden movements, and perform your examination from distal to proximal. Be aware that dressings or bandages may cause tactile sensory

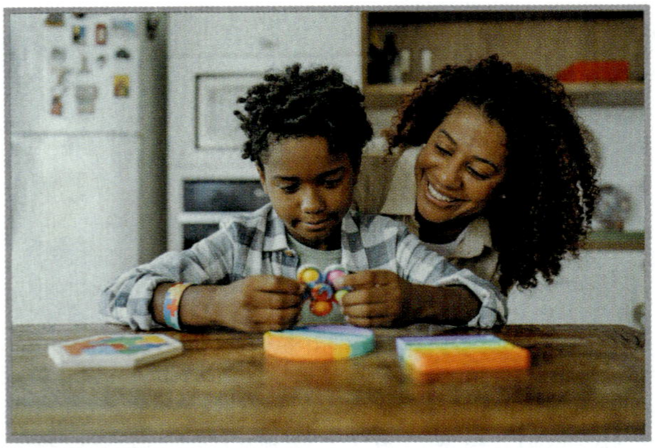

FIGURE 11–3 Children with ASD may have sensory aids that assist them in self-soothing.

andreswd/iStockPhoto.com

sensitivities. Other strategies for ensuring a successful patient encounter include conducting your assessment in a quiet area whenever possible; avoiding any unnecessary physical contact with the patient; and, when physical assessment is necessary, offering simple explanations before and during the assessment. Throughout treatment and transport, continue to reassure the child and parent and use any special comfort adjuncts, such as stuffed animals or blankets, that may help calm and soothe the child during times of increased stress (**FIGURE 11–3**). If a caregiver tells you that a formal diagnosis of ASD has been made, be sure to include the information in your radio and in-person report, along with any approaches that proved successful in your providing care. Otherwise, report the behavior that is witnessed, such as "child is hypersensitive to touch" or "child rocked rhythmically back and forth during the assessment." By modifying your usual pediatric care to include best practices for the patient with presumed or diagnosed ASD, the best possible outcome can be achieved.

> **TIP**
>
> Enlist the caregiver when treating a patient with ASD. They will know ways to approach the child, calming methods that work, and how to avoid causing agitation in the child.

ATTENTION-DEFICIT/HYPERACTIVITY DISORDER

ADHD is the most common behavioral condition in children. It is defined in the *DSM-5* as a constellation of symptoms that are present in more than one setting for at least 6 months and have an onset before 12 years of age (median age of onset, 6 years). Symptoms such as inattentiveness, hyperactivity, and impulsiveness should be inconsistent with the expected developmental findings of the child's chronologic age and need to be significantly impairing function at home or in school for this diagnosis to be made by a mental health professional.

Treatment of ADHD may consist of behavioral modification therapy, pharmacotherapy, or a combination of the two. Behavioral modification therapy includes interventions aimed at changing behaviors using nonpunitive consequences and reward systems. Examples of such interventions are time-outs, positive reinforcements, or withdrawal of privileges. One behavioral intervention that combines all these strategies is a "token economy." In a token economy, children receive tokens in response to desired behaviors and are later able to exchange those tokens for rewards or privileges.

Whereas behavioral modification therapies are preferred in younger patients, pharmacotherapy is considered first-line treatment for children 6 years or older to treat symptoms of inattention, impulsivity, and hyperactivity. Stimulants such as methylphenidate (Ritalin®, Concerta®) or dextroamphetamine (Adderall®) are the usual first-line pharmacotherapy agents offered to patients. Given their rapid onset of action and tolerable side effect profile, stimulants are preferred to other agents. Other nonstimulant medications such as atomoxetine (Strattera®, a selective norepinephrine reuptake inhibitor [SNRI]) and α-2 agonists such as guanfacine (Intuniv®, Tenex®) or clonidine (Catapres®) may also be considered.

Both in the prehospital and in-hospital settings, children with ADHD have difficulty following directions and may be frightened or agitated by medical encounters. Because the parent–child relationship is crucial in children with ADHD, engaging the parent in the interaction with the child will result in a far more productive patient encounter. Children with ADHD respond well to positive reinforcement, minimal distractions, and the use of calming words and movements. Children with ADHD should be encouraged to participate in their own care by being provided with limited choices (for example, "Which arm do you want me to put the blood pressure cuff on?") and encouraging them with positive reinforcement (**FIGURE 11–4**).

> **TIP**
>
> Give a child with ADHD simple instructions and frame questions so that "no" is not an answer. For example, "Which finger do you want me to put the pulse oximeter on?" is better than asking, "Can I put this on your finger?" Reward good behavior with positive reinforcement.

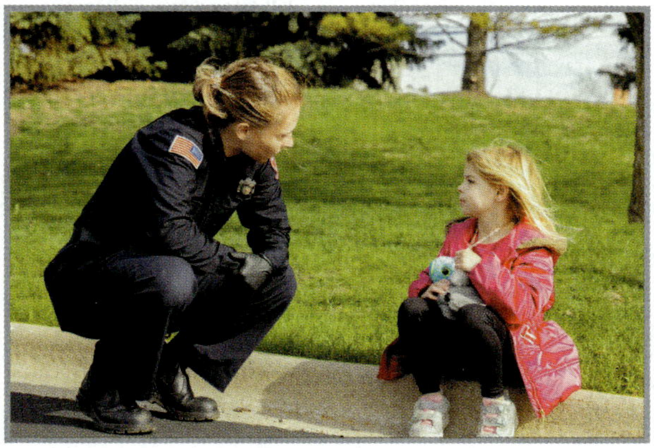

FIGURE 11–4 Children with ADHD should be encouraged to participate in their own care by being provided with limited choices.

BEHAVIOR DISORDERS: OPPOSITIONAL DEFIANT DISORDER AND CONDUCT DISORDER

Oppositional defiant disorder (ODD) and conduct disorder are mental disorders of childhood and adolescence defined in *DSM-5*. Patients with ODD typically exhibit defiant, argumentative, and hostile behavior. These children are often vindictive and frequently disobey rules, argue with authority figures, and blame others for their mistakes or behaviors. These symptoms must persist for at least 6 months and must be negatively impacting the child's functioning for the diagnosis to be made. Oppositional defiant disorder usually starts before age 8 years, but no later than age 12 years.

Conduct disorder is a separate disorder that coexists with ODD in 42% of patients. Conduct disorder is diagnosed by manifestation of aggression or violence toward people or animals and serious violation of rules such as destruction of property, thieving, or deceitful behaviors.

Both ODD and conduct disorder are difficult to treat and require a multidisciplinary approach, with behavioral therapy being the first-line treatment. Examples include parent management therapy, which teaches parents and caregivers how to manage disruptive behaviors and to use collaborative problem solving. Pharmacological therapy may be an adjunct to behavioral therapy. Studies have shown that treatment of comorbid disorders, such as ADHD, diminishes symptoms of ODD and may also help in patients with conduct disorder.

EMS clinicians may be called to transport a patient because of their aggressive behavior. Enlist the caregiver, if possible, to assist with calming the patient. In some cases, law enforcement assistance may be needed to establish scene safety and prevent injury to the EMS clinicians. If calming attempts fail, chemical or physical restraint may be necessary. Use of sedating medications or physical restraints should be guided by the medical needs of the patient and should conform to local EMS protocols (see Assessment and Transport of the Child With a Behavioral Emergency).

CAUTION

The use of restraints is a last resort when transporting an aggressive child.

ANXIETY

When children do not outgrow typical fears, or there are so many worries that they interfere with home, school, or daily activities, a child may be diagnosed with anxiety disorder. Such fears include separation from parents while at school (separation anxiety), fears of a specific situation (phobias), being afraid of places where there are other people (social anxiety), or worry about bad things happening (general anxiety). Anxiety affects 7.8% of children ages 3 to 17 years. Therapy includes behavior therapy, family therapy, or both. In many cases, medication is prescribed, the most common being SSRIs such as fluoxetine (Prozac®), sertraline (Zoloft®), fluvoxamine (Luvox®), and paroxetine (Paxil®) or venlafaxine (Effexor®), an SNRI.

EMS clinicians often encounter anxious children or adolescents with panic disorder. The child may feel as if their heart is beating too fast; they may be dizzy or sweaty, have trouble breathing, or even pass out. Check vital signs, pulse oximeter readings, and bedside glucose levels. Ask if this has happened before. Have the child seated or supine, apply a nonrebreathing mask, speak to the child calmly, and tell them to breathe slowly. Transport decisions should be made on the basis of examination findings and discussion with the parents.

TIP

Lights and sirens are not needed for transporting a patient with a panic attack. This can lead to increased anxiety.

DEPRESSION

Major depression includes a persistent depressed mood or loss of interest or pleasure in daily activities. The patient must also have a specified symptom such as problems with eating, energy, sleep, concentration, or feeling worthless. Approximately 3% of children aged 3 to 17 years have been diagnosed with depression.

Patients with depression typically encounter EMS after episodes of self-harm, suicidal ideation or behaviors, or suicide attempts. These include cutting behaviors, attempts at strangulation, or ingestion of medications or toxic chemicals.

Treatment of major depressive disorder in children and adolescents consists of behavioral therapy and possibly pharmacotherapy. The most commonly used pharmacotherapeutic agents are SSRIs such as fluoxetine (Prozac®), sertraline (Zoloft®), escitalopram (Lexapro®), and citalopram (Celexa®). Abrupt discontinuation of these agents may result in withdrawal symptoms such as worsening anxiety, fatigue, nausea, myalgias, or chills. Therefore, use of these medications should be gradually decreased over time.

Although suicidal ideation and/or suicide attempt is a medical emergency, a child or an adolescent who simply says they are depressed is not. It is important to ask the patient if they have thought about suicide or have a plan. Rapid assessment tools, such as the Ask Suicide Screening Questions (ASQ) and the Columbia Suicide Severity Rating Scale for Pediatrics (C-SSRS), can identify pediatric patients at risk of suicide. These tools are designed to be administered quickly and efficiently by health care providers, allowing for timely intervention and support. They provide valuable information for risk stratification and intervention planning.

Any child with depression needs to undergo a mental health evaluation. The primary focus of EMS clinicians is to keep themselves and their patients safe from harm, using de-escalation techniques whenever possible. Patients who have attempted to harm themselves should be thoroughly assessed for physical injuries, and such injuries should be addressed and treated during transport.

CAUTION

When transporting patients who have expressed suicidal ideation or said they have a plan, ensure that they cannot harm you or themselves during transport.

BIPOLAR DISORDER

Bipolar disorder is a mood disorder previously known as manic-depressive disorder. It is thought to be caused by a chemical imbalance in the brain, usually between dopamine and norepinephrine levels. Adverse childhood experiences can also contribute to the development of bipolar disorder. Bipolar disorder usually has an onset in adolescence or young adulthood and affects males and females equally. A person cannot be diagnosed with bipolar disorder until they exhibit an episode of both mania (increased mood and energy, overconfidence, decreased need for sleep, increased talk and ideas) and depression (unusually sad, sleeping and eating issues, feeling worthless, thoughts of death, irritability, and withdrawal). Children with bipolar disorder may fluctuate between periods of mania, depression, and balanced moods.

EMS clinicians may encounter children in either state of bipolar disorder. The lack of insight and inhibitions and feelings of grandeur in the manic phase can often lead to traumatic injuries. During the depressive

CASE STUDY 2

You are called to the scene of an assault involving a 14-year-old girl. On your arrival, the school nurse reports that the adolescent got into an altercation with another girl that led to hair pulling, but no reported or visible injuries. The adolescent is screaming expletives and telling you to get away. She is picking up books and threatening to throw them at you. She is also yelling, "Get away from me, don't even think about touching me." The nurse tells you privately that the child is in the custody of the state and being fostered by a local family. She was recently placed there because of behavioral issues in a prior school. The patient takes methylphenidate (Concerta®)18 mg, fluoxetine (Prozac®)10 mg, and aripiprazole (Abilify®)5 mg daily for ADHD, conduct disorder, and posttraumatic stress disorder.

Your assessment reveals a female adolescent pacing around the nurse's office threatening to "hurt everyone" and yelling at you and the nurse. You observe the patient from a safe distance initially and note that she is very agitated and appears to be hyperventilating. You are unable to obtain vital signs because of her agitation.

1. What are the key principles in assessing this adolescent?
2. Describe treatment and transport approaches.

phase, children may have nonspecific medical complaints, appear suicidal, or even attempt suicide.

Bipolar disorder is treated with psychotherapy and medications. Mood stabilizers such as lithium (Lithobid) or valproate (Depakote®, Depacon®, Depakene®) are often prescribed. Anticonvulsant medications may be prescribed, even for patients without a comorbid seizure disorder, because these have been found to treat bipolar disorder.

SCHIZOPHRENIA

Schizophrenia is a complex mental health disorder that can be disabling to those affected. It is believed to start with a chemical imbalance in the brain; however, genetic, behavioral, and environmental factors also play a role. Schizophrenia may cause distorted thinking, changes in behavior, and unusual use of language and words. Schizophrenia is not a split-personality disorder as once thought. Because of its similarities to other behavioral health disorders, schizophrenia is commonly misdiagnosed, especially in children and young adults. It is uncommon for children younger than 12 years to be diagnosed with schizophrenia.

Children may develop schizophrenia slowly or with a sudden onset. EMS clinicians may be called when a child has a psychotic episode. Children may exhibit confused thinking, paranoia, distorted perception of reality, hallucinations (auditory, visual, tactile), delusions, moodiness, anxiety, agitation, withdrawal, catatonia, or odd behaviors.

Pharmacologic management may include antipsychotics and mood stabilizers, which are designed to help minimize the severity of delusions and hallucinations and treat the intrusive and disturbing thoughts seen in schizophrenia. Although these medications do not cure the disease, they can help control the symptoms. Psychotherapy, structured activity programs, and support groups can help children and their families cope with this illness.

Suicide Attempt/Intentional Ingestions or Exposures

Suicide is the second leading cause of death in children aged 10 to 14 years and a close third behind homicide for older adolescents. Firearms, hanging, and poisoning are the most common methods used. Firearms are the most common method of suicidal death, whereas medication overdose is the most common method of suicide attempt.

Intentional poisoning may be pharmacological or chemical. Common pharmacological ingestions include acetaminophen, aspirin, ibuprofen, antidepressants, ethanol, and illegal drugs. Common chemical ingestions include bleach, household cleaning products, or industrial adhesives (eg, glue). Ingestions in the context of suicide attempt are discussed in this section. Additional information about toxic ingestions is presented in Chapter 8.

> **TIP**
> The Poison Control Center is available 24/7 and is an invaluable resource regarding treatment for poisonous ingestions or exposures. To reach the Poison Control Center, call 1-800-222-1222.

HISTORY TAKING

When obtaining a medical history in a patient with a suspected harmful ingestion or exposure, there are several important questions to ask:

- When did the ingestion/exposure occur?
- Which medication/substance was taken? If unknown, describe pill size/color/shape.
- Were multiple medications taken?
- How much of each medication/substance was taken? Has the patient used this substance before?

These questions will need to be tailored to the specific circumstances and ingestions.

> **TIP**
> Contact the Poison Control Center at 1-800-222-1222 if you need help identifying the medication(s) involved in an ingestion, as well as for prehospital treatment.

MEDICATIONS ENCOUNTERED IN SUICIDAL INGESTIONS

Acetaminophen

Acetaminophen or paracetamol is an antipyretic (fever reducer) and analgesic that is readily available over the counter. Its widespread accessibility makes it a frequently used medication in intentional ingestions. Additionally, adolescents may not perceive it to be as dangerous or lethal as other medications. Acetaminophen overdoses are often asymptomatic for up to 24 hours after the ingestion. Patients typically develop abdominal pain, nausea, and vomiting 24 to 48 hours after ingestion. Laboratory studies may show elevated liver enzyme levels, abnormal coagulation study findings, and even renal damage.

Acetaminophen overdoses can be fatal as a result of liver failure, usually more than 48 hours after the overdose. Treatment with *N*-acetyl cysteine is successful if given within 8 hours of ingestion. If EMS is called shortly after the ingestion, oral administration of activated charcoal can prevent absorption of acetaminophen by the gut and minimize toxicity. Activated charcoal is harmful if aspirated into the lungs and should only be given to patients who are able to protect their airway.

Aspirin

Aspirin (acetylsalicylic acid) is a common nonprescription analgesic and anticoagulant used primarily in the adult population. However, aspirin is readily available to children and adolescents. In a large overdose, this acid produces a metabolic acidosis and compensatory respiratory alkalosis. Typical signs include fast and deep breathing (hyperpnea) and tachycardia. Patients often have ringing in the ears (tinnitus) and nausea, vomiting, and diarrhea. In severe cases, altered mental status and coma may occur. Patients with aspirin ingestion who are alert and cooperative should be given activated charcoal as soon as possible to prevent absorption of the aspirin by the gut. Activated charcoal is harmful if aspirated into the lungs and should only be given to patients who are able to protect their airway. Hospital treatment of an aspirin overdose is primarily supportive but may include additional doses of activated charcoal, intravenous (IV) sodium bicarbonate to induce alkaline diuresis, or dialysis.

Tricyclic Antidepressants

Tricyclic antidepressants (TCAs) were developed in the 1950s to treat depression. They inhibit the uptake of serotonin and norepinephrine at the presynaptic junction. Although they have largely been replaced by SSRIs, TCAs such as amitriptyline (Elavil®) and nortriptyline (Pamelor®) are still used in some patients. Overdoses of TCAs can be extremely dangerous and even fatal.

Patients with TCA overdoses experience tachycardia, altered mental status, and signs of anticholinergic toxicity (eg, dilated pupils, flushing, and hyperthermia). In severe cases, TCA overdoses result in seizure activity and cardiac arrythmias secondary to QRS prolongation. If the electrocardiogram shows signs of QRS widening, IV sodium bicarbonate can be administered to stabilize the myocardium. If the patient is alert and cooperative, activated charcoal should be administered. Care should be taken with oral administration of activated charcoal because of the potential sudden onset of unconsciousness and seizures. Seizure activity should be treated with benzodiazepines.

Selective Serotonin Reuptake Inhibitors

Selective serotonin reuptake inhibitors (SSRIs) are the preferred agent for the treatment of depression in children. These drugs function by inhibiting the uptake of serotonin into neurons, and act by stimulating serotonin receptors. Although only fluoxetine (Prozac®) and escitalopram (Lexapro®) are approved for pediatric patients, many others (sertraline [Zoloft®], bupropion [Wellbutrin®], paroxetine [Paxil®], and fluvoxamine [Luvox®]) are also used. Consequently, SSRIs are one of the drug types most commonly used in intentional ingestions.

Overdoses of SSRIs are typically mild. Patients may be asymptomatic even after ingesting 30 times the usual dose. Common symptoms include tachycardia, hypertension, vomiting, and drowsiness/lethargy, but more severe symptoms of seizures, respiratory failure, and even death are possible, especially with bupropion. Treatment of SSRI overdoses is primarily supportive, but activated charcoal may be used soon after ingestion to minimize absorption by the gut.

A potentially life-threatening form of an SSRI overdose is serotonin syndrome, which occurs because of increased serotonergic activity in the central nervous system. Serotonin syndrome most commonly occurs when SSRIs are combined with other serotonergic agents such as TCAs, lithium, migraine medications such as triptans, some anticonvulsants (carbamazepine, valproic acid), opioids, or drugs of abuse (cocaine, LSD, methamphetamine). It can also occur in the absence of an overdose. Serotonin syndrome typically presents with severe altered mental status, tremor or hyperreflexia, and autonomic symptoms, as shown in **TABLE 11-2**.

Treatment of serotonin syndrome requires prompt recognition. All serotonergic agents should be discontinued immediately. Agitation and hyperreflexia are managed by sedation with benzodiazepines, and autonomic instability is treated with IV fluid boluses; both can be administered by EMS clinicians. In the hospital, treatment with serotonin antagonists such as cyproheptadine may be required. Rarely, patients with severe hyperthermia ($>41°C$) may require endotracheal intubation, sedation, and paralysis.

TABLE 11–2 Signs and Symptoms of Serotonin Syndrome

Body System	Sign/Symptom
Neurological	Agitated delirium (agitation, hypervigilance, easy startle reflex)*
Neuromuscular	Myoclonus (most common finding) Hyperreflexia* Muscle rigidity (more in legs)* Clonus* Tremor* Akathisia
Autonomic	Tachycardia Hyperthermia* Hypertension that progresses to hypotension Diaphoresis (sweating)* Shivering Diarrhea Dilated pupils

*Used to meet some diagnostic criteria.

Adverse Reactions of Psychiatric Medications

Although many antipsychotics are well tolerated, adverse reactions can occur. Examples of serious adverse reactions include acute dystonic reactions, tardive dyskinesia, and neuroleptic malignant syndrome.

ACUTE DYSTONIC REACTIONS

Acute dystonic reactions are characterized by involuntary muscle tics or spasms that generally affect the head and neck and are most prominent in the tongue and jaw. Acute dystonic reactions are more common with first-generation (typical) antipsychotics such as haloperidol (Haldol) than with second-generation (atypical) antipsychotics. They occur even at therapeutic doses of the medications. Although dystonic reactions are rarely life threatening, symptoms can be very distressing to patients and their families and should be treated whenever possible. One life-threatening adverse effect is laryngeal dystonia, which presents as a choking sensation, difficulty breathing, or stridor. Diphenhydramine is the first-line treatment for patients with dystonic reactions and should be administered by IM, IV, or oral route as soon as possible. If the patient does not experience any relief with diphenhydramine, benzodiazepines may be administered.

NEUROLEPTIC MALIGNANT SYNDROME

Neuroleptic malignant syndrome (NMS) is a rare, but life-threatening complication of antipsychotic medications such as haloperidol and risperidone; mortality rates range from 5% to 20%. Neuroleptic malignant syndrome typically presents over the course of 3 days, and symptoms include altered mental status, hyperthermia (temperature > 41°C), extreme muscular rigidity, and autonomic instability, which generally presents as tachycardia. The most common neurological finding is lead-pipe rigidity. The clinical presentation of NMS is very similar to that of serotonin syndrome, so medication history is important. EMS treatment consists of supportive care to manage symptoms, and hospital treatment may include agents such as dantrolene and bromocriptine. Patients with NMS require monitoring in the intensive care unit and often require mechanical ventilation, cooling measures, IV fluids, antihypertensive agents, and benzodiazepines to control agitation.

Assessment and Transport of the Child With a Behavioral Emergency

When transporting a child with a behavioral emergency, safety is of the utmost importance. EMS clinicians should attempt to establish rapport with the child while assessing the likelihood of violence. Is this child a risk to themselves or others? If the child seems cooperative and gives permission, take a thorough history and begin to perform a physical examination. After assessment, determine the need to transport the child and how to accomplish it. If there is concern about self-harm, check for and remove any sharp objects, weapons, or pills from the patient prior to transport. A caregiver should either ride in the ambulance or follow the ambulance to the hospital.

Consider chemical or physical restraints if the patient cannot be safely transported otherwise. Assist the patient in managing their emotions or regaining control of their behavior. If these do not work, use the least restrictive age-appropriate methods of restraint possible and minimize coercive interventions that may exacerbate agitation.

CASE STUDY 3

You are dispatched to a high school where a 13-year-old student has just admitted to her guidance counselor that she wants to kill herself. On your arrival, she is awake but tearful; she has no increased work of breathing, and her color is pink. Her heart rate is 76 beats/min, respiratory rate is 16 breaths/min, and blood pressure is 106/70 mm Hg. When you take her blood pressure, you note numerous healing horizontal cuts on her left forearm. She has no other injuries. She states she wants to kill herself because she broke up with her boyfriend 2 weeks ago, which is when she cut herself. She says she has not taken any medication.

1. Do you need to take her to the hospital?
2. What additional assessment may be helpful en route?

VERBAL DE-ESCALATION AND RESTRAINT

Verbal de-escalation is the preferred way to reduce aggressive behavior. When verbal de-escalation is inadequate or fails to modify the patient's behavior, restraint may be necessary. Restraint refers to methods of restricting a person's freedom of movement owing to a concern of self-harm or harming others. Restraint can be pharmacological or physical. Recent studies suggest that prehospital restraint use varies between demographic groups, without clear medical indications for that variation. Use of either pharmacological or physical restraints by EMS should be approached cautiously with the primary considerations of patient and crew safety.

Verbal De-escalation

Verbal de-escalation is preferable to restraint. Children experience emotional distress for a variety of reasons, including mental health issues, substance abuse, trauma, or conflict with family or friends. At times, this distress can escalate into aggression. Children voicing threats or warnings should be taken seriously.

Children cannot always communicate their thoughts or emotions clearly. They might not understand what is being said or what is going on around them. It is important to evaluate the situation and try to understand what the child is feeling. This can help when you attempt to de-escalate the situation. Use a nonthreatening approach in both words and body language.

De-escalation techniques from the Youth Mental Health First Aid USA program from the National Council of Behavioral Health provide practical strategies, such as the following:

- Speak slowly and confidently with a gentle, caring tone of voice.
- Invite the young person to sit down if they are standing.
- Use positive words (such as "stay calm") instead of negative words (such as "don't fight"). Ask, "What happened?" rather than, "What's wrong with you?"
- Do not argue with or threaten the young person; it may prompt aggressive behavior.
- Avoid nervous behavior (eg, shuffling your feet, fidgeting).
- Do not restrict the young person's movement (eg, allow them to pace up and down the room).
- Keep your distance from the youth, calculated for their cultural comfort.
- Remain aware that certain acts, such as those involving the police, might exacerbate the situation.
- Consider taking a break from the conversation to allow the young person a chance to calm down.
- If the young person is responsive, ask them if they have a safety or crisis plan in place, and work with them to follow the plan as well as you can.

EMS clinicians can set the tone for how a call goes and create a basis of trust for future EMS interactions the child may have. By remaining calm with relaxed body language and offering a safe personal space, EMS clinicians can model behavior for the child to follow. Take time to learn about resources in your community that can assist youth before, during, and after a crisis.

TIP

When approaching the child or adolescent, clearly introduce yourself and assure them that you are there to keep them safe. Allow caregivers to take part (or remove them if they are inciting). Set firm limits. Offer choices in treatments. Offer rewards for calmer behavior. Use distraction.

Pharmacological Restraint

Pharmacological management should be considered when nonpharmacological interventions fail. Patient restraint and sedation should be used only when the patient's behavior presents a danger to themself or others. Evaluation tools are available to assess the safety risk, such as the Brøset Violence Checklist.

Medication choice should be guided by the etiology of agitation, patient factors, availability, and potential adverse effects. Prioritize medications with evidence-based support and avoid unnecessary polypharmacy. Several medication classes are available for treatment of agitation in youth, including antihistamines, benzodiazepines, and antipsychotics. The use of pharmacological restraint in children may be considered if local protocols exist, with medical direction. A comparison of commonly used options is found in **TABLE 11-3**.

After administering sedating medications, the EMS clinician should closely monitor the patient for airway patency, effective ventilation, and circulatory status. A cardiac monitor and pulse oximeter should be applied prior to transport.

Physical Restraint

Physical restraint involves the use of mechanical devices to limit physical activity. It should be the last

TABLE 11-3 Behavioral Health Emergency Medications

Medication	Indication	Route (Time of Onset)	Dose	Same Syringe Compatibility	Common Side Effects	Precautions
Lorazepam	Agitation Anxiety	IV (2–3 min)	0.05 mg/kg IV or IO over 2–5 minutes; repeat 0.05-mg/kg dose in 5–15 minutes if needed	Haloperidol *alone* Diphenhydramine *alone*	Dizziness Weakness Headache Respiratory depression	Monitor airway and ventilation owing to CNS depression; higher risk when multiple medications used
Midazolam	Agitation Aggression	IM (3–5 min) Intranasal (10–15 min)	IM: 0.05 to 0.1 mg/kg (max total dose, 10 mg) Intranasal: 0.2 mg/kg (max dose < 6 years old, 6 mg; max dose > 6 years old, 10 mg)	—	Akathisia (restlessness) Headache Dizziness Respiratory depression	Monitor airway and ventilation owing to CNS depression; higher risk when multiple medications used
Diphenhydramine	Anxiety Restlessness	Oral (5–30 min) IM (5 min)	Oral/IM: 1-mg/kg dose (max, 50-mg dose)	Lorazepam	Dizziness Dry mouth	When administering haloperidol/lorazepam, give diphenhydramine in a separate syringe
Ketamine	Agitation Aggression	IM (3–5 min) Intranasal (10–15 min)	IM: 4 mg/kg (max, 100 mg) Intranasal: 5-mg/kg dose (half dose in each nostril)	—	Blurred vision Nystagmus Vomiting Jerky movement Dizziness Hallucinations	Monitor airway and ventilation owing to CNS depression
Droperidol	Agitation	IV/IM (3–10 min)	IV/IM: 0.625–2.5 mg	Diphenhydramine	Dystonic reaction/EPS QT prolongation	Avoid use in children receiving other medications that prolong QT

Continued

TABLE 11–3 Behavioral Health Emergency Medications—cont'd

Medication	Indication	Route (Time of Onset)	Dose	Same Syringe Compatibility	Common Side Effects	Precautions
Haloperidol (Haldol®)	Agitation	Oral (30 min) IM (5–15 min)	Oral/IM: < 40 kg, 0.025–0.075 mg/kg; > 40 kg, 2–5 mg	Diphenhydramine *or* lorazepam	Dystonic reaction/EPS Decreased seizure threshold Hypotension	When administering haloperidol/lorazepam, give diphenhydramine in a separate syringe
Olanzapine (Zyprexa®)	Agitation	Oral (30 min) IM (2–5 min)	Oral/IM: < 40 kg, 1.25–2.5 mg; > 40 kg, 2.5–5 mg	—	Paradoxical reaction Sedation	Avoid use within 1 hour of any benzodiazepines
Quetiapine (Seroquel®)	Agitation	Oral (30 min)	Oral: < 40 kg, 6.25–12.5 mg; > 40 kg, 25–50 mg	—	Hypotension QT prolongation	

Drug induced movement disorders (exhibiting involuntary movements, muscle spasms, tremors, and severe restlessness).
Abbreviations: CNS, central nervous system; EPS, extrapyramidal symptoms; IM, intramuscular; IO, intraosseous; IV, intravenous.

resort when the child poses a significant threat. If physical restraints are needed, use the minimum level of physical restraint required.

A method that can be used in younger children is therapeutic holding, in which the caregivers or health care providers hold the child to control the agitated behavior (**FIGURE 11–5**). Similarly, a young child can sometimes be secured in their car seat to provide adequate restraint in a familiar device.

If physical restraint is necessary, explain the need to the patient's caregivers and enlist their assistance. Explain to the patient what you are doing and why,

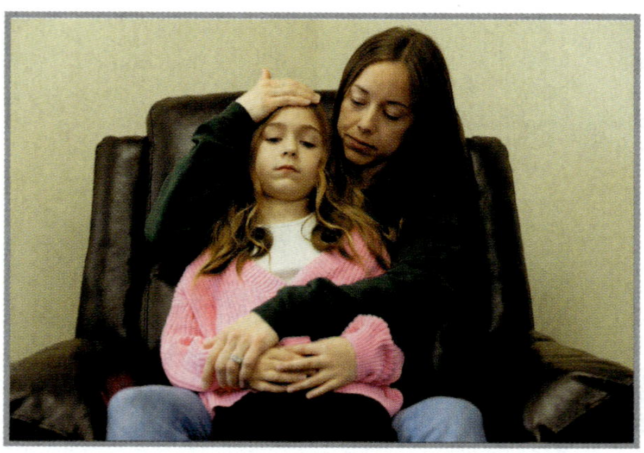

FIGURE 11–5 Therapeutic holding, in which the caregivers or health care providers hold the child to control the agitated behavior, can be used in younger children.

but do not negotiate. Do not attempt restraint placement alone—this often requires 3 to 5 people. Before restraining a child, consider calling law enforcement for support. EMS clinicians should stay near an escape route to avoid the possibility of being injured. If the patient is placed on a stretcher, position supine with the head of the stretcher elevated. Apply restraints to each extremity first, then secure the restraints to the stretcher frame, not to the side rails. Do not cover the patient's face or head except with a mask or other appropriate device to control spitting and/or biting. Document carefully the reasons for and the types of restraints in the run sheet. Perform periodic assessments.

There may be conflict between parents' wishes and the needs of the child. If the child is in immediate danger of self-harm or is an immediate danger to others, notify law enforcement officials to help restrain the patient so they can be transported to the closest appropriate facility.

YOUR EMOTIONAL WELL-BEING

Calls involving children in emotional distress can be especially draining for EMS clinicians. Find opportunities to process your own emotions with peers or any employee assistance program that may be available in your agency. Take care of yourself by getting plenty of sleep, eating properly, and allowing time for reflection and healing.

CASE STUDY ANSWERS

CASE STUDY 1

Assessment of the airway, breathing, and circulation suggests an anaphylactic reaction related to a bee sting. You should ask the child's mother about any history of insect bites and if the child's inhaler is available. Using the child's comfort items to try to calm the child would be beneficial, as intramuscular epinephrine administration is indicated for anaphylaxis and will further agitate the child.

Approach the child calmly and rely on the mother to help answer any questions. Have your partner administer high-flow oxygen while you explain to the mother that, based on symptoms and presentation, her son is going to need an intramuscular epinephrine injection. Suggest that the mother hold the child in his position of comfort, preferably on her lap, and ask her to use the blanket and stuffed animal to comfort the child while you administer epinephrine. Use proper temporary restraint techniques per your agency guidelines and protocol if necessary. Calmly vocalize to the child each intervention you will take and allow extra time, as symptoms allow, for the child to respond.

An albuterol inhaler can be used to help open the child's airways and alleviate respiratory distress. In this case, the parent states that the child's inhaler is available. The child has begun to calm down, but is now rocking back and forth on his mother's lap and is repetitively saying "ouch." The child's father is now at your side with the albuterol inhaler and spacer. The child is agreeable to assisted administration by you and his parents.

The child is now calm, breathing is at a normal rate and rhythm, and the facial swelling is beginning to dissipate. The child begins asking questions about the EMS equipment. You allow the child to try out your stethoscope and blood pressure cuff. After doing so, he lets you obtain his vital signs: blood pressure is 90/56 mm Hg, heart rate is 130 beats/min, respiratory rate is 22 breaths/min, and oxygen saturation is 100% on nasal cannula. You give the patient a trial on room air; the child maintains an oxygen saturation of 98%.

The child is in stable condition, and knowing that noise and flashing lights can aggravate children with ASD, you transport him to the hospital without lights and sirens. You continue to monitor for any change in condition and allow his mother to accompany him in the back of the ambulance. At the ED, you give a full report to the receiving facility, including the diagnosis of ASD, and share the strategies you found successful for soothing the child. The ED is able to place him in a quiet, private room with low lighting. The child is diagnosed with an anaphylactic reaction to bee venom. He remains at the hospital for well over 4 hours of observation and is discharged home in good condition and with a prescription for an epinephrine autoinjector.

Children with autism cannot always be identified by appearance alone, and it is important to remember that some may be nonverbal at baseline or may become nonverbal when stressed. A 3- to 4-second delay from question to answer is not uncommon. If the child does not answer a question, it is often because the child does not understand it, so you should continue to explain interventions calmly. Children with ASD commonly have tactile sensory issues. When assessing these patients, try to avoid any unnecessary or repetitive touching, restrictive bandaging, or use of other confining equipment. These children may also have difficulty with lights and sirens, so use of lights and sirens should be limited whenever possible, as per local protocol.

CASE STUDY 2

While this adolescent clearly needs assistance, scene safety must be paramount throughout the call. Remain vigilant, know your egress routes, and enlist the help of law enforcement or additional EMS personnel as needed to ensure the safety of the patient, yourself, your crew, the school staff, faculty, and other students. At times, less may be more, and additional personnel may further aggravate the patient, but this will vary from situation to situation.

You should remain calm and attempt to verbally de-escalate the situation. Speak calmly and confidently in a caring manner. Do not argue with or challenge the patient.

Do not restrict the patient's pacing, but invite her to sit down. Give clear, calm instructions, such as, "Please put that item down so we may talk," or "Please tell me what happened." Explain that throwing

Continued

CASE STUDY ANSWERS—cont'd

objects is not safe for the patient or those around her. Try to gain the patient's trust by stating that you are there to help her and would like to hear what happened. If the patient can calm down, you may be able to gather information about any potential injuries. You may also be able to obtain a health history and vital signs.

If the patient does not calm down with verbal de-escalation techniques and continues to pose a threat to herself and others, physical and/or chemical restraint may be indicated. You should also attempt to ascertain whether she is an immediate threat to herself or others and requires immediate transport to the ED. If ED transport is chosen and the patient is calm and able, allow her to walk to the stretcher and maintain as much independence and control as you deem safe.

On reaching the ED, the patient became agitated and stated she did not want to go in there because she does not want to be put in the "psych ward." The triage nurse states that she knows the child well from prior ED and inpatient visits for ADHD, ODD, and conduct disorder. The patient became agitated when security guards asked her to remove her shoes, and she began spitting and kicking at the ED nurse. Hospital staff were not able to verbally de-escalate the situation and she was treated with intramuscular injections of haloperidol, lorazepam, and diphenhydramine. She fell asleep shortly thereafter, and when she awoke the following morning was able to complete a mental health crisis evaluation and safety plan. She was discharged home to her foster family.

Attention-deficit/hyperactivity disorder, ODD, and conduct disorder are all classified as behavioral disorders. Children with conduct disorder have difficulty following rules and social norms, which causes them to have difficulty interacting with family and peers; symptoms may be particularly disruptive in the school setting. Physically aggressive behaviors such as theft, vandalism, substance use and abuse, harm to animals, and sexual promiscuity may also be seen in conduct disorder. The cause of conduct disorder is not fully known, but some potential risk factors include early maternal rejection, separation, and neglect; abuse; and domestic violence. Early and continued intervention is important in these children and, many times, the hormonal changes that routinely occur during puberty can exacerbate symptoms.

CASE STUDY 3

Because this adolescent is expressing suicidal ideation and exhibits signs of hurting herself, she does need to have a mental health evaluation. If she is already seeing a mental health professional who can see her now, her parents should be called; if they are able to take her, she can be released to her parents to seek care. If she has no ready access to a mental health professional, she should be transported to the ED where a physical examination and mental health evaluation can occur.

En route, you ensure that the adolescent has no other injuries or signs of an ingestion (see toxidromes in Chapter 8). You engage her in a conversation about how she is doing at school and at home, and about whether there are any other stressors in her life. She does not want to answer you, and that is OK. Just explain that she will need to be on the stretcher, and basic safety measures (straps) are needed for the transport.

At the hospital, the teen is evaluated by a mental health social worker and confirms that she does have daily thoughts of suicide and has a plan to hang herself with a belt she has hidden in her room. She is determined to be at high risk of committing suicide and is admitted to inpatient psychiatry for initiation of medications and safety planning.

Suggested References

TEXTBOOKS

Adirim T, Smith E. *Special Children's Outreach and Prehospital Education (SCOPE)*. Jones and Bartlett Learning; 2006

ARTICLES

Fishe JN, Lynch S. Pediatric behavioral health-related EMS encounters: a statewide analysis. *Prehosp Emerg Care*. 2019;23(5):654–662. PMID: 30612501 doi: 10.1080/10903127.2019.1566423

Hyman SL, Levy SE, Myers SM, et al; COUNCIL ON CHILDREN WITH DISABILITIES, SECTION ON DEVELOPMENTAL AND BEHAVIORAL PEDIATRICS. Executive summary: identification, evaluation, and management of children with autism spectrum disorder. *Pediatrics*. 2020;145(1):e20193448. PMID: 31843858 doi: 10.1542/peds.2019-3448

Mason PJ, Morris VA, Balcezak TJ. Serotonin syndrome. Presentation of 2 cases and review of the literature. *Medicine (Baltimore)*. 2000;79(4):201–209. PMID: 10941349 doi: 10.1097/00005792-200007000-00001

Overberg A, Morton S, Wagner E, Froberg B. Toxicity of bupropion overdose compared with selective serotonin reuptake inhibitors. *Pediatrics*. 2019;144(2):e20183295. PMID: 31278211 doi: 10.1542/peds.2018-3295

Qin L, Wang H, Ning W, Cui M, Wang Q. New advances in the diagnosis and treatment of autism spectrum disorders. *Eur J Med Res*. 2024;29(1):322. PMID: 38858682 doi: 10.1186/s40001-024-01916-2

Riley M, Ahmed S, Locke A. Common questions about oppositional defiant disorder. *Am Fam Physician*. 2016;93(7):586–591. PMID: 27035043

Saidinejad M, Duffy S, Wallin D, et al. The management of children and youth with pediatric mental and behavioral health emergencies. *Pediatrics*. 2023;152(3):e2023063256. doi: 10.1542/peds.2023-063256

Saidinejad M, Foster AA, Santillanes G, et al; ACEP Pediatric Emergency Medicine Committee. Strategies for optimal management of pediatric acute agitation in emergency settings. *J Am Coll Emerg Physicians Open*. 2024;5(4):e13255. PMID: 39183940 doi: 10.1002/emp2.13255

Varigonda AL, Jakubovski E, Taylor MJ, Freemantle N, Coughlin C, Bloch MH. Systematic review and meta-analysis: early treatment responses of selective serotonin reuptake inhibitors in pediatric major depressive disorder. *J Am Acad Child Adolesc Psychiatry*. 2015;54(7):557–564. PMID: 26088660 doi: 10.1016/j.jaac.2015.05.004

Wilms Floet AM, Scheiner C, Grossman L. Attention-deficit/hyperactivity disorder. *Pediatr Rev*. 2010;31(2):56–69. PMID: 20124275 doi: 10.1542/pir.31.2.56

Wolraich ML, Chan E, Froehlich T, et al. ADHD diagnosis and treatment guidelines: a historical perspective. *Pediatrics*. 2019;144(4):e20191682. PMID: 31570649 doi: 10.1542/peds.2019-1682

OTHER RESOURCES

Ask Suicide-Screening Questions (ASQ) Toolkit. Accessed January 13, 2026. https://www.nimh.nih.gov/research/research-conducted-at-nimh/asq-toolkit-materials

Brøset Violence Checklist. Accessed November 22, 2024. https://www.risk-assessment.no/files/bvc-versions/BVC%20English.pdf

Care of the Agitated Patient. EMSC Innovation and Improvement Center. Accessed November 22, 2024. https://media.emscimprovement.center/documents/EMS220128_Agitation24x36_240102.pdf

Glomb N. Safety of Prehospital Medical Clearance for Pediatric Behavioral Health Emergencies. Prehospital Pediatric Readiness Project. Accessed November 22, 2024. https://emscimprovement.center/domains/prehospital-care/prehospital-pediatric-readiness/pprp-toolkit/interactions-systems-care/mental-behavioral-health/pediatric-bhe-presentation/

ImageTrend Collaborate Short Report: Pediatric Behavioral Health Incidents in the Prehospital Setting from 2018 to 2021, Volume 1: Issue 2. Accessed November 18, 2024. https://www1.imagetrend.com/collaborate-short-report-on-pediatric-behavioral-health

National Institute of Mental Health. Statistics. Accessed November 22, 2024. https://www.nimh.nih.gov/health/statistics

National Institute of Mental Health. Suicide. Accessed November 22, 2024. https://www.nimh.nih.gov/health/statistics/suicide

988 Lifeline. Accessed January 13, 2026. https://988lifeline.org/get-help/

Understanding Children on the Autism Spectrum. A Guide for First Responders. Accessed November 22, 2024. https://media.emscimprovement.center/documents/272104_IACP_HomeSafe_First_Responders_508c.pdf

CHAPTER 12

Children and Youth with Special Health Care Needs

Kayla Long, DO, MS, MAPP, FACEP, FAEMS
T.J. Bishop, AS, NRP, NCEE

LEARNING OBJECTIVES

1. **Define and describe 2 examples of cognitive disabilities, physical disabilities, and chronic conditions seen in children.**
2. **List important modifications of field assessment techniques for children and youth with special health care needs (CYSHCN).**
3. **Outline common transport considerations for CYSHCN.**
4. **Describe the most common complications associated with assistive devices (tracheostomy tubes, central venous lines, gastrostomy tubes or gastric feeding tubes, cerebrospinal fluid shunts, ostomies, implantable pacemakers, insulin pumps, and defibrillators) and the emergency management of those complications.**
5. **Describe the use of health information technology, including an emergency information form, for CYSHCN.**

Introduction

Children and youth with special health care needs (CYSHCN) are a diverse group of patients who frequently need prehospital emergency assessment and treatment. According to an article by McPherson, CYSHCN are defined as "those who have or are at an increased risk for a chronic physical, developmental, or emotional condition and who also require health and related services of a type or amount beyond that required by children generally."

This high-user group includes but is not limited to children who were born prematurely; have suffered traumatic or anoxic brain injury; or have chronic diseases/disorders of the heart, lungs, brain, or kidneys. The conditions can be acquired or congenital. Examples of acquired conditions include traumatic brain injury or bronchopulmonary dysplasia. Examples of congenital problems are cyanotic heart disease or spina bifida.

Children assisted by or dependent on technology are a subgroup of CYSHCN who need medical devices for their survival. Common devices include tracheostomy tubes, home ventilators, indwelling central venous lines, feeding tubes, pacemakers, insulin pumps, and cerebrospinal fluid (CSF) shunts.

Many CYSHCN live at home, attend school, work outside the home, and survive to adulthood. They need emergency medical care more frequently than children without special health care needs. Because of their unique baseline status, CYSHCN pose unique challenges in field assessment and treatment. Therefore, prehospital professionals should recognize common types of CYSHCN, incorporate modifications during assessment, and understand management of frequent problems. EMS agencies should develop policies and protocols to assist providers with guidance on transport and care of CYSHCN.

Cognitive and Physical Disabilities

According to the American Association on Intellectual and Developmental Disabilities, an intellectual disability is defined as a "disability characterized by significant limitations both in intellectual functioning (reasoning, learning, problem solving) and in adaptive behavior, which covers a range of everyday social and practical skills." The terms *intellectual disability* and *mental retardation* refer to the same cognitive limitations; however, intellectual disability is less offensive and is the preferred term.

Mental processes, such as judgment, reasoning, memory, and comprehension, are cognitive in nature and develop as the child acquires knowledge. Cognitive impairments are present when there is an alteration in the child's ability to think, reason, learn, and abstract. Intellectual disability results in limited functions of communication, social skills, and self-care. There is significant overlap with disorders of social interaction such as autism spectrum disorder and disorders of attention and impulsivity such as attention-deficit/hyperactivity disorder, both of which are discussed in Chapter 11. Emergency medical services clinicians should consider how a child's cognitive impairments may exacerbate stress and anxiety leading to potential for lack of cooperation.

Physical disabilities may alter the child's mobility or their ability to independently accomplish activities of daily living. This includes physical conditions that may not be obvious such as arthritis, hearing impairment, or visual impairment.

Chronic conditions are present when the child receives ongoing treatment for an injury or illness. Even if the child seems to be healthy, they may be receiving maintenance medications or treatments to prevent complications. Examples of chronic conditions include asthma, cancer, post-transplantation, and congenital heart disease. Additional chronic conditions include the following:

- **Bronchopulmonary dysplasia (BPD)** is a chronic lung condition that develops in preterm infants who require respiratory support after birth. These infants may have pulmonary hypertension and decreased pulmonary function, chronic wheezing, or require supplemental oxygen at home. Children with BPD are at risk of experiencing deterioration with respiratory illnesses.
- **Cerebral palsy (CP)** is a disorder of movement and tone that results from brain injury during fetal development or at birth. These children may have increased motor tone, leading to trouble walking, or difficulty with coordination. They may wear orthotics on their legs to assist with ambulation, or they may be wheelchair users. Some also have intellectual disability, but many do not.
- **Cystic fibrosis** is a congenital disorder that results in lung and digestive disorders due to improper functioning of mucus-producing or exocrine glands. This results in frequent lung infections and pneumothoraces and impaired digestion and absorption of nutrients, resulting in poor growth.
- **Down syndrome** is a congenital disorder in which the child is born with 3 copies of the 21st chromosome, so it is also called trisomy 21. Children with Down syndrome have typical facial features and are at risk of experiencing

CASE STUDY 1

You are called to the scene of a 9-month-old girl with multiple underlying medical problems, including ventilator dependence at night through a tracheostomy tube.

On your arrival, her caregiver states that the girl has had difficulty breathing all day, with a fever and increased tracheostomy secretions. The child has CP with spasticity and a seizure disorder. She depends on a ventilator because of chronic lung disease as a result of prematurity at birth and respiratory distress syndrome. The child receives carbamazepine for her seizures and received her morning dose. Currently, she is receiving feedings through her gastrostomy tube, which is connected to a pump.

Your assessment shows a child who is in bed and connected to a home ventilator via a tracheostomy tube. She does not engage visually and has subcostal retractions and nasal flaring. Her skin is hot to the touch and is pink and dry. She has wheezing and crackles on lung examination. Her heart rate is 130 beats/min, respiratory rate is 60 breaths/min, blood pressure is 85 mm Hg/palp, and pulse oximetry is 90%. Her ventilator is set at 20 breaths/min.

1. What are the key principles in assessing this child?
2. Describe treatment and transport approaches.

congenital heart defects and cervical spine injuries due to cervical spine abnormalities. They also have varying levels of cognitive delay.

- **Hemophilia** is a genetic condition that results in abnormalities in blood clotting. This can lead to prolonged bleeding, and there is a risk of internal bleeding even with minor trauma. These patients require special medication that may not be available at all receiving facilities, such as smaller hospitals or freestanding emergency departments (EDs).
- **Muscular dystrophy** is a genetic muscle disorder that results in muscle weakness and wasting. These children are at risk of experiencing heart failure, aspiration, and pneumonia.
- **Spina bifida** is a congenital anomaly in which the spine has failed to fuse, resulting in protrusion of the spinal cord and meninges at birth, usually in the lumbar region, but it can occur anywhere along the spinal column. Although these lesions can be repaired, the children may have hydrocephalus, impaired lower-extremity strength and feeling, and bowel and bladder issues.

Assessment of CYSHCN

MODIFICATIONS

The most important resource for the prehospital provider is the child's caregiver. They usually know how to care for their child's particular condition and understand the child's equipment. Often, caregivers have forms or cards that outline the child's medical history, medications, and **baseline** general appearance, oxygen saturation, and vital signs.

Begin evaluation of CYSHCN with emergency pediatric assessment techniques adjusted to the child's developmental level, rather than their chronological age. Caregivers usually can provide the child's developmental age, weight, and baseline vital signs. *With children assisted by technology, do not become distracted by their specialized equipment.* Care for the child, not the machinery. Caregivers are often extremely helpful in figuring out the baseline status of CYSHCN or in operating or troubleshooting the equipment. *Ask for assistance from the caregiver!*

The assessment of CYSHCN has the following important modifications:

1. Ask the caregivers what is usual for the child. Most likely, they will know the child's baseline status better than anyone. Rely on the caregivers' opinions: What do they think is wrong? In what ways is the child different from their baseline status?
2. The usual baseline vital signs for a child with special health care needs may be out of the "normal" range compared with a child of the same age who does not have special health care needs. Standard vital signs may have limited value in assessment of these children. Pay more attention to the Pediatric Assessment Triangle (PAT) and observations from the caregiver.
3. If the child is physiologically stable, take a full history on scene. Caregivers usually know the child's medical history, health problems, medications, medical devices, and current complaints. They are also aware of what approaches work best. Ask the caregivers what therapies or interventions have already been undertaken in response to their child's emergency.
4. Talk directly to the child, not only to their caregiver. The child may be slow to answer questions or may be unable to talk. Communicate with the child using developmentally appropriate language, gestures, and techniques, as discussed in Chapter 2.
5. Be vigilant. Seemingly minor illnesses can be life threatening in some CYSHCN. An example is a cold in a child with chronic lung disease who is dependent on a ventilator. The child may have little reserve and can easily become hypoxic.
6. Ask if the child has a form or card with information about their medical problem, normal vital signs, medications, and other important medical data. Look for a bracelet or necklace that might describe the child's condition. An emergency information form (EIF) is available from the American Academy of Pediatrics (AAP) and the American College of Emergency Physicians (ACEP). Some states have created electronic systems for sharing emergency information with EMS such as Missouri's Special Needs Tracking and Awareness Response System (STARS), Oregon's Health Emergency Ready Oregon (HERO) Kids Registry, and Project Austin at Children's Nebraska.
7. Do not assume that a child with communication difficulty is cognitively impaired. Many children with CP, for example, have muscle **spasticity** but do not have cognitive limitations. Discreetly ask the caregiver about the child's typical level of functioning, understanding, and interactions.
8. Be polite and professional. Listen to the caregiver and take their concerns seriously. Keep in mind

the amount of stress caregivers of a CYSHCN may be experiencing. Families of CYSHCN often have had a lot of experience with the medical system. If most of their experience has been positive, they view the prehospital professional as an ally. However, if they have had bad experiences with the medical system, they may be suspicious or aggressive.

9. Try to transport CYSHCN to their "medical home" facility if possible. Always follow local protocol. For patients with particularly specialized needs, agencies and medical directors may develop individualized care plans to guide the care and transport of these patients.

TIP

Sample questions for the caregiver of CHSHCN:

- What is the child's baseline mental and physical function?
- Do you have an EIF or a copy of their care plan?
- What actions have you already taken to manage the situation?
- What hospital is the usual site of emergency care?
- Are you able to ride with the patient to the hospital?
- What equipment or supplies should be taken to the hospital with the patient?

CAUTION

Do not become distracted by the specialized equipment used by children assisted by technology. Care for the child, not the machinery.

PEDIATRIC ASSESSMENT TRIANGLE

The PAT is a good way to look and listen for signs that help determine the type of physiological problem and the urgency of need for treatment. However, because CYSHCN often have altered baseline physiology, there are several limitations and modifications to the PAT.

Appearance

Although the child's overall appearance reflects the adequacy of oxygenation, ventilation, perfusion, and CNS status, this part of the PAT may differ the most in CYSHCN. The underlying medical problem may cause abnormal muscle tone, such as increased tone (spasticity) in a child with CP or the decreased tone seen in children with Down syndrome. Decreased alertness or interactivity is common in a child with brain damage or an intellectual disability. Decreased social responsiveness is common in children with autism spectrum disorder. Look or gaze is helpful because many CYSHCN can recognize their caregiver by looking or by hearing their voice. A CYSHCN may be unable to speak, but the strength and quality of their cry or facial expressions may be a useful sign of health or distress. For example, a high-pitched cry in a child with a CSF shunt may be a sign of shunt obstruction.

Work of Breathing

Many CYSHCN have respiratory problems. Children with chronic pulmonary disease, such as BPD, have rapid respiratory rates and increased work of breathing. When such children have a fever or experience an added respiratory illness or an injury, such as pneumonia or chest trauma, they have less reserve. Therefore, work of breathing in these patients increases rapidly with any acute illness or injury.

TIP

Assess appearance by asking the caregiver about the child's baseline.

CAUTION

Do not assume that a child with a physical disability or communication difficulty is mentally impaired. Many children with CP, for example, have spasticity but not cognitive limitations.

Assess abnormal breath sounds (stridor, wheezing, or grunting) from across the room for the PAT. Some "abnormal" airway sounds may be usual for a CYSHCN. For example, a child with a tracheostomy tube usually has noisy breathing, and an infant with BPD may have slight expiratory wheezing. Children with BPD or congenital heart disease are much more likely to develop viral respiratory infections, such as **respiratory syncytial virus (RSV)** in the winter. They can decompensate quickly. CYSHCN who have an intellectual disability and neurological problems are at high risk of experiencing aspiration, pneumonia, and respiratory failure.

Tripod positioning or head bobbing is an important visual sign of increased work of breathing and hypoxia, and it usually indicates serious breathing problems. For the child who usually has mild retractions, the degree or location of retractions provides clues to increased work of breathing. For example, the baseline retractions may be mild and only **subcostal**, but are now severe and also **suprasternal**. Nasal flaring is an indication of increased work of breathing, especially when associated with tachypnea, grunting, or retractions.

Circulation to Skin

The skin color may appear different in CYSHCN, such as in infants with cyanotic congenital heart disease, chronic lung disease, cancer, or liver failure. A child with cyanotic congenital heart disease or chronic lung disease may have bluish lips and mucous membranes, nail beds, and extremities at baseline. A child with cancer may appear pale, whereas the skin of a child with liver disease may appear yellow. Ask the caregiver to describe the child's baseline color.

ADAPTATIONS IN THE HANDS-ON ABCDEs

After performing the PAT, complete the primary assessment by adjusting the evaluation of the ABCDEs to the child's baseline.

Airway

Open and maintain the airway. Keeping an open airway may be more difficult with CYSHCN. The child may have poor muscle tone and head control, or copious secretions. In children with Down syndrome, the large, protruding tongue may make airway procedures difficult. Achieving, and then maintaining, the correct head position may require several maneuvers: a shoulder roll to correctly position the head in a neutral axis with the airway (align the ear canal to the sternal notch), and a chin lift or jaw thrust to open the airway. Some children with neuromuscular disorders breathe better sitting up. Always have suction available.

Many children with spina bifida have an Arnold-Chiari malformation, in which the base of the brain pushes down through the opening at the base of the skull. Do *not* hyperextend the neck of a child with spina bifida because any pressure on the herniated brain may cause the child to stop breathing. For these children, use in-line stabilization for any airway maneuvers even if no trauma is suspected. Children with Down syndrome carry a higher risk of cervical spine abnormalities and vulnerability to cervical spine injury compared with other children after similar types of trauma.

Special Management in CYSHCN: Tracheostomy Care. A child with a tracheostomy has an artificial airway that is easily blocked by secretions or by dislodgment of the device. The tracheostomy section of this chapter addresses specific management techniques for these children.

Breathing

Count the respiratory rate. Listen to the lungs for **bilateral** air movement and abnormal chest sounds. Listening may not provide accurate results in the CYSHCN who cannot sit still or who has noisy breathing. Keep the child in a position of comfort. Give supplemental oxygen to any CYSHCN with increased work of breathing or an increased respiratory rate by the blow-by method, nasal cannula, face mask, continuous positive airway pressure, or bag-mask device. Obtain pulse oximetry and compare the results to baseline. If the caregiver knows the usual baseline oxygen saturation, give only enough oxygen to achieve baseline levels. Some children with chronic lung disease or congenital heart disease have low baseline oxygen saturations and their condition can worsen if too much oxygen is given. For CYSHCN, the caregiver may know the best way to give oxygen to the child. For infants or children already using home oxygen, increase the flow rate. For a patient with a tracheostomy tube, place the oxygen directly over the tube or stoma.

Special Management in CYSHCN: Bronchodilator Administration. If a CYSHCN has a history of breathing problems or uses bronchodilators at home, give a nebulized bronchodilator when wheezing is present. Consider bronchodilators for those with diminished air movement as well.

Circulation

Assess heart rate, pulse quality, skin temperature, and capillary refill time. These are not usually different in CYSHCN and require no modifications in clinical interpretation. Blood pressure may be difficult to obtain or interpret in very young or uncooperative children, but attempt to obtain a blood pressure during secondary assessment for seriously ill infants and toddlers. EMS clinicians should measure blood pressure at least once in all children older than 3 years. Tachycardia is a common baseline finding in some CYSHCN and by itself does not indicate shock. This is diagnosis dependent, so asking the child's caregiver about the child's usual heart rate can be helpful. Assess heart rate and blood pressure with the other key characteristics of circulation, as outlined in Chapters 1 and 4.

Management of shock in CYSHCN begins with the standard management including oxygen, positioning, fluid administration, and bag-mask ventilatory support as needed. Most CYSHCN have the same fluid requirements as any other child, unless the child has a congenital heart defect and possible heart failure. If the patient is injured or in shock, limit on-scene time and transport to the most appropriate pediatric center. Attempting peripheral vascular access is reasonable, but for a child whose condition is unstable, intraosseous access may be necessary. For most children in shock, 20-mL/kg boluses of crystalloid fluid are used. If a child has a history of chronic heart, lung, or kidney disease, consider smaller boluses of 5 to 10 mL/kg and reassess perfusion and respiratory status after each bolus. Because accurate assessment of CYSHCN may be more difficult, and because vascular access is often troublesome, always transport a child with suspected shock as soon as possible. These patients should be transported to pediatric-ready facilities, if at all possible, with consideration given to transport logistics and patient stability.

Some children with severe, uncontrolled epilepsy may be on a **ketogenic diet**. This regimen eliminates foods and medications that contain glucose and keeps the child in a state of ketosis to control the seizures. For these children, do *not* use any fluids containing **dextrose**. The targeted blood glucose level for these patients is lower than normal (eg, 50 to 80 mg/dL). They should be asymptomatic despite the low glucose levels. Ask the caregiver what plan is established for addressing symptomatic hypoglycemia.

CAUTION
Do not give glucose or glucose-containing fluids to children on a ketogenic diet.

TIP
Bradycardia may be a sign of hypoxia or inadequate brain perfusion. Suspect hypoxia in a child with a chronic cardiac or pulmonary condition whose heart rate is below normal for chronological age. In a child with a ventricular shunt, bradycardia is a sign of increased intracranial pressure (shunt malfunction). Some children with severe intellectual disability have an abnormality in their autonomic nervous system that leads to bradycardia. Ask the caregiver about the patient's baseline heart rate.

Disability

Many CYSHCN often have a compromised baseline neurological status. Assess neurological status by looking at appearance as part of the PAT, and establish the level of consciousness with the Alert, Verbal, Painful, Unresponsive (AVPU) mnemonic. Compare the findings to the child's baseline level. In the assessment of motor activity, assess purposeful movement, symmetrical movement of extremities, seizures, posturing, or flaccidity. Treat altered mental status if there is a change from baseline. The Glasgow Coma Scale may not be applicable for assessment of CYSHCN because many CYSHCN have baseline cognitive and physical challenges that would affect the score. It is better to describe the child's status as being different from their baseline.

TIP
The usual level of consciousness or motor activity for CYSHCN may be out of the "normal" range for the child's chronological age. The Glasgow Coma Scale may not be applicable. It is better to describe the child as being "at baseline" or how their mental status is different from baseline.

Exposure

Be sure to inspect the child's entire body, but respect their modesty. Do not allow the child to become cold. Many CYSHCN have minimal body fat and can become hypothermic quickly.

Summary of Assessment of CYSHCN

Listen carefully to the caregiver when assessing CYSHCN. Ask about the child's baseline status (What is typical for this child?). These children may present a confusing picture, with unexpected behaviors, communication difficulties, extensive medical histories, and complicated equipment. The child's neurological status is often compromised. If the caregiver is not present, look for sources of baseline information, such as a medical information form or a bracelet. Use standard assessment techniques and developmentally appropriate approaches modified by baseline comparisons to evaluate and manage acute problems. Transport early.

Transport

TABLE 12–1 lists key principles of transport of CYSHCN. *Always safely restrain children using approved devices for transport in the ambulance.* These devices include regular gurney straps, child-size modifiers for gurney straps, and approved car seats that can be secured to the gurney. The best type of restraint device and the best method for securing the device in the ambulance depend on the child's size, positioning, and mobility.

TABLE 12–1 Principles of Transport for CYSHCN

1. Transport CYSHCN who are on home oxygen with the oxygen (except for liquid oxygen). If the child has no respiratory distress, continue the same rate of oxygen flow.
2. Transport a child on a home ventilator with the ventilator if there are no equipment problems. If there is a concern about the ventilator, manually assist ventilation. Regardless of the method of ventilation, always secure the child's home ventilator in the ambulance and transport it with the child, so that it can be assessed by hospital personnel for potential problems and appropriate settings.
3. If the child has poor muscle control or increased muscle tone, immobilize the child as needed in a position that is comfortable. If the child has a special seat, wheelchair, or other equipment (eg, feeding pump or suctioning device), transport these items to the ED if they can be safely secured in the ambulance while still allowing enough room to safely care for the child during transport.
4. If the child has contractures or rigid postures, such as scissoring of the legs or an arched back, pad around any open areas when the child is on the stretcher or during spinal motion restriction. Do *not* force the child to conform to the equipment.

Abbreviations: CYSHCN, children and youth with special health care needs; ED, emergency department.

In general, if the child is critically ill or injured, they will be transported on their back secured on a gurney. Try to use a specialized device for spinal motion restriction if the child has experienced an injury to the head or has a suspected spinal injury. Be careful if the child has any contractures or rigid posturing, such as scissoring of the legs or an exaggerated arching of the back seen in children with CP. Pad any open areas and do not force the child to conform to the equipment. Check with the caregiver about positioning and the availability of any special car seat. In some children, the supine position may compromise the airway because of an abundance of secretions, poor tone, or anatomical differences. The child's specially designed child restraint system or car seat may be the best option if it can be secured safely in the ambulance, so long as it was not involved in a collision and has 2 belt paths to secure to the gurney using the gurney straps.

Many CYSHCN have supplemental oxygen and oxygen delivery equipment. Transporting liquid oxygen in an ambulance requires proper handling, storage, and restraints to prevent potential life-threatening hazards. Consider transporting nonliquid (or gaseous) oxygen and the child's personal devices or equipment to the ED.

Summary of Transport

Often, CYSHCN have special transport considerations. Make sure the child is safely restrained in the ambulance. An appropriately sized child safety seat can be used, always facing the rear of the ambulance, if it can be secured appropriately. Parents may have an adaptive restraint, travel vest, or harness that can be used with the car seat. Ensure that belts or harnesses do not interfere with tracheostomies or gastrostomy feeding tubes. Do not use rigid cervical collars to restrain a child's head if they have poor head control, unless deemed necessary because of trauma. Address the issue of transport with the caregiver, and consider bringing ancillary medical equipment (eg, ventilators, feeding pumps) to the ED if it can be safely secured in the ambulance. If a child in a wheelchair cannot be removed from the wheelchair, ideally a transit option chair should be used. If this is not available, the wheelchair should have a metal frame to which tie-down straps and hooks can be attached at frame junctions, and the wheelchair should be secured in a forward-facing direction. If possible, accommodate or coordinate transportation of the caregiver with the patient.

Children Assisted by Technology

Children assisted by technology have devices that may malfunction. The most common devices are **tracheostomy tubes**, **cerebrospinal fluid shunts**, **indwelling central venous catheters**, **insulin pumps**, and **feeding tubes** (buttons). Equipment malfunction can cause a range of problems. Some malfunctions may have minor or no immediate effects, such as loss of a feeding tube or clotting of an indwelling central venous catheter. Other malfunctions may cause serious physiological effects, such as respiratory distress caused by loss of a tracheostomy tube or intracranial pressure elevation caused by obstruction of a CSF shunt.

TRACHEOSTOMY TUBES

A tracheostomy is a surgical opening (stoma) in the front of the neck into the trachea. A tracheostomy tube (sometimes called a "trach tube") is an artificial airway passed through this opening that allows the child to breathe (**FIGURE 12–1**). Infants and children may have a tracheostomy for several reasons, as noted in **TABLE 12–2**.

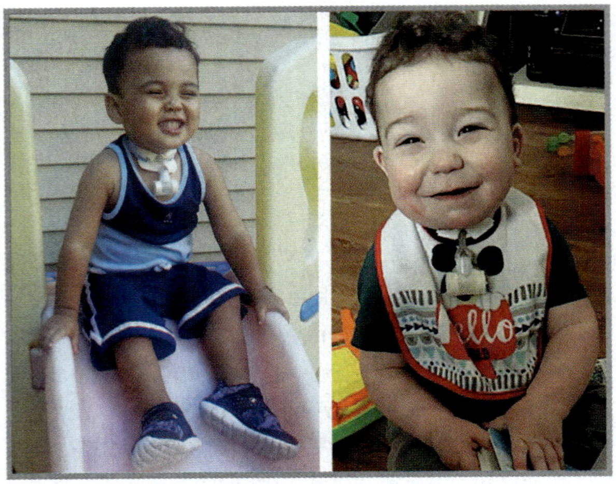

FIGURE 12–1 A tracheostomy. Reproduced with permission from Murray N. Pediatric tracheostomy. In: Schoem SR, Darrow DH, eds. *Pediatric Otolaryngology for Primary Care.* 2nd ed. American Academy of Pediatrics; 2020:450

TABLE 12–2 Indications for a Tracheostomy

To bypass an obstruction in the upper airway caused by trauma, surgery, or a birth defect
To allow clearance of secretions
To provide long-term mechanical ventilation of children with chronic respiratory problems, injuries to the lungs, major CNS deficits, or severe muscle weakness

Abbreviation: CNS, central nervous system.

There are several types of tracheostomy tubes, and they come in many sizes. The size is printed on the wings or flanges of the tube. The size and name (indicating type of tube) are also on the box. The inner and outer diameters are often printed on the wings (**FIGURE 12–2**). The most common pediatric tube sizes are 2.5 to 10 mm (sizes 000–10). A 3.0 tracheostomy tube is the same diameter as a 3.0 endotracheal tube. Tracheostomy tubes have a standard outer opening or hub outside the neck so a bag-mask device can be attached. For some tubes, an adapter may be needed to make this connection.

Types of Tracheostomy Tubes

The main types of tracheostomy tubes are fenestrated, double lumen, and single lumen (**FIGURE 12–3**). Tubes can also come with or without a cuff. These cuffs can be filled with air or foam. All tubes have an **obturator**, which is a solid plastic guide placed inside the tube to make insertion easier. Use the obturator to clear the tube of secretions in an emergency if a suction catheter is not available.

A single-lumen tracheostomy tube has one hollow tube or cannula for airflow and suctioning of secretions. Uncuffed, single-lumen tubes are usually used for neonates, infants, and young children. A double-lumen tube has a hollow outer cannula and a removable (also hollow) inner cannula. Remove the inner cannula for cleaning, and keep it in place to provide mechanical ventilation. Never remove the outer cannula unless the entire tube must be replaced.

A fenestrated tube has holes (fenestrations) for air to flow upward through the vocal cords and mouth. This structure lets the child talk and breathe naturally. Fenestrated tubes have a decannulation plug attached to the outer cannula that blocks airflow through the stoma. If the child cannot breathe through the nose or mouth, remove this plug so breathing is possible through the stoma. In addition, many fenestrated tubes have a hollow inner cannula that must be in place for mechanical ventilation.

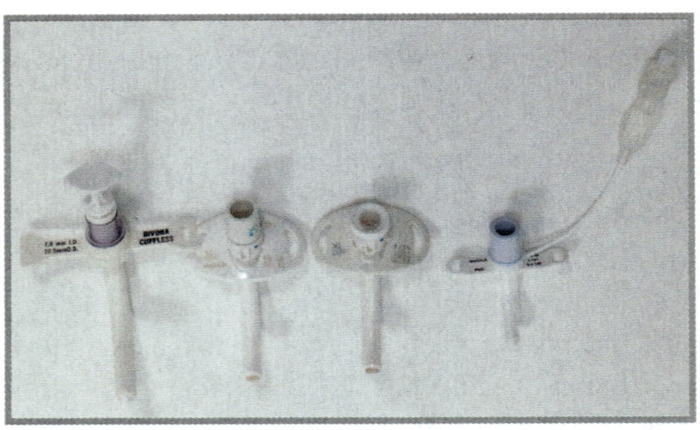

FIGURE 12–2 Sizes and inner and outer diameters are often written on the wings of tracheostomy tubes.

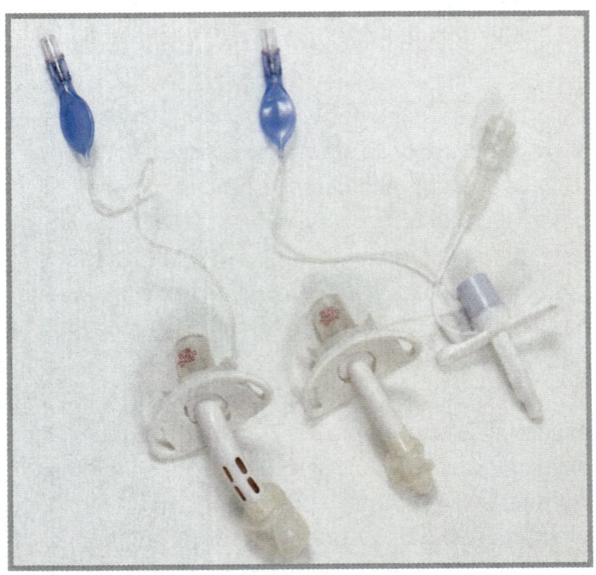

FIGURE 12–3 Fenestrated, double-lumen, and single-lumen tracheostomy tubes (top to bottom).

> **TIP**
>
> If the inner cannula of a double-lumen tracheostomy tube has been removed, a bag-mask device will not secure to the outer lumen of the tube. To ventilate a tracheostomy tube with the inner cannula removed, secure an infant face mask onto the bag, and then cover the tracheostomy tube's opening and seal the face mask on the neck.

Oxygen Delivery and Assisted Ventilation Through a Tracheostomy Tube

A child with a functioning tracheostomy tube can receive oxygen via the blow-by method, by a face mask or tracheostomy mask placed directly over the tube opening, or by manual ventilation with a bag-mask device.

- Provide blow-by oxygen. Place a stoma mask or pediatric face mask a short distance above the tracheostomy tube or stoma and give oxygen at 10 to 15 L/min.
- Secure a face or tracheostomy mask directly over the tracheostomy tube opening and secure the straps around the neck.
- Attach a bag-mask device to a tracheostomy tube adapter. Attach a bag-mask device directly to the outer end of the tracheostomy tube (**FIGURE 12-4**).

For a child who has a stoma (surgical opening in the neck) but no tracheostomy tube, or when a tube cannot be reinserted, apply a seal with a mask over the stoma and ventilate through the stoma; alternatively, cover the stoma with **sterile gauze** and ventilate with a mask to the mouth or mask to the mouth and nose technique. Begin bag-mask ventilation as needed.

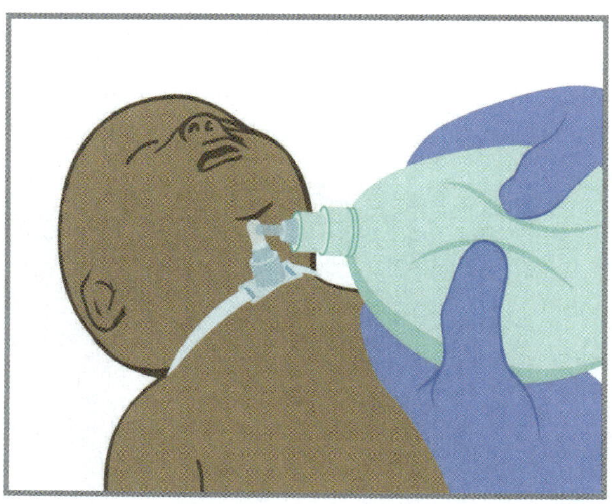

FIGURE 12-4 Bag-mask device attached directly to the external end of the tracheostomy tube.

Tracheostomy Complications: Obstruction

Obstruction of the tracheostomy tube is a life-threatening emergency. Obstruction can be caused by secretions, incorrect insertion (tube malposition), improper positioning of the child's head, or mechanical problems with the tube. Obstruction causes respiratory distress and failure.

Assessment. When a child has an obstructed tracheostomy tube, the child is not ventilating effectively on their own. The PAT shows poor appearance, increased work of breathing, and cyanosis in cases of respiratory failure. The ABCDEs further indicate poor air movement and eventual bradycardia.

> **TIP**
>
> The most common complication of a child with a tracheostomy tube is respiratory distress caused by obstruction of the tube.

Use the DOPE mnemonic to troubleshoot respiratory distress in a child with a tracheostomy.

- Displacement
- Obstruction
- Pneumothorax
- Equipment failure

Treatment: Clearing an Obstructed Tube. To clear an obstructed tracheostomy tube, follow these steps:

1. Position the child's head with a towel roll under the shoulders. Ensure the outer opening of the tube is clear.
2. Check to make sure the tube is in the proper location. The wings or flange should be against the neck, and the obturator should not be in place.
3. If the child has a fenestrated tube, remove the decannulation plug.
4. If the child has a double-lumen tracheostomy tube, remove the inner lumen to clear secretions.
5. If none of these maneuvers works, suction the tube with a suction catheter.

Treatment: Suctioning a Tracheostomy Tube. If efforts to clear the obstruction are unsuccessful, suction the tracheostomy tube using the following procedure (**FIGURE 12-5**):

1. Ask the caregiver if they have suction catheters, equipment, and supplies. If so, use these. Otherwise, choose a suction catheter small enough to pass through the tube. (A size 1.0 [or 3.0-mm] tube will accommodate a size 6 to 8 French catheter.) The caregiver may know

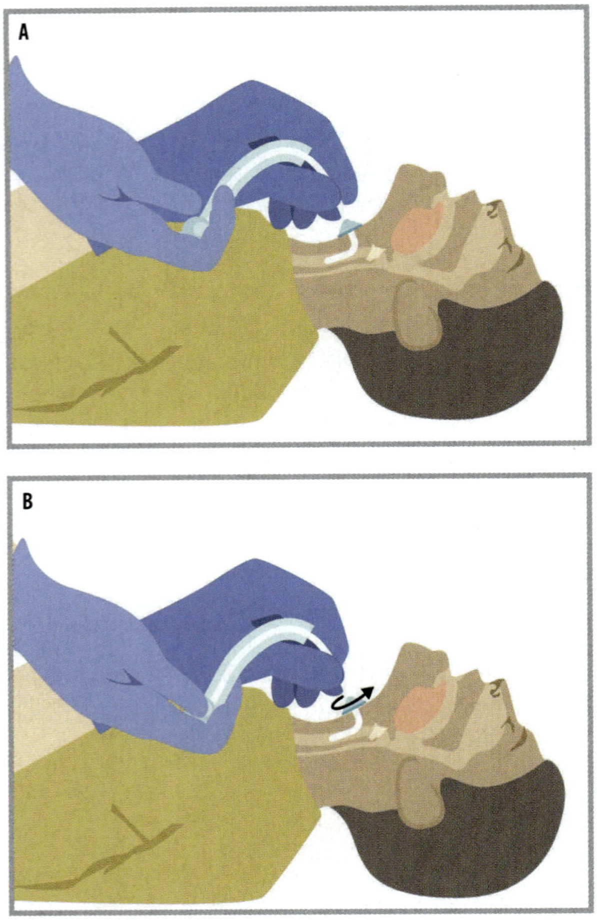

FIGURE 12-5 **A.** Insertion of suction catheter to the proper depth; suction port remains open. **B.** Suctioning the airway in a circular motion as catheter is removed; suction port is closed.

the correct size of catheter. If equipment is not immediately available, insert the obturator to try to clear the obstruction.

2. If using a portable suction machine, set it to negative pressure at 100 mm Hg or less.
3. Preoxygenate using a ventilation bag with a mask.
4. If secretions are thick or sticky, consider placing 1.0 to 2.0 mL of normal saline into the tube.
5. Insert the suction catheter approximately 2 inches (5 cm) into the tube. If the child begins to cough, it means the catheter is through the tube and into the trachea and the insertion is too deep. Do not use suction while inserting the catheter, and never force the catheter.
6. Cover the suction port (hole on the tubing) and suction for 3 to 5 seconds while slowly removing the catheter. Never suction for longer than 5 seconds. Always monitor the child's heart rate and color during this procedure. Stop suctioning immediately if the heart rate begins to drop or the child becomes blue.
7. If the obstruction is removed, and the child can breathe on their own, do not suction further. If additional suctioning is needed, apply oxygen (by blow-by method or direct ventilation) and repeat steps 3 through 6.
8. Always provide supplemental oxygen after suctioning by using the blow-by method or manual ventilations.

Replacing a Tracheostomy Tube

Treatment of a tracheostomy problem usually requires simple techniques to establish a patent airway, such as suctioning or removal of the old tracheostomy tube and replacement with a new tube (**FIGURE 12-6**). Occasionally, it is impossible to ventilate a child through an existing tracheostomy tube because of decannulation or complete obstruction. Under these conditions, the prehospital professional must place a new tracheostomy tube to save the child's life. For a step-by-step explanation of this procedure, see **Procedure 24, Removing and Replacing a Tracheostomy Tube.**

CENTRAL VENOUS CATHETERS

Many children receive nutritional support or medications at home through a **central venous catheter**. This includes children with poor weight gain caused by gastrointestinal or liver problems, children with cancer who require chemotherapy, or children with any other condition that impacts nutritional status.

Many central venous catheters require a surgical incision, but some can be placed percutaneously or through intact skin (called **peripherally inserted central catheter [PICC] lines**). They enter through the skin of the chest, neck, or arm, and the internal end usually lies in or near the **superior vena cava** or right **atrium**. Central lines may be single lumen or double lumen, with 1 or 2 separate external ports.

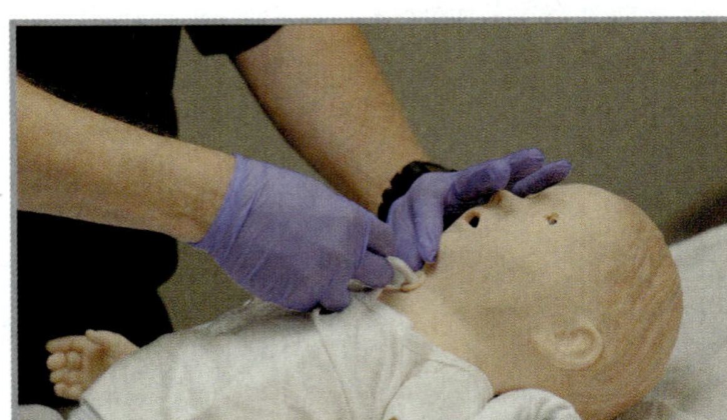

FIGURE 12-6 Replacing a tracheostomy tube.

CASE STUDY 2

You are called to the home of a 6-year-old boy whose central venous catheter has bleeding around the insertion site. His mother panicked because it is a new catheter and she is not used to taking care of it. She tells you that he has a history of short-gut syndrome caused by an infarcted bowel sustained 6 months ago. He also has a gastrostomy tube through which he receives some medications; however, it was accidentally pulled out earlier today.

On arrival, you note a thin 6-year-old boy sitting quietly on the family's couch. He has no increased work of breathing. His skin is yellowish. His respiratory rate is 22 breaths/min, heart rate is 95 beats/min, and blood pressure is 90/50 mm Hg. Pulse oximetry is 98%. There is a tiny ooze of blood from the insertion site of the catheter in the right neck. There is a gastrostomy on his left upper abdomen with no tube in place.

1. What are the key historical points?
2. Outline the assessment and management priorities.

Types of Catheters

Central venous catheters may be inserted into the external jugular, internal jugular, and subclavian veins (**FIGURE 12–7**), or the femoral vein. The skin entry site for the catheter is usually on the chest or arm. This is called a peripherally inserted central catheter (PICC).

Totally implanted devices (ports) are catheters attached to totally implanted injection ports or reservoirs. The catheter is in a central vein, such as the superior vena cava. Instead of coming out of the skin, as with partially implanted catheters, the end is attached to a reservoir (dome or port) that is in a subcutaneous pocket, usually on the chest. Therefore, there are no external parts, just a bulge or bump where the device rests.

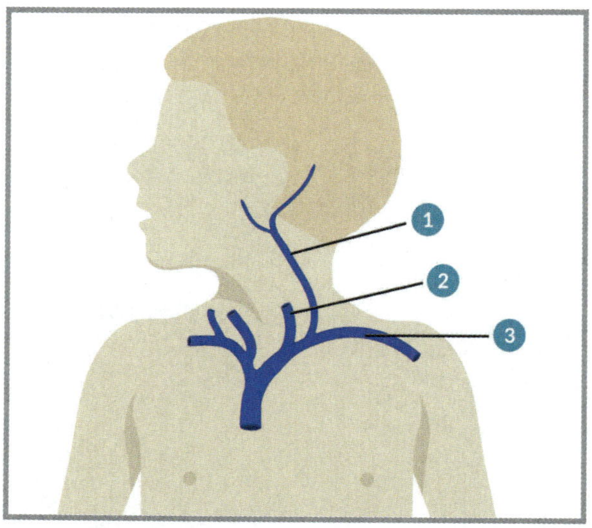

FIGURE 12–7 Possible insertion sites for a central venous catheter. Subclavian, internal jugular, and external jugular sites. 1. External jugular vein. 2. Internal jugular vein. 3. Subclavian vein.

> **TIP**
>
> The most common complication in a child assisted by technology with a partially implanted central venous catheter is a broken or dislodged catheter. If the bleeding is from the catheter and the catheter is in place, inspect the catheter and its end. Apply direct pressure to the bleeding site with sterile gauze. If a cap is missing, replace the cap if possible.

Complications of Central Venous Catheters

TABLE 12–3 lists common complications of central venous catheters. The most common problem with partially implanted devices is a broken or dislodged catheter. Check the site for bleeding. If the catheter is in place but there is bleeding from the entry site, apply direct pressure with sterile gauze. Likewise, if the catheter has been completely pulled out and there is bleeding, apply direct pressure with sterile gauze.

> **ALS**
>
> **Clamping a Leaking Central Venous Catheter. If the child is bleeding through a hole or cut in the catheter, clamp the exposed end. The caregiver usually has a clamp available, but if this has been misplaced, wrap the tips of a hemostat with gauze and apply to the catheter. If no hemostat is available, open the emergency delivery kit, wrap the sharp edges of the umbilical clamp with gauze, then apply to the catheter. Alternatively, attempt to tie off the catheter using suction tubing or oxygen tubing. If bleeding has occurred, estimate the amount of blood loss.**
>
> **Provide appropriate fluid therapy if there are signs of poor perfusion or shock. Do not use the central venous catheter.**

TABLE 12–3 Common Central Venous Catheter Complications

Dislodged or broken catheter
Infection at catheter site
Problems with accessing or flushing the catheter (obstruction)
Air embolism
Medical problems related to **infusion**

Infection at Catheter Site. Infection can occur at the site at which a partially implanted catheter enters the skin or in the pocket in which a totally implanted device is placed. Signs of infection are redness, tenderness, swelling, warmth, or yellow discharge (pus) from the site. Children and youth with special health care needs are at high risk of experiencing sepsis, a blood infection with fever, chills, and shock. In this case, treat for **septic shock**, as described in Chapter 4. If the line might be infected, do not use it for vascular access.

Obstruction. A problem with accessing or flushing the catheter usually means obstruction. This complication can occur with all types of catheters. All that is required is patient assessment and transport. The major concern is a child who depends on parenteral nutrition (intravenous [IV] nutrition) for calories and glucose. If the line is malfunctioning and the child has not received any nutrition, their blood glucose level may be low, so perform a fingerstick check of the blood glucose level.

CAUTION
If the indwelling central venous catheter seems infected, do not use it for vascular access.

TIP
In a child who depends on hyperalimentation for calories and glucose, if the line is malfunctioning and the child has not received any nutrition, their blood glucose level may be low.

Treatment of Hypoglycemia. Perform a fingerstick check of the blood glucose level if there are signs or symptoms of hypoglycemia. For a low blood glucose level, basic life support providers can give oral glucose per local protocol, or advanced life support (ALS) providers can treat with IV dextrose or intramuscular **glucagon,** as described in Chapter 6.

Air Embolism. This complication can occur if air accidentally gets into a central venous catheter when the line is being flushed or if the catheter breaks. Symptoms of air embolism include shortness of breath, chest pain, and coughing. Sometimes there is cardiovascular collapse and cardiopulmonary arrest.

Treatment of Suspected Air Embolism. Clamp the catheter or ask the caregiver to clamp the catheter, provide the child with oxygen, place the child on their left side in the head-down position, and transport to the ED.

Medical Problems Related to Infusion. Because of the various fluids and medications delivered through central venous catheters, several medical problems can develop, such as allergic reactions, abnormal heart rate or rhythms, or respiratory problems. Treat the appropriate problem, and bring the fluids that were being infused to the ED for analysis.

FEEDING DEVICES

A feeding device provides an avenue for nutrition and medications to CYSHCN who are unable to take food or fluids by mouth. This device allows the child to take in enough calories for adequate growth and nutrition and may be used to administer medications.

Types of Feeding Tubes

Some feeding tubes go through the nose (nasogastric [NG]) or, occasionally, through the mouth (orogastric [OG]) and into the stomach or small intestine (nasojejunal and orojejunal, respectively) (**FIGURE 12–8**). These tubes are usually long catheters that are taped in place on the child's face.

Another type of feeding tube goes directly into the stomach from an external site on the abdomen

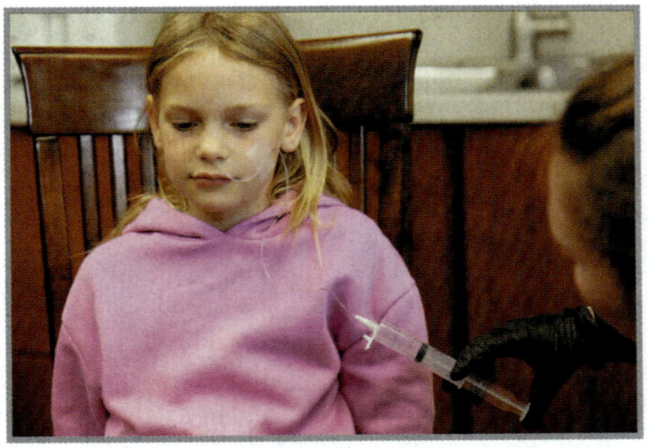

FIGURE 12–8 Nasojejunal catheter taped in place on the child's face.

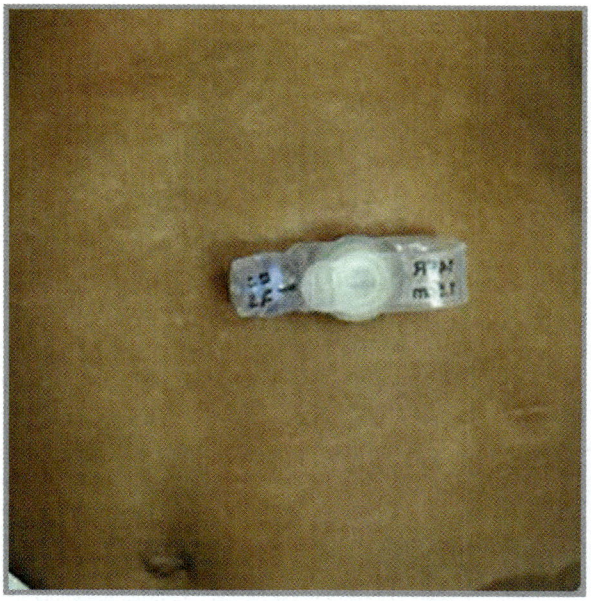

FIGURE 12–9 A G-tube button.

Photo courtesy of Children's Hospital of Philadelphia.

(**gastrostomy tube** or **G-tube** or "**button**") (**FIGURE 12–9**). It has a balloon on the end inserted into the stomach that is similar to the balloon on an endotracheal tube. It is inflated to keep the button in place. There is also a small cap with a valve on the outside to allow access. It can be replaced by the child's caregivers. Another device is called a percutaneous endoscopic gastrostomy, which is a longer tube. Many caregivers prefer a button because there is no tube hanging from the abdomen that could be dislodged during physical activity.

TIP

The main complication of feeding tubes is dislodgment.

Complications of Feeding Tubes

The main complication of a feeding tube is dislodgment. The child may have aspirated fluid if a nasal or an oral feeding tube has come out. For tubes inserted into the abdomen, there may be bleeding or leakage of fluid. A replacement button gastrostomy tube may not fit into the abdominal stoma if it is the wrong size or there was a delay in replacing it. Perform an assessment, paying special attention to the work of breathing, chest auscultation, and pulse oximetry.

Treatment

If an implanted tube (G-tube) comes out, check the site for bleeding and apply direct pressure with a sterile dressing. If the insertion site around the implanted tube seems irritated or infected (the skin seems red, warm, or swollen), apply a sterile dressing to the site.

Whenever a tube dislodges or there is evidence of infection, transport the child to the ED. Ask the caregiver to bring the tube that fell out to the hospital for sizing purposes. If the child was receiving an infusion of fluid or medication, ask the caregiver to disconnect the pump (infusion device) and transport it with the child. If the child has received fluid through a feeding catheter within 30 minutes of EMS arrival, consider transporting the child in a sitting position to prevent reflux, vomiting, and possible aspiration.

ALS

Removing a Feeding Tube. If the NG or OG tube seems to be in place but the child is experiencing respiratory difficulty, ask the caregiver to check its position. If the position cannot be confirmed, remove the tube.

CSF SHUNTS

A CSF shunt is a device that drains excess CSF from the brain. It is usually inserted from a ventricle (in the brain) under the skin, then down the neck into the **peritoneum** of the abdomen (ventriculoperitoneal shunt), the **pleura** of the chest (ventriculopleural shunt), or the heart (ventriculoatrial shunt) (**FIGURE 12–10**). Its path (or track) can usually be felt on one side of the head and down the neck until the

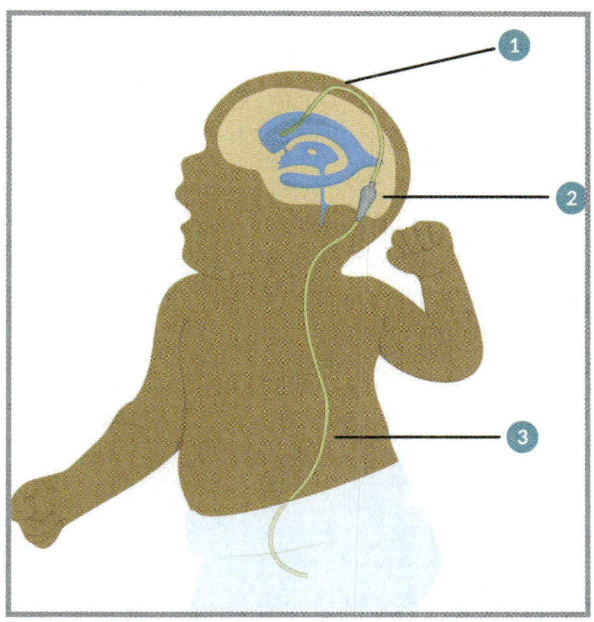

FIGURE 12–10 A CSF shunt directs CSF from a ventricle in the brain to either the abdomen or the heart. 1. Point where shunt dips into ventricles. 2. Reservoir/pump. 3. Point where shunt dips into abdomen.

track reaches a scar on the chest wall or abdomen. A CSF shunt helps a child with **hydrocephalus** maintain normal brain pressure. The hydrocephalus may be caused by a congenital problem or by an acquired condition, such as bleeding, trauma, a tumor, or an infection.

Complications of CSF Shunts

The major complications with a CSF shunt are obstruction and infection. The most common complication is a shunt obstruction/malfunction. **TABLE 12–4** lists key questions to ask during assessment to evaluate the severity of the complaint and the urgency for treatment.

Assessment of a Child With a Possible CSF Shunt Obstruction or Infection

Symptoms of a CSF shunt obstruction are the same as those of increased intracranial pressure and include headache, lethargy, sleepiness, irritability, nausea or vomiting, or trouble walking. Fever is usually a sign of a shunt infection or an intercurrent illness, but it can occur with a shunt malfunction alone. Signs of shunt obstruction are abnormal appearance, high-pitched cry, seizures, or altered mental status. A worrisome finding is Cushing triad (bradycardia, elevated blood pressure, and irregular respirations), which indicates increased intracranial pressure caused by an obstructed shunt.

TIP

Many CYSHCN, especially those with spina bifida, have a sensitivity or an allergy to latex. Always use latex precautions with these patients. Reactions to latex can range from a localized skin reaction to anaphylaxis.

A child with a shunt infection may have a fever, headache, feeding difficulty, or altered behavior. Signs of shunt infection include abnormal appearance, altered mental status, and shock.

TABLE 12–4 Key Questions for Suspected CSF Shunt Malfunction

When was the CSF shunt placed?
Is the child acting the same as the last time there was a shunt problem (obstruction)?
Has the child had a fever?
Has the child complained of a headache, vomiting, or nausea?

Abbreviation: CSF, cerebrospinal fluid.

Treatment

Make sure the child has a clear airway and effective breathing. Supply supplemental oxygen, and transport the patient. Keep the head in midline position and elevate the head of the stretcher to 30 to 45 degrees if possible. If the patient develops the Cushing triad of bradycardia, irregular respirations, and elevated blood pressure, herniation is imminent. Begin bag-mask ventilation, consider hyperventilation to an end-tidal carbon dioxide ($EtCO_2$) level of 35 to 40 mm Hg, and rapidly transport to an appropriate hospital.

ALS

Hyperventilation for Suspected Increased Intracranial Pressure. Hyperventilation is a treatment for children with impending or frank herniation. However, the role of hyperventilation in treating prehospital intracranial pressure elevation from hydrocephalus is not well understood. Hyperventilation, through carbon dioxide reduction and cerebral vasoconstriction, reduces brain perfusion. However, overly aggressive ventilation may dangerously decrease perfusion and cause brain ischemia. If a child with a CSF shunt has signs of impending or frank herniation, use capnography to keep $EtCO_2$ levels at 35 to 40 mm Hg. This is the same treatment outlined for traumatic brain injury in Chapter 9.

OSTOMIES

Some conditions, such as Crohn disease, spinal cord injury, distal ureter or bladder defects, and necrotizing enterocolitis in an infant, interfere with regular elimination of urine and feces. Several types of **ostomies** are created to accomplish this bodily function. With a **colostomy** or an **ileostomy**, an opening in the abdomen is formed when the large or small intestine is surgically brought out to the surface and sutured in place, creating a stoma. This procedure allows the digestive system to continue functioning while bypassing any inflamed or damaged bowel. An external pouch is placed over the stoma to collect digestive waste matter. The intestines below the ileostomy site may not have been removed if there is a possibility of reconnecting the bowel at a later time. Colostomies can also be temporary or permanent. With a **urostomy**, a stoma is surgically created to allow the elimination of urine.

Complications of Ostomies

Complications of ostomies include infection and pouch displacement. Because of an increased risk for dehydration, a child with a colostomy needs to be assessed carefully for clinical signs and symptoms of dehydration and shock, particularly if there is a history of diarrhea or decreased oral intake.

Signs of infection at the ostomy site include red, warm, tender skin spreading away from the stoma site. Ask the child or caregiver if the area is more tender than usual. If the child has signs of infection, transport the child for further evaluation.

Replacing a Pouch

Ask the caregiver to empty the pouch before transport, especially if the pouch is full. Before the pouch is emptied, document the amount of fluid in the pouch. Be sure the pouch is resealed after emptying to prevent leakage. In some instances, the pouch breaks or is torn off. If another pouch is not available, circle the stoma with moist gauze and then attach anything available that can serve as a substitute collection device. If no pouch is available, place several thicknesses of moist gauze over the stoma until a proper replacement is found. Another option is to secure a nonrebreather face mask over the stoma. Remove the valve leaflet, so the reservoir in the mask collects the excreted stool or urine.

Lastly, be respectful of the child's privacy. Keep the site and pouch covered in public.

> **TIP**
>
> Perform a thorough physical examination of stoma pouch devices, especially for displacement and/or damage from trauma, such as a motor vehicle collision or fall.

INTERNAL PACEMAKERS AND DEFIBRILLATORS

Pacemakers are implanted medical devices that regulate the heart rate. Indications include bradycardia that does not maintain adequate perfusion; a previous cardiac arrest; and heart block, especially after open heart surgery. Pacemakers usually include a generator and leads. The generator houses the software and battery and supplies the electrical impulse. The leads are insulated wires that carry the electrical impulse to the heart and carry information about the heart's natural rhythm back to the pulse generator.

Complications of Internal Pacemakers

Several complications can occur for children with pacemakers. Some devices do not allow the child's heart rhythm to go above a certain rate. If the child is in shock or impending shock, the body cannot compensate by increasing the heart rate. Begin treatment and transport to the most appropriate pediatric cardiac facility. With pacemaker malfunction or failure, the child's heart rate becomes too slow to maintain perfusion. Begin treatment and transport to the most appropriate pediatric cardiac facility. In rare cases, such as chest trauma, the leads may become dislodged and the pacemaker firing will cause the child's diaphragm to contract instead of the heart muscle. The respiratory rate will equal the preset pacemaker rate. Monitor the heart rate closely and transport to the most appropriate pediatric cardiac facility.

> **ALS**
>
> **Transcutaneous pacing may be clinically effective in patients with symptomatic pacemaker failure to maintain perfusion.**

Internal Cardiac Defibrillators

An **implantable cardioverter-defibrillator (ICD)** is an electronic device implanted under the skin. Its purpose is to monitor the heart rhythm and slow down or stop excessively fast heart rates that originate in the ventricles. Such rhythms include ventricular tachycardia and ventricular fibrillation.

The mechanical parts of an ICD include a generator and a lead. This generator is a tiny battery-operated electronic device located inside a case that monitors and records the heart rhythm. It sends out shocks or uses bursts of pacing to convert excessively fast heart rates when needed. The computer also records any shocks that it sends to the heart. A lead (or wire) is attached to the generator and is connected to the heart muscle to monitor the heart rhythm and carry shocks to the heart. The battery life for implanted pacemakers and defibrillators is 6 to 12 years.

For any child with a pacemaker or an ICD, prehospital professionals should ask the caregivers the following questions:

- What type of heart disease/disorder does the child have?
- What rate is the child's underlying rhythm?
- What type of pacemaker or ICD does the child have?
  - If a pacemaker, is the child dependent on the pacemaker? What are the settings?
  - If an ICD, what are the settings, at what heart rate does the ICD fire, and how many

shocks has the child felt? In addition, has the child experienced any of the following?

- More than 3 shocks in a row
- Continuation of unusual symptoms after experiencing a shock
- Sensations of dizziness, lightheadedness, and/or palpitations for a period of time, yet has felt no shock

TIP

If using automated or manual defibrillation for a patient with an implanted pacemaker or defibrillator, never place defibrillator paddles, "hands off" defibrillating-pacing patches, or automated external defibrillator patches directly over the internal pacemaker or defibrillator generator. The internal pacemaker can easily be felt near the clavicle or in the abdomen in small children.

VAGAL NERVE STIMULATOR

The **vagal nerve stimulator (VNS)** was approved by the Federal Drug Administration in 1997 for patients with intractable epilepsy. Some children continue to experience seizures despite treatment with conventional medication, surgical procedures, and diet. The VNS provides hope for better seizure control.

The VNS is an implantable device that looks like a pacemaker and is surgically placed by a neurosurgeon just under the skin in the left upper chest. It is programmed to provide baseline intermittent stimulation of the left vagus nerve, which leads directly to the brain. The patient or caregiver activates the device by placing a handheld magnet over it.

When responding to a call involving a CYSHCN with an implanted VNS who is seizing, first assist the caregiver with activation of the VNS. Alternatively, contact medical control for guidance. Children with VNS devices should otherwise be treated as any other patient who is seizing, with attention to airway, breathing, and circulation.

DIALYSIS SHUNTS

Chronic renal failure is progressive and irreversible kidney function inadequacy caused by permanent loss of nephrons. This disease develops over months or years and causes scarring in the kidneys, leading to diminished kidney function and the buildup of waste products and fluid in the blood. **Renal dialysis** is a technique for filtering toxic wastes from the blood, removing excess fluid, and restoring the normal balance of electrolytes. There are 2 types: **peritoneal dialysis** and **hemodialysis**.

In peritoneal dialysis, large amounts of specially formulated dialysis fluid are infused into and drained back out of the abdominal cavity. This fluid stays in the cavity for 1 to 2 hours, allowing equilibrium to occur. It is very effective, yet carries a high risk of peritonitis. Many patients undergo peritoneal dialysis at home after caregivers have received appropriate training. Prehospital professionals usually are not involved in this process.

In hemodialysis, the patient's blood circulates through a machine that functions much like a kidney and requires the use of some type of shunt or surgically created connection between a vein and an artery. External shunts may be located near the wrist, in the upper arm, or on the proximal anterior thigh. Some patients have an internal shunt also known as an arteriovenous (AV) fistula that is usually located in the forearm or upper arm (**FIGURE 12–11**).

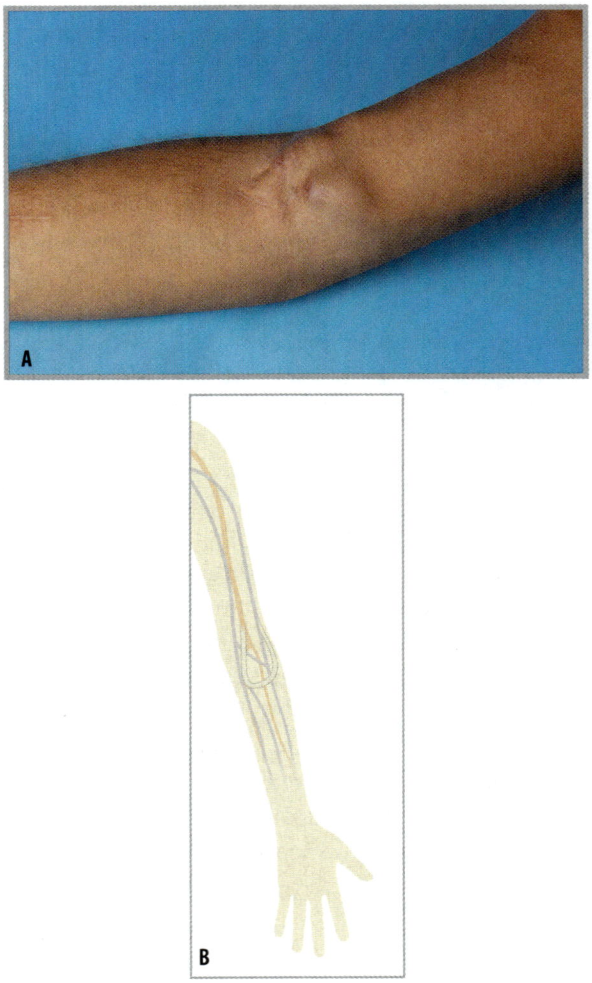

FIGURE 12–11 **A.** Hemodialysis access by an AV fistula or graft that creates a bulge in the skin. **B.** An AV graft creates a raised area that looks like a large vessel.

Vadi Fuoco/Shutterstock.com

CAUTION

Never use an AV fistula for vascular access.

When moving and transporting the patient, make sure the external shunt is protected and is not compromised by any straps. For all blood pressure measurements, use the arm **without** the device. If the patient has an internal shunt or AV fistula, do *not* attempt to access the fistula to draw blood or to infuse any fluids.

INSULIN PUMPS AND CONTINUOUS GLUCOSE MONITORS

Children with type I diabetes may have insulin pumps and continuous blood glucose monitors that help monitor and ensure adequate glycemic control. Insulin pumps are external devices—similar to a pager—that carry several days' supply of insulin in the reservoir and release insulin subcutaneously through a small needle placed in the subcutaneous tissue. Continuous glucose monitors (CGM) are worn on the skin with a subcutaneous needle to measure glucose readings constantly. Often, CGMs are linked with a smartphone that records the glucose readings, and they may be linked with the insulin pump to adjust the insulin dose based on the current glucose reading.

Complications of these devices include skin infections where the device is inserted or malfunction or dislodgement of the insulin pump. Both devices can cause skin infections at the site of insertion. If the site is not changed regularly (every 2–3 days), insulin pumps or CGMs may malfunction and not provide accurate readings; in these cases, patients may present with hypoglycemia or hyperglycemia. Hypoglycemia should be treated accordingly with additional glucose, and the insulin pump should be turned off. The pump can stop delivering insulin if the subcutaneous catheter is dislodged, if the reservoir leaks or runs out of insulin, or if the pump runs out of battery charge. Hyperglycemia or diabetic ketoacidosis (DKA) can result. In DKA, glucose readings are often over 250 mg/dL, and patients experience nausea and vomiting, dehydration, tachypnea, and altered mental status. This is a life-threatening condition. Insulin pumps should be turned off in patients with suspected DKA, and treatment should focus on maintaining the airway, assisting oxygenation and ventilation, and providing IV fluids.

Summary of Children Assisted by Technology

Children assisted by technology may encounter many challenges with their equipment. The prehospital professional must be familiar with the basic purpose, design, and common complications of tracheostomy tubes, central venous catheters, feeding tubes, CSF shunts, pacemakers, insulin pumps, and implantable defibrillators. Always ask the caregiver about the equipment, and transport all devices and infusions with the child to the ED. Ask whether the current problem has ever happened before and, if so, how the situation was handled. Finally, remember that the child may be well versed on the medical device they use. Consider asking the child your questions about the device; in doing so, you may gain their trust, which ultimately leads to better patient care.

The Medical Home for CYSHCN

Care coordination for CYSHCN, who often have involvement of multiple organ systems, is quite complex. A specialist or general pediatrics practice can provide compassionate, comprehensive, and continuous care in a culturally sensitive manner by being the child's family-centered medical home. Information is available at www.medicalhomeinfo.org.

Children and youth with special health care needs usually see multiple physicians, therapists, home care personnel, and other health care providers to manage their chronic conditions. To coordinate that care, these clinicians need to communicate with the medical home and one another in an effective manner. Traditionally, communication has occurred on paper, with hospitals and offices faxing reports or sending copies to one another. This system is flawed in that some of these paper reports are lost, are misfiled, or do not arrive at the office or hospital in time for future visits or procedures. For example, if the child sees a pediatric neurologist who initiates treatment with different medications to manage seizures, the primary care physician may not know about this change and prescribe another medication for an illness, which may cause a dangerous interaction that could be detrimental to the child. In addition to adverse drug reactions, the poor coordination of care may result in unnecessary hospitalizations, duplicate testing, advice from one clinician that contradicts that of another, and poor clinical outcomes.

Electronic health records (EHRs) are one way to improve the quality of care for patients with chronic conditions. By documenting care and treatment in an EHR, the child's medical and surgical histories, medications, allergies, contact information for multiple providers, schedule of preventive services, baseline neurological status, and other information can be immediately available.

Electronic documentation can be beneficial, but sharing that information across systems of care presents yet another challenge. Some areas of the country have developed **health information exchanges (HIEs)** whereby electronic data are shared among hospitals, physician practices, and other entities where patients may be treated. The presence and use of these HIEs are sporadic at best, and many of them do not involve EMS systems.

In an emergency involving a CYSHCN, obtaining accurate medical information is a priority because of the multitude of treatments, medications, and ongoing care. To address this, an electronic version of the EIF, originally developed by the AAP and ACEP, is available (**FIGURE 12–12**).

> **TIP**
>
> Transport a CYSHCN and their caregiver to the child's medical home whenever possible for continuity of care.

Emergency Information Form for Children With Special Needs

American College of Emergency Physicians® — American Academy of Pediatrics

Date form completed	Revised	Initials
By Whom	Revised	Initials

Last name:

Name:	Birth date: Nickname:
Home Address:	Home/Work Phone:
Parent/Guardian:	Emergency Contact Names & Relationship:
Signature/Consent*:	
Primary Language:	Phone Number(s):

Physicians:

Primary care physician:	Emergency Phone:
	Fax:
Current Specialty physician:	Emergency Phone:
Specialty:	Fax:
Current Specialty physician:	Emergency Phone:
Specialty:	Fax:
Anticipated Primary ED:	Pharmacy:
Anticipated Tertiary Care Center:	

Diagnoses/Past Procedures/Physical Exam:

1.	Baseline physical findings:
2.	
3.	Baseline vital signs:
4.	
Synopsis:	Baseline neurological status:

*Consent for release of this form to health care providers

FIGURE 12–12 The AAP/ACEP Emergency Information Form (EIF).

Last name:

Diagnoses/Past Procedures/Physical Exam continued:

Medications:	Significant baseline ancillary findings (lab, x-ray, ECG):
1.	
2.	
3.	
4.	Prostheses/Appliances/Advanced Technology Devices:
5.	
6.	

Management Data:

Allergies: Medications/Foods to be avoided	and why:
1.	
2.	
3.	

Procedures to be avoided	and why:
1.	
2.	
3.	

Immunizations (mm/yy)

Dates					
DPT					
OPV					
MMR					
HIB					

Dates					
Hep B					
Varicella					
TB status					
Other					

Antibiotic prophylaxis: Indication: Medication and dose:

Common Presenting Problems/Findings With Specific Suggested Managements

Problem	Suggested Diagnostic Studies	Treatment Considerations

Comments on child, family, or other specific medical issues:

Physician/Provider Signature: Print Name:

FIGURE 12–12 *(continued)*

Through websites containing EIFs, parents and providers can enter data and then access the data in a secure fashion. This effort is one example of how the care of CYSHCN can be enhanced through health information technology and the electronic exchange of data. In addition, contact with the patient's medical home can provide EMS professionals with important information about the patient.

Additional EMS Considerations for CYSHCN

1. Many CYSHCN, especially those with spina bifida, have a sensitivity or an allergy to latex. Always use latex precautions with these patients. Reactions to latex can range from a localized skin reaction to anaphylaxis.

2. Speak quietly and calmly to the child, and explain what they can expect by using words appropriate for the child's developmental level. This approach decreases the child's anxiety and increases cooperation.
3. Children with musculoskeletal conditions, such as CP or muscular dystrophy, need special care during preparation for transport. Children with CP are often stiff and may have contractures. Do not force movements. Secure these children in their natural position, and pad any open areas. Children with paralysis or muscular dystrophy may not have regular sensation, so special care should be taken to ensure that their limbs are secured on the stretcher and do not extend off the edges of the stretcher.
4. Assess pain in CYSHCN. If the child cannot communicate, then ask the caregiver if the child is in pain. Tachycardia, tachypnea, or hypertension may be the only signs that the child is in pain. Position the child for comfort. Use blankets under vulnerable areas of the body. If local protocols allow, administer medications for pain control after ensuring that the caregivers did not give the child any pain medication before EMS arrival.
5. When leaving the home of a CYSHCN:
   - Ask the parents or caregivers for the child's "go bag." This bag contains all of the supplies necessary (and are not routinely stocked in ambulances) to manage the child's tracheostomy tube, feeding catheter, or central venous line.
   - Ask the parents for the child's daily medical information form or EIF, which contains pertinent medical information regarding the child's medical condition, baseline vital signs, allergies, physicians' names and numbers, medications, therapies, and necessary home support equipment. Ask how you can make the patient most comfortable.
   - Ensure any compressed air or oxygen in the home is turned off before departure.
6. Request the direct caregiver to accompany the child to the hospital to continue assisting with the child's care. The caregiver not only becomes a valuable resource for repeated assessments and interventions, but also provides familiarity and reassurance to the child in the midst of an unfamiliar and a potentially chaotic environment.
7. Recognize when the caregiver is overwhelmed with emotion or exhaustion. In these circumstances, it may be best to offer the caregiver a more passive role in the child's care while allowing them to remain with the child.
8. EMS may be called for CYSHCN with emergencies outside their home, at school, athletic events, or a friend's house. If their usual caregiver is not with them, less medical information will be available and the child may be particularly anxious. If a regular caregiver is not available, attempt to identify a trusted adult with knowledge of the patient's baseline needs.

CASE STUDY 3

A distraught mother calls 9-1-1 because her infant son is having difficulty feeding and appears more blue than usual. She tells you that the 2-month-old infant has Down syndrome and a heart defect. He has been home for a few weeks waiting to grow before undergoing surgery to repair his heart. His mother confirms that he usually has a pulse oximetry reading in the 80s. She hands you a card with the child's medical history, medications, and hospital information and states that he has been vomiting since the day before and has not kept down any of his medications.

You approach the infant and note that he is poorly interactive, has retractions and nasal flaring, and is cyanotic. The chest has crackles, and the pulse oximetry is 75%. His heart rate is 130 beats/min, respiratory rate is 70 breaths/min, and blood pressure is 86 mm Hg/palp.

1. What is the likely physiological problem?
2. What are your primary interventions?

CASE STUDY ANSWERS

CASE STUDY 1

Assessment of the airway, breathing, and circulation suggests respiratory distress. Ask the child's caregiver about her baseline vital signs and activity level. Ask if there have been any changes and, if so, what is different.

Take the child off the ventilator and manually ventilate with a bag to the tracheostomy tube. Determine the ease of air entry through the tracheostomy tube and determine if aided respirations help the child's respiratory distress. Ask the caregiver when the last tracheostomy tube change was and about the frequency of suctioning. Suction the tracheostomy to determine if this helps the child's breathing. Consider a tracheostomy tube change if there are copious secretions or there is difficulty with air entry during manual ventilations.

Consider an albuterol nebulizer treatment. Albuterol can open the child's airways to alleviate distress. In this case, the parent states that he has had to suction more frequently than usual and that he has already changed the tracheostomy tube that day. He states that he thinks the child is getting sick and that her older sister has had a cold for the last few days. This history makes an exacerbation of the child's chronic lung disease more likely, and a mucous plug obstructing the tube less likely.

You decide to transport the child to her medical home hospital and continue the albuterol nebulizer treatment through her tracheostomy tube en route. You ask the caregiver to disconnect the feed through the gastrostomy tube to prepare for transport.

At the hospital, the child is diagnosed with a viral respiratory infection (rhinovirus) and tracheitis. She is admitted to the hospital for antibiotic treatment and frequent suctioning of her tracheostomy. She is discharged a few days later back to her baseline ventilator support.

CASE STUDY 2

This boy is in no distress. The PAT findings are normal. His vital signs are stable. He is totally dependent on this central venous catheter for his nutrition and hydration. Ask the caregiver how long the catheter site has been bleeding. Check the catheter for dislodgement or breakage. Apply direct pressure to the site to stop the bleeding. Ask the caregiver to disconnect the catheter if it is still connected. Prepare the child for transport, preferably to his medical home hospital, so that the catheter can be repaired or replaced. If the child has not received nutrition for 1 to 2 hours, check the blood glucose level.

Another common problem is dislodgement of a feeding catheter. This is especially true if the child is totally dependent on the gastrostomy tube (G-tube or button) for all nutrition and hydration. Also, the longer the tube is out, the more difficult it is to replace. Ask the family to bring the dislodged tube to the hospital, and if they have a replacement tube, to bring that as well. Not all hospitals have the proper size tubes for children, so either call ahead to the local ED or transport the child to his home hospital.

Short-gut syndrome results when a large section of the bowel has been removed. This phenomenon is more likely to occur in preterm children, but can also occur in children who experience shock or hypoxemia to the bowel due to infections, obstruction of the intestines, or trauma. These children often receive their nutrition through feeding catheters, as this child did; however, if they have lost a significant amount of their bowel, they may need their nutrition (hyperalimentation and lipids) delivered through a central venous line. This boy could no longer receive all of his feedings through the gastrostomy tube and needed supplementation through his central venous catheter.

A young child who misses many hours of fluids may be tachycardic and have signs of dehydration, such as dry mucous membranes and no tears, in the early stages of hypoperfusion. Interventions include oxygen supplementation, keeping the child warm, covering the stoma site with a dry gauze, and transporting the G-tube that was dislodged (along with any special adaptors) for sizing purposes.

ALS interventions include a 20-mL/kg crystalloid fluid bolus via peripheral IV in a child who seems dehydrated with a G-tube out or dislodged or a broken central venous line. If the glucose level is low, treat with IV dextrose.

You arrive at the hospital and give the old G-tube to the hospital staff. They locate a new tube of the same size and are able to replace the tube and resume enteral feeding. The child is discharged home later that day in good condition.

Continued

CASE STUDY ANSWERS—cont'd

CASE STUDY 3

Assess airway, breathing, and circulation. You decide that this infant needs assisted ventilations and begin to manually ventilate with a bag-mask device. As your partner looks for an appropriate IV site, she notes that the child has pedal edema. You then consider that this child is in congestive heart failure and decide not to administer IV fluids without advice from medical control. Because blood pressure and perfusion are adequate, do not start a pressor drug. Transport immediately to the most appropriate pediatric ED.

Children with Down syndrome are at increased risk of experiencing medical complications. Some of the organ systems affected include the cardiovascular, sensory, endocrine, orthopedic, gastrointestinal, neurological, and hematologic systems. People with Down syndrome are developmentally delayed and often have intellectual disabilities.

Cardiovascular defects are a leading cause of neonatal death in Down syndrome as a result of congenital abnormalities. When an infant is born with a severe cardiac anomaly, interventions are primarily directed toward home health care until definitive surgery can be performed, or toward supportive treatment in the home of a child whose defect cannot be surgically repaired.

The infant's respiratory distress improves after a minute of assisted ventilations and you transition him to oxygen by nasal cannula. You transport the infant to the hospital while he receives supplemental oxygen titrated to keep his saturations at 85%, which is his baseline. At the hospital, it is determined that his heart failure is worsening and he is admitted for diuresis in preparation for surgical repair of his heart defect.

Suggested References

TEXTBOOKS

Adirim T, Smith E. *Special Children's Outreach and Prehospital Education (SCOPE)*. Jones and Bartlett Learning; 2006

ARTICLES

American Academy of Pediatrics, Council on Children With Disabilities. Care coordination in the medical home: integrating health and related systems of care for children with special health care needs. *Pediatrics*. 2005;116(5):1238–1244. doi: 10.1542/peds.2005-2070

Burton LC, Anderson GF, Kues IW. Using electronic health records to help coordinate care. *Milbank Q*. 2004;82(3):457–481. doi: 10.1111/j.0887-378X.2004.00318.x

Callahan JM, Baldwin S, Bodnar C, et al; Committee on Pediatric Emergency Medicine; Council on Clinical Information Technology; Council on Children and Disasters; American College of Emergency Physicians, Pediatric Emergency Medicine Committee. Access to critical health information for children during emergencies: emergency information forms and beyond. *Pediatrics*. 2023;151(3):e2022060970. doi:10.1542/peds.2022-060970

Kaziny BD. The prehospital care of children with special health care needs. *Clin Pediatr Emerg Med*. 2014;15(1):89–95. doi: 10.1016/j.cpem.2014.02.001

McPherson M, Arango P, Fox H, et al. A new definition of children with special health care needs. *Pediatrics*. 1998;102(1)137–139. doi:0.1542/peds.102.1.137

O'Neil J, Hoffman B, Agran PF, et al; Council on Injury, Violence, and Poison Prevention. American Academy of Pediatrics Council on Injury, Violence, and Poison Prevention. Transporting children with special health care needs. *Pediatrics*. 2019;143(5):e20190724. doi:10.1542/peds.2019-0724

Singh T, Wright JL, Adirim TA. Children with special health care needs: a template for prehospital protocol development. *Prehosp Emerg Care*. 2003;7(3):336–351. doi: 10.1080/10903120390936545

OTHER RESOURCES

Children with special health care needs. EMSC Emergency Medical Services for Children–New York. Accessed November 22, 2024. https://www.health.ny.gov/professionals/ems/pdf/referencecard.pdf

Facts, myths & truths about Down syndrome. National Down Syndrome Society. Accessed November 22, 2024. https://ndss.org/myths-truths

Medical home overview. American Academy of Pediatrics. Updated June 11, 2025. https://www.aap.org/en/practice-management/medical-home/medical-home-overview/

CHAPTER 13

Child Maltreatment

Kathleen Adelgais, MD, MPH, FAAP, FAEMS
John A. Erbayri, MS, NRP, CHSE

LEARNING OBJECTIVES

1. **Discuss the known signs, causes, and complications of child maltreatment.**
2. **Define the terms physical abuse, emotional abuse, sexual abuse, and child neglect.**
3. **Explain the role of child protective services in management of suspected child maltreatment.**
4. **Distinguish features in the scene size-up, in the history and physical assessment, and in the caregiver's behaviors that suggest child maltreatment.**
5. **Describe appropriate communication with caregivers of suspected victims of maltreatment.**
6. **Outline the emergency medical services clinician's legal responsibility to document and report suspected child maltreatment.**
7. **Identify clues to human trafficking.**

Introduction

Consideration of possible child maltreatment begins with the first contact with medical teams. Emergency medical services (EMS) clinicians must know when to suspect **child maltreatment**. Although providing emergency medical care is always the top priority, EMS clinicians also provide valuable scene documentation and are often the first step in the reporting process of suspected cases of maltreatment. All of these actions are critical in protecting vulnerable children and breaking the cycle of maltreatment. When caring for a pediatric patient who has suffered obvious trauma, EMS clinicians need to remain vigilant in looking for potential signs of abuse.

Unfortunately, child maltreatment is common. It is one of the leading causes of death in infants younger than 12 months. Physical abuse and neglect are often detectable, but sexual abuse, emotional abuse, and child neglect may not be so obvious. Some children who die as a result of maltreatment are known to local **child protective services (CPS)**. These deaths are sometimes preventable. Abused or neglected children have a high probability of being maltreated again. Early recognition is important to prevent future injury or death. Government agencies responsive for CPS use many different names (eg, Department of Social Services [DSS], Department of Children and Family Services [DCFS]) but are established in every community to respond to reported cases of child abuse and neglect.

Background, Cost, and Definition

In 2022, there were 2.1 million referrals reported to CPS organizations in the United States through the National Child Abuse and Neglect Data System. Of those, 558,900 children were determined to have been abused or neglected. The highest prevalence is seen in infants from birth to 1 year (22.2 cases per 1,000). For each case of child maltreatment reported, it is estimated that there are 1 to 2 cases that go unrecognized. In addition to being at higher risk of experiencing abuse, ***younger children are at higher risk of experiencing fatal abuse and neglect***. In 2022, an estimated 1,990 children died of abuse or neglect, which is more than 4 children every day. Approximately 71.8% of maltreated children who die are younger than 3 years, and more than 49% are younger than 1 year. Approximately one-half of

CASE STUDY 1

9–1-1 is called for an unresponsive infant. On arrival, you find a 10-month-old male infant who is unresponsive, has irregular respirations, and is pale. The mother is at work; the mother's boyfriend tells you that he found the baby in this condition when he went to get him up from his nap. You note that it is 7 pm. The boyfriend is not holding the infant, and when you pick the baby up from the crib, you also note that there is no muscle tone and the infant is flaccid. During your assessment and treatment, you note bruises on both upper arms.

1. What are your initial patient care priorities?
2. What concerns you about the history reported by the boyfriend and the infant's injuries?
3. What do you suspect is the primary injury?

these deaths occur in children who are known to CPS agencies as current or prior clients. It has been estimated that child maltreatment costs the United States $220 million every day.

Among survivors, there are significant negative outcomes of child maltreatment. Child abuse and neglect is a severe form of what are now known as adverse childhood experiences (ACEs). Long-term outcomes of individuals with ACEs include many negative health and mental health outcomes, including substance abuse, chronic disease, and early death. **TABLE 13–1** lists some long-term complications.

TABLE 13–1 Potential Long-Term Complications of Maltreatment

Low self-esteem and underachievement
Psychological disorders or psychiatric symptoms
Abnormal growth and development
Permanent physical or neurological damage
Poor school performance
Early sexual initiation and teen pregnancy
Social withdrawal
Eating disorders
Substance abuse
Negative learned behavior
Criminal behavior beginning in young adulthood
Vulnerability to further abuse
Suicidal tendencies
Increased survivor health care costs to family and society
Death

Definition of Child Maltreatment

Child maltreatment is a general term that includes all types of abuse and neglect. Yearly, approximately 75% of substantiated maltreatment is classified as neglect, 17% as physical abuse, and 8% as sexual abuse. The remaining types include emotional abuse, medical neglect, or combinations of the different types.

PHYSICAL ABUSE

Physical abuse occurs when a person inflicts injury, or allows injury to be inflicted, on a child younger than 18 years or on a mentally disabled child younger than 21 years that causes or results in risk of death, disfigurement, or distress.

EMOTIONAL ABUSE

Emotional abuse occurs when there is an ongoing and consistent pattern of behavior that interferes with the normal psychological and social development of a child. This includes unreasonable, excessive, or aggressive demands on the child that are not age appropriate; setting tasks that are beyond the child's physical ability; or the caregiver's failure to provide the nurturing, guidance, and psychological support critical for the growth and development of a healthy child. Verbal attacks such as belittling, insults, rejection, and constant criticism are a few examples of emotional abuse.

SEXUAL ABUSE

Sexual abuse occurs when an older child or adult engages in sexual activities with a dependent, developmentally immature child or adolescent for the older person's own sexual excitement or for the enjoyment of other persons (eg, child pornography or prostitution).

A common misconception is that child sexual abuse is perpetrated by strangers; however, in most cases of sexual abuse, the perpetrator is an adult who knows the child. According to the American Psychological Association, an estimated 60% of sexual abuse perpetrators are known by the child but are not a family member, 30% are family members, and only 10% are strangers.

Sexual abuse usually does not occur as a single incident. It does not always involve violence and physical force and commonly leaves no visible sign. The perpetrator may use the power of adult–child authority or the parent–child bond instead of force or violence. The child may be manipulated into thinking that "it's OK" and a normal behavior or that the child is "special" for making the perpetrator feel good. The child may also be made to feel deeply ashamed and powerless or may even be kept silent by threats from the perpetrator. The insidious nature of this abuse makes it difficult to detect unless the child discloses the information to a confidant or the EMS clinician.

CHILD NEGLECT

Child neglect occurs when a child's physical, mental, or emotional condition is harmed or endangered because the caregiver has failed to supply basic necessities or engages in child-rearing practices that are inadequate or dangerous. Child neglect may involve a caregiver's misuse of drugs or alcohol, or it may take the form of child abandonment. Neglect is the failure to act on behalf of a child and is an act of omission. Neglect may not have visible signs, and it usually occurs over a period rather than as a discrete episode.

Neglect may be physical or emotional. **Physical neglect** is a failure to meet the requirements basic to a child's physical development and safety, such as supervision, housing, clothing, medical attention, and nutrition. Some social service agencies subdivide this category into more specific acts of omission, such as medical neglect, lack of proper supervision, or educational neglect. Some states include an exception for cases of extreme poverty. **Emotional neglect** is failure to provide the support or affection necessary for a child's psychological and social development.

> **TIP**
>
> The difference between abuse and neglect is that abuse represents an action against a child, whereas neglect represents a lack of action for the child. In abuse, a physical or mental injury is inflicted on a child. In neglect, there is a failure to meet the basic needs of the child.

High-Risk Groups

Child maltreatment involves risk factors and lapses in child protection at the individual, family, community, and societal levels. Child maltreatment is reported more commonly among single-parent, nonwhite, and low-income families. The reasons for this are complex and include various social determinants of health and the social infrastructure, which leads to reporting. However, no geographic, ethnic, or economic setting is free of child maltreatment. The incidence rates of sexual abuse are similar for urban, suburban, and rural communities, and the EMS clinician must consider maltreatment whenever circumstances suggest it, regardless of the family's race, ethnicity, or socioeconomic status.

Other risk factors for child maltreatment, besides being a nonverbal toddler or infant, include situations in which there are additional stressors but insufficient resources available to the parents or caregivers. Children and youth in these situations include those with special needs (mental and physical disabilities and developmental issues) and those with chronic medical conditions—all of which involve increased responsibilities in caring for the child and a financial impact that may also affect the level of stress in the home.

Maltreatment happens for many different reasons. Child maltreatment can be perpetrated by any person who has care, custody, or control of the child. This can include the child's parents, relatives, teachers, babysitters or child care staff, institution staff, bus drivers, playground attendants, coaches, religious leaders, caregivers, or boyfriends or girlfriends of the caregiver. Often, the perpetrators genuinely care for the child but lack the resources or the skills to deal with children of different developmental states, a situation that can lead to frustration. It is important to know that at the time the child is seen by EMS, they may or may not be with a caregiver who perpetrated the injury. For example, children with abusive head trauma will experience seizures, apnea, or critical illness, often after repeated injury. This caregiver may be unaware of the abuse or in denial and unable to believe that the child has been harmed.

> **TIP**
>
> The caregiver with the child at the time of the 9-1-1 call or EMS arrival may not be the individual who injured the child.

TABLE 13–2 Assessment Factors Associated With Maltreatment

Does the history change over time?
Was there unnecessary delay in seeking care?
Does the history of the injury fit the child's developmental level?
Is the interaction between child and the caregivers appropriate?
Do the findings of the head-to-toe examination fit the history given?
Does the injury fit the history?
Are there any other signals that make you doubt the safety of the patient or siblings?

For more information on the Escape tool, see Louwers et al (2012).

TABLE 13–3 Duties of the Emergency Medical Services Clinician in Suspected Maltreatment

Recognition of suspicious circumstances at the scene
Physical assessment of the child
Assessment of the history given by the caregiver
Communication with the caregiver and family
Careful documentation
Notation of other children living at the scene
Reporting of maltreatment concerns to the proper authority

Rarely does the EMS clinician have sufficient information to determine with certainty when or if maltreatment has occurred. Information gathered in the field, however, is critical in the eventual confirmation of maltreatment. **TABLE 13–2** lists questions posed by the Escape child abuse screening tool (Louwers, 2012) in the clinical history that may be suggestive of maltreatment. Particularly important is the documentation of the exact history given by the caregiver in cases of presumed injury. A changing story is one of the most common hallmarks of maltreatment. Recognizing and reporting suspected child maltreatment is one of the most important ways the EMS clinician can prevent childhood injury.

Duties of the EMS Clinician

The EMS clinician has an extremely important role at the scene. In addition to providing high-quality medical care to the child, the EMS clinician must ensure accurate and complete documentation of the history and scene assessment. Child protective services and health professionals in the emergency department (ED) rely on this information in the setting of suspected child maltreatment. **TABLE 13–3** lists the EMS clinician duties in suspected maltreatment cases.

MANDATORY OBLIGATION TO REPORT

In most states, licensed health care professionals, including EMS clinicians, have a legal obligation (mandate) to report suspected child maltreatment. In other states, the duty of the EMS clinician is to ensure that a report is filed with the receiving hospital, law enforcement, or a designated state office. States with maltreatment laws may require health care providers to independently report suspected maltreatment to either law enforcement or CPS.

Although no law can forbid the filing of civil or criminal charges, most state laws protect the reporter of suspected child maltreatment from any decision or award in a lawsuit, if the report was made in good faith. *However, failure to report suspicion of child maltreatment may result in legal action against the mandated reporter.*

In small communities, especially when the EMS clinician knows the individuals involved, reporting suspected child maltreatment may have significant social implications. In many states, anonymous reports can be filed, and the identity of the person who reports maltreatment is protected. A report of suspected child maltreatment is not an attempt to harm or punish a family, but rather an attempt to help the child.

> **TIP**
> Emergency medical services clinicians should know the obligation-to-report laws in the state in which they practice.

DOCUMENTATION

Emergency medical services clinicians must approach each encounter with a focus on the care of the child and gathering the information available to them. Scene safety for the team and for the patient is critical. *Avoid confrontations with caregivers at the scene, even if there are suspicions of maltreatment.* Such an approach at the scene may delay care, endanger the child, and create a hostile and dangerous situation for the EMS clinician. Note the presence of alcohol or drugs in the EMS report, and document any and all statements from the caregiver. Watch and document interactions among the caregivers. Report what you see and hear, and do not make judgments or interpret intent in the written documentation. Document with exact quotes any comments made by the child about how they were hurt.

Be sure to document your findings of the scene assessment related to possible safety concerns. Make a note of the child's position and location when you first encountered them. It is also recommended to document who else is at the scene (eg, caretakers) and their relationship to the child. When documenting the history and physical assessment, be thorough but objective. Interjecting feelings or interpreting the facts may make the documentation inadmissible in court. For example, write, "palms show a 1-cm circular burn" instead of "cigarette burn to hand." Use objective, clear, specific terminology. Place in quotation marks and note in the records any statements from caregivers (eg, father states that child "climbed into the hot bathtub").

TIP

Document physical findings objectively. The facts speak for themselves in court.

Communicating With the Child and Caregivers

Communicate with the child in an age-appropriate manner. When assessing a stable child about whom there is concern regarding maltreatment, transport the child to the safe environment of the ED for full evaluation as soon as possible.

TIP

Communication with the caregiver of whom child maltreatment is suspected is sometimes challenging for the EMS clinician. Do not make accusations or take a judgmental tone. Focus on the medical treatment of the child and trust any investigation to be handled by other professionals.

Sometimes a caregiver may refuse to cooperate in further assessment, decline transport, or attempt to leave the scene with the child. If you believe the child to be in danger, immediately contact law enforcement for assistance. Never attempt to physically restrain a caregiver or to forcibly take possession of a child, because this may put everyone in danger. If the scene is chaotic but not dangerous, contact medical control, who may be able to speak with the caregiver to permit treatment and transport.

Patient Assessment

SCENE ASSESSMENT

First, ensure that the scene is safe for the child and for the EMS clinicians. If you suspect maltreatment, make a mental note of any conditions at the scene, because you need to document the conditions in the patient care report (**FIGURE 13–1**). Record remarks or specific conversations with the caregiver and document specifics about the environment in which injuries reportedly occurred. For example, note the approximate height of furniture off which an infant rolled, the floor surface, or the location and condition of the sink or room in which a child was burned.

Consider child maltreatment in every pediatric trauma call and every pediatric cardiac arrest situation in children younger than 1 year. Suspicious circumstances in the environment, behavior of the child or caregiver, history, or physical examination may also raise concerns about abuse in responding to calls for unrelated complaints. For example, a torn frenulum in an infant should raise concern for inflicted injury (**FIGURE 13–2**). Look for dangerous home conditions such as the presence of guns or drug paraphernalia, or other unsafe care situations.

If the scene is safe, assess the child using the Pediatric Assessment Triangle and provide appropriate medical care. If an infant with suspected maltreatment has an abnormal appearance (eg, listlessness, inconsolability, weak cry) or altered mental status

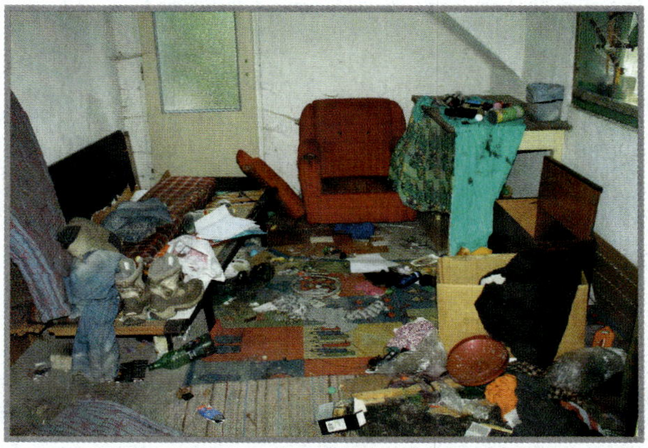

FIGURE 13–1 Document scene conditions that might support suspicion of maltreatment.

sangriana/IStockPhoto.com.

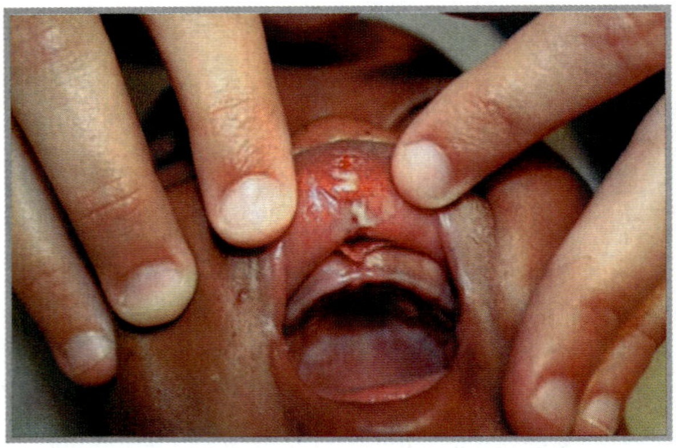

FIGURE 13–2 Torn frenulum in an infant should raise concern regarding inflicted injury.

(abnormal response to verbal or painful stimuli), assess for a traumatic brain injury.

> **TIP**
> Consider child abuse in every injury case, as well as illness cases with suspicious circumstances in the environment, behavior of child or caregiver, history, or physical examination findings.

One serious cause of traumatic brain injury in children is **abusive head trauma**, formerly called shaken baby syndrome. Abusive head trauma can cause intracranial hemorrhages; the symptoms and physical findings in abusive head trauma vary depending on the amount of trauma to the brain. These range from lethargy, irritability, and vomiting to seizures, coma, apnea, or death. **Petechiae** or hand-grip patterns on the arms or chest may also be found in abusive head trauma, but their absence does not exclude it. The incidence of permanent neurological damage resulting from abusive head trauma is high. Seizures, learning disabilities, blindness, and other handicaps are common. The fatality rate in abusive head trauma is 20% to 30%.

If the child with suspected maltreatment has significant injuries, begin transport after the primary assessment and stabilization. If the scene is unsafe for the child or EMS clinician, call for law enforcement back-up and move to the ambulance to complete the assessment and initiate treatment. Transport every child with suspected maltreatment, even if the injuries are trivial.

> **CAUTION**
> **Never leave a suspected victim of child maltreatment. Transport every child, even if the injuries are trivial.**

TABLE 13–4 Focused History: Questions and Considerations in Evaluating Suspected Child Maltreatment

Question	Considerations
How did the injury occur?	Is the caregiver's explanation plausible? For example, is the child developmentally able to roll and fall? Do the physical conditions at the scene support the reported mechanism of injury? How high was the fall, to what type of surface, etc.?
When did it happen?	Was there a long delay before 9–1–1 was notified? Does the injury appearance match the time frame?
Who witnessed the event?	Do all of the caregivers' or witnesses' stories match? Was there adequate supervision?
What is the child's medical history?	Are there pre-existing psychosocial, developmental, or chronic problems?
Does the child have a physician?	When was the last visit?

ADDITIONAL ASSESSMENT

Stay on scene for additional assessment only if the child is stable and the scene is safe. Take a careful history, using the questions suggested in **TABLE 13–4**. Pay close attention to and document in detail the caregiver's description of all events leading to the call. Consider the developmental capabilities of the child. Note when the history does not account for the observed injuries (**FIGURE 13–3**), if the caregiver's history changes over the course of the interview, or the mechanism of injury described is not plausible given the developmental level of the child.

If the injury is described as accidental in nature, determine the mechanism. For example, if the caregiver reports that the child fell, determine the distance, the stopping surface, and the initial reactions of the child (**TABLE 13–5**). The information obtained by EMS at the scene is an important part of the entire investigation into possible maltreatment and evaluation of the child.

PHYSICAL EXAMINATION

The physical examination may reveal the suspicious patterns and physical findings of child abuse.

Specifically, the EMS clinician may note sentinel injuries in the physical examination of the child. About half of physical maltreatment victims have some kind of skin injury. Sentinel injuries are minor injuries that may reflect a more serious pattern of physical abuse. Therefore, early detection of sentinel injuries may provide the opportunity to identify and intervene before more serious injuries occur. In cases of suspected sexual abuse, defer a genital examination to providers with specialized training.

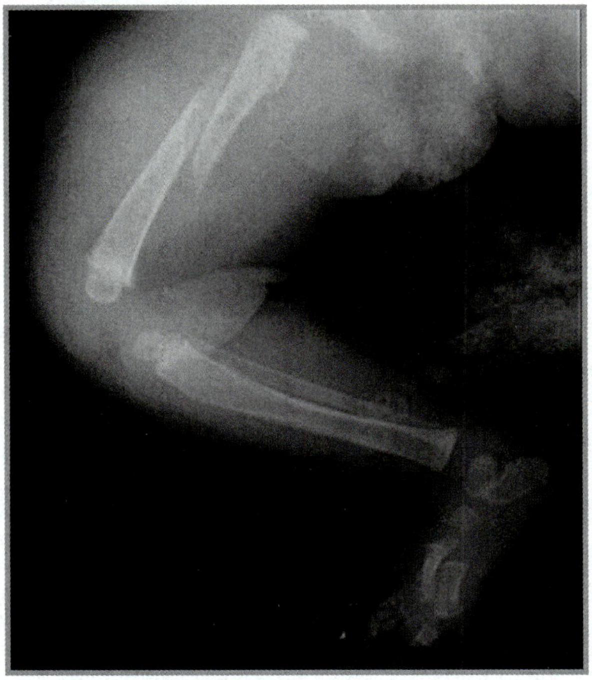

FIGURE 13–3 Children who are not yet walking should not have long bone fractures. History of "fell off the couch" is not consistent with a femur fracture in a nonambulatory child. When the history provided does not match the injury seen, the clinician should consider the possibility of inflicted injury.

Courtesy of James D. Anderst, MD, FAAP.

TABLE 13–5 Distinguishing Fact From Common Fiction

History	Fact
"He fell off the couch, and then seized."	Fewer than 1 in 1,000 falls of 4 feet (1.2 m) or less result in serious injury.
"My 1-month-old rolled off the bed."	Most infants cannot roll over until 3–4 months of age.
"He must have bruised himself."	Bruises are rare in infants who are not yet pulling to a stand; even in those who can do so, bruises in certain places, such as the pinna (ear), buttocks, and back, should raise concern regarding abuse.
"I found him with his leg stuck in the crib slat."	Without an external force, either intentional or accidental, infants do not sustain fractures.

Bruises: Location and Patterns

A recent clinical decision rule for detecting bruising consistent with abuse uses the mnemonic TEN-4-FACES-P (Torso-Ear-Neck, 4 months/4 years, Frenulum-Auricular-Cheek-Eyelid-Sclera Pattern) to help clinicians recognize bruising associated with child maltreatment in children younger than 4 years. Therefore, bruises that suggest inflicted injury include the following:

- Bruises located on soft tissues, such as neck, thighs, genitalia, or buttocks
- Bruises on or behind ears
- Any bruises in a child aged 4 months or younger
- Facial bruises (**FIGURE 13–4**)

Differentiating bruises resulting from maltreatment versus normal wear and tear depends on the child's appearance, location, and developmental age. Bruises over bony prominences, such as the elbow, forehead, or below the knees, are the common result

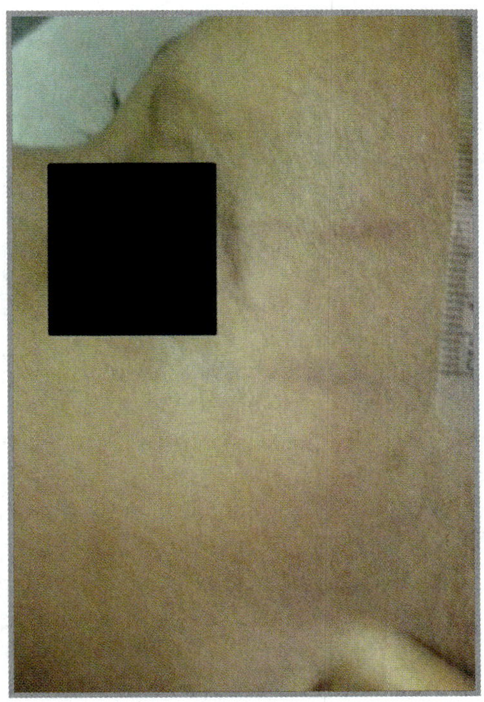

FIGURE 13–4 The face is a common target for physical abuse.

Courtesy of Jamie Hoffman-Rosenfeld, MD.

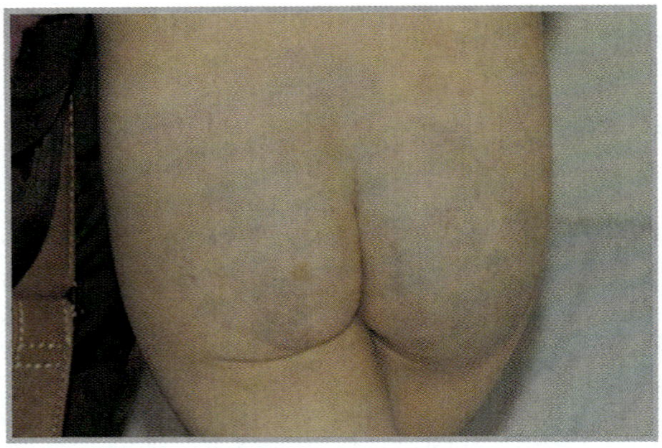

FIGURE 13–5 Bruises on the buttocks are usually inflicted injuries.

Courtesy of Jamie Hoffman-Rosenfeld, MD.

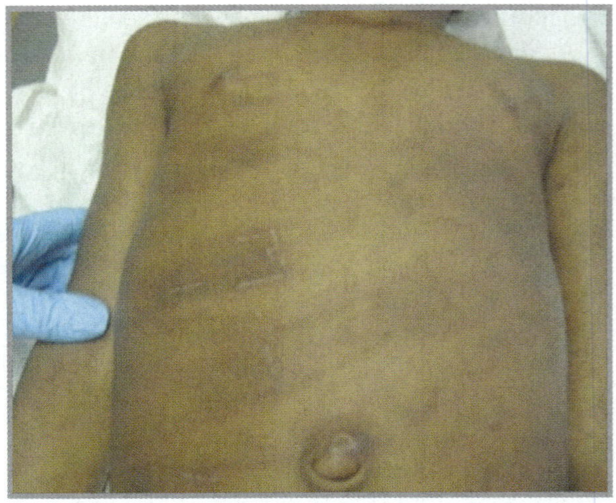

FIGURE 13–6 Bruises with identifiable patterns are highly suspicious of inflicted injury. Demarcated edges are clearly seen here.

Courtesy of Jamie Hoffman-Rosenfeld, MD.

of play injuries in children. However, bruises over soft tissues, such as the thighs, buttocks, cheeks, or ears, or on the back are less common and should raise suspicions of inflicted injury (**FIGURE 13–5**).

Any bruising in an infant who is not yet mobile may suggest inflicted injury. Most children are able to roll over by 4 months of age and able to pull to a standing position and cruise by 9 months of age. A child who is not yet cruising should not have unexplained bruises or fractures—*no cruising means no bruising*. As children become older and increasingly mobile, bruises and abrasions caused by normal activity become more common.

> **TIP**
>
> "If they don't cruise, they shouldn't bruise." In a child who cannot yet pull up to stand and walk while holding onto furniture (cruise), bruising or injury is rare. Most infants do not start cruising until they are about 9 months of age.

Any bruise with an identifiable pattern is almost certain to have been inflicted. Common items wielded in abuse include belts, cords, and hands. When an object hits the skin with high velocity, the edges leave an outline of petechiae. If a very thin object, such as a switch or a cord, hits the skin, parallel **petechial** lines form as an outline of the object (**FIGURE 13–6**).

Bruises resolve at differing rates according to their location and the mechanism of injury, and bruises of different colors can result from injuries sustained in one event. Therefore, the presence of bruises of different colors cannot determine the timing of the injury. It is important, however, to provide a complete description of the injuries sustained, including the size, shape, location, and colors of all bruises.

Burns: Location and Patterns

Inflicted burns are usually caused by immersion in hot water (scalds) or by forced contact between the child and a hot object. Adult skin can develop a full-thickness burn from 2 seconds of exposure to 65.5°C/150°F water; children may burn even faster. Accidental scald burns typically have varying depths and irregular borders, with a "flow" pattern evident. They are rarely symmetrical (ie, both hands or both feet) and occur infrequently in the preambulatory child. In contrast, scalds resulting from deliberately dipping a child in hot water are clearly **demarcated**, in a stocking/glove distribution, sparing **flexural creases** (eg, the creases behind the knees or inside the elbows) because these areas are "protected" when the child reflexively tries to withdraw. "Donut burns" with sparing of the buttocks occur in children who have been dipped into hot water, but whose buttocks are pushed firmly down against the relatively cooler surface of the tub or sink (**FIGURE 13–7**). Children with inflicted burns may also have arm or leg bruises where they were restrained.

Pattern burns that are an even thickness throughout should create strong suspicion regarding maltreatment. Remember that any **acute** burn can be extremely painful. Advanced life support

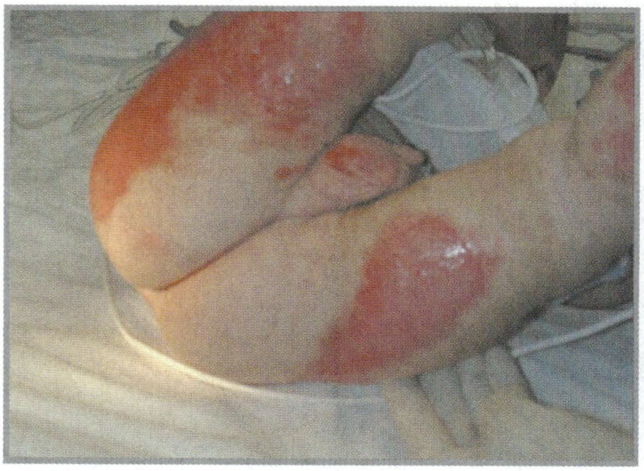

FIGURE 13–7 Donut burn.

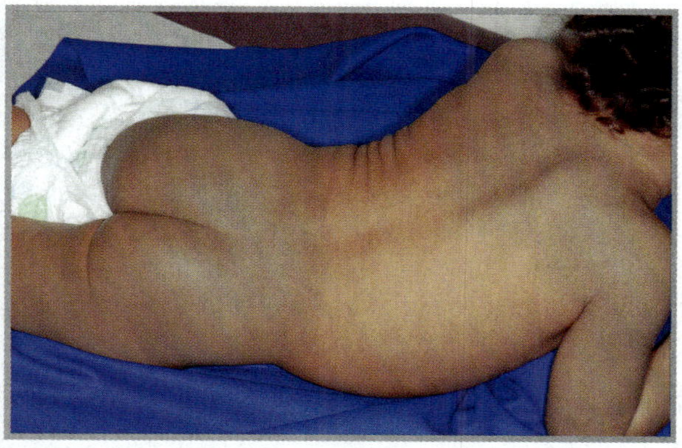

FIGURE 13–8 Congenital dermal melanocytosis spots appear on the buttocks, back, and extremities of many infants.

(ALS) providers should consider the administration of an analgesic as local protocol allows.

Fractures

Fractures are difficult for prehospital providers to detect. Any known fracture in a child who is not yet ambulatory should raise suspicion regarding maltreatment. Although an infant who is being carried and is unintentionally dropped may sustain a fracture, it is not plausible that an infant who is only crawling or cruising could develop sufficient energy on their own to fracture a bone. A history of **osteogenesis imperfecta** or problems causing decreased bone calcification may increase fracture occurrence in some children. Include these conditions in the documentation of the child's history.

Skin Signs That May Be Mistaken for Abuse

Sometimes, normal physical findings are mistaken for an inflicted injury. For example, **congenital dermal melanocytosis** is a birthmark frequently seen in children with darker skin tones (eg, Black, Asian, Latino) that is often mistaken for a bruise (**FIGURE 13–8**). These birthmarks often take the form of large, flat areas of blue, green, or slate-gray hyperpigmented skin, most commonly found on the low back or buttocks.

Certain disease states, such as **leukemia**, **vasculitis**, **meningococcemia**, or bleeding disorders (eg, **hemophilia**), cause bleeding into the skin, producing skin findings that can look like bruises resulting from trauma. Skin infections, such as impetigo, can appear to be burns, but are much less painful. Insect bites in some children can cause redness and blistering. Distinguishing intentional injuries with certainty is sometimes impossible in the field.

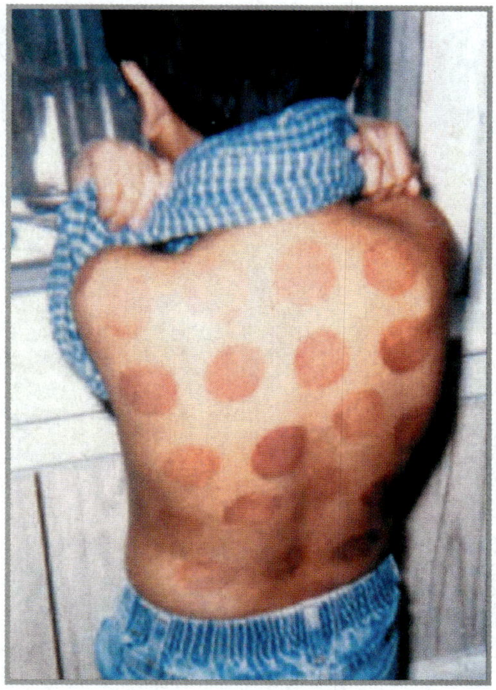

FIGURE 13–9 Cupping is the cultural practice of placing warm cups on the skin to pull out illness from the body. The red, flat, rounded skin lesions are often more intensely red at the borders.

Another benign skin finding that may be mistaken as abuse is the pattern of lesions produced by cultural rituals/traditional healing practices. The most common of these patterns are associated with practices called **cupping** (**FIGURE 13–9**) and **coin rubbing** (**FIGURE 13–10**). These superficial lesions have distinctive rounded edges. Caregivers of these children can explain the purpose for such practices—information that can help distinguish injuries intended to help from inflicted injuries intended to harm.

CASE STUDY 2

You arrive at an apartment at 3 am in response to a call about a baby who is not breathing. On arrival, a woman meets you at the door carrying an unresponsive 6-month-old infant who has apnea and cyanosis and has no pulse. Your partner begins cardiopulmonary resuscitation, and you are able to determine that the woman is the grandmother, who is supposed to be watching her grandchild while the baby's mother is working an overnight shift. The grandmother tells you that she and the infant must have fallen asleep on the couch, and she woke up "next" to the baby and found the baby this way. You also notice several beer cans in the room. There are at least 3 blankets and a pillow piled up on the couch.

1. What are the red flags for maltreatment?
2. What are your medical and legal responsibilities?

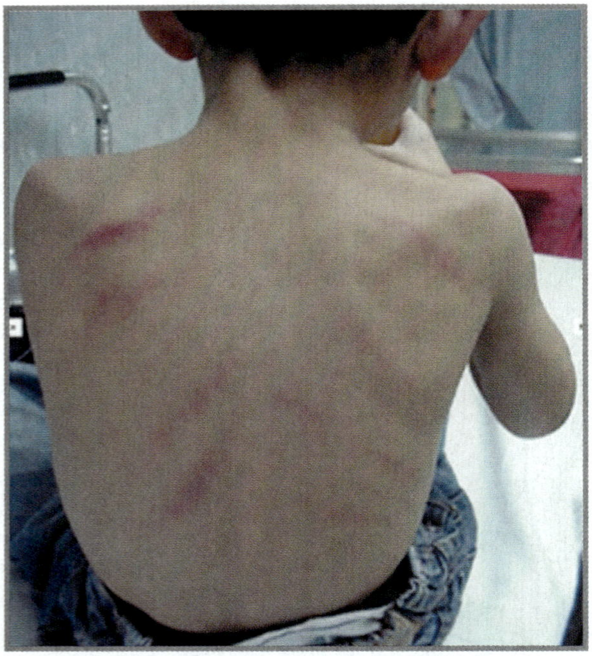

FIGURE 13–10 Rubbing hot coins, often on the back, produces rounded and oblong red, patchy, flat skin lesions.

Summary of Duties, Communication, and Assessment in Suspected Maltreatment

When child maltreatment is suspected, the EMS clinician faces a very challenging situation. A professional, nonjudgmental approach is always necessary. Document conditions in the environment, the child's and caregiver's behaviors, the history, and relevant physical findings that may suggest maltreatment. The EMS clinician has a moral and legal duty to report suspected cases of maltreatment to the proper authorities.

The EMS clinician is in a unique position to recognize signs of possible child maltreatment. The initial principles of field care are the careful scene size-up, history taking, and physical assessment for physiological abnormalities or anatomical patterns of inflicted injuries. Additional assessment and identification of "red-flag" child and caregiver behaviors are sometimes extremely important to maltreatment investigations. The diagnosis of child maltreatment is rarely possible in the field. All cases require a complete investigation by the local agencies responsible for child maltreatment (eg, CPS, law enforcement).

Legislation, Principles, and Protocols

CHILD PROTECTIVE SERVICES

The CPS agency is a legal community organization responsible for protection against child maltreatment and for initial investigations of suspected maltreatment. They must make complicated and important decisions about the maltreatment accusations, provide support services to keep families intact, or at times remove children from the home while investigations are under way. Child protective services has the legal authority to temporarily remove children from the home if they are at risk of experiencing injury or neglect and to secure out-of-home placement if necessary. **TABLE 13–6** lists the initial actions of the CPS when a report is filed. Child protective

TABLE 13-6 Initial Child Protective Services (CPS) Actions

When a report of child abuse or neglect is received, from either a health care professional or a law enforcement agency, the protocols of the receiving agency determine the timing and scope of the initial response.
The facts are reviewed to determine if a home visit is appropriate and, if so, which members of the team will be involved.
The CPS caseworker assesses risk to the child, the family's ability to provide safety, and supportive resources available to the family.
After the investigation and assessment, a reported incident is determined to be founded, unfounded, or unable to be determined because of lack of information.

CAUTION

Judging or confronting caregivers or attempting to intervene in issues of dysfunctional parenting may interfere with patient care or a subsequent maltreatment investigation. The caregiver may in fact not know how the child was injured or by whom. Your interventions may put you at risk, and a confrontation does not help the child.

services may work in concert with law enforcement to investigate the facts and determine who is responsible for maltreating the child. Ultimately, the judicial system determines if an accused individual is "guilty." Although emotions may run high when the EMS clinician suspects child maltreatment, it is neither appropriate nor safe to confront caregivers with these concerns at the scene.

The EMS clinician can provide scene information that helps CPS determine safe placement of the patient. When maltreatment is suspected, always note the presence of other children in the home. If a determination is made that an environment may be unsafe, contact law enforcement or CPS to evaluate the safety of any other children who are present, based on local EMS protocol. When a patient is transported to a hospital, communicate any concerns about maltreatment to hospital staff, who also have a mandatory obligation to report.

Another resource to know and be familiar with is the Child Abuse Prevention and Treatment Act (CAPTA). This federal law provides funding, resources, grants, and guidance to states and organizations to protect children from child maltreatment. This law, among many other items, provides for a national data collection agency, the National Clearinghouse on Child Abuse and Neglect Information; establishes the federal Office on Child Abuse and Neglect; and coordinates activities and programs that serve this particular population. Other national resources of note include the Never Shake a Baby campaign of the National Center on Shaken Baby Syndrome (www.dontshake.org) and Healthy Families America (www.healthyfamiliesamerica.org), which provides education and support to expecting and new parents to help with the arrival of a newborn in the family.

CAUTION

Never attempt to physically restrain a caregiver or to forcibly take possession of a child. Call law enforcement if the scene is unsafe.

TIP

Note and report the presence of other children in situations suggestive of maltreatment.

TIP

Even in the face of probable maltreatment, remain nonjudgmental with the caregiver; maintain control of the scene and transport.

CONTROVERSY

The on-scene role of law enforcement in suspected child maltreatment is controversial. In most cases, it is prudent to transport a child to the ED for physician and CPS evaluation. If the scene is not safe or caretakers are refusing transport, the EMS clinician must call law enforcement for protection and assistance.

CONTROVERSY

It is the duty of the EMS clinician to ensure a CPS report is filed when abuse is suspected. Depending on state law, this duty may be legal or it may be ethical. In some jurisdictions, a single report from hospital personnel is sufficient, whereas in others the EMS clinicians must file their own report.

Pediatric Human Trafficking

Human trafficking is an international problem that has proliferated in the United States. It is estimated that there are more than 40 million victims globally, with almost 30% of them children. Considered modern-day slavery affecting both sexes, it is an international crime and is defined by the United Nations as the "recruitment, transportation, transfer, harboring or receipt of persons, by means of the threat or use of force or other forms of coercion, of abduction, of fraud, of deception, of the abuse of power or of a position of vulnerability or of the giving or receiving of payments or benefits to achieve the consent of a person having control over another person, for the purpose of exploitation." Human trafficking of children includes both sex trafficking and labor trafficking, and children subjected to both types may interface with EMS clinicians, who must be able to detect the signs and report to appropriate authorities. Several risk factors for both forms of trafficking are similar among children and are explained in more detail below.

LABOR TRAFFICKING

Internationally, it was estimated that 4.5 million children around the world were subjected to forced labor in 2016. It is unclear how this number may have changed after the COVID-19 pandemic. Child victims of labor trafficking are involved in work including construction, domestic work, hospitality, health and beauty, agriculture, sales work, and even illicit activities such as theft and drug trafficking. Victims are often trafficked internationally and must pay back what they "owe" to their employer in exchange for their new life.

CHILD SEX TRAFFICKING AND COMMERCIAL SEXUAL EXPLOITATION OF CHILDREN

In the United States, the average age at which the child enters the commercial sex industry is 12 to 14 years; however, infants and toddlers are not immune from this crime. Very young children may be exploited in prostitution or the production of child sexual material such as photographs or videos. It is not uncommon for an adult who is trafficked to be coerced or forced into having their children be trafficked as well.

Minors may be more easily coerced and controlled and are less likely to recognize they are victims. Very young children may lack verbal skills to disclose their plight, and emotional outbursts or change in sleeping patterns may be the only sign. Although physical abuse or restraint may occur, it is not a necessary component of trafficking, because perpetrators use manipulation and prey on the vulnerability of the child, particularly those with minimal support systems. These can include, but not be limited to, runaway youth, homeless children, lesbian/gay/bisexual/transgender/queer youth, and those within the foster care system. Additionally, physical, emotional, or sexual abuse is a common precursor. These children are often isolated and threatened with violence, making escape difficult. The trafficker may destroy forms of identification, change the child's appearance, or change location frequently to avoid detection by authorities.

INTERACTIONS WITH THE HEALTH CARE AND PUBLIC SAFETY SYSTEM

Researchers have found that among adult and adolescent female survivors of trafficking, almost 90% of them encountered a health care professional, including EMS clinicians, during the time they were being exploited. Of those, 63% were seen in the ED. Forty percent of trafficking survivors said that a physician could have done or said something to help them while they were in that situation but did not. None was asked by EMS personnel, nurses, or physicians about their situation or was identified as being trafficked; thus, they remained unidentified, and the result was a missed opportunity to rescue the individual. It is imperative that EMS clinicians perform screening to identify and begin treatment for trafficked children.

Identifying an EMS patient as a victim of trafficking can be challenging, but there are some notable characteristics that can be helpful. It is incumbent on the EMS clinician to ensure the child is alone, separated from others, before asking them questions. The trafficker will likely be very rehearsed, well spoken, and very presentable so as not to arouse suspicion. They also may appear very parental, caring, and sympathetic. The child may not be permitted to answer any questions, and the "friend" or "family member" may not allow the child to be alone with a medical professional. Developmental considerations must be recognized, because the very young child may not know their address, for example, but an older child who does not know their address, or what city or state they are in, should raise concern (see **TABLE 13–7**).

A child victim of trafficking has suffered significant emotional trauma, and it is important for

TABLE 13–7 Human Trafficking Red Flags

History	Physical Assessment of Child
Adult/Trafficker ▪ Has multiple children with unclear relationship ▪ Reluctant to leave child alone with medical professional ▪ Provides inconsistent or vague history ▪ Angry if law enforcement is mentioned **Child** ▪ May not know address or how to get home upon discharge ▪ May have no identification or personal belongings ▪ History of suicide, suicide ideation, depression, mental health issues or substance abuse, posttraumatic stress disorder, shame, and guilt ▪ Inappropriate dress for venue or weather conditions ▪ Sexualized behavior ▪ Working while sick ▪ Untreated chronic illness ▪ Possession of fake identification or with children and hotel keys ▪ Trauma bonding (Stockholm syndrome: a condition that causes hostages to develop a psychological alliance with their captors as a survival strategy during captivity) ▪ Expensive items, such as clothing, handbags, or shoes; large amounts of cash (or, in the very young child, any cash at all) ▪ Forced drug use ▪ Refers to boyfriend as "Daddy" ▪ History of running away (especially > 3 times over past year) or homelessness ▪ Angry if law enforcement is mentioned ▪ Child has older boyfriend/girlfriend (> 4 years older)	▪ Chronic lack of care ▪ Failure to thrive, malnutrition, eating disorders ▪ Disheveled appearance ▪ Sexually transmitted infection ▪ Urinary tract infection ▪ Use of street slang, references to "the life" or "the game," use of signs of gang affiliation ▪ Foreign objects in vagina or rectum ▪ Patterned injury (rope, lighter, electric cord, handprint, etc.) ▪ Trauma to vagina, scrotum, penis, or rectum ▪ Cigarette, iron, or acid burns ▪ Dental caries/rotting teeth/bottle mouth ▪ Injuries to frenulum (from hand being clapped over mouth or bottle being forcefully shoved into mouth) ▪ Jaw and neck pain caused by strangulation ▪ History of abortions or miscarriages ▪ Ligature marks on neck, wrists, ankles ▪ Tattoos, especially with male name, branding, symbol of money, initial, slogan, or barcode, could indicate trafficking; often on back of neck, lower back, groin area, or feet as permanent mark or ownership and of being someone's "property" ▪ Hyperstartle reflexes ▪ Self-injury (cutting and scratching, hitting, biting, picking at skin, pulling out hair)

all professionals to understand the principles of trauma-informed care. Questions must be asked in a developmentally appropriate, culturally sensitive, and child-centered manner. The EMS clinician should build trust, convey respect and patience, ensure the child's safety, and empower the child to participate in their own care and rescue. Ensure that basic needs are met while the child is in your care; in addition to assuring the child that they are safe, ask the child if they are warm enough, hungry, or thirsty. If applicable, allow the child to have choices when possible. Do not allow anyone other than an official and approved translator to interpret for the child. Remember the importance of sitting down or getting down to the child's eye level. The EMS clinician may discover what is self-soothing to the child—such as thumb sucking, certain music, a stuffed animal, or position of comfort—and make every attempt to allow the child to use them.

Just 1 or 2 red flags should create enough suspicion for the EMS clinician to communicate findings to ED staff. Summoning law enforcement or appearing to collaborate with police might cause the trafficker and/or the patient to refuse treatment or transport, placing the child in further jeopardy. When trafficking is suspected, a helpful question to ask (in age-appropriate words) is "Have you ever been made to do something that you didn't want to do?" Other questions are outlined in **TABLE 13–8**.

The EMS clinician has a unique advantage of assessing the scene and the persons present during the call. By knowing the red flags and asking the right questions, EMS clinicians are in an ideal position to identify and begin processes to rescue the child from human trafficking. As mandated reporters of child maltreatment, EMS clinicians should adhere to state laws and follow departmental policies when reporting suspected child human trafficking. The EMS clinician can be the intersection between the child and the outside world, making this single interaction life-changing for the child.

See **TABLE 13–9** for helpful resources and phone numbers.

CASE STUDY 3

9–1-1 is called by a babysitter because a child has been burned. On arrival at the scene, the EMS crew finds a teenage girl holding a sobbing 2-year-old boy. The teenager states that the child has been fussy and crying for the 2 hours he has been in her care. On changing the child's diaper, the sitter noted what looked like burns on the buttocks and, on her mother's advice, called 9–1-1.

The child is alert but upset and is not easily consolable by the babysitter. There is no increased work of breathing; the skin color is pink. There are areas of denuded skin on the buttocks covered with diaper rash cream, with one unpopped blister near the sacrum. The centers of both buttocks, and the gluteal cleft, do not appear to be injured. Extremity examination shows no bruises or other abnormalities.

1. Does this injury raise concern regarding abuse?
2. What interventions are indicated?

TABLE 13–8 Questions to Ask Potential Victims of Human Trafficking

Using age- and developmentally appropriate language, ask the following questions:

- Is it okay for you to be talking to me now? Will there be any problem with so-and-so if you and I are talking alone for a bit?
- Can you tell me what it is that makes it not okay to talk to me alone? Is there something we can do to make it all right, so you can feel comfortable talking to me?

Housing and Personal Relationships Questions

- Have you ever run away from home? (If yes: How many times have you run away? How long is the longest time you've been gone from home? Where did you stay?)
- Can you come and go whenever you please?
- Has anyone at home physically harmed you?
- Have you ever been denied food, water, sleep, or medical care?
- Has anyone threatened your family?
- Has anyone ever taken away your identification papers or cards?
- Do you use drugs or drink alcohol?
- Has a boyfriend, a girlfriend, or anyone else ever asked you or forced you to have sex with them or another person?

Workplace Questions

- It is not uncommon for young people to stay in risky work situations because they have no other options. Have you ever worked in a place that made you feel scared or unsafe?
- Do you have to ask permission to eat, sleep, or use the bathroom? Can you come and go whenever you want?

TABLE 13–9 Resources

National Center for Missing & Exploited Children **1–800–843–5678** If you have information about a missing child or suspected child sexual exploitation, report it by calling or visiting their website (https://www.missingkids.com/).
National Human Trafficking Hotline **1–888–373–7888** The National Human Trafficking Hotline is a national antitrafficking hotline and resource center serving victims and survivors of human trafficking and the antitrafficking community in the United States. The toll-free hotline is answered live 24 hours a day, 7 days a week, 365 days a year. For more information, visit humantraffickinghotline.org.
The National Runaway Safeline 1–800-RUNAWAY The National Runaway Safeline (NRS) serves as the federally designated national communication system for homeless and runaway youth. Through hotline and online services, NRS provides crisis intervention, referrals to local resources, and education and prevention services to youth, families and community members throughout the country 24 hours a day, 365 days a year. For more information, visit www.1800RUNAWAY.org.
U.S. Immigration and Customs Enforcement **1–866–347–2423 (United States & Canada)** **1–802–872–6199 (International Calls)** Immigration and Customs Enforcement runs a hotline to report suspected child predators and any suspicious activity. Call or complete an online tip form (https://www.ice.gov/webform/ice-tip-form).

CASE STUDY ANSWERS

CASE STUDY 1

This child is in critical condition. His appearance is altered (low tone and minimal responsiveness), his breathing is irregular, and his color is pale. He might have an isolated head injury, multisystem trauma, or a medical condition that is not an injury at all.

Be alert for the signs of abusive head trauma in any infant or small child with a sudden onset of altered mental status and irregular respirations. Remember that grab bruises and marks may be found on children who are held and shaken, and the presence of such marks should be documented. Carefully document the scene, the comments of the caregiver, and the reported events leading to the injury.

Immediate transportation after stabilization to the extent possible is critical. One common complication of inflicted head injury is the Cushing triad of bradycardia, elevated blood pressure, and irregular respirations, which can lead to respiratory failure or apnea as a result of elevated intracranial pressure and compression of the medulla (respiratory center in the brainstem). Be prepared to provide respiratory support.

You initiate supplemental oxygen via face mask, and the baby continues to breathe spontaneously but irregularly. His oxygen saturation remains 99% during transport. You share your concerns about possible inflicted injury with the ED staff. The ED staff note the bruises on the baby's arms and confirm that they will be initiating a child maltreatment report. In the course of the ED evaluation, the baby is found to have swelling of the brain parenchyma, multiple areas of bleeding inside the brain, and a large amount of blood in the subdural space. He is also found to have several fractures of his posterior ribs. The baby is admitted to the intensive care unit for ongoing care of his severe brain injury. An investigation by a child protective services team is under way.

Continued

CASE STUDY ANSWERS—cont'd

CASE STUDY 2

This case may be the result of the grandmother's accidentally suffocating the infant. Co-sleeping, especially with a caregiver who is under the influence of alcohol or drugs, can have deadly consequences. Adults may roll over on top of infants and not realize it because of their intoxicated state. Infants do not have the strength to push back or to get the adult to notice that they are lying on them. Make a note of the scene and call law enforcement. Your attention needs to be focused on resuscitation efforts for the child.

You and your partner perform cardiopulmonary resuscitation (CPR) for 30 minutes, but return of spontaneous circulation is not achieved. The baby is noted to be cold and stiff, and with the monitor still showing asystole, you and your partner call online medical control for a discontinuation-of-resuscitation order. At this point, law enforcement is on scene. The grandmother notes that you are discontinuing CPR and begins to wail, "Oh, no—they think I killed the baby."

This case will require the involvement of the medical examiner. It is unclear if the grandmother was criminally neglectful or if this is simply a tragic case of co-sleeping. Treat the grandmother with compassion. Inform her that the baby's heart and breathing stopped sometime before you arrived and despite maximal efforts of CPR, they did not restart. Tell her the baby is dead. Do not assign blame. Ask if there is anyone you can call to come to the house. You leave when law enforcement and the medical examiner are ready to take control of the scene. You document the details of the scene factually and thoroughly in the patient care report.

CASE STUDY 3

This child has obvious signs of an inflicted scald injury. The lack of burn in the creases and the center of the buttocks (donut burn) may indicate the child was forcibly held in hot water. There is no way for the EMS clinician to know who inflicted the injury, nor is establishing responsibility part of their role.

Provide analgesia if possible. Large burns can lead to significant fluid losses, so ALS providers should start an intravenous line and begin fluid resuscitation and pain medication. Document the scene size-up, the child's and caregiver's behaviors, and the history. Transport this child to an ED for burn care as well as an evaluation for inflicted injury. Treatment at a burn center may ultimately be necessary.

The child is seen at the pediatric burn center and undergoes débridement of the burns and extensive wound care. During the hospital stay, several caregivers are interviewed by child protective services, and the mother's boyfriend confesses to holding the child in a tub of hot water owing to frustration with the child's bed wetting. The child is discharged home with his mother and a safety plan stipulating that he will no longer live with the perpetrator. The scald burns heal over several weeks.

Suggested References

TEXTBOOKS

Miller S. The child with a suspicious presentation. In: *Provider Manual 6th Edition Emergency Nursing Pediatric Course.* Emergency Nurses Association; 2023:255–256

Laskey A, Sirotnak A, eds. *Child Abuse: Medical Diagnosis and Management.* 4th ed. American Academy of Pediatrics; 2019

ARTICLES

American Academy of Pediatrics Committee on Child Abuse and Neglect. American Academy of Pediatrics: distinguishing sudden infant death syndrome from child abuse fatalities. *Pediatrics.* 2001;107(2):437–441. PMID: 11158487 doi: 10.1542/peds.107.2.437

Asnes AG, Leventhal JM. Managing child abuse: general principles. *Pediatr Rev*. 2010;31(2):47–55. PMID: 20124274 doi: 10.1542/pir.31.2.47

Escobar MA Jr, Wallenstein KG, Christison-Lagay ER, Naiditch JA, Petty JK. Child abuse and the pediatric surgeon: a position statement from the Trauma Committee, the Board of Governors and the Membership of the American Pediatric Surgical Association. *J Pediatr Surg*. 2019;54(7):1277–1285. PMID: 30948199 doi: 10.1016/j.jpedsurg.2019.03.009

Greenbaum J. Child labor and sex trafficking. *Pediatr Rev*. 2021;42(12):639–654. PMID: 34850175 doi: 10.1542/pir.2020-001396

Greenbaum VJ, Dodd M, McCracken C. A short screening tool to identify victims of child sex trafficking in the health care setting. *Pediatr Emerg Care*. 2018;34(1):33–37. PMID: 26599463 doi: 10.1097/PEC.0000000000000602

Hoehn EF, Wilson PM, Riney LC, Ngo V, Bennett B, Duma E. Identification and evaluation of physical abuse in children. *Pediatr Ann*. 2018;47(3):e97–e101. PMID: 29538781 doi: 10.3928/19382359-20180227-01

Kempe CH, Silverman FN, Steele BF, Droegemueller W, Silver HK. The battered-child syndrome. *JAMA*. 1962;181(1):17–24. PMID: 14455086 doi: 10.1001/jama.1962.03050270019004

Louwers ECFM, Korfage IJ, Affourtit MJ, et al. Effects of systematic screening and detection of child abuse in emergency departments. *Pediatrics*. 2012;130(3):457–464. PMID: 22926179 doi: 10.1542/peds.2011-3527

Pierce MC, Kaczor K, Lorenz DJ, et al. Validation of a clinical decision rule to predict abuse in young children based on bruising characteristics. *JAMA Netw Open*. 2021;4(4):e215832. PMID: 33852003 doi: 10.1001/jamanetworkopen.2021.5832

Sheets LK, Leach ME, Koszewski IJ, Lessmeier AM, Nugent M, Simpson P. Sentinel injuries in infants evaluated for child physical abuse. *Pediatrics*. 2013;131(4):701–707. PMID: 23478861 doi: 10.1542/peds.2012-2780

OTHER RESOURCES

American Academy of Pediatrics. *Visual Diagnosis of Child Abuse*. 4th ed. [CD-ROM]. Itasca, IL: American Academy of Pediatrics; 2016

Centers for Disease Control and Prevention. About adverse childhood experiences (ACEs).Accessed November 18, 2024. https://www.cdc.gov/aces/about/index.html/

Children's Trust of South Carolina. Recognizing child abuse and neglect. https://scchildren.org/recognizing-child-abuse-and-neglect/ Accessed November 22. 2024

Face It: A Movement to End Child Abuse. TEN-4-FACESp Bruising Rule Infographic. https://faceitabuse.org/wp-content/uploads/2023/03/TEN-4-FACESp-brochure.pdf Accessed April 3, 2025

Polaris. Human trafficking facts. https://polarisproject.org/myths-facts-and-statistics/ Accessed April 3, 2025

US Department of Health & Human Services, Administration for Children and Families, Administration on Children, Youth and Families, Children's Bureau. Child maltreatment. https://acf.gov/cb/data-research/child-maltreatment Accessed April 3, 2025

HOTLINES AND ORGANIZATIONS

National Center for Missing and Exploited Children. 1–800–843–5678

National Human Trafficking Hotline. 1–888–373–7888 www.Humantraffickinghotline.org/en

National Runaway Safeline. 1–800-RUNAWAY. www.1800RUNAWAY.org

U.S. Immigration and Customs Enforcement. 1–866–347–2423 (United States and Canada) 1–802–872–6199 (international)

CHAPTER 14

Emergency Birth and Newborn Resuscitation and Stabilization

Jonathan P. Carolla, BSc, NRP, FPC
Franscesca Miquel-Verges, MD

LEARNING OBJECTIVES

1. **Describe the components of the patient history and physical examination that would identify pregnant patients at risk of experiencing emergent birth of a newborn infant outside a hospital setting.**
2. **List potential maternal, fetal, and newborn infant risk factors that may adversely affect the health of the parent or newborn infant during or immediately after birth.**
3. **Compare and contrast when it is appropriate to initiate transport of a pregnant patient to a hospital for birth of a newborn infant versus when it is appropriate to prepare for imminent birth of a newborn infant in the prehospital setting.**
4. **Describe how to prepare for a birth, perform a birth, and provide post birth care to the parent and newborn infant.**
5. **Recognize the conditions and identify the correct interventions when complications jeopardize the health of the parent or newborn infant during childbirth.**
6. **Explain the indications and technique for assisting ventilation in a newborn infant.**
7. **Identify situations in which a newborn infant might require vascular access for drug and fluid administration.**

Introduction

Emergency medical services (EMS) clinicians may be called to assess a patient in labor, assist with childbirth, and perform neonatal resuscitation in the prehospital setting. Historically, childbirth occurred in the home, often without the presence of trained medical personnel. Gradually, childbirth has evolved into a highly specialized area of medicine. Despite the majority of births occurring in health care facilities, the number of home births in the United States has risen and is at the highest level since 1990.

In the United States, among planned home births, 30% involve a certified nurse midwife, and the remainder are attended by certified professional midwives or other noncertified attendants. Certified nurse midwives and certified professional midwives are trained in the care of both the parent and the newborn infant in the birth setting. One quarter of out-of-hospital births are unplanned. For these patients, an EMS clinician may be the only person trained to care for both parent and newborn infant. EMS clinicians may also encounter pregnant patients in a variety of prehospital settings. They may be called to assist with transport of a pregnant patient who is in labor or who has developed a complication of pregnancy such as **pre-eclampsia**. They may be required to assist with childbirth even when labor or pregnancy is unrecognized or concealed, when a transportation misadventure prevents a patient in labor from reaching a hospital in time, when unexpected complications develop during a planned out-of-hospital birth, or when labor or precipitous birth occurs in another prehospital setting.

Obstetric Birth in the Prehospital Setting

EMS CAPABILITIES, SCOPE OF PRACTICE, AND LEGAL PITFALLS

Childbirth is not a common prehospital emergency, so the level of anxiety it creates in both the laboring patient and the EMS clinician is often high. Most newborn infants require only minimal assistance to make the transition to life outside the uterus. EMS clinicians should remain aware that although most newborn infants require minimal resuscitative efforts, complications during birth have the potential to cause devastating, lifelong neurological impairments. Limited training, experience, scope of practice, and equipment may prevent EMS clinicians from recognizing serious complications of pregnancy or birth until it is too late to prevent injury to the parent or newborn infant. Although assisting a patient during an uncomplicated childbirth is arguably a basic life support (BLS)–level skill, many neonatal or maternal complications outlined in this chapter require advanced life support (ALS) interventions. Optimally, ALS clinicians and/or clinicians with training in maternal and infant health should be dispatched.

ETHICAL CONSIDERATIONS AND EMS PROFESSIONALISM

The goal of every obstetric birth is a healthy parent and newborn infant. Not every childbirth attended by EMS clinicians produces a viable, healthy newborn infant. Extreme prematurity and latent fetal demise each create situations in which full resuscitative efforts may not be appropriate. EMS clinicians periodically encounter these situations without the benefit of prior diagnosis and often without the opportunity to discuss resuscitation decisions with the child's parents in a controlled environment. When faced with this situation, EMS clinicians should contact medical control and delicately balance ethical responsibilities to the patient(s) with the professional requirement to adhere to EMS laws and regulations pertaining to initiation and termination of resuscitation.

Complications During Pregnancy

A wide variety of conditions can adversely impact the health of the parent and fetus during pregnancy. These conditions have the potential to create complications for the parent or newborn infant during or after birth. EMS clinicians should consider these conditions when weighing the risks and benefits of pausing to assist in a birth in the prehospital setting versus initiating prompt transport to a health care facility for birth. Many complications, such as certain breech presentations or placenta previa, should not be managed in the prehospital setting. When known complications exist that are beyond the ability of EMS clinicians, it is often better to begin transportation immediately.

UMBILICAL CORD PROLAPSE

Disruption of the oxygen and nutrients supplied to the fetus through the umbilical cord can cause devastating injury to the fetus, including fetal death. On rare occasions, the umbilical cord may enter the vaginal cavity before a birthing fetus. The umbilical cord becomes compressed, and the fetal blood supply is compromised. During assessment, the umbilical cord will be visible at the vaginal opening. When recognized in the prehospital setting, only one treatment option is available. The patient is placed into a knee-chest position (**FIGURE 14–1**), and the EMS clinician inserts a gloved hand into the vagina and elevates the head or presenting fetal body part out of the pelvis to relieve the pressure on the umbilical cord. Transportation should commence immediately to a facility capable of performing an emergency cesarean delivery. The patient should remain in the knee-chest position during transport, and the EMS clinician should continue to elevate the presenting fetal part out of the pelvis using the hand in the vagina. Umbilical cord prolapse is more common in patients with premature rupture of membranes, premature birth, multiple gestation, multiparity, and fetal breech presentations.

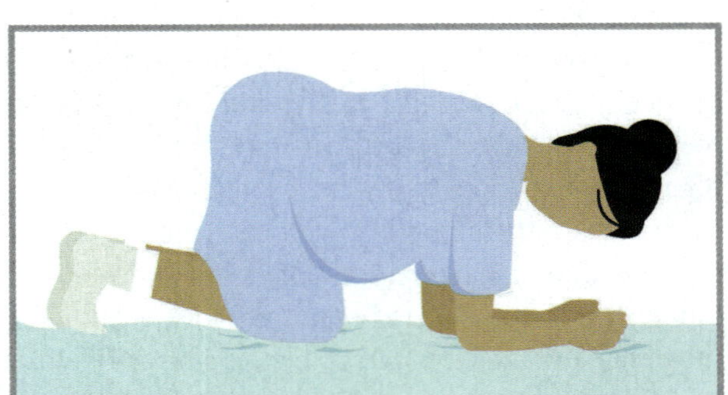

FIGURE 14–1 The knee-chest position.

Preterm Labor

Preterm labor refers to labor beginning before the 37th week of gestation. Treatment of a patient in preterm labor is largely supportive until definitive care can be reached. EMS clinicians should expect complications roughly proportional to the degree of prematurity. Technological advances allow newborn infants as young as 22 to 24 weeks' gestation to survive, although a significant number have life-long complications. Newborn infants born before 22 weeks' gestation have a low chance of survival, although there are isolated case reports of infants between 21 and 22 weeks' gestation surviving with minimal or no long-term complications. Between 24 and 37 weeks, each additional week of gestation reduces the impact or severity of complications for the newborn infant. EMS clinicians may encounter patients in labor at <22 to 23 weeks' gestation; in many instances, these infants will not survive an out-of-hospital birth. Follow local protocols regarding neonatal resuscitation, but be aware that many protocols call for no resuscitation in neonates <22 weeks with no signs of life after birth. If the gestational age is unknown and the newborn infant shows signs of life, contact medical control. Additionally, certain findings on physical examination may aid in determining the approximate gestational age. For example, very thin gelatinous skin that is dark in color, visible veins with no lanugo (hair), and fused eyelids all suggest an extremely premature newborn infant. When in doubt, provide resuscitative measures and transport.

MULTIPLE GESTATIONS

Most multifetal (more than one fetus) pregnancies are diagnosed during prenatal care. Every maternal assessment should include questions about the possibility of a multiple gestation, especially if birth is believed to be imminent. EMS clinicians should consider every multifetal pregnancy a high-risk pregnancy. Breech presentation, umbilical cord prolapse, premature labor, and a variety of other maternal and fetal conditions are more common in multiple gestations.

PLACENTA PREVIA

During gestation, the placenta may become implanted either partially or completely over the cervical os (opening) at the base of the uterus. This condition is known as placenta previa (**FIGURE 14–2**). If placental rupture occurs as a result of either cervical dilation or mechanical perforation, bleeding can be massive and is usually painless. Patients with a placenta over or close to the cervical os (opening) require a cesarean delivery. Profound hemorrhage

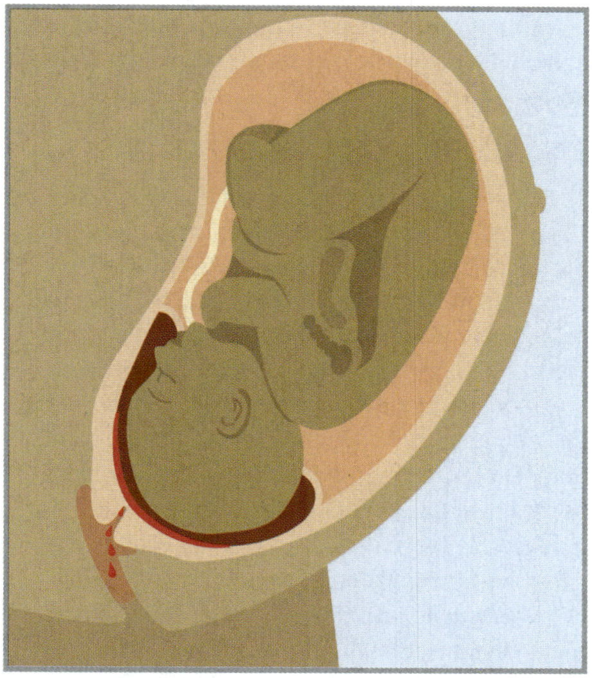

FIGURE 14–2 Placenta previa.

CASE STUDY 1

Emergency medical services are requested to respond to a local mall for a 32-year-old patient reported to be in labor. The patient reports that they are 38 weeks pregnant and this is their fourth pregnancy. They have been having contractions for 30 minutes, starting just after their "bag of water broke," but they are now becoming more frequent and intense. They state they were in labor for 3 hours with their last child.

1. What questions will help you determine whether to transport immediately or perform a birth at the scene?
2. What physical findings would tell you to prepare for birth on scene?

can be fatal for the parent and fetus. These patients cannot safely birth a newborn infant vaginally with EMS attendance in the field. Prompt transport of patients with placenta previa or painless vaginal bleeding should begin immediately.

PLACENTAL ABRUPTION

EMS clinicians may also encounter patients with a placental abruption (abruptio placentae). In these patients, the placenta has either partially or completely detached from the uterine wall, causing significant bleeding. In contrast to placenta previa, patients with placental abruption tend to have abdominal pain with darker vaginal bleeding. Other symptoms include uterine contractions, abdominal tenderness, and signs of fetal distress. Prehospital management is focused on restoring circulating fluid volume and immediate transportation to a facility capable of fetal monitoring and definitive management. The fetus is at high risk of demise in cases of complete placental abruption.

KNOWN BREECH PRESENTATION

The ideal fetal position for a vaginal birth is head down, facing the parent's back (cephalic presentation, occiput anterior). However, when the fetus presents with the buttocks, feet, foot, or other body part aside from the head, this is called a breech presentation. This occurs in 3% to 4% of all term deliveries and more frequently in preterm deliveries, in multiple gestations, and when fetal abnormalities are present. Some presentations require minimal manipulation as the fetus is birthed. Other presentations, such as a transverse breech, require a cesarean delivery or extensive manipulation by a trained physician to allow a vaginal birth. EMS clinicians should expedite maternal transport when a breech birth is known or suspected. There is a variety of techniques and maternal positions that may optimize conditions for certain types of breech deliveries. Online medical control may be a valuable source of guidance if a breech birth begins in the prehospital setting.

POSTTERM PREGNANCY

The normal gestational period lasts from 37 to 42 weeks. As a fetus remains in the uterus past 42 weeks, the uterus and placenta are unable to support the physiological and environmental needs of the growing fetus. The fetus may become distressed and expel stool (meconium) while still within the amniotic sac and uterus. If the fetus inhales the amniotic fluid containing meconium while in the uterus, the meconium may cause respiratory distress after birth. In a patient who is post-term or has meconium-stained fluid leaking from the vagina, EMS clinicians should provide supportive care to the parent and be prepared for possible complications, including the need for neonatal resuscitation.

Triage of a Patient in Labor

EMS clinicians must be capable of deciding whether a patient can safely be transported to a hospital for childbirth or when they must prepare for an imminent birth outside the hospital. The goal of every EMS response should be to transport the patient in labor to a hospital before childbirth occurs. Physicians, midwives, and nurses who are experienced in labor and birth have the training, diagnostic equipment, and procedural skills necessary to intervene in many situations that cannot be adequately managed in the prehospital setting. In instances when labor has progressed or birth is imminent, EMS clinicians may be forced to assist with childbirth outside the hospital. Transport time, type of health care facilities available, EMS capabilities, anticipated complications, and ultimately the patient presentation guide the decision regarding whether to transport or assist with childbirth on scene.

MATERNAL HISTORY

EMS clinicians should obtain a brief, focused patient history when assessing a patient suspected to be in labor. Many factors help determine whether birth is imminent or if complications should be expected. Ultimately, the answer to 3 questions helps determine whether EMS clinicians should anticipate a prehospital birth (**TABLE 14–1**):

1. How many times has the patient given birth? Typically, the time in active labor is longer for first-time parents (primiparas) than for parents who have had prior deliveries (multiparas). If this is not a first-time birth, ask the patient the length of their previous labors. A history of short labor with prior pregnancies may repeat itself. Unless there is a long period between pregnancies, expect each successive labor to be shorter than the previous.
2. Does the patient feel the need to push? Most pregnant patients experience this sensation as birth becomes imminent, usually within 30 minutes and often sooner. Patients with the

TABLE 14–1 Determining If Birth Is Imminent

Questions
Is this your first birth?
If you have birthed before, how long was the labor?
Do you feel the urge to push?
Physical Findings
Is the infant's head crowning?
Is the head or scalp visible at the perineum during contractions?

urge to push require immediate inspection of the perineum and preparation for birth.

3. Do anatomical conditions allow for a successful prehospital birth? Such conditions as placenta previa or transverse breech presentation mean that birth cannot be safely facilitated in the prehospital setting. Transportation should begin immediately.

As time permits, EMS clinicians should inquire about maternal medical history (including medications and allergies), whether abnormalities were identified during prenatal care, previous complications during birth, and gestational age of the fetus. The gestational age or the due date may be calculated from the last menstrual period or the estimated date of birth. Other factors, such as rupture of membranes and the color of the fluid (eg, bloody or green [indicating meconium]), the possibility of multiple gestations, and known newborn infant anomalies should also be included when obtaining a patient history. History may be obtained while simultaneously performing a physical examination or preparing the ambulance and equipment for birth.

> **TIP**
>
> High-risk complications that may be noted by EMS clinicians include premature birth (24–36 weeks or >3 weeks prior to due date), multiple births (>24 weeks' gestation), bleeding disorder in the parent, blood thinner use during pregnancy, and known or suspected placental abruption or placenta previa. These conditions likely require transport to a facility capable of handling high-risk obstetrical patients.

MATERNAL PHYSICAL ASSESSMENT

Every patient encountered by EMS requires a primary assessment to identify any immediate threats to life. This assessment includes airway patency, the quality of respirations and perfusion, and an assessment of level of consciousness. In many instances, immediate threats to life can be excluded if a patient is awake, is speaking appropriately in full sentences, and has normal skin color and strong pulses. Any deviation from these findings suggests a potential threat to life and must be further evaluated before proceeding to a more focused assessment related to the pregnancy.

The EMS clinician needs to perform a brief physical assessment of the perineum if an imminent birth is suspected. Look for **crowning**—the visible appearance of the fetal head at the **vaginal introitus** (**FIGURE 14–3**). Crowning is a sign that birth is imminent.

If the child's head is not immediately visible, inspect the parent's perineum during a contraction and note if the head becomes visible. If the infant is crowning or if the head is visible at the perineum with contractions, prepare for birth unless the transport time is extremely brief (<5 min). Assessment of the perineum should be deferred if imminent birth is unlikely and the patient is able to reliably report the absence of any pressure, unusual sensation (including urge to defecate), or fluid discharge (blood or amniotic fluid) in the vaginal area. The presence or suspicion of any of these items requires a visual inspection of the perineum by the EMS clinician.

Amniotic fluid, released from the vagina before birth, should be examined for meconium (fetal stool), a dark green or mustard-colored viscous substance visible in the normally clear amniotic fluid.

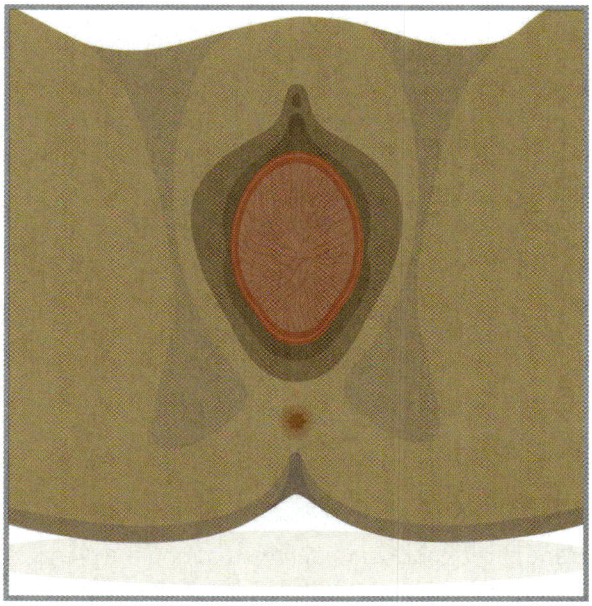

FIGURE 14–3 Use the presence or absence of crowning to help decide whether to transport or to prepare for birth.

The presence of meconium is often a sign of fetal distress, increasing the likelihood that the resuscitation will be required after birth. Some newborn infants born in the setting of meconium may develop meconium aspiration syndrome, a condition treated with respiratory support in a newborn special care unit.

Uterine contractions provide valuable clues regarding the likelihood of a prehospital birth. Most patients in active labor demonstrate obvious contractions readily identifiable through simple visual observation. The patient may show periods of discomfort, exhibit panting respirations, and often verbalize that a contraction is occurring. Gentle palpation of the abdomen reveals a uterus that becomes noticeably firm during a contraction and relaxes between contractions. When contractions increase in intensity and duration while becoming closer together (<3 min from the start of one until the start of the next and lasting at least 60 seconds), labor is considered active, and birth of the newborn infant could occur within a short time. It is always possible for patients to experience subtle contractions (occasionally described as back pain), an urge to defecate, or even abdominal or menstrual cramping. The absence of classic, obvious uterine contractions does not exclude the potential for imminent prehospital birth.

BREECH DELIVERIES

Three to 4 percent of term deliveries are breech deliveries (**FIGURE 14–4**). Inspection of the perineum does not show a head crowning, but rather another anatomical part, such as the feet or buttocks. In this situation, transport the patient immediately to the nearest emergency department that has labor and birth capabilities. Given the risk of complications and the potential need for an emergency cesarean delivery to safely birth the infant, initiate transport to the hospital as soon as a breech presentation is identified, even if birth seems imminent. If the feet are presenting first, support the body while the head is birthed. However, if the head fails to birth, do not pull or apply traction to the body, because this could result in head entrapment. Instead, encourage the parent to push with the next contraction.

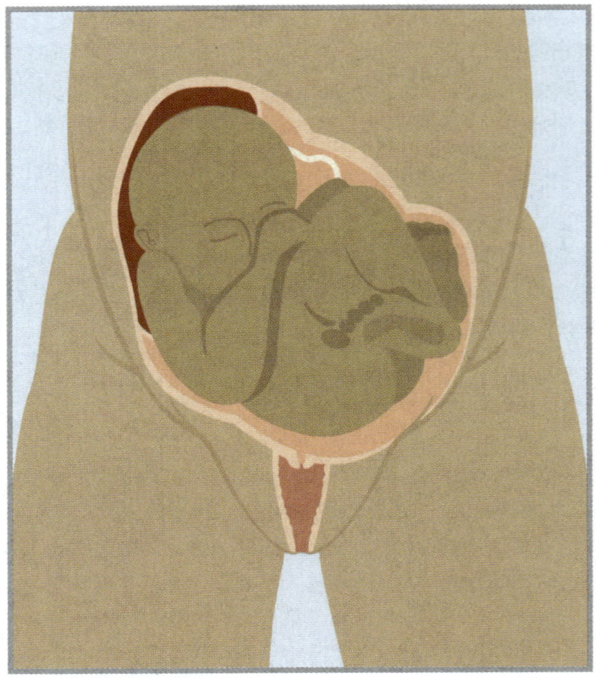

FIGURE 14–4 Breech birth.

ADDITIONAL COMPLICATIONS

Many of the conditions identified during the prenatal period or through the maternal history and physical examination prompt EMS clinicians to anticipate complications. Some complications can be mitigated by the skills and experience of EMS clinicians, but many complications require specialized care, techniques, and equipment not available in the prehospital setting. When potential or certain complications are identified, EMS clinicians must carefully consider whether the risks and benefits of birthing on scene (**TABLE 14–2**) exceed the risks and benefits of initiating prompt transportation (**TABLE 14–3**).

TRANSPORT CONSIDERATIONS FOR THE PATIENT IN LABOR

Patients in labor who have not birthed before transport may require a wide range of services at the destination hospital. This is also true when an infant has been born and complications are present. The destination decision for EMS clinicians is based on a combination of patient preference, geographic location, and the type of services required by the parent and newborn. When complications are expected and birth is not imminent, it may be much better to bypass a smaller community hospital and transport the patient to a health care facility with high-risk obstetric services or neonatal intensive care unit capabilities. Conversely, it may be in the patient's best interest to transport them directly to the closest available facility where the parent or newborn infant can be stabilized before a longer transport to a tertiary care center. EMS clinicians should consult with online medical control when required by protocol or

TABLE 14–2 Risks and Benefits of Birthing on Scene

Benefits	Risks
▪ At least one additional EMS clinician to assist with birth ▪ Nobody is needed to drive the transport vehicle at this time	▪ No progress toward definitive care if complications develop or additional trained personnel or equipment are needed
▪ Possible helpful assistance from patient's family or bystanders	▪ Bystanders or patient's family may interfere with patient care, disrupt privacy, or otherwise distract EMS clinicians from providing optimal care
▪ No vehicle movement, noise, or road hazards to undermine patient care	▪ The scene may pose safety hazards to EMS personnel or patient; may not have adequate climate control for newborn care
▪ Possibly more room to assess patient and birth newborn	▪ Scene may have less room, more obstacles, or poor lighting, which make assessment and newborn birth more difficult

Abbreviation: EMS, emergency medical services.

TABLE 14–3 Risks and Benefits of Initiating Prompt Transportation

Benefits	Risks
▪ Movement toward definitive patient care setting where trained personnel, specialized equipment, and a controlled environment are available	▪ One fewer EMS clinician to assist with patient care (this may be mitigated in certain situations if an alternate trained driver is available)
▪ Patient may have increased privacy in the transport vehicle, without detrimental interference from bystanders or family members	▪ Limited or no assistance available from family or bystanders
▪ May avoid safety risks and uncontrolled environmental temperature that may have been present on scene	▪ Vehicle movement, noise, and road hazards may undermine patient care efforts
▪ May have more room to assess the patient and deliver the newborn than was available on scene, with better lighting and immediate access to resuscitation equipment.	▪ May have less room or less access to the patient for assessment and newborn birth

when the appropriate destination choice is not clear. Providers should also make efforts to understand the obstetric capabilities of the various destination hospitals within their coverage area. Not every hospital has labor and birth services. In many locations, obstetric physicians are not always in the hospital. Early notification provides hospitals the opportunity to activate essential resources when they are not immediately available 24 hours a day, 7 days a week. If possible, efforts should be made to keep the parent-newborn infant dyad together at a facility able to care for both.

Routine care for patients in labor includes skills frequently performed by EMS clinicians. Patients in labor who have hypoxemia should receive supplemental oxygen to prevent or mitigate fetal hypoxemia. The routine use of oxygen in the absence of maternal hypoxemia is controversial. Consult local guidelines or online medical control regarding oxygen use in these situations. Intravenous (IV) fluids may be administered to patients in active labor to prevent dehydration or hemoconcentration and maintain a favorable fluid volume status, as dictated by local protocols. Alternatively, patients in active labor may be provided clear fluids.

Vital signs remain a valuable part of any prehospital patient assessment and should be monitored at appropriate intervals during patient care. The taking of vital signs may be temporarily deferred in patients in active labor if birth is imminent, personnel are limited, and the primary assessment does not suggest any likelihood of abnormality.

Because of the position of the vena cava, pregnant patients are at risk of experiencing hypotension when placed in a supine position. In the supine position, the uterus can compress the inferior vena cava, which may decrease preload to the heart and result in decreased cardiac output. This is primarily a complication during the third trimester. Whether placed on an ambulance stretcher or backboard,

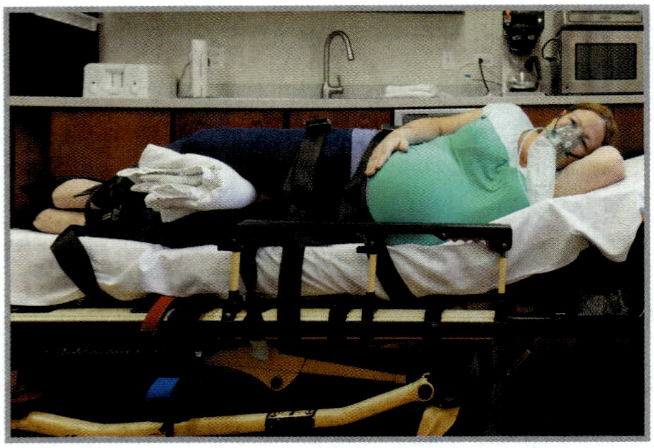

FIGURE 14-5 A pregnant patient tipped in a left lateral recumbent position.

the pregnant patient should be positioned on an angle to one side or the other to displace the uterus off their inferior vena cava and promote optimal blood return to their heart (**FIGURE 14-5**). The left lateral recumbent position is preferred, but this may not be possible in certain transport vehicles when continuous airway monitoring is needed. Stretcher and backboard straps should not be placed over the pregnant patient's gravid abdomen. Place straps or seat belts above and below the patient's abdomen during transport.

TIP

The urge to push experienced by most women at the end of labor is a sign that birth is near, usually within 30 to 60 minutes.

Summary of Triage of Patient in Labor

The responses to the 3 previously asked questions (**TABLE 14-1**), along with visual assessment of the perineum, provide essential information to triage a laboring patient in the field. Known breech births, umbilical cord prolapse, and patients diagnosed with placenta previa require immediate transport, regardless of whether or not birth is imminent. Other findings obtained from the maternal history and physical examination influence the decision whether to initiate transport or prepare for birth on scene.

CAUTION

Never try to birth a newborn infant with a breech presentation in the field. Initiate transport to the hospital as soon as a breech presentation is identified, even if birth seems imminent.

Preparation for Birth

RESUSCITATION-ORIENTED HISTORY

Many factors in the parent's medical history affect the outcome of the newborn infant and help predict the need for resuscitation of the newborn. However, once the decision has been made to birth on scene, only 5 questions are pertinent for the immediate safety of the newborn infant (**TABLE 14-4**):

1. What is the gestational age? The EMS clinician can ask the patient: "What is your due date?" A significant number of out-of-hospital births are preterm (<37 weeks' gestation), and the further from the expected birth date, the greater the chances the newborn infant will require resuscitation. Knowing the due date is important for preparing the appropriate resuscitation equipment for airway management and breathing support. For example, for an expected preterm birth, ensure the appropriately sized mask (preterm), laryngoscope (0 blade), and endotracheal tube (sizes 2.5 and 3.0) are ready (**FIGURE 14-6**).

TABLE 14-4 Resuscitation-Oriented History: Five Essential Questions

What is the gestational age?
Is the amniotic fluid clear?
How many babies are expected?
What is the plan for umbilical cord management?
Are there any risk factors?

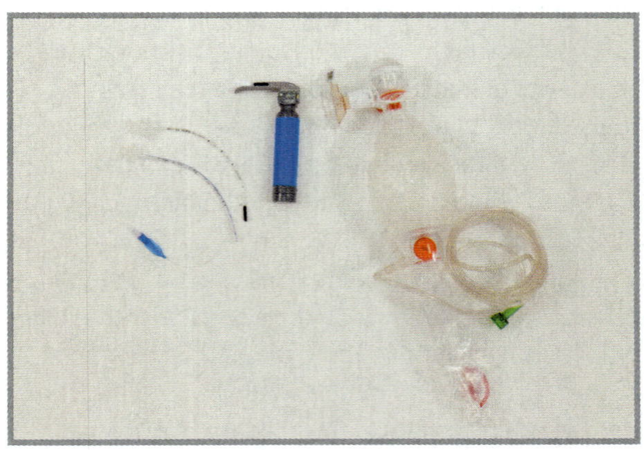

FIGURE 14-6 Special equipment for premature infant resuscitation: bag-mask device with small mask, size 0 laryngoscope blade, and endotracheal tubes sizes 2.5 and 3.0.

2. Is the amniotic fluid clear? Greenish color in the amniotic fluid is a sign of passage of **meconium**, which is fetal stool. Meconium is released by the fetus during periods of intrauterine stress, especially hypoxia. If meconium is observed, be prepared to deal with a depressed newborn infant or airway obstruction. Suctioning of the newborn infant's mouth, oropharynx, and nose to clear the airway of thick meconium may be necessary.
3. How many babies are expected? If twins or multiple newborns are expected, prepare for more than one birth. This may mean finding extra equipment, preparing an additional warm environment, and planning the care of the first newborn infant while birthing the second. This usually requires calling for a second ambulance. In tiered EMS systems, an ALS ambulance should be requested.
4. What is the plan for umbilical cord management? For most vigorous term and preterm newborns, the umbilical cord clamping should be deferred for at least 60 seconds.

TIP

Many out-of-hospital deliveries are preterm, and the need for resuscitative efforts rises with the number of weeks of prematurity.

5. Are there any risk factors? This can include gestational hypertension (**pre-eclampsia**), maternal diabetes, or maternal drug use. If the parent has pre-eclampsia, this puts them at risk of experiencing seizures. Infant of a parent with diabetes tends to be large, especially if postterm. If the parent has a drug addiction, the infant may be born depressed (nonvigorous) and require assisted ventilation.

TIP

If the parent has seizures, she has transitioned from pre-eclampsia to eclampsia. In cases of eclampsia or severe pre-eclampsia (sustained blood pressure >160 systolic or 110 diastolic or an increase of 30/15 mm Hg from baseline, severe headache, blurred vision, significant right upper quadrant or epigastric pain, and reports of having elevated protein in the urine), administration of magnesium sulfate may be indicated for prevention or treatment of seizures. Dilute 4 g in at least 100 mL of water and administer it intravenously over 20 minutes. If the patient is not seizing, deep tendon reflexes should be assessed to check for magnesium toxicity.

PREPARING FOR NEONATAL RESUSCITATION

If the triage decision is to birth on scene, it is important for EMS clinicians to perform a quick team briefing to determine the plan and gather and check the appropriate equipment. **TABLE 14–5** lists the essential ambulance equipment, best organized in a portable **obstetric** pack (**FIGURE 14–7**). Ideally, every birth should be attended by 1 person whose only responsibility is the care of the newborn infant.

TABLE 14–5 Contents of a Portable Obstetric Pack for Vaginal Birth

Number	Item
1	Sterile disposable scalpel or scissors
3	Disposable towels
1	Receiving blanket
1	Sterile disposable bulb syringe
2	Sterile umbilical clamps or ties
1	Large plastic bag with twist tie (to store the **placenta**)
2	Plastic-lined underpads
1	Disposable plastic apron, mask, and protective eyewear

CASE STUDY 2

You are called to a residence by a patient in labor who has no transportation to the hospital. On arrival, you find the patient lying on the floor screaming, "It's time!" They tell you that this is their sixth birth, and the last one was "really quick." Their water broke 30 minutes ago, and it was clear. Your examination shows the newborn infant is crowning and the patient has an urge to push.

1. What 4 questions are most appropriate to ask at this time to best prepare for birth?
2. What equipment should be prepared for birth?

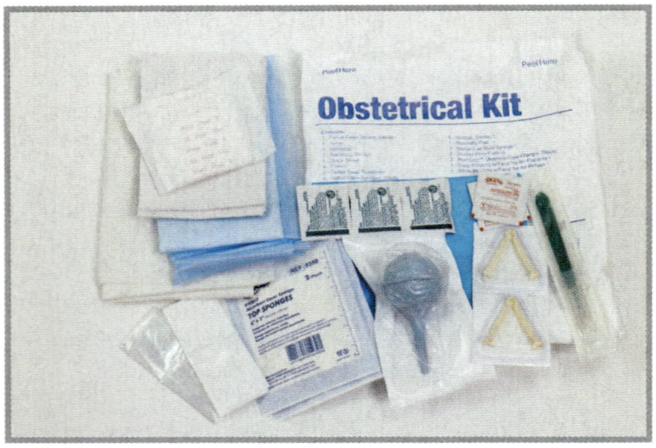

FIGURE 14–7 Obstetric pack.

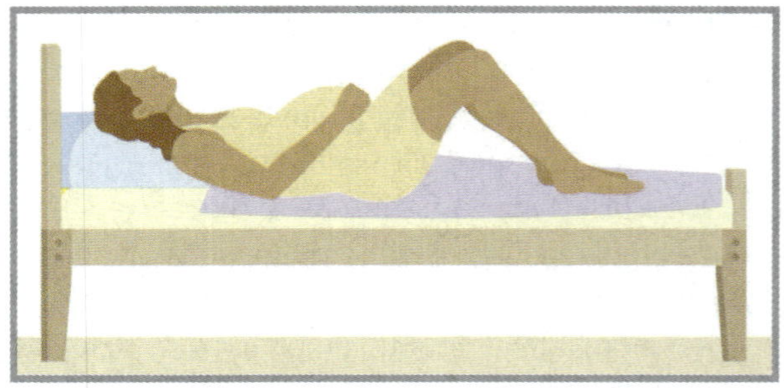

FIGURE 14–8 A safe position for birth is with the parent lying supine tilted to the left side of the bed, allowing them to birth the newborn infant onto the bed with minimal handling.

WARMING THE ENVIRONMENT

Avoiding hypothermia is an important part of newborn infant care. Before birth, make the room or ambulance as warm as possible. Turn up the heat until it is uncomfortable for an adult. Air blowing across the newborn infant can lead to heat loss, so turn off all fans. Drying the newborn infant, providing skin-to-skin contact with the parent, and placing a dry towel over the infant are usually sufficient to prevent heat loss. Premature newborns <32 weeks' gestation are at higher risk of experiencing hypothermia and should be immediately placed feet first in a polyethylene plastic bag with the head out of the bag. If using a reclosable bag, you may cut the bottom open, slide the baby into the bag through the cut side, and close the bag below the baby's feet.

POSITIONING THE PARENT

Although it is a medical emergency for the patient and the family, the birth of a newborn infant is also a highly personal and emotional event. Establish a plan for positioning for birth with the parent, but before birth let them stay in a comfortable position and covered.

The squatting position optimizes the space in the pelvis and birth canal. This position can be achieved in a bed propped up on pillows, on one's side in the Sims position, or at the edge of the bed with feet supported by family members or other birth attendants. Some patients may also prefer to push and birth on their hands and knees.

A safe position for the birth is lying supine (tilted on the left side) on a bed. Allow the parent to birth the newborn infant onto the bed with minimal handling (**FIGURE 14–8**). The current recommendation is to avoid routine suctioning of the newborn infant's mouth and nose, even in the presence of meconium.

Another safe position is the **Sims position**, in which the parent lies on their side with their back toward the attendant and their knees drawn toward their chest (**FIGURE 14–9**). The parent's perineum is still over the bed, so birth onto the bed with minimal handling is still possible.

A third position to consider involves the patient lying supine and positioned sideways on the bed, with each foot on a separate chair and their perineum at the edge of the bed (**FIGURE 14–10**). The disadvantage of this position is the lack of a supportive surface under the perineum, so that the EMS clinician must "catch" the newborn infant.

SELECTING A CLEAN BIRTH SURFACE

Select a surface that is as clean as possible to conduct the immediate care of the newborn infant. Make sure everyone involved in the newborn infant's care has washed their hands and wears gloves.

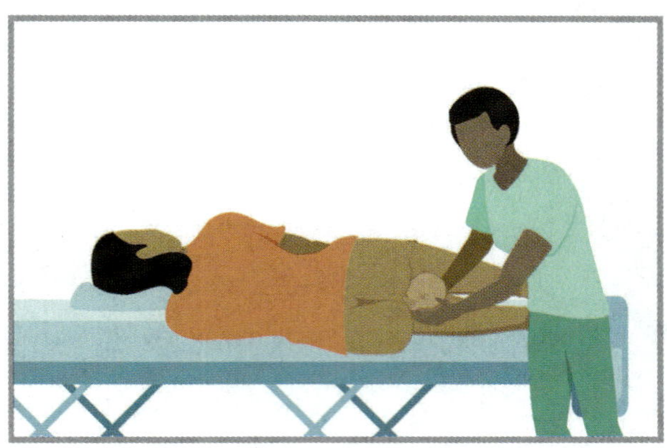

FIGURE 14–9 In the Sims position, the parent is on their side with their back toward the attendant and their knees drawn toward their chest.

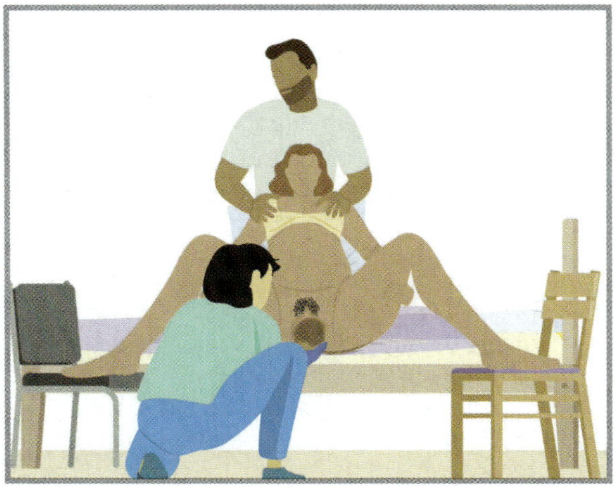

FIGURE 14-10 Alternate birth position. The patient is perpendicular to the bed with each foot on a separate chair and their perineum at the edge of the bed.

Assisting With the Birth

Most newborn infants are birthed vaginally without assistance, especially if the laboring parent is lying supine or in the Sims position in bed. Although the EMS clinician may attempt to control the birth as described next, only minimal interference with this natural process is necessary in most cases.

Use the following sequence for all deliveries:

1. Allow the parent to push the head out of the vaginal opening. You may need to place gentle pressure on the infant's head as it comes out to prevent too rapid a birth.
2. Next, with one finger, feel the infant's neck for the **umbilical cord** (**FIGURE 14-11**). If it is there, gently lift it over the newborn infant's head. Do not pull hard on the cord, because it may lead to **avulsion** of the cord with severe hemorrhage.

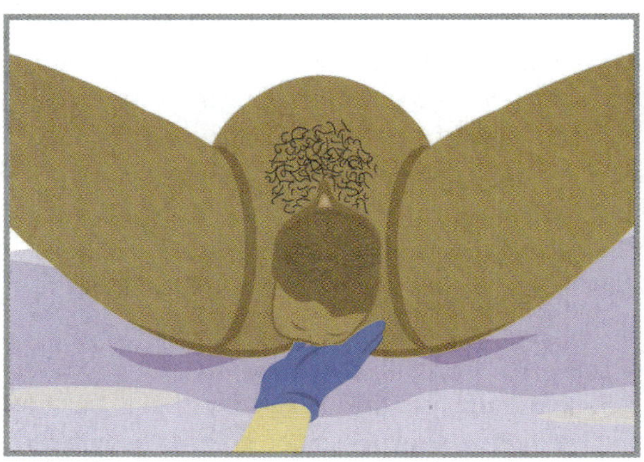

FIGURE 14-11 Ensure the umbilical cord is not wrapped around the newborn infant's neck.

3. If the patient is birthing in bed, let the birth proceed without intervention. Cradle the infant's head in one hand **posteriorly**. Place the other hand gently on the head anteriorly (**FIGURE 14-12**). On occasion, the infant's anterior shoulder needs to be gently moved posteriorly to clear the parent's **symphysis pubis**. If this occurs, direct assistants to help the parent pull their knees up toward their shoulders and apply gentle downward pressure to release the anterior shoulder (**FIGURE 14-13**).
4. For an infant (term or preterm) who is vigorous, position the infant skin to skin on the parent's chest, dry and warm the newborn infant, and delay cord clamping for at least 60 seconds. If the infant is not vigorous, or if there is concern regarding placental abruption, clamp the cord and begin resuscitation.
5. Place the newborn infant skin to skin on the parent's chest. Dry and warm the newborn infant with clean, warm towels. This removes amniotic fluid, prevents heat loss, and stimulates the newborn to breathe. Gently clear the airway with bulb suction, if necessary. Remove damp towels or blankets from around the newborn infant and replace them with clean, dry ones. If there are no complications, place the newborn infant skin to skin on the parent's chest and cover both with a blanket. If the newborn infant is <32 weeks' gestation, immediately place him/her in a

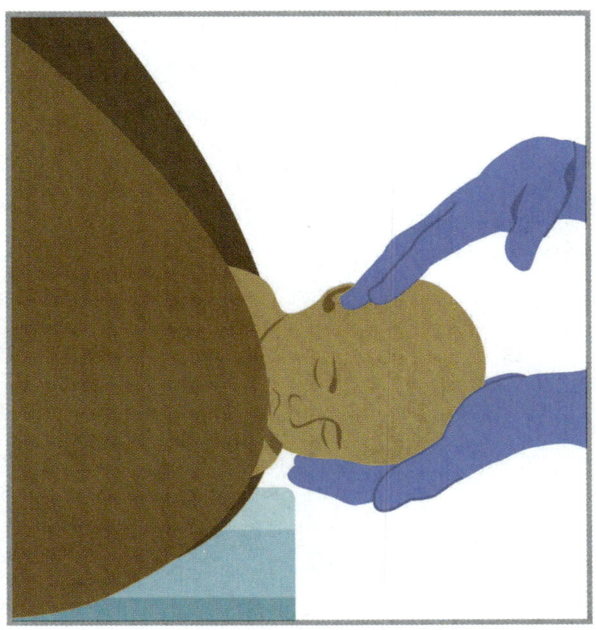

FIGURE 14-12 Cradle the infant's head in one hand posteriorly. Place the other hand gently on the head anteriorly.

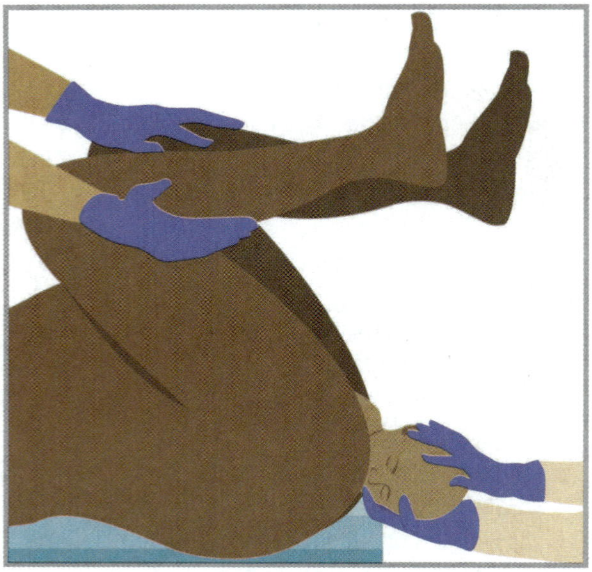

FIGURE 14–13 On occasion, the infant's anterior shoulder may need to be pulled posteriorly to clear the parent's symphysis pubis. This can be accomplished by having assistants help the parent pull their knees up toward their shoulders while placing a hand on either side of the infant's head and gently pulling downward.

polyurethane plastic bag with the head out of the bag; there is no need to dry the infant. If a newborn hat is available, place it on the infant's head. If none is available, cover the head with a warm blanket, but ensure the infant's nose and mouth are not covered.

6. Tie or clamp the cord in 2 places, approximately 3 to 4 inches from its connection to the newborn infant. Cut the cord between the 2 ties (**FIGURE 14–14**). This is considered a low priority and can be done after the placenta has birthed.

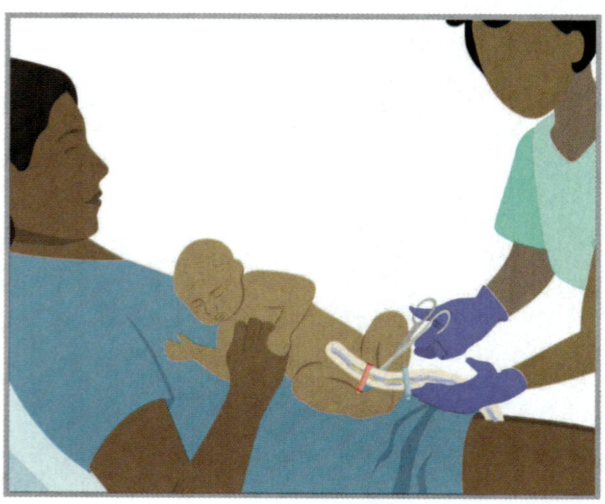

FIGURE 14–14 Tie or clamp the cord in 2 places (approximately 3–4 inches from its insertion into the newborn infant). Cut the cord between the 2 ties or clamps.

7. The last step in the birth process is the birth of the placenta. This generally occurs spontaneously 10 to 15 minutes after birth. Birth of the placenta is not an emergency procedure and must not delay the transport of the parent and infant. Do not pull on the umbilical cord to hurry the process.

TIP

Recent research has shown benefits from deferred cord clamping, especially in preterm infants. Although recommended times vary, at least 60 seconds is now recommended for vigorous term and preterm infants.

Separation of the placenta from the uterus is often signaled by a uterine contraction accompanied by a gush of blood from the vagina. After the placenta has separated from the uterine wall, gentle pulling on the cord removes it from the vagina. Pulling too much before it has separated naturally may lead to uterine inversion or avulsion of the cord and bleeding. Place the placenta in a plastic bag and transport it with the patient for pathologic evaluation. Place your hand on the parent's abdomen at the level of the umbilicus and massage the uterus to expel any remaining blood clots.

TIP

Birth of the placenta is a natural act that requires no assistance in the field. Do not pull on the cord.

MATERNAL AND NEWBORN INFANT COMPLICATIONS DURING VAGINAL BIRTH

Nuchal Umbilical Cord

During the birth, EMS clinicians should assess for the presence of a nuchal cord, which is the umbilical cord wrapped around the neck of an infant as it is born. Although it is more common that the umbilical cord is wrapped around the newborn infant's neck only once, it is possible for the umbilical cord to wrap around the neck multiple times. To reduce a single-wrapped nuchal cord, simply slide the umbilical cord from around the newborn infant's neck. When the cord is wrapped too tightly around the neck and preventing birth, EMS clinicians should apply 2 clamps across the cord, then cut the cord between the clamps. Cutting the umbilical cord will stop blood supply to the fetus, so this should be done with caution. Multiple-gestation pregnancies create a noteworthy hazard regarding nuchal umbilical cords, because it is possible for the umbilical cord of one fetus to strangle another fetus. Use extreme caution when considering whether to clamp and cut a nuchal cord when multiple gestation has not been excluded.

Meconium

Meconium is fetal stool passed in the uterus. It can be thin and watery or thick and sticky. If the newborn infant is vigorous (normal respiratory effort, muscle tone, and a heart rate >100 beats/min), no intervention is needed. Evidence does not support routine intrapartum oropharyngeal or nasopharyngeal suctioning, because these interventions do not prevent or alter the course of meconium aspiration syndrome. *Immediate endotracheal intubation and deep tracheal suctioning are no longer recommended when meconium is present and the infant is not vigorous* (see the procedure in the Specific Newborn Infant Complications section). This is a significant change from previous versions of this text and other longstanding recommendations for resuscitation of newborn infants. If the airway appears obstructed by secretions, simply use a bulb syringe or large-bore suction catheter (12F or 14F catheter) to clear the secretions and any meconium from the mouth and nose and perform resuscitation as needed. Avoid using deep suctioning in newborns.

Shoulder Dystocia/Cephalopelvic Disproportion

Shoulder dystocia is the mechanical entrapment of the anterior shoulder under the parent's pubic symphysis (anterior aspect of their pelvis) after the fetal head has successfully emerged from the vaginal introitus (**FIGURE 14–15**). Maternal diabetes, fetal macrosomia, maternal obesity, and postterm pregnancy are risk factors for this condition. A relatively large or disproportioned fetus may not birth smoothly through the vaginal canal without assistance from EMS clinicians. One or both fetal shoulders may become stuck within the maternal pelvis, typically against the symphysis pubis. The initial treatment is the McRoberts maneuver (**FIGURE 14–16**), in which 2 assistants sharply hyperflex the maternal thighs toward the parent's shoulders onto the abdomen, straightening the maternal sacrum relative to the lumbar spine by rotating the pelvis anteriorly. This position resolves many episodes of shoulder dystocia. Some clinicians recommend combining suprapubic pressure (just above the pubic symphysis) to dislodge the fetal shoulder and allow it to enter the vaginal canal with the McRoberts maneuver (**FIGURE 14–17**).

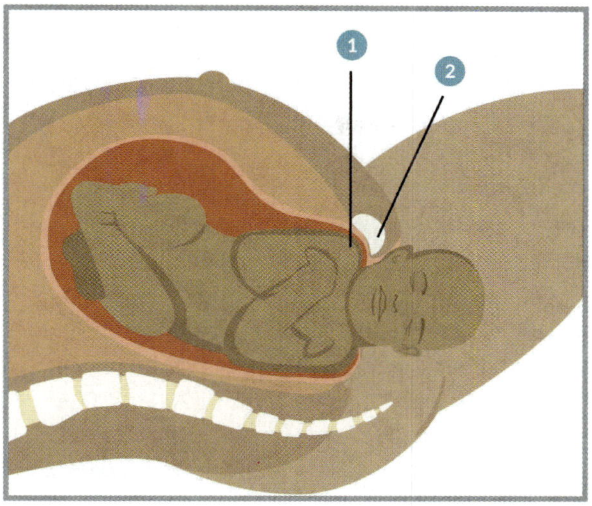

FIGURE 14–15 Shoulder dystocia. 1. Shoulder, 2. Pubic symphysis.

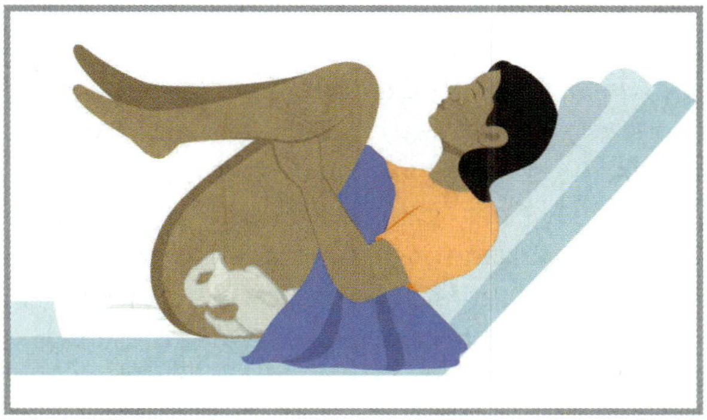

FIGURE 14–16 The McRoberts maneuver.

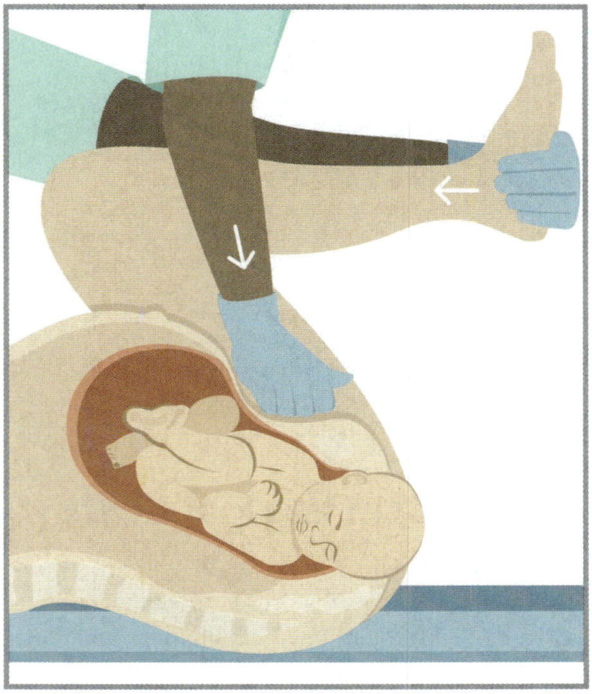

FIGURE 14–17 McRoberts maneuver with suprapubic pressure.

If this fails, an additional "rescue" technique is to attempt birth of the infant's arm or shoulder that is closest to the parent's rectum. This technique is likely to relieve the dystocia of the anterior shoulder.

Postpartum Hemorrhage

The most common **postpartum** parental complication and leading cause of parental death is excessive bleeding after birth. Usually, pregnant women lose 500 mL of blood with a vaginal birth. Symptoms such as tachycardia and orthostatic hypotension begin to appear in the parent with 1,200 to 1,500 mL of blood loss. Because estimating blood loss is difficult, one must monitor the postpartum parent's vital signs carefully.

If a postpartum parent has excessive vaginal blood loss, perform uterine massage (**FIGURE 14–18**). To massage the uterus, place one hand with fingers fully extended just above the parent's pubic bone and use the other hand to press down into the lower abdomen and vigorously massage the uterus until it becomes firm. This should take from 3 to 5 minutes. As the uterus firms up, it should feel about the size of a softball or large grapefruit. If the infant is stable, encourage breastfeeding, which causes the posterior pituitary to release oxytocin that, in turn, causes the uterus to contract and slows uterine bleeding.

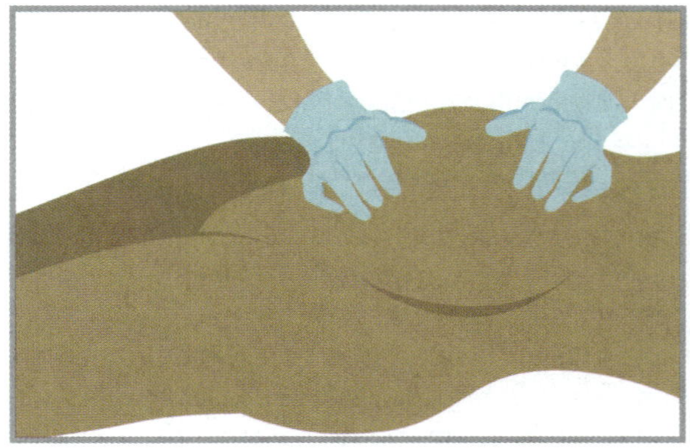

FIGURE 14–18 To massage the uterus, place one hand with fingers fully extended just above the parent's pubic bone and use your other hand to press down into the lower abdomen and vigorously massage the uterus until it becomes firm.

ALS

Treatment of Postpartum Hemorrhage. Begin volume resuscitation with crystalloid fluid in the parent who continues to bleed after the placenta is birthed and has dizziness, pallor, tachycardia, or low blood pressure. There is some evidence to suggest use of tranexamic acid may be beneficial in postpartum bleeding. Usual dosing is 1 g IV over 10 minutes initially, followed by an additional 1 g if bleeding continues or restarts after 30 min. Maternal stability determines the rate and amount of IV fluids needed. In severe situations, massive amounts of IV fluids and blood products may be required. Persistent hemorrhage requires uterine exploration, surgical intervention, or uterotonic medications not generally available to EMS clinicians.

Summary of Vaginal Birth

Birth is a natural process that usually does not require much intervention. In most cases, the birth attendant must simply control the environment to avoid things happening too fast and prepare for neonatal resuscitation if required. A history of preterm labor, multiple fetuses, prenatally diagnosed congenital anomalies, or meconium-stained amniotic fluid suggests higher probability of a newborn infant who requires resuscitation. Review the steps for performing a vaginal birth while on the way to the scene. Have the proper equipment ready, control the temperature of the environment, and position the parent to facilitate childbirth and care of the newborn. Control postpartum bleeding with uterine massage and encouragement of breastfeeding.

TIP

Encourage the parent to breastfeed the active, vigorous infant, keeping the infant skin to skin with the parent to maintain normothermia.

Immediate Care of the Newborn

A well-organized plan guides EMS clinicians through the optimal care of the newborn. **TABLE 14–6** lists the essential steps in caring for every newborn infant in every setting. EMS clinicians should keep every infant warm and dry, maintain a patent airway, and support newborn respiratory and circulatory function when indicated. Most term newborn infants do not require any ALS interventions.

The rapid assessment to determine if a newborn requires routine care or further interventions are as follows:

1. Is the newborn infant full-term?
2. Is the newborn infant's tone normal?
3. Is the newborn infant breathing/crying?

This assessment gives providers an immediate indication of the clinical status of a newborn infant

TABLE 14–6 Organized Approach to Assessment and Care of the Newborn

Dry and warm the newborn infant
Clear the airway, if necessary
Assess breathing
Assess heart rate
Assess color

and guides the approach to resuscitation. If the answer to these 3 questions is "Yes," the newborn infant can undergo routine care. However, if the answer is "No," the newborn infant will require further assessment and resuscitation.

The APGAR score (**TABLE 14–7**) is a numerical representation of the newborn infant status obtained at 1 min and again at 5 min after birth, after supportive and resuscitation measures are initiated. Although this score may be requested on hospital arrival, EMS clinicians must *not interrupt critical resuscitation procedures to obtain or calculate an APGAR score* on an unstable newborn.

TIP

Perform the initial steps of warming and maintaining normal temperature, positioning, and drying (which provides stimulation) on all newborns, whether active or depressed.

ROUTINE CARE

If the answer to the 3 rapid assessment questions is yes, the newborn infant should be placed on the parent's chest, positioned to avoid airway obstruction, dried, and suctioned only if necessary. The newborn infant should be monitored continuously until arrival at the accepting hospital.

DRY AND WARM THE NEWBORN INFANT

At birth, the newborn infant is covered in amniotic fluid and can quickly lose heat. Heat loss drastically increases the metabolic demand and oxygen consumption. Remove wet towels or blankets from around the newborn infant after drying and replace them with clean, warm, dry towels. Place a hat on the newborn, if one is available. This should take no more than 5 to 10 seconds. Premature newborns $<$32 weeks' gestation, who have thinner skin and higher insensible losses, should immediately be placed in a polyurethane plastic bag with the head outside the bag without being dried first.

POSITION THE HEAD/CLEAR THE AIRWAY

During routine care when the newborn infant is crying/breathing, they can remain on their parent's chest with the newborn infant's head positioned to the side against the parent's chest so that the airway is not compromised. Newborn infants who require more than routine care should be placed supine on a firm surface with the head in a neutral to slightly extended position. A towel may be placed under the newborn's shoulders to maintain a neutral head position.

Routine suctioning of the vigorous newborn infant is not necessary. If secretions are seen or heard and the newborn infant is not breathing or is breathing with difficulty, gently suction the mouth and then the nose with a bulb syringe or suction tubing. Avoid aggressive or deep suctioning. When meconium is present, EMS clinicians should anticipate the need for additional resuscitation measures. Routine endotracheal intubation and deep suctioning are no longer routinely recommended, even in nonvigorous newborns.

TABLE 14–7 APGAR Scoring

Sign	0	1	2
Appearance: Color	Blue or pale	Acrocyanotic	Completely pink
Pulse: Heart rate	Absent	$<$100 beats/min	$>$100 beats/min
Grimace: Reflex irritability	No response	Grimace	Cry or active withdrawal
Activity: Muscle tone	Limp	Some flexion	Active motion
Respiration	Absent	Weak cry; hypoventilation	Good, crying

Reproduced with permission from American Academy of Pediatrics, Committee on Fetus and Newborn; American College of Obstetricians and Gynecologists; Committee on Obstetric Practice. The Apgar score. *Pediatrics*. 2006;117(4):1444–1447. doi:10.1542/peds.2006-0325.

CASE STUDY 3

On arriving at the home of a family who had called 9-1-1 for labor, you find a woman lying on the floor who has just birthed an apparently full-term female. The newborn infant is being held by the father, still attached to the umbilical cord. She is not moving or crying, is cyanotic, and appears limp.

1. What are the steps in the resuscitation of this newborn infant?
2. What is the role of vascular access?

Stimulate

Drying the newborn infant usually provides enough stimulation, but if the newborn infant has not started breathing or is premature and has been placed in a polyurethane bag and thus not dried, gently rub the newborn's back, trunk, or extremities to stimulate them.

ASSESS BREATHING

Most newborn infants will be crying, indicating adequate respiratory effort. Breathing effort may be slightly irregular in normal newborns. Gasping is a sign of respiratory failure in a severely compromised newborn infant and should be treated with **assisted ventilation**. Grunting may be subtle or significant and is a sign of respiratory distress that may require additional assistance but also may be transient. If the newborn infant is otherwise vigorous and pink, grunting may not require any intervention until arrival at the hospital.

An **apneic** newborn infant, with no visible respiratory effort, requires immediate treatment. Most apneic newborns start breathing simply with tactile stimulation. If the newborn infant is completely apneic or has only gasping respiration after drying and suctioning, further stimulation is not likely to improve respiratory effort. Begin assisted ventilation via bag-mask device at a rate of 30 to 60 breaths/min. The AAP recommends starting initial resuscitation without supplemental oxygen (21%) attached to the bag-mask device for infants >35 weeks' gestation. For those born at 32 to 34 weeks' gestation, start with a low oxygen concentration (21%–30%) and titrate oxygen according to pulse oximetry reading. For infants <32 weeks' gestation, start with at least 30%. Do not expect newborns' oxygen saturation to be >85% to 95% until 10 min after birth. This represents a huge paradigm shift from decades of resuscitation procedures.

ALS

Treatment of an Infant Born to a Parent Addicted to Opiates. A special situation occurs when the EMS clinician encounters a newborn infant with respiratory depression after birth by a narcotic-addicted parent. Do not give naloxone (Narcan) to the newborn infant if the parent is addicted to narcotics. Reversal of narcotics may precipitate acute withdrawal symptoms and seizure activity. Assist ventilation with a bag-mask device and follow the guidelines for care of a depressed newborn. Consider inserting a supraglottic airway, depending on local protocols, if the infant requires prolonged ventilation or continued resuscitation measures.

TIP

Do not expect a newborn's pulse oximetry result to be 85% to 95% until 10 min after birth.

TIP

Place the pulse oximeter on the right hand or wrist of the newborn, because the blood in these locations is preductal blood and better represents the blood supplied to the brain and heart. The oxygenation target is a preductal saturation of >80% to 85% by 5 min after birth.

ASSESS HEART RATE

The normal heart rate for a newborn infant is 100 to 205 beats/min while awake and 90 to 160 beats/min while sleeping. Bradycardia in a newborn infant is usually caused by hypoxia, not primary cardiac disease, and thus the intervention most likely to help the newborn infant is ventilation. This is the most important difference between newborn infant resuscitation and resuscitation in pediatric patients and adults, in whom the focus of resuscitation is on chest compressions and not ventilation.

The crying, active newborn infant usually has an adequate heart rate. Assess heart rate carefully in a newborn infant who is not active or who requires assisted ventilation. The heart rate is best assessed with a stethoscope over the left side of the chest.

In the past, the AAP recommended palpation of the umbilical cord; however, this method has been found to be less accurate than auscultation. In addition, place a pulse oximeter on the infant's right hand, which will help determine not only the heart rate but also oxygenation.

> **TIP**
> You may encounter pregnant patients who are addicted to drugs. If the pregnant patient is "high," so is their newborn infant. In such patients, it can be difficult to determine the parent's medical history, the gestational age, or how long the patient has been in labor. Be prepared for anything.

> **CAUTION**
> **Do not give naloxone to the newborn infant if you suspect the parent is addicted to narcotics.**

Treat heart rate of <100 beats/min for >1 min after birth with bag-mask ventilation, even if the respiratory effort seems normal. Bradycardia usually responds rapidly to effective bag-mask ventilation, in which case no further treatment is necessary. Tachycardia (heart rate >160 beats/min) may also be present in a newborn. Severe physiological stress, such as maternal infection or newborn infant hypovolemia, may cause an increased fetal heart rate. When providing bag-mask ventilation for a preterm infant, use a pressure of 20 to 25 centimeters of water pressure (cm H_2O) (if the bag has a manometer) and 25 to 30 cm H_2O for a term infant. If the heart rate is increasing, you do not need to achieve chest rise. If heart rate is NOT increasing, assess your ventilation technique and ensure the newborn infant's chest is rising. If there is no chest rise, it is important to reposition the mask (over mouth and nose), ensure that the patient's head is in a neutral position and not hyperextended, suction the mouth or nose if obstructed by secretions, open the mouth if needed, and consider increasing the pressure slightly.

ASSESS COLOR

Skin color assessment in newborns has several unique features. **In utero**, the fetus depends on placental delivery of oxygen, and blood oxygen concentrations are low compared with conditions after birth. Therefore, before the initiation of respiration after birth, the infant appears cyanotic.

If the cyanotic newborn infant is apneic, immediately begin bag-mask ventilation. If the newborn infant is breathing but appears blue, determine if the cyanosis is central (on the trunk and face) or peripheral (limited to the hands and feet). This difference helps with decision making and therapy. If **central cyanosis** is present, a pulse oximeter with an infant probe should be applied to the right hand to confirm hypoxemia. When hypoxemia is present, and the heart rate is >100 beats/min, administer supplemental oxygen and titrate according to pulse oximetry readings. Administer free-flowing oxygen using oxygen tubing or a simple face mask.

Peripheral cyanosis, bluish skin color present only in the extremities, is also termed **acrocyanosis**. This is a common finding in newborns through the first 24 to 48 hours after birth and requires no therapy.

> **TIP**
> Assist ventilation in an infant whose heart rate is <100 beats/min with bag-mask ventilation. Bradycardia usually reflects inadequate respiratory effort. Do not perform chest compressions until effective bag-mask ventilation has been established.

Infant color and pulse quality provide an indication of overall perfusion status. Hypovolemia, shock, and congenital cardiovascular defects may present with **central cyanosis**, poor overall skin color, delayed capillary refill, or absent peripheral pulses. Persistent infant bradycardia, tachycardia, or alterations in perfusion may represent a severe condition requiring intervention and transport to a specialty care center.

Although most nonvigorous newborns respond to effective bag-mask ventilation until they can arrive at a facility able to care for them, a few will require an alternative airway—either a supraglottic airway (SGA) or intubation. Intubation can be difficult in the field given the neonatal anatomy (large head, anterior airway) and may not be warranted in the field, because it will likely delay transport and may not be successful. It is recommended that an SGA be inserted, if patient size allows it, and ventilations be optimized before chest compressions are initiated.

CHEST COMPRESSIONS

Chest compressions are rarely necessary in a newborn infant when effective ventilation can be established. Insert a supraglottic airway if patient size allows and optimize ventilation before initiating chest compressions. If despite effective ventilation the infant's heart rate remains <60 beats/min, initiate chest compressions. Chest compressions should be coordinated with bag-mask ventilation at a rate of 1 breath to 3 compressions. The compressor should place their hands around the newborn's chest and place their thumbs on the center of the sternum just below an imaginary line between the newborn infant's nipples. Compress one-third of the newborn infant's chest. The goal is to provide 3 compressions and 1 ventilation every 2 seconds, for a total of 120 event/min or 30 breaths and 90 compressions/min.

General Principles of Newborn Infant Resuscitation

Most newborns do not require extensive resuscitation. Routine care for the term newborn infant who is breathing or crying and has good tone includes keeping the newborn infant with the parent, drying, stimulating, positioning, suctioning only if needed, and providing ongoing evaluation while keeping the newborn infant warm. If the newborn infant is preterm or not breathing or crying and has poor tone, dry the infant, remove all wet items, and place the newborn infant in the supine position in a warm environment. Gently suction the mouth, then nose, if necessary and position the head in slight extension.

When the newborn infant remains depressed after initial drying, warming, and positioning of the airway, begin resuscitation. Use the following sequence, which is illustrated by the Neonatal Resuscitation Program (NRP) Algorithm (**FIGURE 14–19**):

1. Assess heart rate and breathing. If heart rate is >100 beats/min but the infant has labored breathing or persistent cyanosis, position the infant and clear the airway, apply a pulse oximeter, and provide supplemental oxygen as needed. If able to provide CPAP, this is recommended. If the heart rate is <100 beats/ min or if respiratory effort is absent or gasping, start bag-mask ventilation at 30 to 60 breaths/min (**FIGURE 14–20**). When a pressure manometer is available, start ventilations using 25 cm H_2O. Place a pulse oximeter on the infant's right hand.
2. Assess heart rate after 30 seconds of ventilation. If <100 beats/min but >60 beats/min, then check that ventilation technique is resulting in adequate chest rise. If the heart rate is <60 beats/min and there is chest rise with ventilation, begin chest compressions. If the heart rate is <60 beats/min and there is no chest rise, perform corrective steps first (adjust mask, adjust head/neck, suction airway, open mouth, increase pressure) and re-assess heart rate after 30 seconds of *effective* ventilation. Compressions should be delivered at a depth of one-third the anteroposterior diameter of the chest. The "two-thumb encircling hand" technique—2 thumbs positioned on the lower one-third of the sternum (just below the nipple line), with fingers encircling the chest and supporting the back—is preferred because it generates superior coronary arterial perfusion pressure while also causing less fatigue in the clinician. Deliver 90 compressions and 30 ventilations (120 events) per minute with a 3:1 compression-to-ventilation ratio. When compressions are begun, increase oxygen to 100%.
3. Reassess heart rate after 60 seconds. Continue compressions and assisted ventilation with 100% FiO_2 until heart rate is >60 beats/min. When the pulse oximetry signal is considered reliable, titrate the FiO_2 according to the target saturation table. Positive-pressure ventilations should be continued until the heart rate is >100 beats/min and the newborn infant is spontaneously breathing. If the heart rate remains <60 beats/min, consider placement of a supraglottic airway or intubation. You may need to continue bag-mask ventilation until arrival at a facility with a higher level of care.

The endotracheal route of epinephrine administration is less effective. This route may be considered

ALS

Endotracheal Intubation and Epinephrine Administration. Check the heart rate after 30 seconds of effective ventilation. If <60 beats/min, prepare for either SGA insertion or endotracheal intubation as allowed by local protocol. If an invasive airway is not available, chest compressions are reasonable. Intravenous or intraosseous (IO) access should be obtained as soon as possible. The preferred route for epinephrine administration is IV. The recommended IV/IO dose of epinephrine is 0.01–0.03 mg/kg (equal to 0.1-0.3 mL/kg) of a 0.1 mg/mL (or 1 mg/10 mL) concentration. Flush with 3 mL of normal saline. You may need to estimate the newborn's weight.

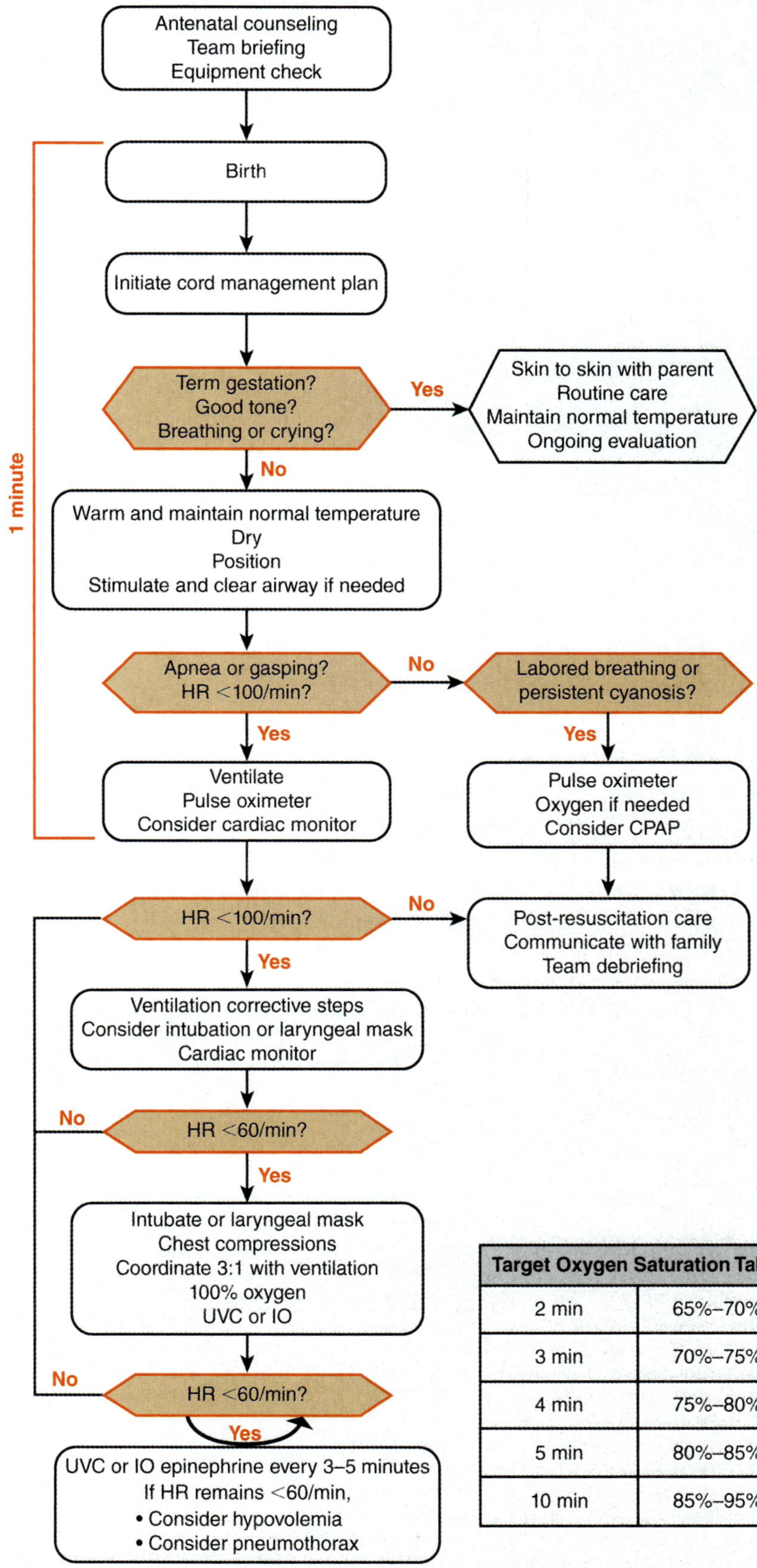

Target Oxygen Saturation Table	
2 min	65%–70%
3 min	70%–75%
4 min	75%–80%
5 min	80%–85%
10 min	85%–95%

FIGURE 14–19 The Neonatal Resuscitation Program (NRP) Algorithm.

Reproduced with permission from American Academy of Pediatrics, American Heart Association. *Textbook of Neonatal Resuscitation*. Weiner GM, Cooper C, Lee H, eds. 9th ed. American Academy of Pediatrics; 2025.

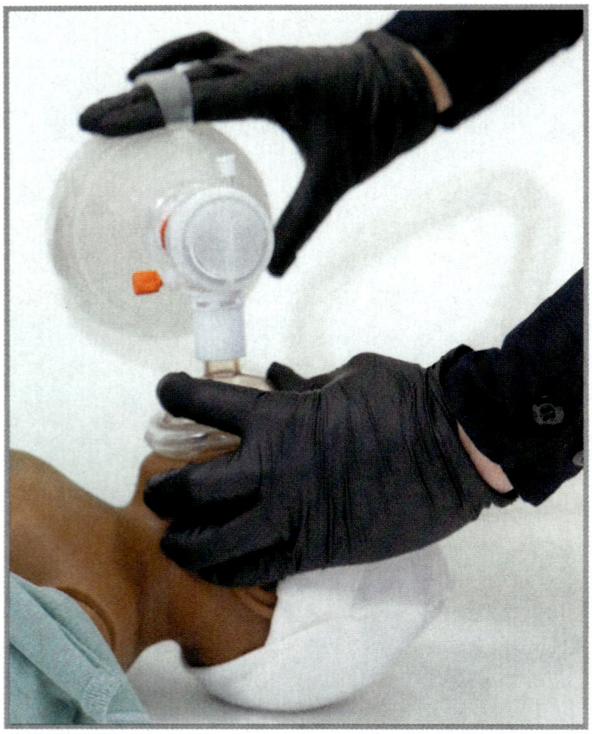

FIGURE 14–20 Using a bag-mask device on a newborn.

while vascular access is obtained. Provide a dose of 0.05-0.1 mg/kg (equal to 0.5-1 mL/kg) of the 0.1-mg/mL (1 mg/10 mL) concentration. Be sure to follow drug delivery by providing ventilations. *No* flush is recommended. Note that the same concentration of epinephrine is used for both endotracheal and IV administration in neonatal resuscitation. This differs from concentrations used in pediatric resuscitation.

Continue chest compressions and administer repeated doses of epinephrine every 3 to 5 min until heart rate is >60 beats/min.

Monitor blood glucose concentrations, especially if the infant has received prolonged or aggressive resuscitation measures. If a serum glucose level of <40 mg/dL is documented in a depressed newborn, and an IV or IO line can be established during transport, give 10% **dextrose** in a 2-mL/kg bolus. Initiate prompt transport to a health care facility capable of neonatal stabilization. If there is no IV or IO access, glucose gel may be administered at a dose of 0.5 mL/kg (200 mg/kg) using an oral syringe. Dry the buccal mucosa and massage the dextrose gel into the inner cheek with a gloved finger.

The Inverted Pyramid. The inverted pyramid (**FIGURE 14–21**) illustrates the relative need for interventions in depressed newborns.

> **TIP**
> Good ventilation usually reverses bradycardia.

Basic life support is usually all that is required during deliveries and therefore constitutes the largest area at the top of the inverted pyramid. In contrast, chest compressions and ALS interventions, such as intubation and medication administration, are rarely

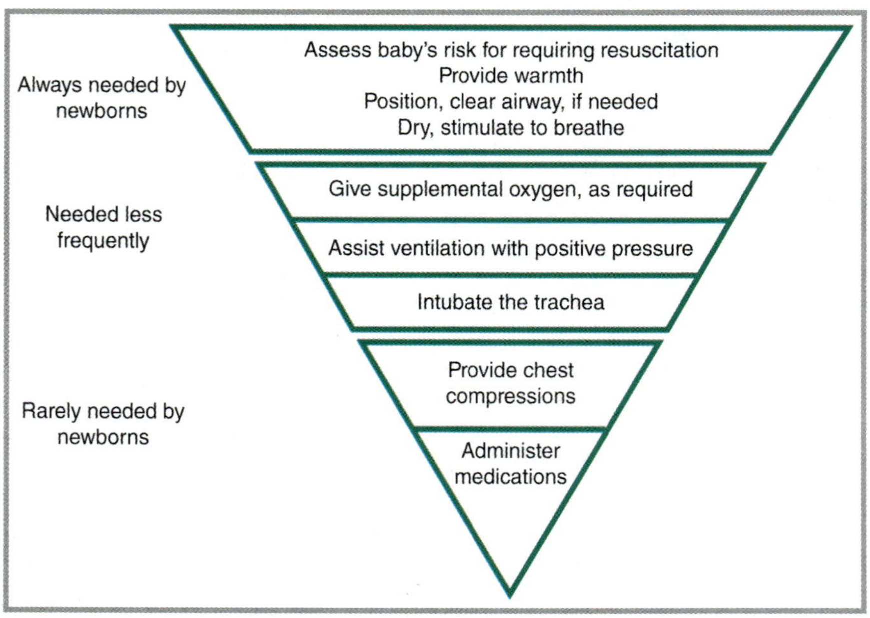

FIGURE 14–21 The relationship between resuscitation procedures and the number of newborn infants who need them.

required and constitute the smallest area at the bottom of the inverted pyramid.

Specific Newborn Infant Complications

MECONIUM ASPIRATION

A newborn infant born with meconium-stained amniotic fluid who appears active and without respiratory distress needs no suctioning or only gentle oral then nasal suctioning as necessary, along with routine care of the newborn. Evidence does not support routine intrapartum oropharyngeal or nasopharyngeal suctioning, because these interventions do not prevent or alter the course of meconium aspiration syndrome. Routine suctioning is not recommended, even for infants born through meconium-stained fluid. Suctioning is necessary only if airway obstruction is suspected. Overly aggressive suctioning may cause vagal stimulation and lead to bradycardia. Previous guidelines recommended endotracheal intubation and tracheal suctioning of nonvigorous newborns born through meconium-stained fluid; *this intervention is no longer recommended*. Provide assisted ventilation for the nonvigorous newborn infant even if meconium is present.

PRETERM INFANTS

Premature infants are at risk of experiencing a vast array of complications, which increase in likelihood and severity as the degree of prematurity increases. EMS clinicians need to provide the warmest environment possible during resuscitation and transport. For newborns <32 weeks' gestation, the AAP recommends placing the newborn infant feet first in a polyethylene plastic bag with the head outside the bag immediately after birth to aid with thermoregulation. If possible, also place a hat on the premature newborn infant's head. Support ventilations as needed with bag-mask ventilation for those with apnea, labored breathing, cyanosis, or heart rate <100 beats/min.

CONGENITAL DISORDERS

Choanal Atresia

Infants are rarely born with a complete nasal obstruction. In severe, untreated cases, this condition may cause newborn infant death caused by hypoxia. Unless crying, newborn infants breathe exclusively through their nasal passages. Patients with choanal atresia may experience profound respiratory distress that resolves during crying episodes. If you suspect this condition, place an oral airway or endotracheal tube into the posterior pharynx (it does not need to enter the trachea). The respiratory distress should improve. A more presumptive diagnosis may be made in EMS systems that carry small suction catheters capable of being placed into the infant's nose. If the catheter cannot pass through either nasal passage into the posterior pharynx, **choanal atresia** is presumed (**FIGURE 14–22**). Do not use excessive force to try to pass a nasal suction catheter. A number of different devices, such as a modified pacifier (with the tip removed) or oropharyngeal airways and endotracheal tubes, can be partially inserted into an infant's mouth to keep the airway open while the patient is being transported.

Pierre Robin syndrome (also known as **Robin sequence**) is another potential cause of airway obstruction in newborn infants (**FIGURE 14–23A and B**). An underdeveloped mandible causes the tongue to obstruct the posterior pharynx. This can be treated in the prehospital setting by placing a suction catheter or endotracheal tube into the infant's nasal

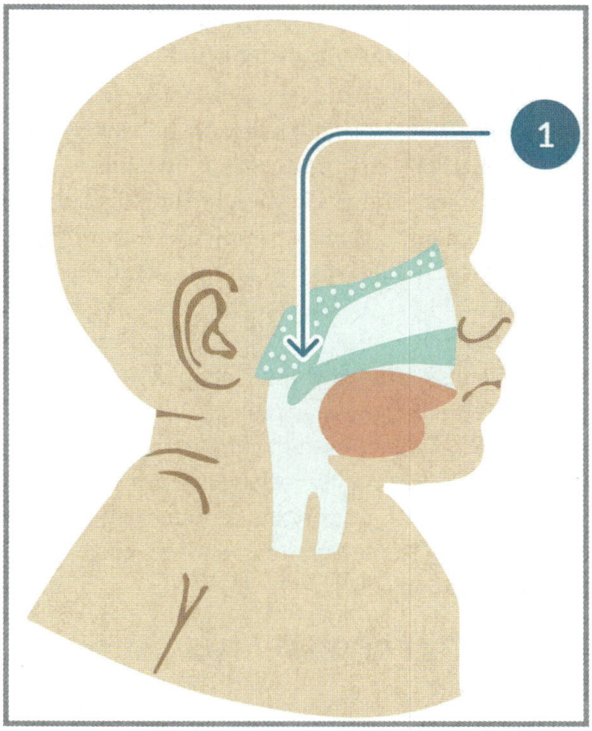

FIGURE 14–22 1. Congenital obstruction of posterior nasopharynx.

Reproduced with permission from American Academy of Pediatrics, American Heart Association. *Textbook of Neonatal Resuscitation*. Weiner GM, Cooper C, Lee H, eds. 9th ed. American Academy of Pediatrics; 2025.

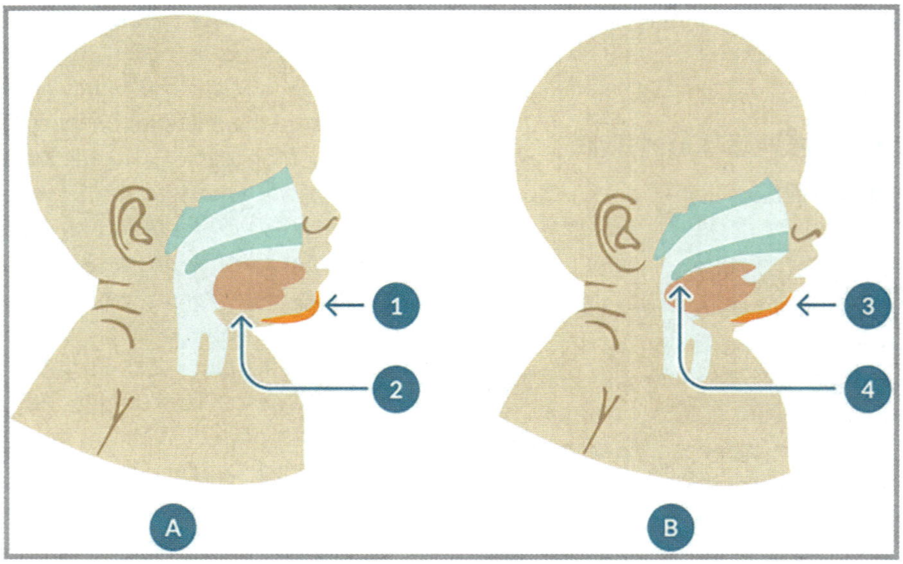

FIGURE 14–23 **A.** Newborn with normal anatomy: jaw (1) and (2) tongue. **B.** Newborn with Pierre-Robin syndrome: abnormally small jaw (3) and tongue displaced against posterior pharynx (4).

passage with the tip in the posterior nasopharynx beyond the base of the tongue, but not inserted into the trachea, and placing the infant in a prone position, as long as resuscitation is not needed.

Congenital Diaphragmatic Hernia

It is possible for infants to be born without an intact diaphragm. The stomach or intestines and liver may migrate into the chest cavity, collapsing lungs or inhibiting ventilation. EMS clinicians should suspect **congenital diaphragmatic hernia** when an infant has a flat (scaphoid) abdomen and respiratory distress (**FIGURE 14–24**). Prolonged bag-mask ventilations force additional air into the infant's stomach, worsening respiratory distress. Treatment in the prehospital setting requires prompt insertion of a supraglottic airway or endotracheal intubation and decompression of the stomach with a gastric tube if available. Prompt transport and cautious bag-mask technique may be the only intervention available to clinicians providing BLS.

CONGENITAL CARDIOVASCULAR DEFECTS

Approximately 1% of infants are born with a congenital cardiovascular defect. These include minor, clinically insignificant defects. Critical congenital heart defects occur in approximately 2 per 1,000 newborns. Defects may involve several different parts of the heart and one or more of the great vessels in the chest. Diagnosis is often impossible without the assistance of a pediatric cardiologist or similar specialist, but certain clues may alert EMS clinicians to newborns with these conditions. Cyanosis, shock,

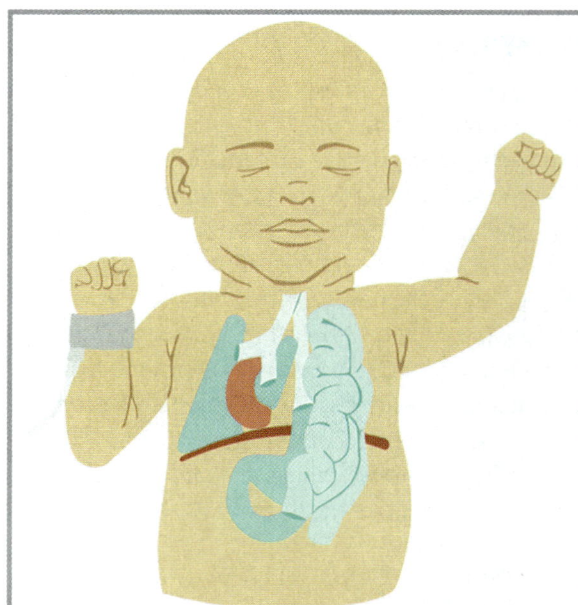

FIGURE 14–24 Congenital diaphragmatic hernia. The defect in the diaphragm allows abdominal contents to herniate into the left chest.

pulmonary edema, and altered peripheral pulses occur in infants with cardiovascular anomalies and may present across the full spectrum of severity. EMS clinicians should initiate immediate transport to a specialized facility capable of neonatal stabilization whenever a congenital cardiovascular defect is suspected. Many types of defects present with persistent cyanosis that cannot be corrected in the prehospital setting, even with optimal resuscitation measures. Conversely, resuscitation with high concentrations of oxygen may actually worsen many of these conditions by altering the pulmonary circulation and vascular resistance. EMS clinicians are often limited to basic supportive care and prompt transport of newborns with suspected cardiovascular defects.

SHOCK

Shock at birth is most commonly caused by **asphyxia** (severe hypoxia in the uterus or during birth) and **acidosis**. Blood loss during birth caused by umbilical cord avulsion or fetal-placental transfusion is an uncommon cause of shock in the newborn. Signs and symptoms of shock, whatever the cause, include abnormal appearance (lethargy, hypotonia), abnormal skin color (pallor, mottling), tachycardia or bradycardia, and prolonged capillary refill time. Hypothermia may also mimic these findings.

ALS

Treatment of Shock. Because intrauterine or perinatal asphyxia is the most common cause of depression in the newborn, initial resuscitative efforts should ensure adequate oxygenation and ventilation. Volume resuscitation is rarely needed. In exceptional circumstances in which hypovolemic shock is suspected, consider placing an IV or IO line. Isotonic crystalloid solution is recommended at a dose of 10 mL/kg. Fluid resuscitation should be cautiously performed in premature infants, because giving fluids too rapidly has been associated with intraventricular hemorrhage.

Vascular Access. Vascular access is rarely needed in newborn infants in the field, because resuscitation is largely focused on airway management and ventilation. In reality, establishing vascular access is challenging in infants, and its benefits must be carefully weighed against prolonged on-scene time and potential complications. Intravenous access may be attempted in the **antecubital fossa** or the **saphenous vein** at the ankle. Tibial IO access, using a manual IO technique, is an alternative.

Hypoglycemia. The depressed newborn infant or prematurely newborn infant is at risk of experiencing hypoglycemia. If transport time is prolonged, measure a bedside glucose level approximately 30 min after birth, or immediately in any newborn infant who has an acute change in responsiveness or perfusion. If the serum glucose level is $<$40 mg/dL, glucose gel can be administered. To administer glucose gel to a newborn infant for hypoglycemia, draw up the prescribed dose (0.5 mL/kg, 200 mg/kg) into an oral syringe, dry the newborn infant's buccal mucosa, and then massage the gel into the inner cheek with a gloved finger. Alternatively, if glucose gel is not available, an IV or IO line can be established in transport and 10% dextrose administered in a 2-mL/kg bolus. Recheck serum glucose level every 30 min during long transports. If the infant has documented hypoglycemia but is active, is in no respiratory distress, and has a suck reflex, allow the infant to breastfeed or offer the infant 20 to 30 mL of formula, breast milk, or 5% dextrose by bottle.

When there is no IV or IO access, some resuscitation medications, such as lidocaine, epinephrine, atropine, and naloxone (identified by the mnemonic LEAN), can be administered through the endotracheal tube. Do not administer other solutions, such as dextrose or sodium bicarbonate, through the endotracheal tube.

CAUTION

Umbilical vein catheterization is a controversial field procedure. Although this route of vascular access is widely used in the neonatal intensive care unit, there are very few opportunities for the EMS clinician to practice and maintain this skill, and serious complications can occur.

TIP

Intraosseous infusion may be preferable if vascular access is clearly necessary for resuscitation and a peripheral IV line cannot be placed.

Summary of Resuscitation of the Newborn

Many newborn infant conditions present with airway, respiratory, or cardiovascular compromise. The primary treatment of the depressed newborn infant involves reversal of hypoventilation and hypoxia with immediate bag-mask ventilation. If the infant does not improve, begin chest compressions and provide oxygen. Consider a supraglottic airway or endotracheal intubation per local guidelines if bag-mask ventilation is ineffective. Shock is rare and is most commonly the result of asphyxia. Hypovolemia is an uncommon cause of shock in the newborn. If hypovolemic shock is suspected, transport immediately and initiate volume resuscitation via IV or IO line.

Transport Considerations

EMS clinicians may need to transport healthy infants who have had an uncomplicated birth or critical infants in continued cardiopulmonary arrest. The degree of monitoring and ongoing intervention depends entirely on the clinical status of the patient(s). All neonates require a warm environment. Every neonate needs to be secured during transport in a manner that will not cause devastating injuries if the transport vehicle is involved in a collision during the transport (see Chapter 18).

HEALTHY INFANT

The active term infant requires no intervention or electronic monitoring during transport. Be sure the infant is restrained as per local EMS system policy. Encourage the parent to breastfeed the active infant if possible. This may prevent hypoglycemia and promote maternal–infant bonding, uterine contractions, and decreased uterine bleeding.

NEWBORN INFANT WITH COMPLICATIONS

Oxygen Therapy

Excessive oxygen can be harmful to newborns, particularly preterm infants or those with congenital heart defects. Most newborn infant conditions do not require any supplemental oxygen, provided that the infant's heart rate and oxygen saturation can be continuously monitored and remain stable. In the event that a newborn infant is having respiratory distress, carefully monitor the patient's condition and provide only the oxygen necessary, according to pulse oximetry readings.

Monitoring

After resuscitation, reassess the status of the infant throughout transport. Place cardiac leads in the same position as in an adult. A heart rate between 120 and 160 beats/min is normal in a newborn. If the heart rate decreases or increases unexpectedly, search for possible causes, which often include airway or respiratory compromise.

In newborn infants, the most accurate location for pulse oximetry sensor placement is the right hand or wrist because of alterations in blood flow related to the ductus arteriosus in the aorta. The pulse oximetry reading on the right upper extremity is termed the preductal pulse oximetry reading. Healthy newborn infants have initial oxygen saturations between 60% and 65% immediately after birth, slowly increasing over the next 10 min. Oxygen saturations between 85% and 95% are normal after the first 10 min following birth. Although there are negative effects of **hyperoxia** in the newborn infant, if the newborn infant is distressed, the goal in the field should be to ensure adequate oxygenation through administration of supplemental oxygen and assisted ventilation when needed. Any supplemental oxygen should be titrated carefully to the infant's condition and targeted oxygen saturation according to the results of pulse oximetry and the number of minutes since birth.

Hypothermia

Hypothermia develops rapidly in newborn infants. Oxygen demand triples when skin temperature drops by 1 degree. Signs of hypothermia are similar to those of shock. Keep the newborn warm during transport. Have a small knit cap available to cover the infant's head. Turn on the heat in the ambulance, even at the risk of discomfort to the parent and crew. Before transport, place the newborn infant on the parent's bare chest (skin-to-skin contact) and cover both of them to maintain the infant's temperature. Clear occlusive plastic bags (polyethylene plastic), such as trash bags and food storage bags, are a very effective way to minimize hypothermia in preterm and low-birth weight newborn infants, particularly in high-risk (cold) environments or when the infant cannot be held at the parent's chest during transport. The AAP recommends placing the premature newborn infant <32 weeks' gestation in one of these bags immediately after birth to decrease hypothermia. The infant's torso and extremities, *not the head*, are placed in the bag, which is rolled loosely around the infant's neck. These bags also minimize the risk of dehydration from evaporative losses through the infant's skin. Use clear bags to allow continuous visual monitoring of the infant. Palpation of chest movement and auscultation can both be performed through the bag when needed.

TRANSPORT DESTINATION

It is impossible to account for all potential variables when discussing transport destination. When choosing a receiving hospital, EMS clinicians should consider the condition of the parent and newborn, patient preference, transport times, and the obstetric and neonatal capabilities of the potential receiving hospitals. In many situations, it is appropriate to bypass a smaller community hospital to take the infant to a larger tertiary care center where specialty obstetric and neonatal services are immediately available. In other instances, EMS clinicians should transport to the closest facility available where the newborn infant can be stabilized for later transport. Contact online medical control when required by protocol or when the destination choice is not entirely clear. If allowed by local protocol, attempt to transport the parent-infant dyad to the same facility able to care for both.

SPECIALTY CARE TEAMS

Many regions of the country have specialty high-risk obstetric or neonatal transport teams, often comprising a physician, nurse, respiratory therapist, advanced practice nurse, and/or specially trained paramedics. Consider activating these resources early when maternal, fetal, or newborn infant complications are present or expected. Prompt access to specialty care dramatically improves the outcome for many critical parent or newborn infant patients.

Summary

EMS clinicians are in a unique position to provide assistance to women in labor outside the hospital setting, assist with birth, and provide immediate lifesaving care to compromised parents and newborns. Decisions and interventions performed by EMS clinicians have a potential to impact the health and lives of a pregnant parent and their child.

CASE STUDY ANSWERS

CASE STUDY 1

First, decide whether to transport the parent to the nearest hospital or to prepare for birth of the newborn infant. She tells you this is her fourth pregnancy and her last birth took 3 hours. Does the parent feel the urge to push? If the parent feels the urge to push, then examine for the presence of crowning. If crowning is not visible, wait and examine again during the next contraction.

If you decide to birth at the scene, obtain a resuscitation-oriented history. Are twins present? What is the due date? What color was the amniotic fluid when the membranes ruptured? Are there any risk factors? These questions assist you in preparation.

If the newborn infant is crowning at the perineum, prepare the obstetric birth pack, familiarize yourself with the contents, and make sure all necessary equipment is present. Warm the environment and obtain clean towels to dry the newborn infant. Find a clean birth surface for the newborn infant. Obtain or make a cap to place over the child's scalp to reduce heat loss from the head once birthed and dried.

Crowning was evident during your examination, and there were no red flags noted in your resuscitation-oriented history. A healthy full-term girl was birthed on scene with APGAR scores of 9 and 10 at 1 min and 5 min, respectively. The infant was warmed and dried. Postpartum bleeding was controlled via uterine massage. The parent and newborn infant were transported to the hospital, and both were released in good health the next day.

CASE STUDY 2

If time allows, review the procedure for a vaginal birth while on the way to the scene. On arrival, first plan for appropriate positioning of the patient. Discuss the position with the patient ahead of time so that they understand the plan for birth. The patient should be lying supine with an object (eg, stack of towels or a phone book) under their hips. Alternatively, they can lie on their side facing away from you with their knees drawn toward the chest (Sims position).

Obtain a resuscitation-oriented history. Are twins present? What is the due date? What color was the amniotic fluid when the membranes ruptured? Are there any risk factors?

Clear amniotic fluid implies there is no meconium. Meconium is fetal stool, which occurs in conditions of stress. Although the presence of clear fluid does not rule out the possibility of a depressed newborn infant, it is a reassuring sign and increases the chances of an active newborn infant who will need only the initial measures of standard newborn infant care.

Continued

CASE STUDY ANSWERS—cont'd

Equipment prepared should include the obstetric birth pack. Neonatal resuscitation equipment should be readily available.

A full-term boy was birthed with some difficulty related to shoulder dystocia. Pulling the anterior shoulder posteriorly facilitated birth. Initially, the infant was apneic. Drying and stimulation resulted only in weak gasps, so ventilation was initiated at 50 breaths/min using room air. Heart rate was initially 60 beats/min but increased rapidly to >100 beats/min after ventilations were started. The newborn infant began crying at 4 min and remained alert and spontaneously breathing during transport. The parent was hospitalized for 1 day, and their son remained in the hospital for 3 days to treat elevated bilirubin levels.

CASE STUDY 3

The newborn infant is in acute distress and needs immediate intervention. Thoroughly dry the newborn infant, position them on their back, tie or clamp the umbilical cord at 3 inches and 4 inches from the newborn infant, and cut it in between the clamps. Quickly begin bag-mask ventilation at 30 to 60 breaths/min and observe for chest rise. After 30 seconds of assisted ventilation, assess the heart rate. If the heart rate is <60 beats/min, ensure you are providing effective bag-mask ventilation and the chest is rising. If this is not the case, then improve your bag-mask ventilation. If despite improved bag-mask ventilation the heart rate remains <60 beats/min, then place a supraglottic airway; if that is not available, prepare to intubate. If you are unable to intubate, then begin chest compression and increase oxygen delivery to 100% FiO_2. Chest compressions should be alternated with ventilation at a 1 ventilation–to–3 compressions ratio (90 compressions and 30 breaths/min with 100% oxygen). Administer 3 compressions followed by 1 bag-mask ventilation. Optimal cardiopulmonary resuscitation requires 3 individuals: 1 to assist ventilation, 1 to administer chest compressions, and 1 to prepare for intubation and possible administration of epinephrine. If only 2 EMS clinicians are present, as is frequently the case, get help from another adult to perform chest compressions if possible.

If the heart rate remains <60 beats/min despite 60 seconds of chest compressions coordinated with ventilation, epinephrine may be administered. Epinephrine 0.1 mg/mL concentration (1 mg/10 mL) can be administered at a dose of 0.02 mg/kg (0.2 mL/kg) via IV or IO. The endotracheal dose is 0.1 mg/kg (1 mL/kg). Chest compressions and ventilations should be continued, with epinephrine administered every 3 to 5 minutes, until the heart rate is >60 beats/min.

Although vascular access is not usually needed for newborn infant resuscitation, vascular access should be obtained when chest compressions are required or transport time is prolonged. Attempt an IV or IO line in transport. Check the serum glucose at 30 min after birth and treat with 10% dextrose in water at 2 mL/kg if the glucose is <40 mg/dL. Because further resuscitation may be necessary, secure the newborn infant to the stretcher and transport with continuous electrocardiographic and oxygen saturation monitoring. Consider transport to a facility with a neonatal intensive care unit, because this newborn infant is likely to need ongoing critical care.

The newborn infant was resuscitated on scene following 5 minutes of cardiopulmonary resuscitation. During transport, 10% dextrose in water was administered IO to treat a serum glucose level of 15 mg/dL. The infant was admitted to the neonatal intensive care unit for targeted temperature management for hypoxic ischemic encephalopathy and remained hospitalized for 4 weeks.

Suggested References

TEXTBOOKS

American Academy of Orthopaedic Surgeons. *Emergency Care and Transportation of the Sick and Injured.* 12th ed. Jones and Bartlett Learning; 2021

American Academy of Pediatrics, American Heart Association. *Textbook of Neonatal Resuscitation.* 9th ed. American Academy of Pediatrics; 2025

ARTICLES

Brenner A, Ker K, Shakur-Still H, Roberts I. Tranexamic acid for post-partum haemorrhage: what, who and when. *Best Pract Res Clin Obstet Gynaecol.* 2019;61:66–74. doi:10.1016/j.bpobgyn.2019.04.005

Committee Opinion No 689: Delivery of a newborn with meconium-stained amniotic fluid. *Obstet Gynecol.* 2017; 129(3):e33-e34. doi:10.1097/AOG.0000000000001950. Reaffirmed 2024

Euser AG, Cipolla MJ. Magnesium sulfate for the treatment of eclampsia: a brief review. *Stroke.* 2009;40(4):1169–1175. doi:10.1161/STROKEAHA.108.527788

Gregory ECW, Osterman MJK, Valenzuela CP. Changes in home births by race and Hispanic origin and state of residence of mother: United States, 2018-2019 and 2019-2020. *Natl Vital Stat Rep.* 2021;70(15):1–10. doi:10.15620/cdc:110853

Isayama T, Mildenhall L, Schmölzer GM, et al. International Liaison Committee on Resuscitation Newborn Life Support Task Force. The route, dose, and interval of epinephrine for neonatal resuscitation: a systematic review. *Pediatrics.* 2020;146(4):e20200586. doi:10.1542/peds.2020-0586

Leadford AE, Warren JB, Manasyan A, et al. Plastic bags for prevention of hypothermia in preterm and low birth weight infants. *Pediatrics.* 2013;132(1):e128–e134. doi:10.1542/peds.2012-2030

Lee HC, Strand ML, Finan E, et al. Part 5: Neonatal Resuscitation: 2025 American Heart Association and American Academy of Pediatrics Guidelines for Cardiopulmonary Resuscitation and Emergency Cardiovascular Care. *Pediatrics.* 2026;157(1): e2025074352. doi:10.1542/peds.2025-074352

Mateos Rodriguez AA, Benito Vellisca MAB. Management of eclampsia in the prehospital setting. *Emerg Med J.* 2007;24(7):504. doi:10.1136/emj.2007.047209

Roberts I, Brenner A, Shakur-Still H. Tranexamic acid for bleeding: much more than a treatment for postpartum hemorrhage. *Am J Obstet Gynecol MFM.* 2023; 5(2 suppl):100722. doi:10.1016/j.ajogmf.2022.100722

Vali P, Weiner GM, Sankaran D, Lakshminrusimha S. What is the optimal initial dose of epinephrine during neonatal resuscitation in the delivery room? *J Perinatol.* 2021;41(7):1769–1773. doi:10.1038/s41372-021-01032-7

OTHER RESOURCES

Centers for Disease Control and Prevention. Congenital heart defects (CHDs): data and statistics. Accessed June 20, 2025. https://www.cdc.gov/heart-defects/data/index.html

Oyelese Y, Ananth CV. Acute placental abruption: management and long-term prognosis. *Up to Date.* Accessed June 20, 2025. https://www.uptodate.com/contents/acute-placental-abruption-management-and-long-term-prognosis

CHAPTER 15

Sudden Unexpected Infant Death, Brief Resolved Unexpected Event, & Death of a Child

Rehman Chowdhry, MD, FAAP
Aaron Bates, NRP

LEARNING OBJECTIVES

1. **Describe the common clinical presentations and risk factors for sudden unexpected infant death (SUID).**
2. **Discuss the actions of the emergency medical services (EMS) clinician in the setting of suspected SUID.**
3. **Define a BRUE, and discuss assessment, management, and transport considerations.**
4. **Recognize responses of the family to the death of an infant or a child.**
5. **Recognize emotional responses of EMS clinicians to the death of an infant or a child.**
6. **List community resources for support after the unexpected death of an infant or a child.**

Introduction

The death of a child is an extremely difficult, emotional experience for the emergency medical services (EMS) clinician. **Sudden unexpected infant death (SUID)** was the fourth leading cause of death in infants between 1 month and 1 year of age in 2024 in the United States. Like other causes of infant mortality, rates of SUID are disproportionately higher in non-Hispanic Black and indigenous populations compared to non-Hispanic White infants.

The death of an infant or a child is an unparalleled event that creates emotional trauma for the primary caregivers, as well as the EMS clinician. These events occur at variable locations (home vs friend or relatives) under different circumstances and with different care providers (parent, babysitter, child care facility). Absence of the primary caregiver(s) may complicate field management and interactions at the scene.

DEFINITION OF SUID

Sudden unexpected infant death is the unanticipated death of an infant younger than 1 year whose cause of death is not immediately obvious before investigation. The Centers for Disease Control and Prevention (CDC) defines sudden infant death syndrome (SIDS) as "the sudden death of an infant <1 year that cannot be explained after a thorough investigation, including a complete autopsy, examination of the death scene, and review of the clinical history."

Sudden unexpected infant death is a broader term, encompassing SIDS, accidental suffocation, and infant death from unknown causes. Therefore, SUID is the preferred terminology for EMS clinicians and emergency department (ED) use in unanticipated out-of-hospital infant deaths.

SUID Epidemiology

Sudden unexpected infant death is the fourth leading cause of death in infants aged 1 month to 1 year. A report published by the CDC in 2022 demonstrated that 41.5% of SUID cases were due to SIDS, 28.1% were due to accidental suffocation/strangulation in bed, and in 30.5% of cases, the cause was unknown. Published reports suggest that environmental and socioeconomic factors, including low income, crowded living conditions, and use of drugs and/or alcohol, may increase the risk of SIDS and SUID.

The medical examiner can sometimes identify a specific illness or injury as the cause of SUID. Unfortunately, the cause is sometimes child maltreatment, as discussed in Chapter 13. It is not the EMS clinician's job to determine the actual cause of death. Treat every caregiver with compassion for their grief. *Never discuss child maltreatment as a possible cause of death while on scene*. To help identify deaths that may not be from natural causes, the EMS clinician can note details of the death scene and record observations in the patient-care report. For example, dangerous or unclean home conditions, bruises or burn marks on the child's body, or a changing or implausible story may raise red flags for child maltreatment that require further investigation, as discussed in Chapter 13.

Key information about the mechanism of suffocation includes co-sleeping (adults and infants sharing a bed), soft bedding, and wedging or entrapment of the infant between 2 objects (eg, bed and wall). Information provided by EMS clinicians can assist in the later determination of the cause of death, so the scene survey and thorough documentation of findings are imperative.

TIP

Sudden unexpected infant death is the second leading cause of infant death from age 1 month to 1 year.

A thorough scene survey by the EMS clinician describing the location and position of the child can assist forensic reviewers in the determination of the cause of death.

CAUTION

Do not discuss child maltreatment as a possible cause of death on the scene.

Common Clinical Presentation of SUID

When evaluating an unresponsive infant, a thorough scene assessment is imperative. The EMS clinician should be prepared for a variable range of emotions—including the potential for hostility—from individuals present at the scene, especially family members. Given the profound nature of the unexpected death of an infant, the EMS clinician must constantly survey the scene for hazards.

In the setting of SUID, the infant will be unresponsive, pulseless, and apneic on arrival, and cardiopulmonary resuscitation (CPR) may be in progress. The EMS clinician should evaluate central pulses. Pupils may be fixed and dilated. The advanced life support (ALS) EMS clinician will also note asystole on the cardiorespiratory electrocardiogram (ECG) monitor, which should be confirmed in a minimum of 2 leads. Additional ECG strips may be required to hand over to the coroner/medical examiner. Along with the signs described previously, the EMS clinician may note lividity or rigor mortis. Lividity is reddish-blue mottling, caused by venous pooling, noted on the face and the dependent portion of the body. **TABLE 15-1** describes the clinical appearance of infants who died of SUID. These signs may differ depending on how long the infant has been dead, and some cases of SUID do not involve any of these signs.

TABLE 15-1 External Appearance of Infants Who Died of SUID

Cold skin
Frothy or blood-tinged fluid in the mouth and nose
Lividity or dark, reddish-blue mottling on the dependent side of the body
Rigor mortis
Vomitus (uncommon)
Normal hydration and nutrition

Abbreviation: SUID, sudden unexpected infant death.

CASE STUDY 1

You are dispatched for an infant who is not breathing. On arrival, you find a 4-month-old boy in his mother's arms, with dark purplish bruising on his face and chest. He has pink frothy sputum around his mouth and nose, and he is cold, pulseless, and apneic. His arms and jaw are stiff. His mother is weeping. "I think he is dead."

1. Is this a SUID death?
2. What can you do to assist the family with the death of their child?

A comprehensive assessment of environmental factors by the EMS clinician is part of a thorough scene survey. This includes, but is not limited to, how the baby was typically positioned during sleep (on their back, on their side, or prone). Note where the baby was sleeping, and whether another person was co-sleeping with the child. Note unusual conditions such as high or low room temperature or odors. Note whether there is any bodily fluid or other debris on or around the child or on the bedding.

TIP

The typical SUID scenario is an apparently healthy infant, younger than 1 year, who is found dead in their bed after having been seen alive a short time before.

TABLE 15–2 Key Questions in Focused History Taking in Sudden Unexplained Infant Death

What happened?
Who found the infant and where?
What did the caregiver do?
Has the infant been moved?
What time was the infant last seen alive?
Had the infant been sick?
Was the infant receiving any medications?

*When asking these questions, use the infant's name rather than "the infant."

The EMS clinician should note the time the infant was found, the position in which the infant was found, and the last time the infant was known to be responsive by the caregivers. Count the number of pillows and plush toys in the sleeping quarters. The EMS clinician should also note if the infant had a blanket over their head or if there was soft or loose bedding.

Get a focused history at the scene if the child is not transported to the ED. Be careful to avoid judgmental or leading questions. **TABLE 15–2** gives examples of key questions to ask. Always ask the baby's name at the beginning of the interview. Using the baby's first name in discussions with the caregiver is extremely helpful during these stressful encounters.

A thorough history is important for identifying potential causes of the infant's death. The EMS clinician should pay close attention to the patient's medical history, which may include recent illnesses, potential birth defects, or any other complications. When possible, the infant's prenatal history and the maternal gestational history should also be noted in detail.

CAUTION

Avoid asking judgmental or leading questions that suggest the caregiver may be at fault for the infant's death.

Actions in Suspected SUID

The EMS clinician's first actions when SUID is suspected must always be to assess and treat the baby. If the child is in cardiac arrest, begin resuscitation if indicated, using local treatment protocols consistent with the American Heart Association Guidelines. However, in many SUID cases, the infant has easily recognizable signs of death that meet local EMS system criteria for determination of death in the field. If resuscitation is indicated, encourage the family to remain present during the resuscitative attempt, whenever possible. Should the infant or child respond to resuscitative measures, transport as soon as medically appropriate, as discussed in Chapter 18.

TIP

In all cases of cardiopulmonary arrest, immediately begin resuscitation using standard treatment protocol, unless the infant meets local EMS criteria for death in the field.

TABLE 15–3 Pros and Cons of Transporting Infants Suspected of Dying of SUID

Pros	Cons
ALS capability in ED	Caregiver concern about infant's body
Facilitation of autopsy	Disruption of scene investigation by medical examiner
More medical personnel to manage infant and caregivers	High costs in dollars, personnel, and equipment
Physician involvement in management	Possible violation of family's culture
Abiility to conduct religious services	Removal of family from familiar setting
Social services for grief counseling	Transport liabilities, especially ambulance crashes and adverse bystander reactions

Abbreviations: ALS, advanced life support; ED, emergency department; SUID, sudden unexpected infant death.

If the infant has recognizable signs of death such that resuscitation is considered to be futile on the EMS clinician's arrival at the scene or if the initial response to CPR is unsuccessful, it may be appropriate to halt life-saving measures and allow the coroner or medical examiner to facilitate the death investigation at the scene. In such a case, the EMS clinician should not leave the scene after a child has died until appropriate authorities have arrived. Notify medical oversight when there is uncertainty about treatment or transport. **TABLE 15–3** lists the pros and cons of transporting infants suspected of having died of SUID. Because the EMS clinician cannot distinguish a child with SUID from any other child in cardiopulmonary arrest, use standard principles of treatment and transport for children in cardiopulmonary arrest, as discussed in Chapter 5.

ALS

The value of immediate or delayed hospital transport when a child does not respond to resuscitation is controversial. The chances of neurological survival of a child in the ED after failed ALS resuscitation in the field are almost zero, unless rare extenuating circumstances (eg, profound hypothermia, barbiturate overdose) are present.

Sometimes, the child meets the EMS system's criteria for death in the field or resuscitation is not successful, but grief counseling is not available at the scene. In this situation, consider transporting the baby to the hospital in a controlled transport mode (no lights or siren) with the caregiver, if possible. Transporting with lights and siren is the most dangerous transport that EMS clinicians perform, and successful resuscitation on prompt transport for pulseless infants after failed ALS is extremely rare. The risks generally outweigh the benefits of lights-and-siren transport. Allow the caregiver to touch or hold the child before transport. This may be the last time the caregiver is able to be with the child. This may not be possible if the scene is related to a crime, but it can be helpful in the grieving process.

TIP

Encourage the family to be present during the attempted resuscitation.

The EMS clinician's emotional support for the caregivers is extremely important. When possible, have one person stay with the caregiver to provide information and support. Let family or caregivers stay with the child and do not separate them, even during attempted resuscitation and transport. If the family chooses to ride with the patient, ensure that they remain restrained with a seat belt according to the manufacturer's recommendations and local protocols. *Be clear that the child is dead.* Do not use euphemisms such as "Your child has left us" or "They have gone to a better place." Well-intentioned but inappropriate remarks such as "You can always have other children," "I know how you feel," or "You will get over this in time" should be avoided. **TABLE 15–4** suggests

TABLE 15–4 Communicating About an Unexpected Death of a Child

Use the child's name.
Show **empathy** and express condolences.
Ask questions in a nonjudgmental manner. Never become hostile or angry.
Use a calm and directive voice.
Be clear with instructions and answers to questions.
Provide explanations to the caregivers about treatment and transport.
Repeat statements when necessary.
Avoid well-intentioned but inappropriate remarks.
Allow the caregiver to accompany the baby if possible.

specific ways to communicate with caregivers when there is an unexpected death of a child.

It is vital that EMS clinicians create a clear picture of the events that occurred through their documentation, which should be as objective as possible. Any pertinent statements made at the scene should be captured with quotation marks when possible. This patient-care report should be extremely detailed and include dispatch information, a scene assessment, a thorough head-to-toe assessment, interventions, response to interventions, transport decision and reasoning, and transfer of care. Also note any communication that occurs with the family, coroner, law enforcement, medical control, or any other entity involved. Inadequate documentation can create significant difficulty later on and possibly affect the determination of the cause of death. The SUID Investigation Reporting Form is a template freely available from the CDC to guide documentation in these cases.

COMMUNITY OUTREACH AND RISK REDUCTION ACTIVITIES

Aside from providing high-quality care when in service, EMS clinicians can also play a key role in community outreach by educating parents in ways to decrease the risk of SUID. This includes active support of the American Academy of Pediatrics (AAP) recommendation to place infants on their backs to sleep. Although side sleeping is several times safer than prone sleeping, the risk of SUID for the side sleeping position is still double the risk for the supine position. EMS clinicians can participate in community risk reduction by advocating for firm, flat mattresses in safety-approved cribs and avoidance of soft or bulky blankets or comforters and overheating in the infant's sleeping area. Recommendations for reducing the risk of SUID are presented in **TABLE 15–5**.

Support of antismoking campaigns is important. Recent research shows that the risk of SUID doubles among infants exposed to cigarette smoke after birth and triples for those exposed both during pregnancy and after birth.

CAUTION

Use clear, unambiguous language when discussing the death of the child with the family.

EMS clinicians can also become involved in local or state child fatality review teams. These teams meet to discuss the community trends in infant and child deaths. They often review all sudden and unexpected deaths in children younger than 2 years to improve the accuracy of SUID as a diagnosis versus other natural and nonnatural causes, especially child maltreatment.

TABLE 15–5 Recommendations for Reducing the Risk of SUID

Always place the baby on their back to sleep.
Always place the baby on a firm sleeping surface.
Keep any objects that could increase the risk of entrapment, suffocation, or strangulation out of the crib. This includes soft objects, loose bedding, pillows, blankets, and bumper pads.
Place the baby to sleep in the same room where you sleep, but not in the same bed.
Breastfeeding is strongly encouraged.
Schedule and complete all well-child visits.
Keep the baby away from smokers and places where people smoke.
Do not let the baby become too hot.
Offer a pacifier at naptime and bedtime.
Do not use home cardiorespiratory monitors to help reduce the risk of SUID.
Do not use products that claim to reduce the risk of SUID, such as wedges and positioners.

Abbreviation: SUID, sudden unexpected infant death.

Summary of SUID

Sudden unexpected infant death is the fourth most common cause of infant death. Determining the cause of death requires an autopsy. The EMS clinician cannot "diagnose" SUID in the field, and the emergency physician cannot diagnose SUID in the ED. There are, however, common clinical signs and important risk factors that may be helpful in identifying probable SUID cases.

When faced with an infant in cardiopulmonary arrest, begin, continue, or cease CPR according to the local EMS system policies. In some EMS systems, policy permits withholding or discontinuing resuscitation and focusing on the important tasks of talking to the family and helping them with their grief. **FIGURE 15–1** provides a typical sequence of events when there is a suspected SUID case. **TABLE 15–6** lists the responsibilities of the coroner, medical examiner, and local health department in a case of suspected SUID.

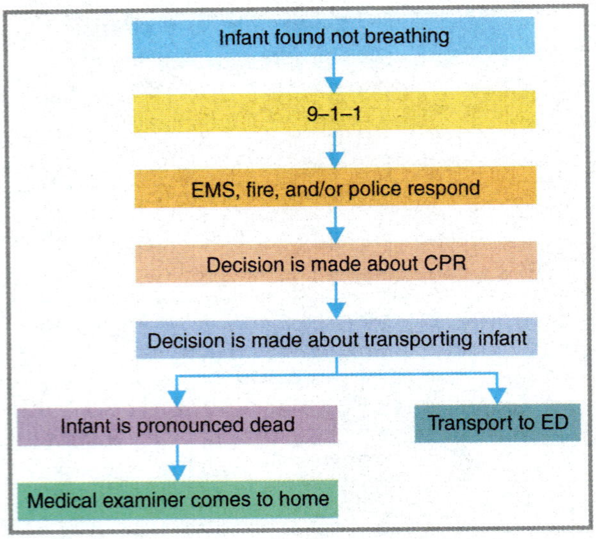

FIGURE 15–1 Flowchart of what to do in suspected SUID cases.

TABLE 15–6 Medical Examiner/Coroner and Local Health Department Responsibilities in Suspected SUID Cases

Medical Examiner/ Coroner Responsibilities	Local Health Department Responsibilities
Performs death scene investigation	Provides information and counseling
Performs autopsy	Provides referral information for peer support
Notifies local health department	Provides information to state program
Notifies state program	Performs periodic follow-up
Signs death certificate	Provides community education (with peer group)
Notifies parents of cause of death	

Abbreviation: SUID, sudden unexpected infant death.

DEFINITION OF BRIEF RESOLVED UNEXPLAINED EVENT

Formerly called an apparent life-threatening event (ALTE), a brief resolved unexplained event (BRUE) is an episode in a patient younger than 1 year characterized by at least one of the following: (1) cyanosis or pallor; (2) absent, decreased, or irregular breathing; (3) marked change in tone (hypertonia or hypotonia); or (4) altered level of responsiveness. In some cases, the observer fears that the infant has died, and the call may initially be dispatched as a cardiac arrest. Avoid terminology such as *apparent life-threatening event*, *aborted crib death*, or *near-miss SIDS* to reduce confusion between BRUEs and SUID.

TIP

Brief resolved unexplained event is defined as a sudden, brief, and now resolved episode that includes one or more of the following features: (1) cyanosis or pallor; (2) absent, decreased, or irregular breathing; (3) change in tone; or (4) altered level of consciousness.

CAUTION

Use only the term brief resolved unexpected event to describe infants with transient events of color change, breathing irregularity, or unresponsiveness. Using the term apparent life-threatening event (ALTE) is not accurate or appropriate. Terms such as ALTE or near-miss sudden infant death syndrome are misleading and frightening.

Common Clinical Presentation of BRUEs

Similar to SUID, BRUEs generally present with a stressful scene. A thorough scene assessment should be performed when evaluating scene safety. Primary assessment begins with the Pediatric Assessment Triangle, noting the patient's appearance, breathing, and circulation. The EMS clinician should assess airway patency and evaluate breathing, including rate, depth, and quality. Circulation should be assessed by palpating pulses for rate, regularity, and quality; assessing capillary refill; and assessing skin color, temperature, and condition. In infants, this is best done by palpating the brachial pulses.

A thorough history should be assessed using the SAMPLE mnemonic (refer to Chapter 1, Table 1–10). Attempt to establish a timeline of the event and anything that made the patient's symptoms better or worse. The baby's entire medical history is pertinent. This includes any medications the baby is taking and, for breastfed babies, any medication the nursing parent is taking. Identifying the time of the infant's last feeding and the events leading up to the BRUE may help point toward a potential diagnosis.

Vital signs (heart rate, respiratory rate, pulse oximetry) and blood glucose levels should be assessed in all patients with suspected BRUE. A thorough head-to-toe assessment should be performed, and any abnormalities should be noted.

Actions in Suspected BRUEs

CLINICAL INTERVENTIONS

Most BRUEs resolve before arrival of EMS clinicians, and it is common for an initial assessment to be unremarkable (**FIGURE 15–2**). *Do not* be misled by the normal appearance of the patient. The caregiver may imply that an evaluation is no longer needed because the child is fine. The EMS clinician should be clear that BRUE can be a sentinel event for an underlying issue, and an evaluation at an ED or a hospital is necessary. Serious illnesses in newborn and young infants may be intermittent and/or subtle, making detection difficult. **TABLE 15–7** lists many of the potential causes of BRUEs.

If the child's condition appears to be unstable or the child needs urgent treatment, complete the assessment en route to the hospital. The EMS clinician should pay attention to and protect the patient's airway. Supplemental oxygen should be provided if the child has an altered mental status, respiratory distress, or hypoxia. Provide assisted ventilations early if indicated. The ALS provider should be prepared to obtain intravenous access and provide fluid resuscitation or cardiac medications if indicated. The infant must be transported to an ED even if the complete assessment reveals no abnormalities.

TIP

Every child with a reported BRUE must undergo evaluation in the ED or hospital for a potentially serious underlying problem.

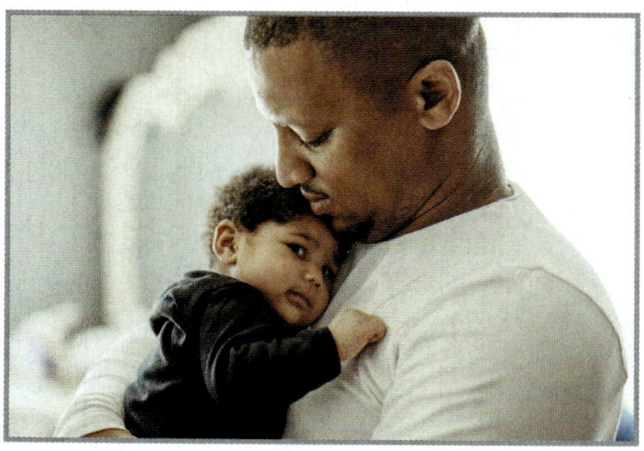

FIGURE 15–2 Most BRUEs resolve before arrival of EMS clinicians, and it is common for the infant to appear normal on assessment.

LumiNola/iStockphoto.com.

TABLE 15–7 Serious Conditions That May Present With BRUEs

Cardiac: Arrythmia, congenital heart disease, cardiomyopathy or myocarditis
Child maltreatment: Abusive head trauma, purposeful suffocation, poisoning
Gastrointestinal: Gastrointestinal reflux disease (GERD), dysphagia, tracheoesophageal fistula
Genetic conditions: Inborn errors of metabolism, hypoglycemia
Hematologic: Anemia
Infections: Sepsis, meningitis, pneumonia, urinary tract infection, respiratory viruses (eg, RSV), pertussis
Neurologic: Seizure, structural brain abnormalities, progressive neurologic disease, infantile spasms
Pulmonary: Upper or lower airway obstruction, congenital central hypoventilation syndrome, pneumonia, aspiration pneumonitis

Abbreviations: BRUE, brief resolved unexplained event; RSV, respiratory syncytial virus.

Summary of BRUE

A BRUE is a special clinical condition of infants involving a sudden and transient change in appearance, respiratory effort, or perfusion. Examples of BRUE presentations include sudden loss of muscle tone, cyanosis, or cessation of breathing. Although sometimes no cause is found despite hospital workup, a BRUE may be an indicator of serious **occult illness** or injury that cannot be diagnosed in the field. Perform a standard assessment and treat any demonstrable physiological or anatomical problems. In most cases, transport alone is the most important field intervention.

RESPONSES TO AN INFANT'S DEATH

Caregiver's Response

The EMS clinician is often the first medical responder on the scene following the discovery of an infant who has died. Responses of the caregiver to the sudden and unexpected death of an infant are not predictable and may vary from numb silence to rage. Common reactions include denial, anger, hysteria, withdrawal, intense guilt, or no visible response. The caregiver may or may not accept that the infant is dead and that resuscitation is not possible. The caregiver may cling to the hope that the EMS clinician can do something to save the infant, even though the child is obviously dead.

The death of a child is likely the most stressful and tragic event in the life of a parent or caregiver. It is not uncommon for caregivers in this situation to make "demands" of the EMS clinician. Remember, this is the individual's last chance to fulfill their role as protector and caregiver for the infant. Respond to the caregiver gently and professionally. The caregiver may do any of the following:

- Ask repeated questions
- Request that you not start care or that you stop resuscitation efforts
- Request to be alone with the infant
- Want to know the cause of death
- Physically interfere with care
- Insist on continuation of care or that resuscitation efforts begin

TIP

Be prepared for a wide variation in, and unpredictability of, the caregiver's response to the sudden and unexpected death of an infant or a child. Reactions may vary from numb silence to rage.

The EMS clinician may have unrealistic expectations regarding how the caregiver should behave and respond or may believe that the caregiver was responsible for the baby's death. These feelings can become obstacles to communication, as outlined in **TABLE 15–8**. When the caregiver or family expresses their preferences or asks difficult questions, use a calm and professional approach. Keep explanations simple. Be honest and direct with family members. Follow EMS system protocol for death in the field and maintain an empathetic and nonjudgmental attitude.

TABLE 15–8 Responses of EMS Clinicians That Hinder Communication With Caregivers After an Unexpected Death

Having stereotyped expectations of how the caregiver should respond to the event
Judging a caregiver who did not initiate CPR
Distrusting a caregiver who has recognized the infant is dead and does not want resuscitation
Misunderstanding the mourning and grief behaviors of persons of different cultures or religious beliefs

Abbreviations: CPR, cardiopulmonary resuscitation; EMS, emergency medical services.

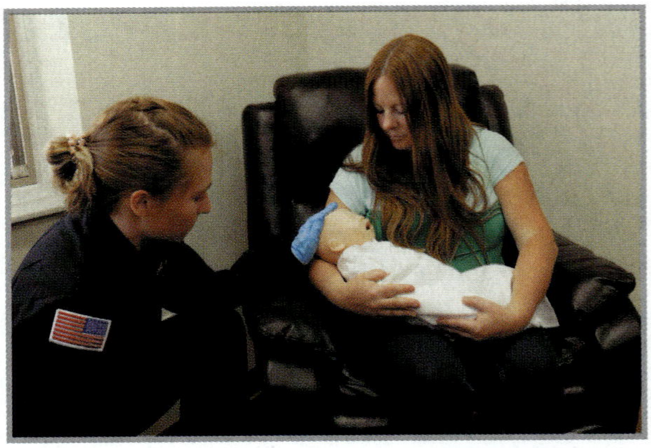

FIGURE 15–3 Caregivers can react to the death of a child in many ways, but all need support. Attempt to contact identified individuals who might provide comfort.

Allow room for the family to grieve. Be respectful of the family's religious beliefs, customs, or traditions.

If there is no indication to attempt resuscitation, while awaiting arrival of the medical examiner or coroner at the scene, ask the family member or caregiver if someone can be called to give them additional support (**FIGURE 15–3**). This may be friends, relatives, clergy, or public agencies to help care for other children or pets in the home. If the scene is a child care setting, inclusion of law enforcement may be necessary to assist with other children and to contact the child's caregivers or the caregivers of other children present.

EMS Clinician's Response

The EMS clinician has a difficult and sometimes agonizing role in the setting of an unexpected death of an infant or a child. After death is declared, comfort the parents. Never place blame on the parents or caregivers. Offering compassionate support to the family and gathering accurate information in a nonthreatening manner can help family members. This is often challenging, because the EMS clinician may be struggling with overwhelming emotional responses related to the loss of a patient.

Sometimes there are cultural or language differences between the EMS clinician and the caregiver. There may be unfamiliar rituals and behaviors pertaining to how death is regarded or how grief is expressed. This presents another important challenge. *Respect cultural diversity. This is necessary to communicate effectively.* When cultural or language differences arise, attempt to find an interpreter to explain and translate.

CASE STUDY 2

You are called to an apartment complex that is home to a large number of immigrant families. On arrival, there is a large, agitated group congregated at the doorway to the apartment, speaking in a language that you do not understand. You enter the apartment to find a mother and father sitting on a couch, quietly weeping. They gesture toward a bassinet, where a stiff, cold 3-month-old infant with dependent lividity lies covered in a pile of blankets. Through a neighbor who speaks English, you explain that the baby is dead and ask if they would like to hold her. They decline and seem offended by the proposal.

1. How should you react?
2. What steps do you take from this point?

Talking to the family or caregivers can be difficult. However, there are techniques that may improve the quality of these interactions:

- Use the child's name. This acknowledges the child as an individual rather than a "patient" and the unique, intensely personal nature of this child's death.
- Try to find a quiet area to talk to the caregivers. Often, the scene becomes noisy with activity. Finding an area where the caregiver can concentrate on your conversation helps to keep your message clear.
- Use concrete terms. The use of euphemisms to soften the news can make it harder for the caregiver to understand what has happened. "Your child has died" has a definite meaning, whereas "Your child is in a better place" has infinite possibilities (the hospital is a better place).
- It is okay to show emotion. Parents whose child has died often comment on how meaningful it was to them that a health care provider clearly was concerned. Expressing your emotions is appropriate in such tragic circumstances, so long as the focus remains on the family and child, and you are able to fulfill your professional duties at the scene.

TIP
Ask the name of the child and use it in discussions with the caregiver.

The EMS clinician's responses to the sudden and unexpected death of an infant may include one or more of the following:

- Anger or blame
- Identification with the caregiver
- Withdrawal
- Avoidance of the caregiver
- Self-doubt (if resuscitation is attempted and the child does not recover)
- Sadness and depression

TIP
The unexpected death of an infant or a child is one of the most stressful experiences for the EMS clinician.

CRITICAL INCIDENT STRESS MANAGEMENT

Stress is an unavoidable part of the EMS clinician's job. The death of a child may be the most stressful situation in the EMS clinician's career (**FIGURE 15–4**). The acknowledgment and processing of emotions is key to successfully coping with stress and maintaining a healthy mental attitude. **TABLE 15–9** lists the frequent signs and symptoms of stress.

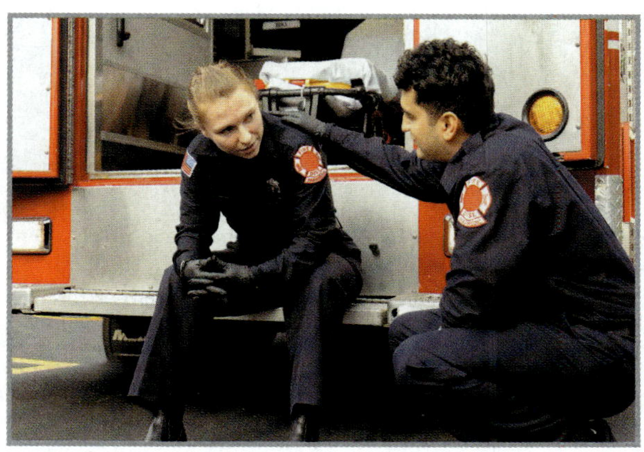

FIGURE 15–4 Stress is an unavoidable part of an EMS clinician's job. The death of a child can be agonizing.

TABLE 15–9 Signs and Symptoms of Critical Incident Stress

Anger and irritability
Changes in eating habits
Changes in sleeping patterns
Depression
Excessive alcohol consumption
Inability to concentrate
Mood changes and emotional instability
Physical illness
Recurring dreams or frightening images
Withdrawal

There are many ways to decrease the impact of stress related to the death of an infant or a child. Critical incident stress management (CISM) is an important technique that can be helpful for coping with the emotional toll of a sudden unexpected death of an infant or a child. Other techniques to help decrease stress include the following:

- Talk to field supervisors and experienced EMS clinicians to share feelings.
- Maintain a well-balanced lifestyle outside of work. Exercise, plan leisure time, and limit overtime hours.
- Get adequate rest and eat a balanced diet.
- Avoid excessive alcohol or drugs.
- Write a personal journal.
- Obtain religious or peer counseling.
- Request professional psychological assistance.

COMMUNITY RESOURCES

Community resources available to caregivers and EMS clinicians to help them cope with the unexpected death of a child include the following:

- Local support groups
- Local public health departments
- First Candle/SIDS Alliance (1-800-221-SIDS)
- American SIDS Institute (https://sids.org)
- Professional counseling
- Emergency services chaplain

TIP

CISM is an important technique that can be helpful in coping with the emotional toll of a sudden unexpected death of an infant or a child.

CONTROVERSY

The value and appropriate timing of CISM are not known. Although the EMS clinician experiences predictable stress after the death of a child in their care, how and when such intervention should take place has not been studied.

CONTROVERSY

Risk reduction and risk counseling are important community prevention activities. Further research must be conducted to help define the appropriate educational role of the EMS clinician at the scene of an injury or a death.

TIP

EMS clinicians can play a key role in educating parents in the community on ways to decrease the risk of SUID.

CASE STUDY 3

You are dispatched to a coworker's home where a grandmother is weeping and largely incoherent. She leads you to a bedroom where a 3-month-old boy lies motionless in his crib, face down on a sheepskin. He is apneic and pulseless, has lividity on his chest and face, and is stiff. In between sobs, the grandmother tells you she put the baby to sleep 4 hours ago and found him this way when she checked on him 10 minutes ago. She asks you if he is dead.

1. What are your key medical actions?
2. How should you deal with the grandmother? The coworker?

CASE STUDY ANSWERS

CASE STUDY 1

The infant has many findings commonly associated with a SUID death. Sleeping prone (indicated by the lividity on the chest and face), the pink frothy sputum, and the absence of traumatic injuries are the initial clues to a SUID death. However, remember that SUID is a diagnosis of exclusion made by a medical examiner or coroner at autopsy and cannot be made in the field.

In this setting, provide a direct and calm explanation to the parent that the child is dead. Find out the child's name and use it. Do not ask questions in a way that suggests blame. Use controlled and supportive language with the parent. If the child is not transported, try to obtain grief counseling for the parent, contact the medical examiner or coroner from the scene, and consider CISM for yourself and your partner. Gather family support resources.

CASE STUDY 2

Different cultures have different beliefs about death, afterlife, and the proper handling of a dead body. There may be rituals or taboos with which you are unfamiliar, and different ways of coping with loss. Because there is no medical intervention that will help this child, your focus must be on providing support to the survivors. Obtaining a professional interpreter, where available, is an important aspect of the scene management and death investigation. Through an English-speaking neighbor, you can inquire about family needs, whom they might want you to contact, and any way that you might assist them at the scene. Remember that even with an interpreter present, concepts may be difficult to translate and the family may have a very different belief system from yours with regard to illness, health care, and cause of death. If you cannot communicate the rationale for your treatment or nontreatment to the family, transport.

CASE STUDY 3

In most EMS systems, this child would meet criteria for death in the field and would not require any resuscitation attempt. If you are uncertain about whether resuscitation is indicated, begin CPR and call medical oversight to clarify treatment options.

The grandmother may need to be medically evaluated if she cannot be calmed down. Provide a calm and controlled environment. Do not place blame.

Try to minimize radio communications if your coworker may be listening. If the employee is at work, have a supervisor contact the coworker and provide safe transportation to the scene. Contact other family members, friends, or clergy if the situation warrants. Watch for symptoms consistent with that of critical incident stress and initiate CISM if indicated.

Suggested References

ARTICLES

Goldstein RD, Trachtenberg FL, Sens MA, Harty BJ, Kinney HC. Overall postneonatal mortality and rates of SIDS. *Pediatrics*. 2016;137(1):e20152298. PMID: 26634772 doi: 10.1542/peds.2015-2298

Merritt JL II, Quinonez RA, Bonkowsky JL, et al. A framework for evaluation of the higher-risk infant after a brief resolved unexplained event. *Pediatrics*. 2019;144(2):e20184101. PMID: 31350360 doi: 10.1542/peds.2018-4101

Moon RY, Carlin RF, Hand I; American Academy of Pediatrics Task Force on Sudden Infant Death Syndrome and Committee on Fetus and Newborn. Sleep-related infant deaths: updated 2022 recommendations for reducing infant deaths in the sleep environment. *Pediatrics*. 2022;150(1):e2022057990. PMID: 35726558 doi: 10.1542/peds.2022-057990

Parks SE, Erck Lambert AB, Hauck FR, Cottengim CR, Faulkner M, Shapiro-Mendoza CK. Explaining sudden unexpected infant deaths, 2011–2017. *Pediatrics*. 2021;147(5):e2020035873. PMID: 33906930 doi: 10.1542/peds.2020-035873

Shapiro-Mendoza CK, Camperlengo L, Ludvigsen R, et al. Classification system for the sudden unexpected infant death case registry and its application. *Pediatrics*. 2014;134(1):e210–e219. PMID: 24913798 doi: 10.1542/peds.2014-0180

Tieder JS, Bonkowsky JL, Etzel RA, et al. Clinical Practice Guideline: brief resolved unexplained events (formerly apparent life-threatening events) and evaluation of lower-risk infants. *Pediatrics*. 2016;137(5):e20160590. PMID: 27474014 doi: 10.1542/peds.2016-0590

OTHER RESOURCES

Centers for Disease Control and Prevention. Sudden unexpected infant death and sudden infant death syndrome. Accessed April 12, 2025. https://www.cdc.gov/sudden-infant-death/?CDC_AAref_Val=https://www.cdc.gov/sids/index.htm

Centers for Disease Control and Prevention. SUID Investigation Reporting Forms. September 17, 2024. https://www.cdc.gov/sudden-infant-death/php/suidrf/?CDC_AAref_Val=https://www.cdc.gov/sids/SUIDRF.htm

Centers for Disease Control and Prevention. Trends in SUID Rates by Cause of Death 1990–2022. September 17, 2024. https://www.cdc.gov/sudden-infant-death/data-research/data/sids-deaths-by-cause.html#toc

Department of Health and Human Services, Center for Disease Control and Prevention, National Center for Health Statistics. National Vital Statistics System. National Vital Statistics Rapid Release. Accessed January 7, 2026. https://cdc.gov/nchs/nvss/vsrr/infant-mortality-dashboard

CHAPTER 16

Children in Disasters

Debra L. Bell, MS, CCEMTP, EMT-T, NJ-CEM
Claire Gahm, MD, MPH, FAAP

LEARNING OBJECTIVES

1. **Define disaster and mass-casualty incident, and list the phases of disaster response.**
2. **Discuss the modifications of the triage systems used by EMS clinicians to accommodate the special needs of children during disasters and mass-casualty incidents.**
3. **Discuss the role of EMS in managing pediatric patients during both manmade and natural disasters.**
4. **Recognize the anatomical, physiological, and psychological features specific to children that increase their vulnerability and place them at special risk when disasters occur.**
5. **Identify specific actions that emergency medical services (EMS) agencies can take to enhance pediatric-focused disaster preparedness.**
6. **Recognize the importance of critical incident stress management in supporting EMS personnel exposed to traumatic pediatric cases.**

Children in Disasters

Disasters occur with little or no warning and can have devastating effects on communities. Children are particularly vulnerable during these events because of their physiological, emotional, and developmental needs. Effective disaster preparedness requires a comprehensive understanding of how to respond to mass casualty events, including school shootings, and how to provide appropriate care for pediatric patients. Despite the limited data on pediatric injuries and illnesses during disasters, it is clear that thorough planning and preparation are imperative. This chapter focuses on the importance of pediatric disaster preparedness and the role of emergency medical services (EMS) agencies in improving outcomes for children in crises.

What Is a Disaster?

Disasters pose a significant local impact but also may have a countywide, statewide, or regional impact. The definition of a disaster varies by the size and location of the event. For example, a bus crash in a large city will not have that much of an impact on its EMS system, but the same incident in a small, rural town may exceed the response capabilities. Therefore, a disaster is an event or a series of events that overwhelms the capabilities of the local emergency system and its mutual aid agreements.

Disasters disrupt normal community functioning and threaten citizen safety. Because the US emergency care system primarily addresses adult needs, the infrastructure for managing pediatric care during disasters is often inadequate, with fewer hospital beds and specialists trained in pediatric critical illness and injury.

There are 2 types of disasters: natural and manmade. **TABLE 16–1** lists common examples.

TABLE 16–1 Common Natural and Manmade Disasters

Natural	Manmade
Earthquake	Hazardous material spill
Hurricane	Structural fire
Tornado	Biological exposure
Flood	Chemical exposure
Blizzard	Nuclear exposure
Wildland fire	Structural failure
Disease epidemic	Mass shooting

Natural disasters are events caused by environmental perturbations, such as earthquakes, severe storms, flooding, wildfires, and pandemics. Manmade disasters result from human errors such as toxic spills or structural collapses, or from malevolent intent such as terrorism or mass shootings. Regardless of their origin, disasters typically cause a significant increase in the incidence of pediatric injuries and illnesses.

What Is a Mass-Casualty Incident?

A mass-casualty incident (MCI) is a disaster event that overwhelms the local health care system in that the number of casualties vastly exceeds the local resources and capabilities in a short time. A lower-level MCI occurs when local medical resources are available and adequate, and regional backup resources may be put on alert. A moderate-level MCI requires multijurisdictional medical mutual aid. Mutual aid agreements should be in place to provide backup for jurisdictions stripped of their local resources. The highest-level MCI involves activation of the state disaster plan. Requests for federal assistance may be necessary.

In responding to an MCI, prehospital clinicians need to identify the type of MCI and be aware of the presence of pediatric patients. The categories of MCI include the following:

- Planned (sporting event, concert)
- Conventional (transportation incidents)
- Chemical, biological, radiological, nuclear, explosives
- Catastrophic (explosion, shooting, major earthquake, pandemic)

There are critical pediatric considerations in disasters and MCIs, including the lack of a universally accepted response and management plan for children. Each state and territory has its own regional oversight of EMS, leading to diverse operating procedures among first responders. This variability impacts the coordination of care, the implementation of pediatric management protocols, and the guidelines for interfacility transfers. When EMS systems are inadequately supplied for pediatric care or lack pediatric training resources, their ability to care for children in disasters is hindered.

Roles of the EMS Clinician in a Disaster

DISASTER PREPAREDNESS

EMS plays a crucial role in disaster preparedness and response. Before a disaster occurs, EMS professionals may assist with evacuations from hospitals, nursing homes, and skilled care facilities, as well as provide medical staffing for evacuation shelters. After an MCI occurs, they act as incident command on scene, perform search and rescue operations, conduct triage, provide medical care, and provide timely information to the public on response.

Effective planning and preparation is essential for success. Because pediatric calls are a small portion of EMS work (about 10% of 9-1-1 calls), the unique needs of children are often overlooked in disaster preparedness plans. To address this gap, it is vital to involve pediatric health care experts in the planning process.

> **TIP**
>
> The federal Administration for Strategic Response funded 3 Centers of Excellence (The Gulf-7 Pediatric Network, WRAP-EM, Region V for Kids) for pediatric disaster preparedness. They have subsequently formed the Pediatric Pandemic Network in conjunction with EMS-C (EMS for children) to improve national preparedness for children.

EMS agencies can support community preparedness by participating in local disaster planning and activities. With about 67 million children in schools or child care centers during the week and countless activities on the weekend, it is crucial to consider strategies that will mitigate the effect of disasters on children (**TABLE 16–2**). To meet this challenge, agencies can use resources and guidelines provided by the National Prehospital Pediatric Readiness Program and EMS for Children (EMS-C).

EMS-C is a federally funded program aimed at ensuring that children receive state-of-the-art care in an emergency through prehospital and in-hospital education, and development of pediatric protocols, guidelines, policy statements, and educational resources for the triage and treatment of children.

Incorporating Pediatric Scenarios Into Disaster Drills

- Scenario Development: Develop disaster scenarios that specifically address pediatric emergencies, such as school shootings, natural disasters, or chemical spills.

TABLE 16–2 Emergency Medical Services Preparedness Checklist

▪ Know your community's incident command system (ICS), when and how it is activated, and what your role is at a disaster or hostile event
▪ Plan responses to schools or buildings and become familiar with the various rooms, sports fields, and blueprints of a school campus
▪ Know which agencies take the lead in evacuation and the ICS for multijurisdictional disasters
▪ Be aware of children and youth with special health care needs in your area and the accommodations they require (ie, technology dependent)
▪ Identify a process for patient tracking
▪ Maintain the supply of pediatric supplies and be aware of the supply chain should a disaster hit that requires additional resources
▪ Be proficient in the agency's public information and outreach plans

- Child Actors: Use child actors to simulate pediatric patients during drills. This will help EMS clinicians practice their skills in a realistic setting.
- Pediatric Experts: Involve pediatric experts in the planning and execution of drills to ensure that the scenarios are realistic and that EMS clinicians are receiving appropriate training.
- Debriefing and Feedback: Conduct thorough debriefings after drills to identify areas for improvement and provide feedback to EMS clinicians.

Phases of Disaster Management

Disaster management can be divided into 4 phases. The first phase is preparedness activities, such as training before a disaster occurs. The response phase begins when a disaster occurs and includes initiation of the incident command system (ICS), scene assessment, search and rescue, triage, stabilization, and transport of the injured. This is followed by the recovery phase to restore normal operations and postincident debriefing functions. Finally, the mitigation phase takes lessons learned to guide activities to reduce the effects of future disasters (**FIGURE 16–1**).

OVERALL RESPONSE STRATEGY

Disasters can overwhelm EMS clinicians in the EMS system, necessitating activation of a response plan within a unified command structure. The National Incident Management System provides a scalable framework for coordinated responses among various agencies, ensuring integration of facilities, personnel, and communication. The goal is to maximize assistance for the greatest number of victims while maintaining efficient management of the event.

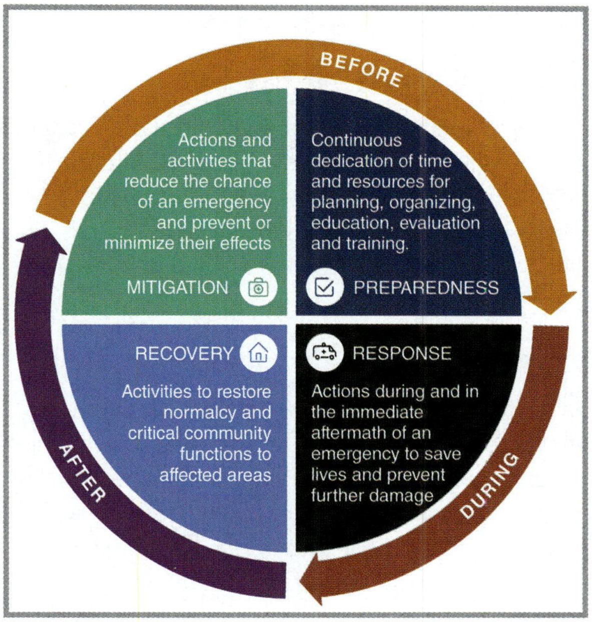

FIGURE 16–1 The disaster management cycle.

EMS clinicians must refrain from rushing on scene until it is deemed safe, to avoid the risk of becoming patients themselves. This task is even more daunting when children are involved, given the powerful impulse to help them. Appropriate safety gear and personal protective equipment (PPE) should be used on every call. Chemical, biological, and radiological incidents require specific and specialized equipment. Level C respiratory protection (a face mask with a canister filtration system) may be adequate for most conventional disasters; however, higher levels of protection may be required to meet the specific circumstances of the incident.

EMS clinicians must also exercise the highest degree of vigilance in securing communication between patients and families. This is especially important for children during disaster triage, treatment, and transport.

CAUTION
EMS clinicians must refrain from rushing onto an unsafe scene. Always assess scene safety to avoid becoming a victim yourself.

Pediatric Response Considerations

Disaster response requires foresight and planning long before the disaster occurs. After the initial recognition and response to a disaster, there are 4 specific components: (1) staging, (2) triage, (3) treatment, and (4) transport, with attention to disaster preparedness planning.

PLANNING

Before a disaster occurs, it is important to have the appropriate resources and training to treat pediatric patients. Response vehicles should stock pediatric supplies, including a range of pediatric airway equipment, pediatric-sized cervical collars, intraosseous needles, smaller-gauge intravenous (IV) catheters, and methods to control hypothermia. Additionally, tracking and reunification systems should be well publicized for the agency.

STAGING

Staging occurs when ambulances and personnel arrive on the scene of a disaster. EMS clinicians should meet in designated locations and await instructions from the staging officer. This ensures an efficient, systematic deployment. For the ICS to function properly, all EMS clinicians must coordinate their efforts to ensure appropriate and timely patient care.

TRIAGE

Triage is the process of prioritizing patients according to the severity of their injuries and the resources available, particularly in disaster settings. The goal of triage is to quickly assess and mobilize patients while managing resource constraints and providing a framework to ease the mental burden on responders. The pediatric population presents unique challenges, because many children may be nonverbal, frightened, or separated from their families, often with injuries that are difficult to identify. Effective triage of pediatric patients relies on use of standardized triage algorithms to ensure appropriate care and prioritization.

START and JumpSTART

The simple triage and rapid treatment (START) system is used to triage adults. The START triage system categorizes patients by color and allows the EMS clinician to quickly classify each patient according to physiological status and urgency of need for treatment. There are limitations in using START to triage young children, given the use of adult vital signs and clear communication.

JumpSTART triage is a pediatric-specific triage system designed for use in mass casualty incidents. It builds on the principles of the START system but is tailored to the unique needs of children (<8 years old or <100 lbs [45.4 kg]). The JumpSTART method focuses on quickly assessing and categorizing pediatric patients according to their ability to walk, respiratory status, and level of consciousness and relies less on specific vital signs (**FIGURE 16-2**).

Decision points (green, yellow, red, black) include the following: ability to walk (except infants), presence of spontaneous breathing, respirations less than 15 breaths/min or greater than 45 breaths/min, palpable peripheral pulse, and appropriate response to painful stimuli on the **alert-verbal-painful-unresponsive (AVPU) scale**. One of the distinguishing features is the administration of rescue breaths along with airway repositioning to apneic children.

SALT

Another triage system is the sort, assess, lifesaving interventions, and treatment and/or transport (SALT) system (**FIGURE 16-3**). The SALT triage system is designed to be efficient and adaptable, enabling responders to make rapid decisions and optimize resource allocation during high-stress emergency situations. This guideline has the advantage of being applicable in adults and children, and it is often used in international disaster assessments given its adaptability.

1. Global **S**orting of patients using voice commands: This often works for older children who can follow a command, but may not be effective in younger children because of developmental limitations
2. Individual triage: **A**ssessment and assignment of a triage category for those unable to respond during global sorting
3. **L**ifesaving intervention(s): Must be applied quickly, may include tourniquets, needle decompression, or rescue breaths for children who do not respond to repositioning of the airway
4. **T**reatment or transport

Despite the variety of published triage algorithms, there are currently no standardized pediatric tools. All EMS clinicians should be familiar with the method used by their EMS system and regularly practice it

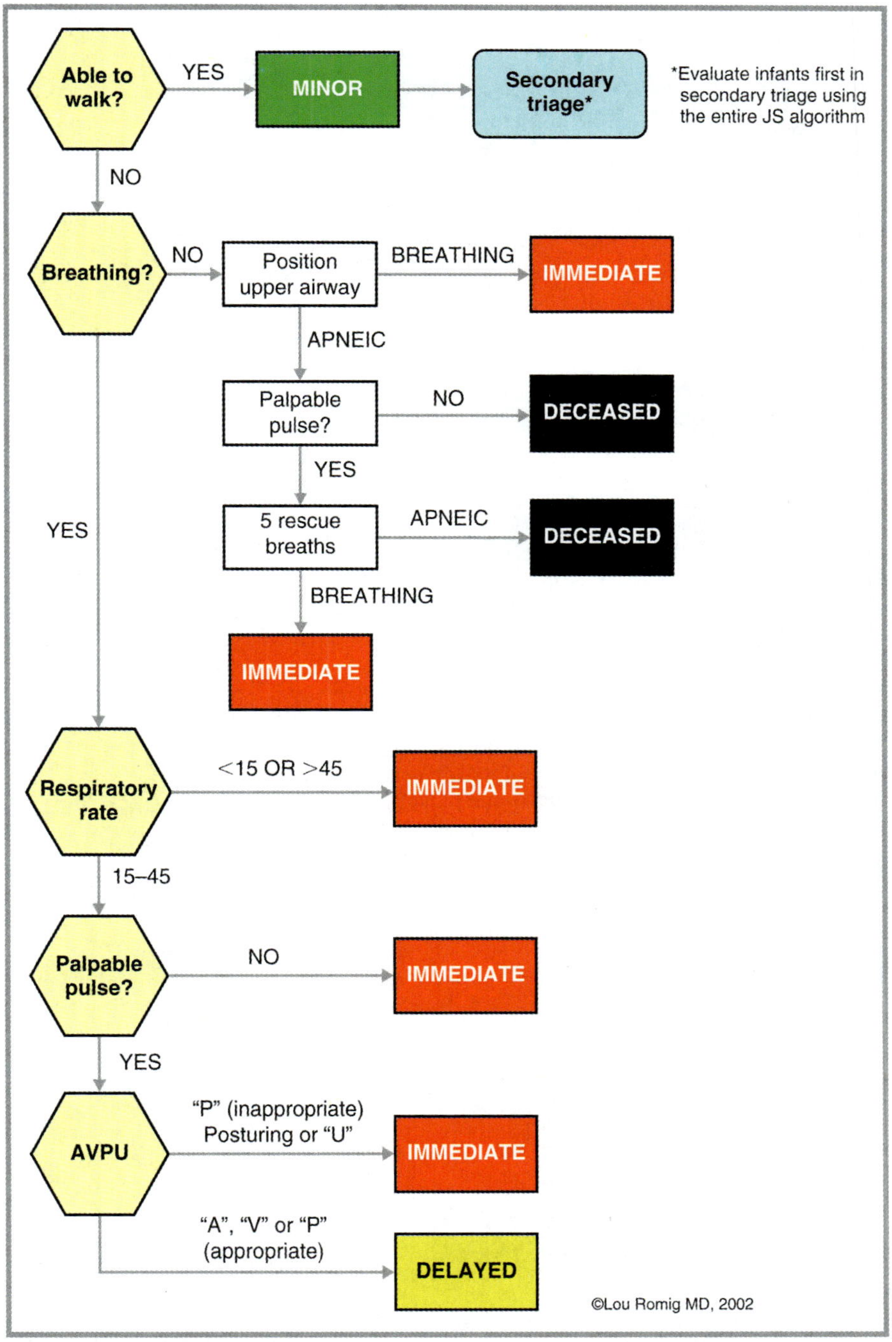

FIGURE 16–2 The JumpSTART (JS) triage system. Abbreviations: A, alert; P, pain; U, unresponsive; V, verbal.

during drills that provide a scenario specific to children in disasters.

TREATMENT

Treatment of pediatric patients in disaster situations is highly variable, influenced by the nature of the disaster, patient exposure, and resource availability. The first priority is to remove the patient from the threat source, with due considerations for the hot zone (contaminated area), warm zone (where full decontamination occurs), and cold zone (safe area); secondary threats; and the EMS clinician's safety.

Once in a safe location, perform decontamination if necessary to remove harmful substances from the

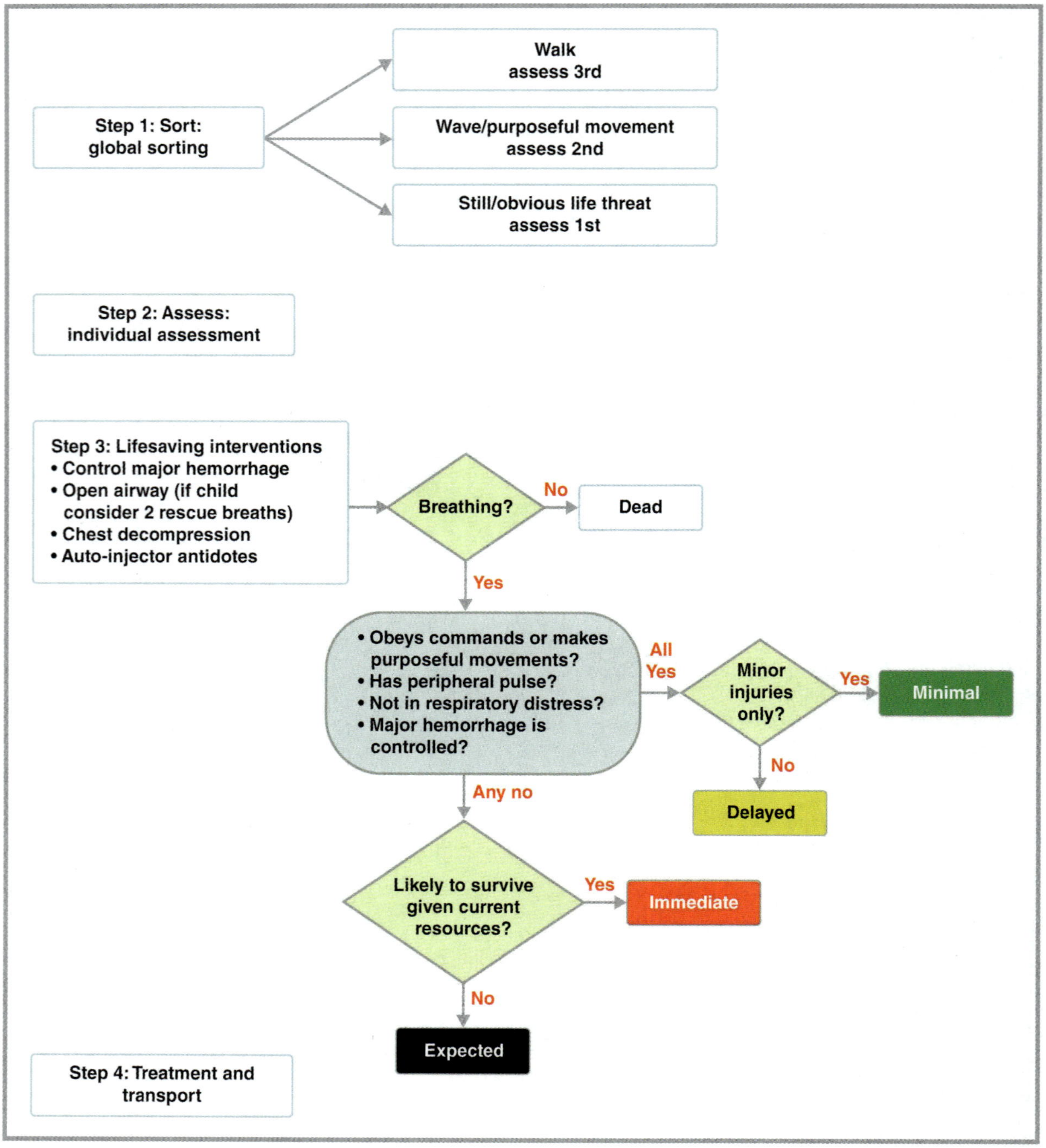

FIGURE 16–3 The SALT triage system.

patient. This process is vital for children, who have a higher risk of systemic toxicity because of their relatively larger body surface area and more permeable skin. Rapid decontamination decreases the risk of absorption and prevents contamination of rescuers. Special care is needed to prevent hypothermia in children during decontamination, necessitating the availability of warm water, warming equipment, and appropriately sized clothing. Every effort should be made to keep families together during decontamination and treatment when feasible.

In scenarios in which patient numbers exceed transport resources, designated treatment areas should be established. A secondary triage should follow to reassess patients' conditions on arrival to designated treatment areas. Areas should be stocked with medical equipment for ongoing stabilization before transport to definitive care.

TRANSPORT AND TRACKING

Early identification of patients in combination with patient tracking technology is an important part of every disaster plan. Coordination with regional resources (eg, EMS agencies, hospitals, and emergency management personnel) is critical to ensuring compatibility and access.

The transport officer's duty is to funnel patients into ambulances routed to designated hospitals in collaboration with dispatch. EMS clinicians should be cognizant of destination policies and guidelines to ensure young children are transported to appropriate trauma centers, preferably with a pediatric trauma designation when available and rapidly accessible. Pediatric patients who are in stable condition should not be given priority for transport over critically injured or ill adults simply because of their age. Assign transport priority on the basis of the patient's condition and available on-scene resources.

FAMILY REUNIFICATION

Family reunification is crucial for children during disasters, because it mitigates the emotional and psychological impacts of trauma. If parents and guardians are not involved in the disaster themselves, they will be anxious to access their child and receive updates on their care. In some cases, children may be orphaned by a disaster, leading to prolonged and challenging reunification processes as other guardians are identified and the child's safety is prioritized. Children are particularly vulnerable during disasters. They face risks of permanent separation from their caregivers; failure to be properly identified owing to significant injuries, burns, or young ages; and a high risk of experiencing abuse or trafficking. Hurricane Katrina in 2005 is an example of child displacement across state lines that posed considerable challenges to reunification. Years later, children were still in the process of being reunited with family members. Social media has been instrumental in easing this process, but it also creates new risks to child safety following a disaster. The stress and chaos can lead to confusion and fear, making it essential for EMS personnel and hospitals to have structured processes in place to facilitate reunification.

Steps and Processes for Family Reunification That Can Be Implemented by EMS Personnel and Hospitals During a Mass-Casualty Incident

1. Initial Assessment: Assess the needs of children and prioritize their care while ensuring they remain in a safe environment.
2. Identification: Use wristbands or tags for children that include vital information, such as their name, age, and emergency contact information.
3. Communication: Establish clear communication channels with families, keeping them informed about the situation and where to find their children.
4. Triage and Treatment: Ensure that children receive prompt medical attention and are triaged according to their needs.
5. Designated Reunification Areas: Set up specific areas for family reunification where families can be directed to find their children. Family reunification should not take place at the active disaster or hostile incident scene. All areas should include psychological first aid personnel.
6. Establish a pediatric safe area, where children who are medically cleared but unable to

CASE STUDY 1

An Expanded Fujita scale 4 tornado has struck the outskirts of a major city. Multiple families are affected, and several children have been separated from their caregivers. EMS teams are dispatched to assist with triage. One team encounters a 7-year-old girl who has a broken arm and is visibly distressed, calling for her mother.

While assessing her injuries, the EMS team learns that an adult matching her mother's description has been transported to a hospital for critical injuries.

1. How can EMS clinicians effectively communicate with this child about her mother?
2. What protocols should EMS teams follow to ensure the safe and timely reunification of children with their caregivers after a disaster?
3. In what ways can EMS personnel collaborate with other agencies to facilitate family reunification in disaster situations?

be reunited with caregivers can be supervised and supported. Activities and necessary supplies, including games and snacks, should be included.

7. Documentation: Maintain accurate records of all children treated, including their status and location, to assist in the reunification process.
8. Collaboration With External Resources: Engage with local community resources—including child protective services, social work, law enforcement, school boards, and other child safety personnel—to coordinate reunification efforts and provide additional support.

External Resources

Involving external resources is essential for effective reunification. Child protective services can help ensure the safety and welfare of children, whereas social workers can provide emotional support to families. Law enforcement can assist in identifying and safeguarding children, preventing potential trafficking. School boards and child safety personnel can facilitate reunification by providing additional information and support systems.

By implementing these steps and collaborating with external resources, EMS clinicians and hospitals can significantly enhance the safety and well-being of children during disasters, ensuring a smoother reunification process for families.

Natural Disasters

EARTHQUAKES

Although ground movement itself rarely causes direct injuries, most earthquake-related harm arises from falling debris, flying glass, and collapsing structures. The damage from earthquakes can be severe, often resulting in blunt and multisystem trauma and triggering illnesses such as asthma due to environmental dust. Additionally, children may face exposure to environmental hazards, including stray animals, insects, and hazardous materials, because of inadequate shelter. The psychological stress following an earthquake can also lead to increases in domestic violence and child abuse.

> **TIP**
>
> A natural disaster or an environmental disturbance, such as an earthquake, often causes a major increase in pediatric respiratory ailments, especially asthma.

Floods

Several environmental events cause flooding, including heavy rains, rapid snow melt, and coastal storm surges (**FIGURE 16–4**). Unlike earthquakes, flooding is usually somewhat predictable and typically develops more gradually. Therefore, evacuation can be anticipated with plans in place to avoid the separation of families. An additional public health consequence of flooding is contamination of drinking water and disease outbreak. Children are at a greater risk of experiencing dehydration due to vomiting and diarrhea associated with contaminated water.

Weather-Related Disasters

Severe storms differ from one geographic region to another. Coastal areas are subject to hurricanes, whereas inland regions may experience more tornado activity (**FIGURE 16–5**). Many regions are also susceptible to wildfires, blizzards, heavy rains, or high winds, all of which can severely impact communities. EMS clinicians should be aware of the increased risk of extreme temperature–related emergencies in pediatric patients. Infants and young children lose heat more rapidly than adults, leading to hypothermia. On the other end, they lose considerable water and electrolytes in extreme heat, making them prone to hypovolemia and heat stroke. Smoke exposure due to wildfires may lead to increased pediatric respiratory disease over a broad region.

Hurricanes, tornadoes, and severe storms can cause structural damage, power outages, and communication failures, potentially leading to flooding. EMS clinicians must coordinate with local

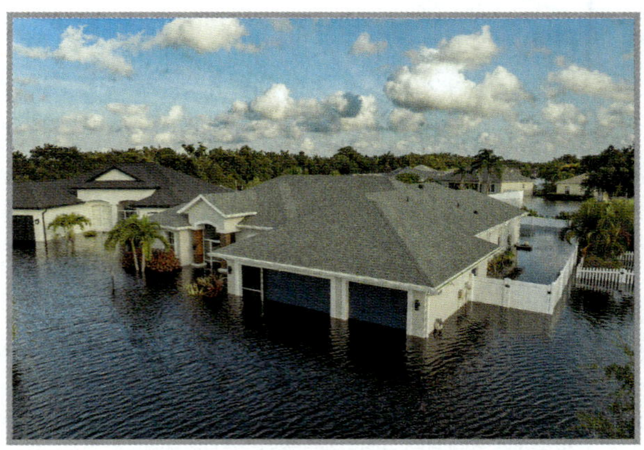

FIGURE 16–4 Flooding is a yearly concern in many areas of the country.

Bilanol/Shutterstock.com

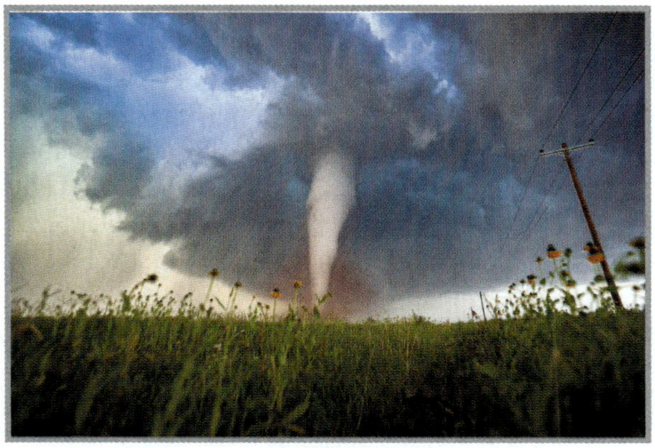

FIGURE 16–5 Inland regions experience tornadoes.

Xiyu Zhang/iStockphoto.com.

agencies, such as search and rescue, to assist children and elderly individuals who are vulnerable to injuries due to environmental conditions and structural collapse. Because children may be concentrated in schools and child care facilities during such events, it is crucial for EMS systems to anticipate their needs.

> **TIP**
> EMS systems must anticipate psychological trauma in children who are separated from their families during a disaster. They must have a reunification plan in place as well as staff and resources to care for children without medical needs during the reunification process.

Epidemics and Pandemics

The entire world experienced the effects of the COVID pandemic, but every year there are significant communicable disease outbreaks. In 2022, a convergence of respiratory syncytial virus, influenza, and COVID disproportionately affected young children and led to severe respiratory illness, with a national shortage of pediatric hospital beds. Annual outbreaks are a reminder of our vulnerability to epidemics and the need to remain vigilant when in contact with infected patients.

Manmade Disasters

Manmade disasters include hazardous material incidents, structure failures, and malicious intent events, such as shootings or acts of terrorism. These events can have an extensive impact on children, including those not directly involved in the disaster, causing post-traumatic stress disorder (PTSD) or anxiety.

HAZARDOUS MATERIALS EXPOSURES

In daily life, hazardous materials are everywhere (**TABLE 16–3**). Examples include chemicals used in cleaning, refrigeration, and swimming pool maintenance; fuels; and agricultural products. Many of these materials are present in schools, other public facilities, and homes. Additionally, illegal activities, such as methamphetamine laboratories, involve the use of materials that are highly explosive and toxic, which may cause burns and serious injuries to bystanders, including children.

> **TIP**
> Children have a proportionally greater body surface area and thinner skin than adults, which make them more susceptible to injury from burns, chemicals, and absorbable toxins. In addition, they are more susceptible to heat and water loss through their skin, putting them at risk of experiencing hypothermia and dehydration.

Structural Failures

Buildings, bridges, and platforms can fail. These collapses typically cause multiple injuries. Children can be the primary victims, especially when structural failures involve schools, bus transport, or recreational facilities.

Terrorism

Terrorism is a threat in all regions of the world. Children may be targets, sometimes precisely because of the psychological impact of death and injury of vulnerable individuals by the perpetrators.

Mass Shootings

Mass shootings have become a common disaster in the United States, and school shootings are one of the most common disasters disproportionately affecting children in the United States. These pose unique difficulties because of the inherent safety issues for EMS clinicians, demands of mass-casualty triage, communication requirements, emotional responses,

TABLE 16–3 Examples of Common Hazardous Materials

Diesel fuels	Insecticides
Gasoline	Fertilizers
Motor oil	Propane
Herbicides	Natural gas

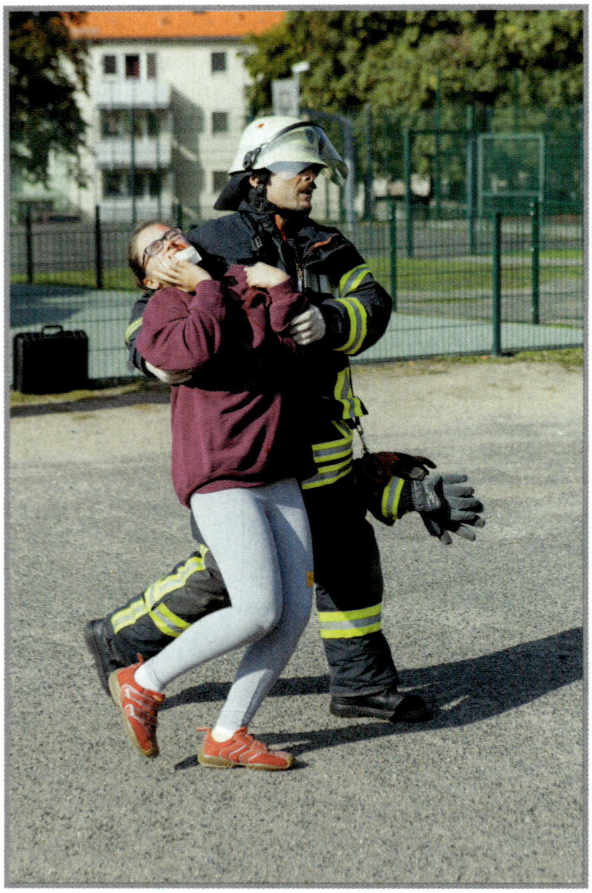

FIGURE 16–6 Evacuating children from a school.
ollo/iStockphoto.com.

and overextension of emergency resources. Uninjured children and anxious parents may require significant EMS resources. A coordinated plan for family reunification is an essential element to preparedness for a school shooting MCI (**FIGURE 16–6**).

Special Focus: EMS Preparation for a School Shooting Mass-Casualty Incident

EMS ROLES AND ACTIONS IN SCHOOL SHOOTING EVENTS

Mass-casualty incidents with large numbers of children, such as school shootings, present unique challenges for EMS clinicians. Children are particularly vulnerable to the physical and psychological effects of these events because of their smaller bodies, immature physiology, and limited coping mechanisms.

Preparation and Training

- Specialized Training: EMS agencies should provide specialized training that focuses on pediatric emergency care, trauma response, and the psychological impact of mass-casualty events on children. This training should cover child-specific assessment techniques, communication skills, and strategies for dealing with pediatric trauma.
- Collaboration with Local Schools: Establish partnerships with schools to conduct drills that include both EMS and school personnel. This collaboration ensures that everyone understands their roles during a crisis and fosters effective communication.

Specific EMS Roles and Actions

- Rapid Response: EMS clinicians must respond quickly to mass shooting incidents to minimize casualties and optimize patient outcomes. This involves coordinating with law enforcement to ensure scene safety and expedite medical care.
- Triage and Prioritization: EMS clinicians must rapidly assess the severity of injuries and prioritize patients according to their immediate need for care. This process is particularly challenging in school shootings because of the potential for multiple casualties and the emotional distress of children and their families.
- Trauma Care: EMS clinicians must be prepared to manage a variety of trauma injuries, such as gunshot wounds, bleeding, and fractures. This may involve applying tourniquets, controlling bleeding, and providing pain relief.
- Psychological Support: EMS clinicians should be trained to recognize and address the psychological needs of children and their families. This compassionate care includes providing comfort and reassurance.
- Coordination With Hospitals: During a mass shooting, EMS clinicians must coordinate with hospitals to ensure that pediatric patients are transported to appropriate destinations to receive the care they need. This may involve communicating patient information, determining whether or not the child needs a trauma center, and prioritizing patients for transportation.
- Postevent Support: EMS clinicians may be involved in postevent activities, such as assisting with disaster recovery efforts.

Unique Challenges in Caring for Children in School Shootings

- Mass-Casualty Incident Management: The chaotic nature of school shootings can make it difficult for EMS clinicians to effectively manage multiple casualties and prioritize care. Identify your incident command immediately on arrival to the scene.
- Separation From Caregivers: Children are likely to be separated from their parents or guardians during the event, which can exacerbate their distress.
- Limited Communication: Children may have difficulty communicating their needs or understanding instructions owing to fear, anxiety, or language barriers.

Pre-Event Planning for Effective Care

- Specialized Training: EMS clinicians should receive specialized training in pediatric emergency care and disaster response.
- Pediatric Equipment: EMS vehicles should be equipped with appropriate pediatric medical equipment.
- Communication Tools: Using age-appropriate communication tools can help bridge language and developmental barriers.
- Mental Health Support: Mental health support should be available for both children and EMS responders.
- Disaster Planning: EMS systems should work with local school districts to develop plans for responding to school shootings and other school based MCIs involving children.
- Postincident Debriefing and Support for EMS Clinicians

Postincident Debriefing and Support

- Critical Incident Stress Management (CISM): Following a school shooting, EMS personnel may experience vicarious trauma from witnessing the effects of violence on children. Implementing CISM programs can provide essential support to first responders, allowing them to process their experiences.
- Community Support and Resources: Collaborate with mental health professionals and community organizations to ensure that affected children and families receive ongoing support and counseling after the incident.

By addressing these challenges and implementing effective strategies, EMS clinicians can improve their ability to care for children in school shooting events and minimize the long-term consequences of these traumatic experiences.

> **TIP**
>
> The American College of Surgeons and the Federal Bureau of Investigation created a set of critical actions—THREAT—to maximize the survivability of mass shootings on scene.
>
> - T: Threat suppression
> - H: Hemorrhage control
> - RE: Rapid Extrication to safety
> - A: Assessment by medical providers
> - T: Transport to definitive care

Physiological and Psychological Characteristics That Make Children Vulnerable in Disasters

Children face unique challenges during disasters because of their unique anatomy and physiology that can impact their health and safety. Their physiological differences, such as higher respiratory rates, thinner skin, and smaller body mass, make them more susceptible to the effects of traumatic injuries and chemical

CASE STUDY 2

You are the first EMS clinician to arrive on scene of a reported shooting at an elementary school. Dispatch conveyed that at least 4 people have been shot and one perpetrator has been apprehended. It is not clear if there is still another perpetrator inside the school. When you arrive on the scene, law enforcement has not secured the area. Three students in the cafeteria and one adult on the second floor in the principal's office are seriously injured.

1. As you pull your gear from the ambulance, what are your first considerations?
2. What pediatric issues are important to consider?

TABLE 16–4 Characteristics That Put Children at Risk During Disaster

Pediatric System or Aspect	Physiological or Psychological Vulnerability
Respiratory	Smaller airway easily obstructed by edema or secretions Higher RR increases fluid loss, leading to dehydration Higher minute volume increases risk resulting from exposure to inhaled agents Nuclear fallout and heavier gases settle low to the ground and may affect children more severely
Cardiovascular	Smaller circulating blood volumes and higher heart rates can lead to rapid progression in hemorrhagic or hypovolemic shock
Gastrointestinal	Risk of experiencing dehydration due to vomiting and diarrhea
Skin	Higher body surface area increases risk of skin exposure Evaporative loss is higher when skin is wet or cold, so hypothermia more likely Skin is thinner and more susceptible to injury caused by burns, chemicals, and absorbable toxins
Endocrine	High risk of experiencing hypoglycemia owing to low body glucose stores, especially in the setting of prolonged fasting period during the response
Developmental	Communication, mobility and understanding of the disaster event compromise safety and provide challenges for EMS clinicians
Psychological	Prolonged stress due to critical incidents; susceptibility to separation anxiety
Special Considerations	Rapid metabolism of many medications, compared with that in adults Children and youth with special health care needs may have chronic conditions that require health-related services, including technology-dependent care requiring a source of power or an oxygen supply

Abbreviations: EMS, emergency medical services; RR, respiratory rate.

and biological agents. Additionally, children may experience heightened anxiety and trauma, as well as developmental regression after disasters. Children and youth with special health care needs, especially those with technology-dependent care, require a source of power or oxygen supply during a disaster. These factors necessitate a tailored approach to disaster preparedness and response. **TABLE 16–4** summarizes the physiologic and psychological characteristics of children that put them at increased risk during disasters.

EMOTIONAL RESPONSES OF CHILDREN

Children who experience disasters are at high risk of experiencing psychological trauma, including PTSD, anxiety, and depression. Children who witness violence may experience traumatic memories and nightmares. Reunification is an important step in addressing the emotional responses from both parents and children. These responses may include fear, anxiety, depression, grief, and post-traumatic stress symptoms, with children being particularly susceptible to PTSD. Mental health professionals with pediatric expertise play a vital role in providing stress management and counseling services after a disaster.

If children require temporary shelter during a disaster response, considerations for pediatric needs are essential, especially if children are separated from their caregivers. Each child's reaction to a disaster will vary according to age, maturity, previous experiences, and cultural background, yet all children are likely to experience anxiety.

Psychological Needs

- Safety and Security: Children need to feel safe and have a stable environment.
- Supportive Relationships: Establishing trust with caregivers is crucial for emotional recovery.
- Open Communication: Children benefit from age-appropriate discussions about the disaster to help them process their experiences.
- Routine and Normality: Maintaining or restoring daily routines can provide a sense of stability.

Current Research

- Early interventions, including psychological first aid and trauma-informed care, can significantly reduce long-term psychological effects in children.

- Targeted mental health resources and interventions are required to address the unique needs of children affected by disasters, with an emphasis on timely support, which can mitigate the severity of traumatic responses.

In summary, children's emotional responses to disasters are profound and multifaceted, necessitating immediate and sustained psychological support tailored to their specific needs.

Effects of Chemical, Biological, Radiation, Nuclear, and Explosive Disasters on Children

CHEMICAL AGENTS

Millions of chemicals pose risks to human health (**TABLE 16–5**), especially as they are transported on a daily basis with a potential for unintentional or deliberate population exposure. Chemical spills require the response of officials who are trained to work with **hazardous materials (hazmat)**. They provide skills and expertise in identification of the toxicity, relative risk, decontamination procedures, and specific treatments required.

ASSESSMENT AND TREATMENT OF SPECIFIC CHEMICAL AGENTS

Nerve Agents

Nerve agents are highly toxic with rapid onset of effects. Examples include tabun, sarin, soman, VX, and organophosphate pesticides. They may occur as gas, aerosol, or liquid and can enter the body via inhalation, skin contact, or ingestion in contaminated food. These agents overstimulate the parasympathetic nervous system by blocking the breakdown of the neurotransmitter acetylcholine. Children are at greater risk because of their faster respiratory rates, short stature, thin skin, and larger surface area; children often show symptoms sooner than adults.

Early symptoms may include headache, eye pain, pupil constriction, runny nose, vomiting, diarrhea, excessive sweating, and respiratory distress. Bradycardia is typical (although tachycardia may occur). Severe exposure can lead to dehydration, seizures, apnea, paralysis, and coma.

TIP

Remember the mnemonic DUMBELS for symptoms associated with nerve gas exposure: diarrhea/diaphoresis, urination, miosis, bradycardia/bronchorrhea/ bronchospasm, emesis, lacrimation, salivation.

Treatment of nerve agent exposure begins with donning of PPE by EMS clinicians, followed by immediate decontamination. Children may be frightened by clinicians whose faces are covered by PPE.

Treatment for nerve agents includes atropine, pralidoxime, and benzodiazepines.

- Atropine dosage for children is 0.05 to 0.1 mg/kg IV or intramuscular (IM), with repeat doses every 2 to 5 minutes as needed to treat symptoms. Patients with nerve agent exposure often require many doses of atropine, with available stockpile being the limiting factor.
- Pralidoxime dosage is 25-50 mg/kg IV over 5-30 minute, then 10 mg/kg/hr or repeat load after 1 hour (max dose 2 g/dose). IM 15 mg/kg (up tp 600 mg), repeat as needed every 15 minutes to a maximum of 45 mg/kg.
- Benzodiazepines are indicated for patients with seizure after nerve agent exposure. The dosage may be simplified for mass-casualty events, but the range does not differ from standard pediatric seizure dosing.

CAUTION

Patients with nerve agent exposure often require extraordinary dosing of atropine. If there is concern regarding potential nerve agent exposure, notify incident command of the need for additional stores of atropine to adequately treat symptomatic patients.

Cyanide

Cyanide is a rapidly acting and potentially lethal chemical available in various forms, including colorless gas and crystallized solids. Although it can sometimes be detected by its bitter almond smell, not everyone is able to perceive this odor. Exposure

TABLE 16–5 Common Chemicals Detrimental to Human Health

Alcohols	Drain and oven cleaners
Ammonia	Hydrocarbons (gasoline, paint thinner)
Asbestos	Hydrofluoric acid
Bleach (laundry)	Pesticides
Chlorine	Sulfuric acid

can occur through inhalation, ingestion, skin contact, or contaminated soil; breathing cyanide gas is particularly harmful. Cyanide disrupts the body's ability to use oxygen, primarily affecting the heart and brain, which are more oxygen dependent. Symptoms of cyanide exposure in children can manifest rapidly and may include tachypnea, restlessness, dizziness, and nausea. Severe exposure can lead to convulsions, hypotension, loss of consciousness, and respiratory failure, potentially resulting in death.

Treatment begins with decontamination and administration of 100% oxygen to help mitigate cellular oxygen deprivation. The antidote hydroxocobalamin (vitamin B_{12}) binds cyanide into cyanocobalamin, which is excreted in the urine. It is administered by IV infusion over 15 minutes. The hydroxocobalamin dose for children is 70 mg/kg, with a maximum (adult) dose of 5 g. Adverse effects include hypertension and red discoloration of skin and mucous membranes.

The EMS clinician must determine if the exposure in question was to a nerve agent or to cyanide, given the different immediate antidotes required in each scenario. One important distinction is that patients exposed to nerve agents are more likely to have cyanosis, altered vision with miosis, copious secretions, and bronchospasm.

Pulmonary Intoxicants

Pulmonary intoxicants produce pulmonary edema. The most widely known agents are phosgene and chlorine. Patients typically exhibit eye and airway irritation, dyspnea, and chest tightness. In most cases, patients develop shortness of breath caused by pulmonary edema hours after the exposure. Without supportive treatment, including decontamination and advanced airway management with intubation if necessary, patients may progress to respiratory failure.

Vesicants

Vesicants are chemicals that cause blistering of the skin, irritation and inflammation of the eyes and airways, and vomiting and diarrhea. Exposure to vesicants can occur through inhalation, absorption, or ingestion. The most common vesicants are sulfur mustard (mustard gas) and lewisite. Treatment for these chemical exposures includes decontamination with large volumes of warm, soapy water at low pressure; eye irrigation; airway control; and oxygen administration. Bandage wounds with dry dressings.

BIOLOGICAL AGENTS

Biological agents, ranging from common pathogens such as influenza to lethal agents such as plague, pose significant threats to human health, particularly in the context of potential terrorist attacks. These agents can be weaponized because of their availability and, in some cases, high transmissibility, which poses a unique risk to children in settings such as schools and child care facilities.

Description of Biological Agents

- Anthrax: A bacterial spore that can be inhaled or ingested, leading to severe illness, pneumonia, or death; the serious forms of human anthrax are inhalation anthrax, cutaneous anthrax, and intestinal anthrax
- Botulism: A potentially fatal illness caused by toxins from bacteria, leading to muscle paralysis and respiratory failure
- Influenza: A common respiratory viral illness that is spread through aerosolized particles, leading to severe illness, especially in vulnerable populations such as children
- Plague: A bacterial infection transmitted by fleas, known for causing severe respiratory illness, septic shock, and rapid death if untreated
- Ricin: A highly toxic protein derived from castor beans that can cause severe respiratory symptoms when inhaled and bloody vomiting/diarrhea when ingested, ultimately leading to hallucinations, seizures, and death
- Smallpox: A highly contagious virus causing severe flu-like illness; in 30% of cases it can lead to death (**FIGURE 16–7**)
- Tularemia: A bacterial infection that can cause serious respiratory issues

Biological agents can have unique and severe impacts on pediatric patients because of children's

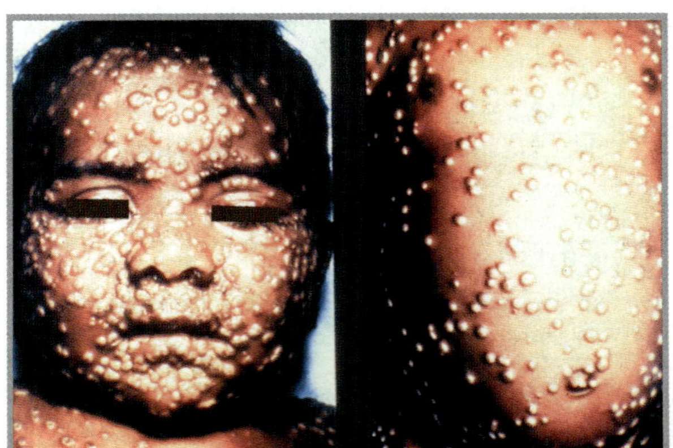

FIGURE 16–7 Smallpox. Courtesy of Paul Wehrle, MD.

TABLE 16–6 Medical Management of Bioterrorism Infections

Pre-exposure Vaccine	Treatment Postexposure *With* Symptoms	Postexposure *Without* Symptoms
Anthrax, inhalation Anthrax vaccine, 0.5 mL IM or SQ at weeks 0 and 4 and months 6, 12, and 18, then annual boosters This vaccine is *not* recommended for use in those aged <18 years	Ciprofloxacin, 15 mg/kg IV twice daily (max, 1 g/d) *or* Doxycycline ▪ < 45 kg child: ▪ Load with 4.4 mg/kg IV once, then ▪ Continue with 2.2 mg/kg IV every 12 hours ▪ Stepdown once clinically stable and able to tolerate PO: ▪ 2.2 mg/kg/dose PO every 12 hours ▪ ≥ 45 kg child: ▪ Load with 200 mg IV once, then ▪ Continue with 100 mg IV every 12 hours ▪ Stepdown once clinically stable and able to tolerate PO: ▪ 100 mg PO every 12 hours	Ciprofloxacin, 15–20 mg/kg (max, 1 g/d) orally twice a day for 60 days *or* Doxycycline ▪ < 45 kg child, 2.2 mg/kg/dose PO every 12 hours ▪ ≥ 45 kg child, 100 mg PO every 12 hours
Smallpox Smallpox vaccine No vaccine for those aged <12 months Not recommended for those aged ≤18 years for pre-event vaccination	No current treatment other than supportive care	Vaccination within 96 hours of exposure
Plague, pneumonic Vaccine is not available	Ciprofloxacin, ▪ 10 mg/kg IV every 8 to 12 hours (max, 400 mg/dose) If able to take PO, 15 mg/kg every 8 or 12 hours (max 500 mg/dose every 8 hours; max 750 mg/dose every 12 hour *or* ▪ Levofloxacin If < 50 kg, 8 mg/kg IV or PO every 12 hours ▪ If > 50 kg, 500 to 750 mg IV or PO once daily Doxycycline ▪ If <45 kg, 2.2 mg/kg IV twice daily (max, 250 mg daily) for 10 days ▪ If >45 kg, 100 mg IV twice daily	Doxycycline ▪ If <45 kg, 2.2 mg/kg orally twice daily (max, 200 mg daily) for 7 days ▪ If >45 kg, 100 mg twice daily *or* Ciprofloxacin, 15 mg/kg orally every 12 hours (max, 500 mg/dose *or* Check CDC recommendations

Abbreviations: IM, intramuscular; IV, intravenous; SQ, subcutaneous.

developing immune systems, higher susceptibility to respiratory illnesses, and the potential for rapid spread in communal environments. **TABLE 16–6** summarizes the specific treatment of diseases caused by biological agents, including pediatric doses, although these medications are not typically carried by EMS clinicians.

Radiation and Nuclear Disasters

Radiation disasters can occur wherever radioactive materials are used, stored, or transported. Nuclear power plants, hospitals, universities, research laboratories, industries, major highways, railroads, and shipping yards are all possible sites. Growing children are more susceptible to radiation injury because of their rapidly dividing cells. Individuals exposed to high levels of radiation may or may not develop symptoms of radiation sickness, but should be decontaminated and treated at Radiation Injury Treatment Network (RITN) centers. Most children's hospitals with dedicated oncology wards serve as RITN sites for pediatric patients and their families.

A **dirty bomb**, also known as a radiological dispersal device, consists of a conventional explosive, such as dynamite, packaged with radioactive material that is meant to scatter when the bomb explodes. A dirty bomb can kill or injure by means of the initial blast of the conventional explosive or by airborne radiation and contamination (hence the term *dirty*).

A nuclear bomb uses the power of nuclear fission or fusion to produce an intense pulse or wave of heat, light, air pressure, and radiation. In a nuclear blast, injury or death may occur as an immediate result of the blast itself or later from radiation exposure.

Protection from radiation exposure can be attained by using a shield, minimizing exposure time, and maximizing the distance from the source. Shielding varies depending on the type of radiation, with α particles stopped by a sheet of paper, β particles by a layer of clothing, and gamma rays requiring more than 6 feet of concrete. Because PPE cannot protect against radiation associated with most radiation emergencies, first responders should wear direct-reading personal radiation dosimeters to monitor radiation doses and stay within recommended dose limits. External decontamination of radioactive particulate can be accomplished by removal of all clothing, warm soap water irrigation, wound débridement with foreign body removal, oral rinsing, and eye and ear irrigation. Care should be taken to avoid the contamination of vehicles and equipment through on-site decontamination, and hospitals should not be used as decontamination centers.

TIP

Perform a full decontamination of an individual whenever exposed to a hazardous substance. Decontaminate yourself and your space if affected as well.

CAUTION

Children may require assistance with decontamination, depending on their age. It is important to prevent hypothermia after decontamination by drying immediately and giving them warm clothes.

Explosives

Explosive devices are frequently used for terrorism. Children are at risk for blast injury because of their size and susceptibility to head and abdominal injuries. Injuries from the blast wave, flying debris, and impact from being thrown may be fatal.

Critical Incident Stress Management

Critical incident stress management is a structured approach designed to mitigate the psychological impact of traumatic events on EMS professionals, especially during pediatric disasters. The CISM framework for crisis intervention includes education, support, and debriefing, helping first responders process their experiences and emotions in a supportive environment.

Recent research emphasizes the importance of CISM in enhancing resilience and reducing the risk of PTSD among EMS personnel. Studies have shown that early intervention through CISM can significantly improve mental health outcomes for responders involved in pediatric disasters, in which the emotional toll can be particularly severe. For instance, data indicate that CISM programs can lead to decreased levels of distress and improved coping mechanisms in first responders.

Moreover, a 2021 study found that EMS agencies implementing CISM protocols reported better mental health outcomes, including lower rates of burnout and improved job satisfaction among personnel. These findings underscore the necessity for ongoing training and integration of CISM in EMS operations, particularly in high-stress situations like pediatric emergencies.

Summary

Children are uniquely vulnerable during disasters because of their physiological and psychological needs. To prepare for the needs of children in disasters, EMS agencies should prioritize pediatric training, develop age-specific protocols, and conduct realistic drills. Effective triage (JumpSTART, SALT), interagency coordination, and family reunification strategies are essential in managing mass-casualty events involving

CASE STUDY 3

You are dispatched to a gymnasium at the local high school. On arrival, you find 20 adolescents and 4 adults still inside. They all have eye irritation, respiratory distress, chest tightness, and coughing. The pool is next door, and there is a cloud above the pool.

1. What is the likely agent?
2. How would you treat and transport these patients?

children. Disaster preparedness for children requires participation from a broad coalition of emergency management, EMS, law enforcement, public health officers, and school systems, as well as extensive community engagement. In this coalition, EMS agencies can significantly enhance their preparedness for pediatric responses during disasters and ensure the safety and well-being of the youngest victims in critical situations.

Critical incident stress management teams play a crucial role in supporting EMS clinicians exposed to disasters involving children. Principles of trauma-informed care are important for both the children we care for and ourselves.

CASE STUDY ANSWERS

CASE STUDY 1

During your assessment of the child, determine the severity of injuries and triage her using an appropriate standardized technique such as the JumpSTART triage system. You splint her injured arm and provide pain medication. Provide psychological support by remaining calm and reassure her you will make sure she is safe while you do your best to find out what happened to her mother. Keep your reassurance vague but comforting. The adult matched the description of her mother but has not been confirmed to be her mother, so you should not share any additional information. Furthermore, it is usually best to delay sharing any traumatic news about family members until the child has been transferred to a safe location with support services readily available.

You work with incident command to establish identifiers for the child and clearly document triage and transport destination. On arrival at the hospital, teams will often take photos of children including distinguishing clothing, birthmarks, and other features to assist in reunification.

Social services, schools, law enforcement, and child protective services will provide additional resources.

When you arrive at your destination hospital, your supervisor contacts you to let you know that incident command has located the child's mother. She was not injured and is coming to the hospital where you transported the girl. They are reunited in the ED, and the mother is able to provide consent for surgical treatment of the girl's broken arm.

CASE STUDY 2

Scene safety must be your primary consideration. Law enforcement is in charge, and you will not be allowed inside the school until the scene is safe. Do not make yourself the next victim. While awaiting clearance, establish incident command and determine staging and triage areas. Request appropriate response of other providers (basic and/or advanced life support) and ensure the availability of transportation or additional resources, such as an aeromedical team.

Determine the amount of pediatric equipment that is available and the level of care that may be needed; request additional resources as needed. Coordinate with dispatch transport destinations that have pediatric trauma care capabilities. Do not forget to institute family reunification protocols and psychological support.

CASE STUDY 3

These students and chaperones likely have been exposed to a chlorine gas leak.

Begin by donning PPE, including gowns, gloves, and masks. Treatment should begin by moving anyone who is able to walk outdoors. Call for a hazmat team to decontaminate the patients; request additional ambulances to provide oxygen, airway management, and hospital transport; and notify the local hospital and law enforcement.

The children are all transported to a nearby children's center where they are evaluated for signs of respiratory distress. One child develops wheezing at the hospital and is admitted for overnight observation. The rest of the children are discharged home in good condition.

Suggested References

TEXTBOOKS

Hogan D, Burstein J. *Disaster Medicine*. 2nd ed. Lippincott Williams & Wilkins; 2007

ARTICLES

Callahan JM, Baldwin S, Bodnar C, et al; Committee on Pediatric Emergency Medicine; Council on Clinical Information Technology; Council on Children and Disasters; American College of Emergency Physicians, Pediatric Emergency Medicine Committee. Access to critical health information for children during emergencies: emergency information forms and beyond. *Pediatrics*. 2023;151(3):e2022060970. doi:10.1542/peds.2022-060970

Freyberg CW, Arquilla B, Fertel BS, et al. Disaster preparedness: hospital decontamination and the pediatric patient—guidelines for hospitals and emergency planners. *Prehosp Disaster Med*. 2008;23(2):166–173. doi:10.1017/S1049023X0000580X

Heffernan RW, Lerner EB, McKee CH, et al. Comparing the accuracy of mass casualty triage systems in a pediatric population. *Prehosp Emerg Care*. 2019;23(3):304–308. doi:10.1080/10903127.2018.1520946

Krug SE, Chung S, Fagbuyi DB, et al; Disaster Preparedness Advisory Council; Committee on Pediatric Emergency Medicine. Ensuring the health of children in disasters. *Pediatrics*. 2015;136(5):e1407–e1417. doi:10.1542/peds.2015-3112

Lerner EB, Cone DC, Weinstein ES, et al. Mass casualty triage: an evaluation of the science and refinement of a national guideline. *Disaster Med Public Health Prep*. 2011;5(2):129–137. doi:10.1001/dmp.2011.39

Lozon MM, Bradin S. Pediatric disaster preparedness. *Pediatr Clin North Am*. 2018;65(6):1205–1220. doi:10.1016/j.pcl.2018.07.015

Owusu-Ansah S, Moore B, Shah MI, et al; Committee on Pediatric Emergency Medicine, Section on Emergency Medicine; EMS Subcommittee, Section on Surgery. Pediatric readiness in emergency medical services systems. *Pediatrics*. 2020;145(1):e20193308. doi:10.1542/peds.2019-3308

OTHER RESOURCES

60 Seconds to Survival: Disaster Triage. Accessed October 15, 2024. https://disastertriagegame.org/index.html

American Academy of Pediatrics. Family Separation and Reunification in Disasters. October 2024. Accessed May 5, 2025. https://www.aap.org/en/patient-care/disasters-and-children/disaster-management-resources-by-topic/family-separation-and-reunification-in-disasters/

American Academy of Pediatrics. Pediatric Tabletop Exercise Toolkit: Preparing for Disasters. Accessed November 22, 2024. https://www.aap.org/en/patient-care/disasters-and-children/pediatric-tabletop-exercise-resource-kit/pediatric-tabletop-exercise-toolkit-preparing-for-disasters/

Cicero MX, Davis NR, Henning AM, Krug S. National Academy of Medicine. Planning for Children in Disasters: Education and Strategies for the Best Outcomes. September 30, 2024. Accessed February 9, 2026. https://nam.edu/planning-for-children-in-disasters-education-and-strategies-for-the-best-outcomes/

Everytown Research & Policy. Mass Shootings in the United States. An Everytown for Gun Safety Support Fund Analysis. Everytown Res Policy. Updated March 2023. Accessed February 9, 2026. https://everytownresearch.org/maps/mass-shootings-in-america/

Mass Shootings in the United States. An Everytown for Gun Safety Support Fund Analysis. Everytown Res Policy. Updated March 2023. https://everytownresearch.org/maps/mass-shootings-in-america/

Pediatric Pandemic Network. Enhance Your Preparedness for Pediatric CBNRE Emergencies. August 27, 2024. Accessed February 9, 2026. https://pedspandemicnetwork.org/our-work/enhance-your-preparedness-for-pediatric-cbrne-emergencies/

60 Seconds to Survival: Disaster Triage. Accessed October 15, 2024. https://disastertriagegame.org/index.html

US Department of Health and Human Services. JumpSTART Pediatric Triage Algorithm. Updated February 21, 2025. Accessed February 9, 2026. https://chemm.hhs.gov/startpediatric.htm

US Department of Health and Human Services. START Adult Triage Algorithm. Updated February 21, 2025. Accessed February 9, 2026. https://chemm.hhs.gov/startadult.htm

World Health Organization, Division of Mental Health. Psychosocial consequences of disasters: prevention and management. 1992. Accessed February 9, 2026. https://iris.who.int/handle/10665/58986

CHAPTER 17

Medicolegal and Ethical Considerations

Kathleen Adelgais, MD, MPH, FAAP, FAEMS
Robert Sharkey, EMT-P, IC

LEARNING OBJECTIVES

1. **Identify prehospital ethical and legal issues unique to pediatric emergency care.**
2. **Discuss the doctrine of implied consent in the prehospital treatment and transport of a minor.**
3. **Understand the different ethical and legal challenges in caring for older children and adolescents.**
4. **Outline the emergency medical services (EMS) clinician's responsibilities when a caregiver may refuse to grant consent to EMS clinicians to treat or transport a minor.**
5. **Review the legal and ethical considerations when faced with a child who has a "Do Not Resuscitate" status.**

Introduction

The emergency medical services (EMS) clinician frequently encounters ethical and legal issues while caring for children. These may include the inability to obtain the legal guardian's permission to treat a child, refusal of consent by parents or legal guardians, challenges of confidentiality, conflicts regarding the care provided, and identification of possible child maltreatment. This chapter discusses these issues and emphasizes the importance of protocols and policies for EMS clinicians to address common pediatric ethical and legal concerns.

Consent

The requirement to obtain **informed consent** from a patient or legal surrogate before delivering medical care is a central feature of American health care law and ethics. A legally competent adult with capacity may not be treated or transported without their consent. **Minors** (individuals younger than 18 years), however, present a special issue because, under most circumstances, they do not have the legal authority to give or refuse consent. Therefore, in most states, a parent/legal guardian must give permission before a minor can be medically treated or transported (**FIGURE 17–1**). Many states have provisions for minor children to consent to medical care for certain types of conditions. These provisions often involve access to reproductive health needs, treatment for sexually transmitted infections, treatment for drug and/or alcohol addiction, and access to behavioral health services. EMS clinicians should consult local protocols or agency/department guidelines for requirements in a particular state or region.

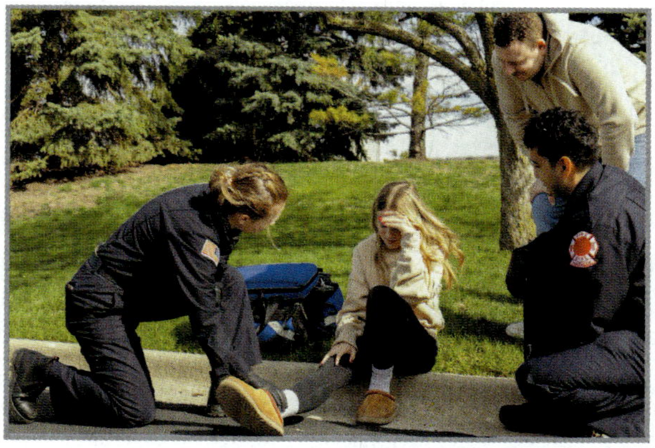

FIGURE 17–1 In most states, a parent or legal guardian must give permission before a minor can be transported.

State laws designate certain minors as "emancipated" and grant these emancipated minors the right to make decisions, including health care decisions. Adolescents who are legally emancipated may give consent for medical treatment and transport; they may refuse medical care or transport; and they may give consent for the treatment and transport of their own minor children. Although emancipated-minor laws vary from state to state, most states recognize minors to be emancipated if they are married, are pregnant, have a child, are economically self-supporting and/or not living at home, or are on active-duty status in the armed services. In most jurisdictions, the actual determination of emancipation is established by court order. You must know your state's laws regarding emancipation of minors to be sure that you are compliant with these requirements.

In situations wherein an unemancipated minor has a medical condition that represents a threat to life or health and a parent/legal guardian is not readily available to provide consent, EMS clinicians can assess the child, provide necessary medical treatment, and transport the child. The legal basis for taking action in an emergency when consent is not available is known as the doctrine of **implied consent**. For EMS clinicians, this means that they can presume consent and proceed with appropriate treatment and transport if all of the following 4 conditions are met:

1. The child is experiencing an emergent condition that places their life or health in danger.
2. The child's parent/legal guardian is unavailable or unable to provide consent for treatment or transport.
3. Treatment or transport cannot be safely delayed until consent can be obtained.
4. The EMS clinician administers only treatment for emergency conditions that pose an immediate threat to the child.

The doctrine of implied consent is based on the principle that all reasonable people want to live and, therefore, would consent to the provision of essential emergency medical care if necessary to save a person's life. Any time a minor is treated without consent, the burden of proof falls on the EMS clinician to justify that the emergency actions were necessary. The EMS clinician must fully and clearly document in the prehospital record the nature of the medical emergency, attempts made to contact the parent/legal guardian, and the reasons the minor required immediate treatment or transport, in addition to the actual care provided.

When possible, EMS clinicians should contact online medical control for assistance when consent is unclear or unavailable. If the parent/guardian is unavailable or cannot be notified, provide information about the destination emergency department (ED) to the most responsible person on scene (in writing whenever possible), with instructions to pass the information on to the minor's parent/guardian.

REFUSAL OF CARE OR TRANSPORT

Guardian Refusal

A special situation occurs when the EMS clinician is faced with a parent/guardian who refuses to give permission for medical treatment or transport of a child with an acute illness or injury. As long as a child's parent/guardian is of sound mind, they have the right to refuse medical care for their child. However, the parent/guardian must act in the best interests of the child.

When a parent/guardian refuses to allow provision of care or transport of a child whose life or health might be threatened, a serious legal and ethical issue arises. In such circumstances, attempt to contact medical control for guidance. The medical control physician may speak directly to the parent/guardian and explain the need for immediate treatment and transport. If medical control agrees that the child's

CASE STUDY 1

You are called to a home where you find a 3-year-old girl in respiratory distress. She is interactive and consolable but has a heart rate of 144 beats/min, a respiratory rate of 42 breaths/min, and a pulse oximeter reading of 87%. Physical assessment reveals increased work of breathing and bilateral wheezing. She is at her home with a 16-year-old babysitter, who tells you that the child's parents are not expected to return for several hours and did not leave information about their destination or contact information.

1. Can the babysitter give you legally valid consent to treat the child?
2. Can you legally provide care and transport this child?

condition requires immediate treatment to prevent serious harm, yet the parent/guardian continues to refuse consent for care, it may be necessary to enlist the assistance of law enforcement in placing the child in **emergency protective custody**. Likewise, when a parent/guardian seems to be intoxicated or impaired, or their decision-making capacity seems to be impacted by another medical condition, involvement of law enforcement officers may be necessary to place a minor in emergency protective custody. Local EMS pediatric guidelines and protocols should guide the EMS clinician's procedure in such situations. Not all law enforcement officers will place patients in protective custody under these circumstances, so you should defer to your local protocols when such conflicts arise.

CAUTION

When a parent/guardian is not readily available to provide consent for a minor, the EMS clinician must provide only treatment and transport for emergency conditions that pose an immediate threat to the child.

Although emergency protective custody may allow the EMS clinician to transport a minor to a medical facility for purposes of medical evaluation, it does not give the EMS clinician the right to treat a minor for medical conditions that are not serious or life-threatening. *An EMS clinician can provide medical treatment without consent only when the child has a medical condition that poses a risk of death or serious harm, only when immediate specific treatment is necessary to prevent that harm, and only when those specific treatments are provided (ie, this does not apply to treatments that are not necessary to prevent harm).* Discuss these situations with medical control before initiating treatment, whenever possible. Document everything completely and clearly about the medical condition of the child, the need for emergency care, the basis for overriding the wishes of the parent/legal guardian, including the involvement of medical control and/or law enforcement, and the reasoning behind any decisions you make.

Every case of unclear consent or refusal requires careful scene management; notification of medical control, when possible; and full and accurate documentation in the prehospital record.

EMS clinicians should never confront a parent/guardian with accusations, moral judgments, or threats when difficult circumstances develop at the scene. It is important to establish whether the parent/guardian refuses all care and transport or only certain aspects of care. For example, some parents/guardians may prefer that EMS clinicians not initiate therapy, but permit the child to be transported to the hospital. If the child can be safely transported without initiating care, the EMS professional should respect the parent/guardian's wishes concerning care. It may be appropriate for the caregiver of a child with a terminal illness or significant disabilities to restrict certain kinds of care for the child. Discuss these difficult situations with medical control.

TIP

Call for law enforcement assistance when a parent/guardian who is intoxicated or impaired or whose decision-making capacity has been impacted by another clinical condition refuses care or transport of an ill or injured child.

TIP

Never confront the parent/guardian with accusations, moral judgments, or threats.

CHILD REFUSAL

There are 3 instances in which a minor has the legal authority to refuse care and make decisions regarding their health care. The first situation is when the child is an emancipated minor, as previously discussed. A second situation in which a minor might have legal status to make decisions arises when a court has declared an individual a **mature minor**. This is different from an emancipated minor. Mature minor status exists in several states, with age limits defined by the state (most commonly teenagers), and recognizes their ability to make some independent decisions, again with limitations defined by state law. **TABLE 17–1** lists the legal circumstances in which pediatric patients can provide or refuse consent for medical care and transport in some states. Unlike the "Emancipated Minor" section in **TABLE 17–1**, which lists different ways to become emancipated (eg., being married OR being in the armed services), the "Mature Minor" list functions as a cumulative checklist that must be satisfied to be considered a mature minor. In the context of prehospital care, mature minor doctrine most often applies to a child with a chronic medical condition who has demonstrated an active, informed role in managing their own care and may involve refusal of care for a life-threatening or terminal illness. The ability of emancipated or mature minors to consent or refuse care is limited to those with decision-making capacity. An emancipated

TABLE 17–1 Characteristics of Emancipated and Mature Minors

Emancipated Minor
Married or,
Pregnant or,
Has a child, or
Has active-duty status in the armed services
15 years or older, economically self-supporting, and living apart from parents
Mature Minor
Meets minimum age required for mature minor by state law (12 to 14 years in most states), and
Declared a mature minor by the state court, and
Is not on a psychiatric hold, and
Demonstrates competency to be involved in their own health care decision-making
Minor With Decision-Making Capacity (Statutory Conditions Recognized in Most US States)
A minor who exhibits decision-making capacity seeking care for any of the following: ▪ Pregnancy ▪ Birth control ▪ Sexually transmitted infections ▪ Drug or alcohol abuse

minor who is being transported for a mandated mental health evaluation or who is unconscious lacks capacity to consent or refuse.

Because these laws vary, the EMS clinician must be familiar with the specifics of emancipated and mature minor laws in the state in which care is being provided.

For children who are not formally emancipated or mature minors, nearly all US states recognize the right of adolescents to independently seek care for certain medical conditions, including pregnancy, birth control, sexually transmitted infections, and substance abuse. The specific parameters vary somewhat by state statute but nearly all include pregnancy, birth control, and substance abuse. A 16-year-old girl in labor would be able to consent for transport to the hospital or to refuse transport so long as she has capacity.

Outside of these state-defined conditions, if a child is not an emancipated or a mature minor, they lack ability to consent or refuse care. Regardless of whether a child has the legal authority to provide or withhold consent, it is prudent to obtain the child's assent to treat and transport, if possible. This approach respects the personal dignity and self-determination of the patient and minimizes confrontation. A willingness to provide the child with some control and some choices may allow for a compromise that helps EMS clinicians achieve a safe transfer. Avoid physical or chemical restraint to transport a child except in those situations in which the child is at risk of serious harm if they are not transported, and only after consultation with medical control.

TIP

A minor child who does not meet the local definition of emancipated or mature minor cannot legally refuse care or transport when essential care is needed.

CAREGIVERS WHO DISAGREE

One rare but confusing situation arises when the EMS clinician is confronted by multiple family members or caregivers who disagree about whether to consent to treatment and transport of a sick or an injured child. In these cases, attempt to establish who the legal decision-makers are for the child. If both parents have legal decision-making authority, the EMS clinician may need to negotiate a plan that both find acceptable. Focus on the child's needs and the common desire to assist the child, while deflecting attention from the disagreement. Medical control may need to be involved to assist the EMS clinician in determining the proper course of action and to determine the need for law enforcement.

Custody Issues and Nontraditional Families

Parents who are legally divorced may disagree about the child's care or access to the child's medical records. One parent may accuse the other of harming the child or otherwise providing substandard care. Perhaps one parent has exclusive legal custody, and the other parent's rights have been terminated. Another parent may refuse transport because they do not want the child's insurance to be billed, because that responsibility rests with the parent who is not available. Stepparents often do not have legal decision-making rights for children they have not legally adopted.

Many children live in nontraditional families in which they are cared for by grandparents, older siblings, same-sex parents, or foster parents. It may not be clear who has the responsibility of consenting for the minor child. In addition, these caregivers may be the only adults involved with the child on a regular basis despite the fact that they may not be legally responsible for that child. State statutes may have various mechanisms to allow caregivers who are neither a parent nor legal guardian to provide valid consent for minors. These caregivers can stand **in loco parentis**, meaning "in place of the parent," with recognized rights to consent for medical care, make educational decisions, and perform other parental functions even though they have no other legal rights to the child. In general, health care providers can place reasonable reliance on statements made by individuals professing to be in an *in loco parentis* role for a child. Conversely, health care providers have a duty to investigate further if a purported caregiver's claims seem suspicious or questionable. Certain states may allow parents/legal guardians to convey certain rights to others through a power of attorney, guardianship, or a caregiver's affidavit without severing their parental/guardianship ties to a child.

In these situations, determining legal authority for treatment and transport may be difficult. If the child is acutely ill or injured, there may not be time to consult legal documents, even when available. Contact medical control for advice and involve law enforcement if the situation becomes violent or may cause harm to the child.

CAUTION

Many children live in nontraditional families, and it may be unclear who has legal responsibility for consenting for the minor child.

Summary of Consent

Laws strictly protect the right of adult patients to accept or reject medical care so long as they have decision-making capacity. Interpreting these consent laws for children in a prehospital setting, however, can pose special challenges. The EMS clinician faces a difficult situation in cases where the parent/guardian refuses to consent or where consent to provide care and transport for a child cannot be readily obtained. Every case requires careful scene management; notification of medical control, if available; and accurate documentation in the prehospital record. EMS systems should provide clear policies, procedures, and protocols based on state law to guide the EMS clinician or medical control. Local EMS policies and protocols on consent should clearly define the following:

- Who can consent and refuse ambulance transport according to state law
- The process for field evaluation, consultation, and documentation
- The method for enlisting law enforcement and medical control when the patient's medical condition and other scene factors warrant these resources

Confidentiality

Medical information is private. Carelessly or inadvertently revealing identifiable information is an ethical and legal risk that EMS clinicians face, because they frequently care for individuals in a public environment. *It is essential to remain aware of the potentially sensitive nature of identifiable information and to take every possible precaution to protect confidentiality.* Conduct all sensitive discussions, when possible, in a setting where bystanders cannot overhear. Avoid using last names, if at all possible, at the scene. Do not share private information with concerned bystanders (other than those legally responsible for the patient).

TIP

EMS clinicians must be aware of the potentially sensitive nature of protected health information and take every possible precaution to protect confidentiality.

Respect for Cultural or Religious Differences

Respect for cultural differences and religious beliefs is an important component of family-centered care. In some instances, these differences and beliefs may present challenges. Although the care of the patient is always of primary concern, the EMS clinician must be sensitive to requests from the family or patient regarding preferences that may originate from their religious or cultural beliefs, especially when these preferences do not interfere significantly with the provision of treatment to the child.

The EMS clinician must always remain nonjudgmental about requests that stem from cultural or religious beliefs; acknowledge the importance of these requests to the family; and attempt to accommodate them when possible. When the EMS clinician cannot accommodate requests that are based on cultural or religious beliefs because those requests would put a child at risk of serious harm, the reasons the requests cannot be accommodated must be respectfully explained and documented. Parents/guardians have great latitude in making medical decisions for themselves based on religious beliefs; however, as in all cases where parents/guardians refuse necessary and lifesaving care and the child is at risk of imminent harm, it is appropriate to contact medical control and law enforcement.

> **TIP**
>
> The EMS clinician must always remain nonjudgmental about cultural or religious beliefs, acknowledge their importance to the family and the community, and attempt to accommodate them whenever possible.

Language barriers may also present a challenge as the EMS clinician attempts to communicate with a child's caregiver. The EMS clinician should be familiar with locally available resources to provide translation in a timely manner. Miscommunication can have a significant impact on patient care, especially if the EMS clinician is unable to obtain information about a child's underlying medical conditions, allergies, current medications, or other factors relevant to their current medical needs. When available, professional interpreter services should be used instead of family members or bystanders. If interpreter services are not available, a family member or neighbor may be asked to assist with interpretation, with the understanding that information may be inaccurate or incomplete. When using nonprofessional interpreters, care should be taken to avoid medical terminology when possible.

Patient Rights and Advocacy

For children, patient rights may depend on the wishes of their parents/legal guardians. However, emancipated minors have the ability to make decisions about their medical care and treatment, even though these decisions may not be accepted by family members or the general public.

The decision to accept or not accept medical treatment may be difficult. Give the parent/guardian or the emancipated minor time to consider what is most appropriate. In some instances, this emergency may be the first time the patient has had to face the reality of their medical condition.

End-of-Life Issues

The parents/guardians of children who are terminally ill, usually in consultation with the primary care physician, may decide on limitations to treatments and interventions. These decisions usually arise from the child's underlying condition and the desire to avoid futile or invasive interventions if the child has little or no hope of recovery. EMS clinicians, in responding to a call about a sick child, may be confronted with a **do not resuscitate (DNR)** order or **physician orders for life-sustaining treatment (POLST)/medical orders for life-sustaining treatments (MOLST)**.

EMS clinicians must know the specifics of DNR and/or POLST/MOLST guidance in their jurisdictions and develop protocols for dealing with them.

A DNR order informs health care providers that cardiopulmonary resuscitation (CPR) or additional resuscitation, such as defibrillation or advanced airway management, should not be initiated in the event of a cardiopulmonary arrest. Do-not-resuscitate orders must be signed by a licensed medical provider to be valid (**FIGURE 17–2**). Some local EMS regions do not recognize DNR orders for children.

A POLST or MOLST form is a comprehensive document indicating goals of care, treatment that is permitted when the patient still has a pulse and is breathing, permissions pertaining to artificially administered nutrition, CPR and airway management permissions, and other directions for care (**FIGURE 17–3**). Endorsement of the POLST/MOLST form varies by state.

> **CASE STUDY 2**
>
> You are called to care for a homeless 15-year-old boy whose friends called because he was not feeling well and was not acting normally. You find the young man lying on the sidewalk, complaining of a severe headache. When you attempt to assess him, he starts cursing, pushes you away aggressively, and demands to be left alone. He screams that he has rights and that he does not have to talk to you. He will not even answer questions that would allow you to assess his level of consciousness and orientation.
>
> 1. What rights does the teenager have to refuse care and transport?
> 2. How can you engage this patient in assessment and care?

CMA PUBLICATIONS 1(800) 882-1262 WWW.CMANET.ORG

EMERGENCY MEDICAL SERVICES AUTHORITY • CALIFORNIA • EMSA

EMERGENCY MEDICAL SERVICES
PREHOSPITAL DO NOT RESUSCITATE (DNR) FORM

CMA California Medical Association

An Advance Request to Limit the Scope of Emergency Medical Care

I, ______________________________, request limited emergency care as herein described.
(print patient's name)

I understand DNR means that if my heart stops beating or if I stop breathing, no medical procedure to restart breathing or heart functioning will be instituted.

I understand this decision will **not** prevent me from obtaining other emergency medical care by prehospital emergency medical care personnel and/or medical care directed by a physician prior to my death.

I understand I may revoke this directive at any time by destroying this form and removing any "DNR" medallions.

I give permission for this information to be given to the prehospital emergency care personnel, doctors, nurses or other health personnel as necessary to implement this directive.

I hereby agree to the "Do Not Resuscitate" (DNR) order.

______________________________ ______________________________
Patient/Legally Recognized Health Care Decisionmaker Signature — Date

____
Legally Recognized Health Care Decisionmaker's Relationship to Patient

By signing this form, the legally recognized health care decisionmaker acknowledges that this request to forego resuscitative measures is consistent with the known desires of, and with the best interest of, the individual who is the subject of the form.

I affirm that this patient/legally recognized health care decisionmaker is making an informed decision and that this directive is the expressed wish of the patient/legally recognized health care decisionmaker. A copy of this form is in the patient's permanent medical record.

In the event of cardiac or respiratory arrest, no chest compressions, assisted ventilations, intubation, defibrillation, or cardiotonic medications are to be initiated.

______________________________ ______________________________
Physician Signature — Date

______________________________ ______________________________
Print Name — Telephone

THIS FORM WILL NOT BE ACCEPTED IF IT HAS BEEN AMENDED OR ALTERED IN ANY WAY

PREHOSPITAL DNR REQUEST FORM

White Copy:	To be kept by patient
Yellow Copy:	To be kept in patient's permanent medical record
Pink Copy:	If authorized DNR medallion desired, submit this form with Medic Alert enrollment form to: Medic Alert Foundation, Turlock, CA 95381

FIGURE 17–2 California EMS do-not-resuscitate form.

MM 3 2013 Page 1 of 2

Maryland Medical Orders for Life-Sustaining Treatment (MOLST)

Patient's Last Name, First, Middle Initial	Date of Birth	☐ Male ☐ Female

This form includes medical orders for Emergency Medical Services (EMS) and other medical personnel regarding cardiopulmonary resuscitation and other life-sustaining treatment options for a specific patient. It is valid in all health care facilities and programs throughout Maryland. This order form shall be kept with other active medical orders in the patient's medical record. The physician, nurse practitioner (NP), or physician assistan t (PA) must accurately and legibly complete the form and then sign and date it. The physician, NP, or PA shall select only 1 choice in Section 1 and only 1 choice in any of the other Sections that apply to this patient. If any of Sections 2-9 do not apply, leave them blank. A copy or the original of every completed MOLST form must be given to the patient or authorized decision maker within 48 hours of completion of the form or sooner if the patient is discharged or transferred.

CERTIFICATION FOR THE BASIS OF THESE ORDERS: Mark any and all that apply.

I hereby certify that these orders are entered as a result of a discussion with and the informed consent of:

________ the patient; or
________ the patient's health care agent as named in the patient's advance directive; or
________ the patient's guardian of the person as per the authority granted by a court order; or
________ the patient's surrogate as per the authority granted by the Heath Care Decisions Act; or
________ if the patient is a minor, the patient's legal guardian or another legally authorized adult.

Or, I hereby certify that these orders are based on:

________ instructions in the patient's advance directive; or
________ other legal authority in accordance with all provisions of the Health Care Decisions Act. All supporting documentation must be contained in the patient's medical records.

________ Mark this line if the patient or authorized decision maker declines to discuss or is unable to make a decision about these treatments. **The patient's or authorized decision maker's participation in the preparation of the MOLST form is always voluntary.** If the patient or authorized decision maker has not limited care, except as otherwise provided by law, CPR will be attempted and other treatments will be given.

1

CPR (RESUSCITATION) STATUS: EMS providers must follow the *Maryland Medical Protocols for EMS Providers*.

________ **Attempt CPR:** If cardiac and/or pulmonary arrest occurs, attempt cardiopulmonary resuscitation (CPR). This will include any and all medical efforts that are indicated during arrest, including artificial ventilation and efforts to restore and/or stabilize cardiopulmonary function.

[If the patient or authorized decision maker does not or cannot make any selection regarding CPR status, mark this option. Exceptions: If a valid advance directive declines CPR, CPR is medically ineffective, or there is some other legal basis for not attempting CPR, mark one of the "No CPR" options below.]

No CPR, Option A, Comprehensive Efforts to Prevent Arrest: Prior to arrest, administer all medications needed to stabilize the patient. If cardiac and/or pulmonary arrest occurs, do not attempt resuscitation (No CPR). Allow death to occur naturally.

________ **Option A-1, Intubate:** Comprehensive efforts may include intubation and artificial ventilation.

________ **Option A-2, Do Not Intubate (DNI):** Comprehensive efforts may include limited ventilatory support by CPAP or BiPAP, but do not intubate.

________ **No CPR, Option B, Palliative and Supportive Care:** Prior to arrest, provide passive oxygen for comfort and control any external bleeding. Prior to arrest, provide medications for pain relief as needed, but no other medications. Do not intubate or use CPAP or BiPAP. If cardiac and/or pulmonary arrest occurs, do not attempt resuscitation (No CPR). Allow death to occur naturally.

SIGNATURE OF PHYSICIAN, NURSE PRACTITIONER, OR PHYSICIAN ASSISTANT (Signature and date are required to validate order)

Practitioner's Signature	Print Practitioner's Name	
Maryland License #	Phone Number	Date

FIGURE 17–3 A Maryland form for medical orders for life-sustaining treatment.

Patient's Last Name, First, Middle Initial	Date of Birth	Page 2 of 2 ☐ Male ☐ Female

Orders in Sections 2-9 below do not apply to EMS providers and are for situations other than cardiopulmonary arrest. Only complete applicable items in Sections 2 through 8, and only select one choice per applicable Section.

Section	Orders	
2	**ARTIFICIAL VENTILATION** 2a. ________ May use intubation and artificial ventilation indefinitely, if medically indicated. 2b. ________ May use intubation and artificial ventilation as a limited therapeutic trial. Time limit________ 2c. ________ May use only CPAP or BiPAP for artificial ventilation, as medically indicated. Time limit________ 2d. ________ Do not use any artificial ventilation (no intubation, CPAP or BiPAP).	
3	**BLOOD TRANSFUSION** 3a. ________ May give any blood product (whole blood, packed red blood cells, plasma or platelets) that is medically indicated.	3b. ________ Do not give any blood products.
4	**HOSPITAL TRANSFER** 4a. ________ Transfer to hospital for any situation requiring hospital-level care.	4b. ________ Transfer to hospital for severe pain or severe symptoms that cannot be controlled otherwise. 4c. ________ Do not transfer to hospital, but treat with options available outside the hospital.
5	**MEDICAL WORKUP** 5a. ________ May perform any medical tests indicated to diagnose and/or treat a medical condition.	5b. ________ Only perform limited medical tests necessary for symptomatic treatment or comfort. 5c. ________ Do not perform any medical tests for diagnosis or treatment.
6	**ANTIBIOTICS** 6a. ________ May use antibiotics (oral, intravenous or intramuscular) as medically indicated. 6b. ________ May use oral antibiotics when medically indicated, but do not give intravenous or intramuscular antibiotics.	6c. ________ May use oral antibiotics only when indicated for symptom relief or comfort. 6d. ________ Do not treat with antibiotics.
7	**ARTIFICIALLY ADMINISTERED FLUIDS AND NUTRITION** 7a. ________ May give artificially administered fluids and nutrition, even indefinitely, if medically indicated. 7b. ________ May give artificially administered fluids and nutrition, if medically indicated, as a trial. Time limit________	7c. ________ May give fluids for artificial hydration as a therapeutic trial, but do not give artificially administered nutrition. Time limit________ 7d. ________ Do not provide artificially administered fluids or nutrition.
8	**DIALYSIS** 8a. ________ May give chronic dialysis for end-stage kidney disease if medically indicated.	8b. ________ May give dialysis for a limited period. Time limit________ 8c. ________ Do not provide acute or chronic dialysis.
9	**OTHER ORDERS** ________	

SIGNATURE OF PHYSICIAN, NURSE PRACTITIONER, OR PHYSICIAN ASSISTANT (Signature and date are required to validate order)

Practitioner's Signature	Print Practitioner's Name	
Maryland License #	Phone Number	Date

FIGURE 17–3 *(continued)*

Even in the presence of a valid DNR or POLST/MOLST order, clarify with the parent/guardian what kinds of interventions they do and do not consider acceptable. For example, oxygen delivery and transport may be acceptable and expected for some children with DNR orders. Parents/guardians generally have the right to revoke a DNR or POLST/MOLST order for a minor; local laws may vary, and EMS clinicians should be aware of local laws with regard to when resuscitation should be performed in a patient with a valid DNR/POLST/MOLST.

RESUSCITATION

Sometimes resuscitation attempts are ineffective for children in cardiopulmonary arrest, and occasionally such attempts are unnecessary, as discussed in Chapter 5. Resuscitation policy should define circumstances in which cardiopulmonary resuscitation must be initiated, when it may be withheld, and when it may be discontinued. Personnel in rural and wilderness situations must also consider the time it takes for a patient to reach definitive care at the hospital. For pediatric patients, the policy should take a patient-focused approach, but allow appropriate withholding of resuscitation to focus on grief management and family interactions.

Local resuscitation policy may allow EMS clinicians to withhold or discontinue resuscitation when a child is clearly deceased, as defined by specific criteria (eg, rigor mortis or injuries incompatible with life). This situation may be emotionally difficult for the EMS clinician. Likewise, it may be difficult emotionally for family members or bystanders if EMS clinicians do not attempt resuscitation. In such cases, the child can be treated with basic life support (BLS) measures only and transported to the ED, where physicians can formally pronounce the child dead. Local protocols vary widely in guidance for such scenarios.

As part of educational and training requirements for field personnel, EMS systems should have a formal training program regarding sudden unexpected infant death (SUID) (see Chapter 15) and sudden unexpected death in childhood. Local EMS policies should clearly establish the responsibility of the EMS clinician at death scenes regarding care of the body, notification of the coroner or medical examiner and law enforcement, and interaction with parents/guardians and other caregivers.

ORGAN DONATION

A major issue in medical ethics involves the potential for patients to donate organs at the end of their life. Donor organs are much needed within the medical system, and many patients wait years or die while waiting for a match (**TABLE 17–2**). Whether a child should be kept alive for the sole purpose of organ donation is an issue that EMS clinicians should discuss with medical control and the local hospital system. The parameters for viable organs should be clearly outlined within the individual EMS system. Understanding state laws regarding organ donation helps the EMS clinician decide how to proceed.

TABLE 17–2 Organ Donation Statistics

▪ As of October 2024, more than 100,000 individuals were waiting for an organ transplant to survive.
▪ Another person needing a transplant is added to the waiting list every 8 minutes.
▪ Each day, approximately 16 people die waiting for a transplant.
▪ In 2023, more than 46,000 organ transplantations were performed.

Another helpful resource is the local organ transplant programs within the EMS service area. They may offer workshops or an in-service to EMS clinicians for continuing education and to increase awareness of organ donation programs, as well as support the development of prehospital protocol.

TELLING THE TRUTH IN DIFFICULT SITUATIONS

EMS clinicians should address children and their caregivers with honesty. It is not unusual for family or caregivers to ask about the condition of a child or request information about a child's "chances of survival." Given the lack of true knowledge of the chance of survival early in resuscitation, EMS clinicians should not speculate; instead, they should inform the family that the team is providing the best care possible. Possible statements are, "We'll take the best possible care of your child," or "Everything is being done to help them."

The EMS clinician may also face situations in which multiple patients have sustained injuries and a parent or child requests information about others involved in the incident. The best course of action is to offer reassurance, such as "I need to focus on taking the best care of you right now. My partners are doing their best to take care of the others." It is appropriate to deflect questions when a definite answer is not known and to avoid delivering particularly distressing information (eg, death of another person in the vehicle) in the back of the ambulance.

CASE STUDY 3

You respond to the scene of a motor vehicle crash where you find a 10-year-old child with facial bruising; a tense, tender abdomen; and an obviously deformed left thigh. The child is wearing a seat belt in the rear passenger seat of the car, which has been struck on the driver's door by a truck. The child seems scared and begins to cry as you begin your assessment. The woman who had been driving the car has obvious head injuries and lacks a pulse. Another team begins work on the adult while you tend to the child. As you stabilize the child for transport, she asks you if her mother is okay.

1. Would it be appropriate to tell the child her mother is okay to enable a safe and efficient transport?
2. How should you respond to this child's question?

PHYSICIAN ON SCENE

Prehospital care is under the authority of EMS medical control. However, when EMS is called to an outpatient medical setting, the patient may simultaneously be under the care of a private physician. State and local laws vary about whether EMS clinicians can or cannot carry out orders from non-EMS–affiliated physicians, including the patient's private physician. These interactions are sometimes controversial. EMS clinicians should know the laws applicable to their practice location and rely on EMS medical control to guide their actions when conflict arises with a physician on scene.

CONTROVERSY

The role of an unaffiliated (non-EMS) physician in on-scene care is controversial. The EMS clinician must provide care according to the local EMS system policy, but an on-scene physician may choose to provide care on their own authority. Always proceed in the best interests of the child. Contact online medical control when clear guidance is needed.

HOSPITAL DESTINATION

The hospital destination policy for children should define the following components:

1. Field triage criteria (which patients with what conditions go where)
2. Designated receiving hospitals
3. Specialized pediatric centers

The appropriate ED for a sick or an injured child may differ from the ED appropriate for an adult with a similar condition. Some EMS systems identify specialized pediatric centers (eg, pediatric trauma centers, general trauma centers with pediatric capability) with protocolized medical direction guidance when making a destination decision for certain pediatric patients. However, not every scenario can be anticipated. For example, should a severely burned child be transported to a regional children's hospital or a nonpediatric hospital with a regional burn center? If the existing destination policy is not clear regarding where a patient with complex medical issues should be transported, it is appropriate to contact online medical control for destination guidance. The EMS clinician and parent/guardian should discuss the destination choice in the context of the EMS agency's destination policy. If a parent/guardian disagrees with the destination choice, contact medical control and have them speak to the parent/guardian. Always document your observations and decision-making objectively.

Pediatric Policies and Procedures

EMS systems should provide clear guidelines for common problems related to ethical and legal issues involving children. In addition, when available, online medical control provides the EMS clinician with the ability to obtain real-time consultation regarding particularly difficult situations, such as the inability to obtain consent, refusal of assent by a child or consent by a guardian, presence of a physician on scene, resuscitation or other clinical decisions, and suspected child maltreatment or sexual assault.

PROTOCOLS, POLICIES, AND PROCEDURES

Operations are the administrative backbone of the EMS system. The goal of **operations** is to manage day-to-day field care with standards established by the EMS system. An important part of operations is the **policies**, **procedures**, and **protocols** that define the **medical responsibility** and **legal authority** of the EMS clinicians and medical director within the EMS system. These written directives assist the EMS clinician in knowing what to do in complicated prehospital situations. These written directives, along with education and training, also help set performance standards.

Because the needs of children differ from those of adults, pediatric-specific protocols, policies, and procedures are necessary tools for a comprehensive EMS system. Protocols define explicit field treatments or the order and type of medical interventions for specific illness and injury conditions. They provide appropriate pharmacologic options, including drug doses, routes of delivery, and methods of administration. Most EMS systems have protocols for prehospital pediatric advanced life support (ALS), medical emergencies, and trauma treatments. Appropriate treatment protocols for prehospital BLS personnel and for first responders are also important. **TABLE 17–3** lists some common EMS pediatric treatment protocols.

Policies and procedures also reflect the expectations of the community for prehospital care, quality management, and system accountability. These forms of regulation consist of clear, written directives to guide EMS clinicians. They are intended to help with decision-making in difficult or legally sensitive pediatric field situations, such as those discussed previously in this chapter. Policies usually explain how the EMS clinician should handle certain situations and the reasoning behind them, rather than specific medical treatment. Procedures describe the sequence of actions for the EMS clinician in applying medical protocols or medicolegal policies. The field policies with the most frequent application to pediatric care include the following:

- Consent for care or transport
- Refusal to consent for care or transport
- Death in the field
- Triage guidelines
- Hospital destination
- Child maltreatment

Each state has statutes that establish basic requirements for local EMS systems; provide guidelines for quality management, accountability, and enforcement; and establish EMS clinician scope of practice. Policies, procedures, and protocols may differ substantially from one EMS system to the next. Mutual aid agreements between bordering geographic areas are especially useful because resources, equipment, and personnel for specialized care of children are not evenly distributed. Specialized trauma care and critical care centers for children are usually only available at major hospitals in large urban areas. In some states, no specialized centers for children exist.

TABLE 17–3 Examples of Pediatric Treatment Protocols

Airway obstruction
Allergic reaction and anaphylaxis
Altered mental status
Bradycardia
Brief resolved unexplained events
Burns
Cardiopulmonary arrest
Hypoperfusion or shock
Neonatal resuscitation
Respiratory distress
Seizures
Tachycardia
Toxic exposures
Trauma

CHILD MALTREATMENT AND SEXUAL ASSAULT

Education of EMS clinicians in identifying possible maltreatment is an essential component of initial education and continuing medical education in pediatrics (see Chapter 13). EMS clinicians are mandatory reporters of child maltreatment. A policy and procedure for reporting suspected cases of maltreatment and for appropriate patient transport to an ED are important components of every EMS system. The EMS clinician must ensure that victims of maltreatment or sexual assault are initially evaluated in a careful, compassionate, and respectful way. When possible, these patients should be transported to an ED staffed by clinicians experienced in working with child victims of maltreatment and/or sexual assault and equipped to provide the appropriate ancillary and follow-up services. Never confront a parent/guardian or others with accusations, moral judgments, threats, or suspicions. Although these situations are emotionally difficult, the immediate goal must always be to provide necessary treatment and ensure the safe transport of the child.

MEDICAL CONTROL FOR PEDIATRICS

Medical control, medical direction, or medical oversight are the mechanisms by which physicians, nurses, and EMS officials supervise field practice. Medical control includes direct and indirect methods.

Online (Direct) Medical Control

Online or **direct medical control** refers to any communication between the EMS clinician and medical control by telephone or radio (**FIGURE 17–4**). This form of medical oversight is required by some local EMS systems for many or all cases involving patients younger than 18 years because decisions about pediatric ALS treatment (eg, intravenous lines, drug routes, and doses), triage, scene control, and transport are often difficult. Online medical control can be very useful in cases of high-risk pediatric refusals of care or transport. Online medical control is often done on a recorded line, and any conversation with the parent/guardian while speaking with medical control can be recorded. In cases of high-risk refusals with a life threat, the medical control physician should speak directly with the parent/guardian via the recorded line. **TABLE 17–4** lists some examples of problems in pediatric field practice that often require online physician input or direct medical control.

Offline (Indirect) Medical Control

Offline or **indirect medical control** involves prospective written guidance. Prospective indirect control consists of planning for anticipated educational and operational requirements within the EMS clinician's scope of practice. Continuous quality improvement (CQI) programs provide accountability through review of individual and overall system performance to guide improvement. **TABLE 17–5** lists common examples of how indirect medical control creates and monitors different types of policies, procedures, and protocols for children.

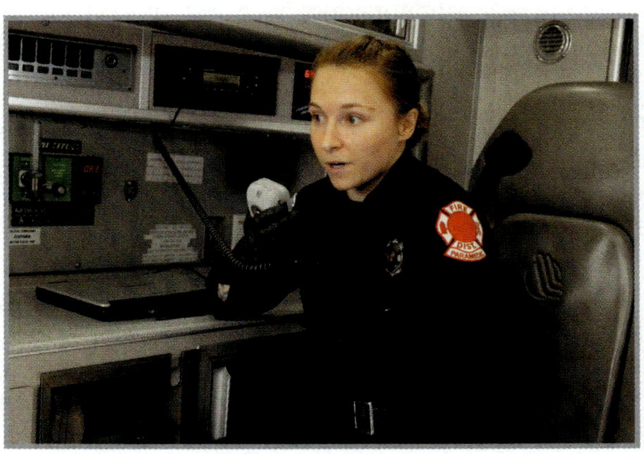

FIGURE 17–4 Direct medical control can be extremely helpful when the EMS clinician confronts medical and legal problems with children.

TABLE 17–4 Possible Pediatric Issues Needing Direct Medical Control

Pediatric Issue	Possible Scenario
Field treatment	Discontinuation of resuscitation
Hospital destination	Appropriate ED for an injured child
Specialized scene control	Hazardous materials exposure in a school
Transport	Guardian reluctant to transport after BRUE

Abbreviations: BRUE, brief resolved unexplained event; ED, emergency department.

TABLE 17–5 Indirect Medical Control and Continuous Quality Improvement (CQI)

Examples of Indirect Medical Control	Examples of Possible CQI Measures
Pediatric seizure treatment protocol	Percentage of patients with seizure receiving benzodiazepine Percentage of patients requiring respiratory support after benzodiazepine use
Pediatric asthma treatment protocol	Percentage of patients with complete respiratory assessment documented Percentage of patients with asthma treated with bronchodilator
Endotracheal intubation procedure	Rate of successful endotracheal intubation
IO needle insertion procedure	Rate of successful IO insertion Locations used for IO in pediatric patients
Field triage or destination guidance	Review of ED or hospital capabilities for the care of children
Refusal of care policy	Monitoring subsequent calls for pediatric patient after transport refusal

Abbreviations: ED, emergency department; IO, intraosseous.

Summary of Rationale for Protocols, Policies, and Procedures

Pediatric-specific guidelines (as defined in protocols, policies, and procedures) help set standards of care for children. Medical control is especially important in the delivery of prehospital services to families and children because of the unusual circumstances that often arise medically and legally.

CASE STUDY ANSWERS

CASE STUDY 1

Although a babysitter (even an adult babysitter) usually cannot provide valid consent to treat, the doctrine of implied consent allows you to treat and transport this child who is in respiratory distress. She is experiencing an emergent condition that places her at risk, her legal guardian is unavailable, and it would be unsafe to delay treatment. If the babysitter has a telephone number for the parents, call them, apprise them of the situation, and ask permission to provide necessary treatment and transport. If there is no way to reach the parents, you should provide treatment for the child's wheezing and respiratory distress with oxygen and a bronchodilator and transport her to an appropriate facility. Follow local policies regarding requirements to involve law enforcement in the transport of the child without a caregiver. Finally, make sure this 16-year-old babysitter is safe, and leave a note with her to give to the child's caregivers that explains what happened and where you have transported the child.

You provide supplemental oxygen and nebulized albuterol en route to the hospital. The child is diagnosed with asthma exacerbation and receives additional albuterol and oral steroids in the ED. Her oxygenation is normal but she continues to wheeze and have mild respiratory distress. The child is a prior patient at the hospital, and the hospital staff finds a telephone number for the mother in her chart. The mother arrives a short time later and the child is observed overnight in the hospital for frequent albuterol treatments.

CASE STUDY 2

Unless you can persuade the child to allow you to deliver care, this will be a difficult situation. Some states would not consider a homeless adolescent to be an emancipated minor without a court order. Even if he cannot legally refuse treatment and transport, every effort must be made to show respect, involve him in decisions, and avoid the use of force. If he persists in refusing to be evaluated, contact medical control. If his combativeness seems to be the result of a medical condition that impairs judgment (eg, meningitis, a head injury, intoxication), call law enforcement to provide assistance in restraining the adolescent sufficiently to allow a safe assessment and transport.

As a practical matter, respect the boy's dignity, but be firm that transport to an ED is necessary. Try to establish rapport and do not be judgmental. If a friend or counselor is available, try to obtain assistance in persuading the teenager to agree to care and transport.

Eventually, you convince the teen to be transported to the ED with the assistance of law enforcement. Hospital social workers determine that he is a runaway from foster care and contact the local department of social services, which is his legal guardian. The patient undergoes medical screening and a mental health evaluation in the ED; he has no medical emergencies and is not a danger to himself or others. He is referred for intensive outpatient mental health services, and the department of social services arranges for a new placement in a group home.

CASE STUDY 3

Carefully consider your answer to this child's question. On the one hand, avoid being dishonest. Because you do not know whether her mother will survive, you should not assure the child that her mother will be okay. On the other hand, it would be appropriate to withhold your concerns and

CASE STUDY ANSWERS—cont'd

suspicions about the mother's condition until the child has been transported safely, more is known about the mother's condition, and there are resources (eg, a social worker) available to assist the child in receiving what may be terrible news. One honest answer might be, "I know you are worried about your mother. My partners are taking good care of her. I need to take good care of you, and I'm going to take you to the hospital. Once we get there, we'll try to find out more about your mother."

When you arrive at the hospital, the child is greeted by her maternal grandparents, who were informed by law enforcement of the mother's death and are eager to check on the condition of their grandchild. The child bursts into tears and reaches out to her grandparents. She asks her grandparents about her mother and they tell her that her mother is dead. Hospital staff, including a social worker and a chaplain, provide comfort and allow the child to grieve with her grandparents.

Suggested References

TEXTBOOKS

American Academy of Orthopaedic Surgeons. *Nancy Caroline's Emergency Care in the Streets*. 8th ed. Jones & Bartlett Learning; 2018

ARTICLES

Anders JF, Fishe JN, Fratta KA, et al. Creating a pediatric prehospital destination decision tool using a modified Delphi method. *Children (Basel)*. 2021;8(8):658. PMID: 34438548 doi: 10.3390/children8080658

Cicero MX, Brown L, Auerbach M, Baird J, Adelgais K. Modified Delphi method derivation of the FAMILY (Family Assessment of Medical Interventions & Liaisons with the Young) EMS instrument. *Prehosp Emerg Care*. 2021;25(5):689–696. PMID: 32940539 doi: 10.1080/10903127.2020.1824052

Larkin GL, Fowler RL. Essential ethics for EMS: cardinal virtues and core principles. *Emerg Med Clin North Am*. 2002;20(4):887–911. PMID: 12476886 doi: 10.1016/S0733-8627(02)00034-2

Schears RM, Marco CA, Iserson KV; ACEP Ethics Committee. "Do not attempt resuscitation" (DNAR) in the out-of-hospital setting. *Ann Emerg Med*. 2004;44(1):68–70. PMID: 15226711 doi: 10.1016/j.annemergmed.2004.01.008

Sharko M, Jameson R, Ancker JS, Krams L, Webber EC, Rosenbloom ST. State-by-state variability in adolescent privacy laws. *Pediatrics*. 2022;149(6):e2021053458. PMID: 35531640 doi: 10.1542/peds.2021-053458

Sirbaugh PE, Diekema DS; Committee on Pediatric Emergency Medicine and Committee on Bioethics. Consent for emergency medical services for children and adolescents. *Pediatrics*. 2011;128(2):427–433. PMID: 21788221 doi: 10.1542/peds.2011-1166

OTHER RESOURCES

Donate Life America. Accessed November 23, 2024. https://donatelife.net

National Association of Emergency Medical Technicians (NAEMT). Code of Ethics. Accessed November 23, 2024.

Ogilvie WA, Moy HP, Goldstein S. EMS Legal and Ethical Issues. In: *StatPearls* [Internet]. StatPearls Publishing; Updated May 8, 2023. https://www.ncbi.nlm.nih.gov/books/NBK519553/

Privileged communication. *Encyclopedia Britannica*. Accessed November 23, 2024. https://www.britannica.com/topic/privileged-communication

SchoolHouse Connection. State Laws on Minor Consent for Routine Medical Care. Accessed November 23, 2024. https://schoolhouseconnection.org/article/state-laws-on-minor-consent-for-routine-medical-care

U.S. Department of Health and Human Services. Summary of the HIPAA Privacy Rule. Updated March 14, 2025. https://www.hhs.gov/hipaa/for-professionals/privacy/laws-regulations/index.html

CHAPTER 18

Transportation Considerations

Chris Coughlin, PhD, NRP
Rudy Kink, MD, FAAP

LEARNING OBJECTIVES

1. **Discuss transport considerations for pediatric encounters in an ambulance.**
2. **List the considerations used to determine the mode of transport for children in an ambulance.**
3. **Discuss advantages and disadvantages of transporting caregivers in the ambulance.**
4. **Identify and discuss current guidelines for child restraint systems in ambulances.**
5. **Identify issues related to choice of destination when making pediatric transport decisions.**
6. **Outline issues involved in transporting multiple children.**

Pediatric Transport

Although pediatric patients make up a small portion of EMS runs, every EMS clinician is faced with the critical decision of when and how to transport a child. Whether the child is a patient or accompanying an adult, the transport decision involves multiple considerations. One must assess current and potential circumstances when determining how, or even if, to transport the child. The EMS clinician must be familiar with local EMS protocols for safe transport of children, state motor vehicle laws regarding child occupants, available local resources and equipment, and EMS regulations governing the treatment of children during transport. Most importantly, the EMS clinician must be prepared to address the urgent and evolving medical needs of the patient while managing operational challenges associated with transport.

The decision regarding whether a child should be transported in the ambulance if they are accompanying an adult patient should be guided by established policies and protocols, which should be determined in advance. If such protocols are not available within the system, it is important to note that ambulances are not designed for the safe transport of pediatric passengers. This design limitation poses challenges even for experienced personnel when determining safe options for nonpatient pediatric passengers.

When the child is the patient and transport is necessary, the position in which the patient is secured typically depends on the child's stability and whether any interventions are required en route. Although rapid transport of any patient is rarely required, it may be considered when there is any of the following circumstances:

- A serious injury or illness that cannot be stabilized in the field
- Significant pain that cannot be controlled
- A time-sensitive condition such as stroke or loss of circulation to a limb

TIP

Many EMS systems have clear policies or protocols that define pediatric transport practices, whether at the local or state level, but not all do. Although there is no regulation, there are national guidelines about safe transport of children in ambulances.

Another important consideration is the choice of destination. Not all areas have pediatric centers and may rely on local hospitals for stabilization. This should be addressed in local EMS protocols when determining transportation destinations. Many states have pediatric hospital designation agreements and

CASE STUDY 1

You arrive on scene to find a 27-year-old mother who fell down the steps in her home. She briefly lost consciousness and sustained a head laceration. Her ankle is also swollen, and she cannot bear weight, so she requires transport. Her 6-month-old daughter is asleep in her crib. The patient agrees to be transported, but not without her child. No other family members or neighbors are available at this time.

1. Is it appropriate to transport the child with the mother?
2. What issues are involved when transporting children who are not patients?

pediatric-specific programs through the Emergency Medical Services for Children program of the US Health Resources & Services Administration.

Ambulance Crashes

Ambulance crashes continue to be the leading cause of on-the-job fatalities among emergency medical services (EMS) personnel. Compared with other emergency vehicles, ambulances have the highest percentage of crashes in which occupants are killed or injured. A 7-year study of ambulance crashes by the National Highway Traffic Safety Administration (NHTSA) cited lack of proper restraint use by both clinicians and patients as a key contributor to ambulance crash fatalities.

How to Begin Transport

IS THE CHILD THE PATIENT?

The first factor in determining how to transport is understanding why the individual is being transported. Is the child the patient, or are they accompanying a caregiver who requires ambulance transport? *Children who are not patients and need transport to accompany a parent or caregiver are best transported properly restrained in a vehicle other than an ambulance.* There are limited safe options for securing a nonpatient child in an ambulance, and transporting any person in an ambulance poses risk of injury. Ambulances are not designed to transport children who are not patients.

CAUTION
Avoid transporting a child who is not a patient in an ambulance.

Many communities have pediatric coalitions that can serve as resources for alternate transport of children who are not patients. Public safety disaster plans and school resources can also help in developing partnerships. Agreements to provide alternative transport options are best established ahead of time. By working with these partners, EMS clinicians can establish a system that offers a range of child restraints and safe vehicles for transport. Providers should explain that ensuring the safe transport of family members may require temporarily separating the family.

WHEN A CHILD IS THE PATIENT

If a child requires ambulance transportation, they should be secured to the stretcher in a supine or **semi-Fowler position** using a size-appropriate **child restraint system (CRS)**. This positioning allows the EMS clinician to safely and effectively perform ongoing assessment and treatment during transport. Car seats designed for passenger vehicles generally cannot be secured to an ambulance stretcher in compliance with the manufacturer's directions. **Never secure a child in their parent's arms.** There are several commercially available CRSs designed to secure children to an ambulance stretcher for transport. In June 2024, the National Association of State EMS Officials (NASEMSO) began crash testing CRSs in ambulances under a grant from the NHTSA Office of Emergency Medical Services.

CAUTION
It is never acceptable to secure a child in a parent's arms.

TIP
Transport a child appropriately secured on a stretcher in a supine or semi-Fowler's position. This provides the safest and most effective position for ongoing assessment, monitoring, and treatment.

Taking Caregivers in the Ambulance

Transporting parents or caregivers in an ambulance is typically governed by local EMS protocols. Often,

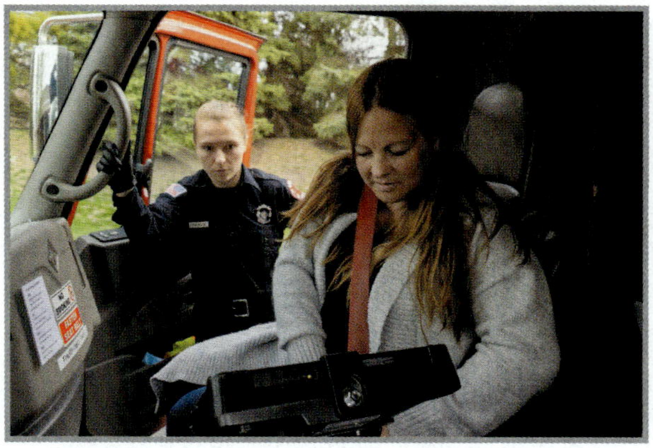

FIGURE 18–1 Allowing a parent to accompany a child may reduce the child's anxiety, but make sure all occupants are safe.

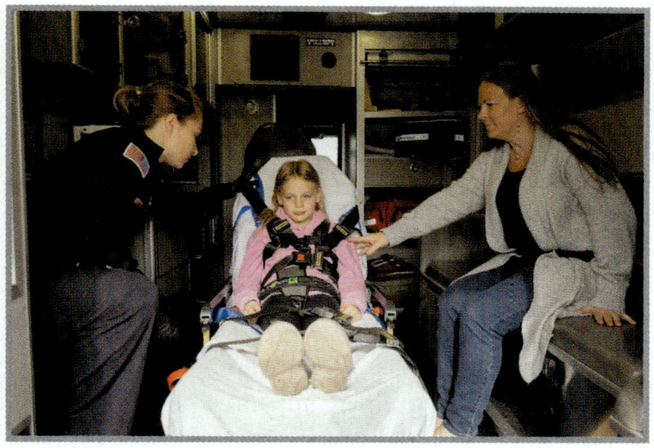

FIGURE 18–2 If caregivers are allowed to ride in the ambulance with the child, make sure all equipment and passengers are securely fastened in.

having the caregiver present can help reduce the child's anxiety during transport, especially for age groups more prone to emotional distress when separated from familiar caregivers. Addressing the emotional distress of children is a critical aspect of prehospital pediatric care and a key component of quality care. Although the impact of a family member or a caregiver on the EMS clinician's effectiveness and comfort level is not well studied, their presence has been linked to higher satisfaction in pediatric care delivery in other settings. Additionally, their presence may help reduce anxiety for both the parent and child (**FIGURE 18–1**).

Some EMS clinicians may feel less comfortable when a caregiver is present in an ambulance during a resuscitation or an advanced procedure, such as endotracheal intubation. One way to reduce this discomfort is by engaging in child advocacy and increasing pediatric training and exposure.

If local EMS policy permits a caregiver to be transported with the child, the policy should specify where both the child and caregiver should be positioned during transport. A common placement for the caregiver is in the front seat of the ambulance, properly restrained. Ensure that the caregiver fastens their seat belt correctly and remains seated throughout transport. Another option is seating the caregiver in the rear of the ambulance, if it is configured with secure seating options for both crew and the caregiver. This allows the child to see the caregiver and receive emotional reassurance, which can be particularly helpful for children with autism. All occupants and equipment must be properly secured, as unsecured items and occupants can pose a significant safety risk in the event of vehicular events (**FIGURE 18–2**).

Child Restraint Systems in Ambulances

DANGERS FACING CHILDREN DURING TRANSPORT

Several factors can help reduce the risk of additional injury to a child during ambulance transport, including

CASE STUDY 2

You arrive at the home of an 18-month-old who has altered mental status. She is limp in her mother's arms and does not respond to your arrival. She is pale but does not seem to have increased work of breathing or noisy respirations. The patient has been sick for 24 hours with nausea and vomiting and could not be awakened from her afternoon nap. The child responds to painful stimuli and is wearing a dry diaper. Vital signs include a heart rate of 160 beats/min, respiratory rate of 40 breaths/min, and blood pressure of 70 mm Hg/palp. The patient weighs 22 lbs (10 kg).

1. Should this child be transported in a car seat?
2. Should the mother be transported with the child?
3. Discuss the possible transport modes and destination for this patient.

how the child is secured, the ambulance's configuration, and the securing of both crew and equipment. The NASEMSO considers safe transport to be a standard of care, akin to airway, breathing, and circulation. Their recommendation is to have CRSs that cover weights ranging from 5 to 99 lbs (2.3–45 kg). This can vary from a car seat to a harness attached to the stretcher, depending on the child's condition.

The first step in deciding how to transport a child is determining the necessary assessment, monitoring, and treatment during transport. The Working Group Best-Practice Recommendations for the Safe Transportation of Children in Emergency Ground Ambulances provide recommendations for 5 situations (**TABLE 18–1**).

If the patient is in stable condition and no interventions are expected, transport the infant or child using a CRS that meets the injury criteria of the Federal Motor Vehicle Safety Standard (FMVSS) No. 213. This includes securing a car seat to the ambulance stretcher with appropriate restraints, if possible. Often, the appropriate restraints needed to secure a car seat are not available on ambulance stretchers. If continuous medical attention or spinal motion restriction (SMR) is required, a car seat would not be appropriate. In this case, use an appropriate CRS directly attached to the stretcher or backboard. If spinal injury is a concern, transport the child using SMR. This could involve an ambulance stretcher, vacuum splint, or similar device. Spinal motion restriction cannot be achieved with the head elevated more than 30° or without securing the child in a manner that restricts neck and spine movement.

TABLE 18–1 Working Group Best-Practice Recommendations for the Safe Transportation of Children in Emergency Ground Ambulances

Situation	Description
1	For a child who is uninjured/not ill
2	For a child who is ill and/or injured and whose condition *does not require* continuous and/or intensive medical monitoring and/or interventions
3	For a child whose condition *requires* continuous and/or intensive medical monitoring and/or interventions
4	For a child whose condition *requires* spinal immobilization and/or lying flat
5	For a child or children who *require* transport as part of a multiple patient transport (eg, newborn with mother, multiple children)

National Highway Traffic Safety Administration. Working group best-practice recommendations for the safe transportation of children in emergency ground ambulances. DOT HS 811 677. September 2012. https://static.nhtsa.gov/nhtsa/downloads/p2017-documents/811677.pdf

Pediatric evidence supports use of a cervical collar for any of the following presentations: neck pain, inability to move neck, neurological deficit, altered mental status, high-risk mechanism (high-speed motor vehicle collision or diving accident), torso trauma, or predisposing condition. If a backboard is used, such as when a child is critically injured or unresponsive, secure the child to the backboard, then secure the backboard to the stretcher with 3 horizontal restraints across the torso (at the chest, waist, and knees) and a vertical restraint over each shoulder. Tether the foot end of the backboard to the stretcher to prevent forward movement during rapid decelerations. To prevent skin breakdown, use backboards for the shortest time possible.

When using a CRS in the ambulance, it is important to decide where to position the device. Car seats are designed to protect a child during a front-end or rear-end collision and provide only moderate lateral stability. This means these seats cannot be secured sideways on a bench seat, which limits the options for a CRS to the rear of an ambulance secured to the stretcher or the EMS clinician's seat at the head of the stretcher.

CAUTION

Rear-facing-only or infant-only CRSs cannot be secured properly to the ambulance stretcher or rear-facing EMS clinician seat because they have only one belt pathway to secure the device and are not engineered to be restrained on a rear-facing seat.

CAUTION

Never secure car seats to a bench seat in the ambulance.

CHOOSING A CHILD RESTRAINT SYSTEM

Although many car safety seats and CRSs are available for use in ambulances, there are no federal regulations and only limited testing of these devices in emergency vehicles. Car safety seats designed for passenger vehicles are tested to meet FMVSS 213. Convertible car safety seats, with weight limits specific to each model (usually up to 40–50 lbs [18–23 kg]), and car beds using 2 belt paths have been tested and meet FMVSS 213 injury criteria. There are a few integrated seats

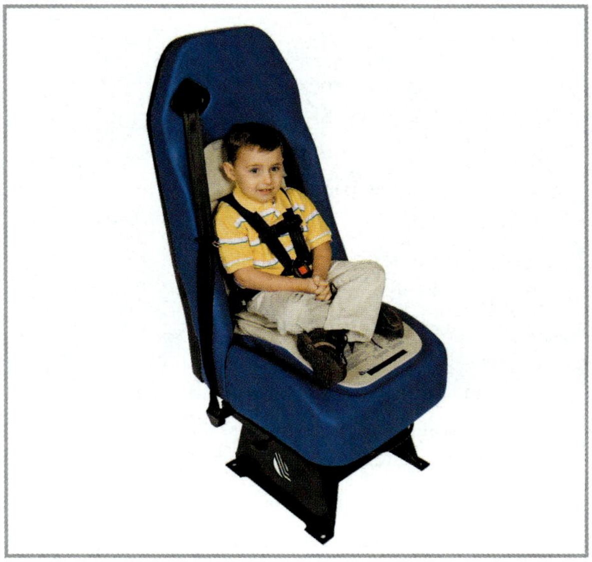

FIGURE 18–3 An integrated child restraint system.

Photo courtesy of EVS LTD.

and restraints that are permanently mounted on the rear-facing captain's chair (**FIGURE 18–3**), and there are some restraint systems designed to be secured on a rear-facing stretcher. These options have varying recommendations for use, and some have been tested to meet FMVSS 213 injury criteria, although no ambulance-specific standards currently exist. Rear-facing-only child safety seats, formerly called infant-only seats, are designed for children weighing from 4 to 5 lbs (1.8–2.3 kg) up to 22 or 30 to 35 lbs (14–16 kg), depending on the model. Convertible car safety seats are designed for children of different ages and weights up to 40 to 50 lbs (18–23 kg); they often feature 2 belt paths for both forward- and rear-facing positions. Some newer seats have increased weight limits up to 80 lbs (36 kg), but none has been tested in children over 40 lbs (18 kg) for use on an ambulance stretcher (**FIGURE 18–4**).

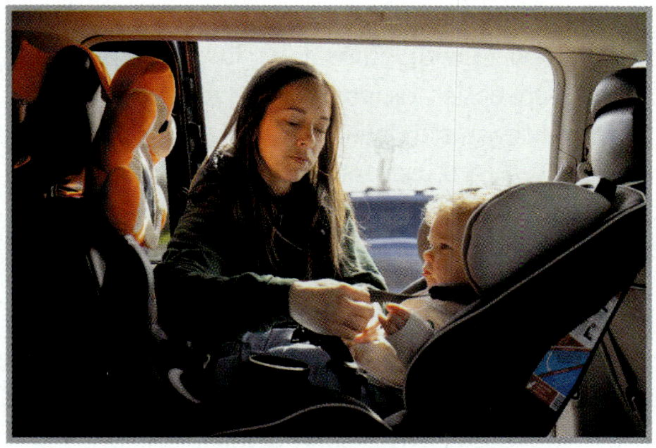

FIGURE 18–4 Convertible child safety seat for children 5 to 40 lbs (2.3-18 kg).

If a booster seat is used, it should only be placed on forward-facing captain's chairs with available lap/shoulder belts. Other specialty restraints, such as vest and harness devices, may be available to specialty crews with additional training on installation and securing patients for transport. Detailed instructions for selecting and installing ambulance restraints are available from EMS clinicians who have completed the EMS training course on child transportation in ambulances.

There are some Food and Drug Administration–cleared neonatal harnesses that secure a newborn to the parent's chest; these may be useful for restraining a healthy newborn during transport. Like other CRSs, these have yet to be tested using FMVSS.

TIP

Practice installing CRS to the stretcher as part of training, or bring in a certified child passenger safety technician with ambulance transport training to help familiarize your team with the installation process.

CASE STUDY 3

You are called to the scene of a vehicle crash involving 2 automobiles that collided at slow speed in a downtown intersection. There are 3 patients. One is the restrained driver of the vehicle that struck another vehicle broadside. The other patients are the restrained driver of the second vehicle and an 11-month-old boy, who was fully restrained in a rear-facing convertible car seat on the opposite side of the point of collision. The airbags did not deploy. The 2 drivers have minor wounds and no significant physiological abnormalities. Assessment of the child reveals a crying infant with no signs of injury.

1. Should the child be transported?
2. Should the child be transported in his own car seat or in an ambulance car seat?

A CRS should be properly cleaned and maintained. Devices with removable pads and wipeable surfaces are easier to clean. Check with the manufacturer for acceptable cleaning materials. If a dedicated ambulance CRS is used, ensure that it complies with EMS policy and that no safety recalls have been issued.

USING CAR SEATS AFTER A COLLISION

If the ambulance does not have a CRS and a child in stable condition requires transport, a dilemma arises when the child's own car seat is available. If local EMS policy permits using the child's personal car seat, ensure that it is fully intact. If the seat shows any signs of damage, it should not be used in the ambulance. The NHTSA recommends replacing child restraints after a moderate or severe crash to maintain a high level of crash protection. However, reuse of a child safety seat after a minor crash is permissible if the crash meets certain criteria; refer to NHTSA guidelines (**TABLE 18–2**).

CAUTION
If a child's personal car seat shows any signs of damage, or does not meet NHTSA criteria, do not use it in the ambulance.

SECURING OLDER CHILDREN TO THE STRETCHER

As mentioned earlier, the NASEMSO recommends having CRSs that cover a minimum weight range from 5 to 99 lbs. When ambulance-specific CRSs that accommodate larger children are available, these children should be transported in an appropriate device secured to the stretcher. If a CRS is unavailable, the child needs to be secured directly to the stretcher, with the stretcher straps adjusted to the size of the patient.

TABLE 18–2 Recommendations for the Use of a Child Restraint System After a Crash

It is safe to reuse a child safety seat that has been involved in a minor crash if
▪ The vehicle was able to be driven away from the crash site.
▪ The vehicle door nearest the safety seat was undamaged.
▪ There were no injuries to any of the vehicle occupants.
▪ The airbags, if present, did not deploy.
▪ There is no visible damage to the safety seat.

Car seat use after a crash. National Highway Traffic Safety Administration. Accessed February 3, 2026. https://www.nhtsa.gov/car-seats-and-booster-seats/car-seat-use-after-crash

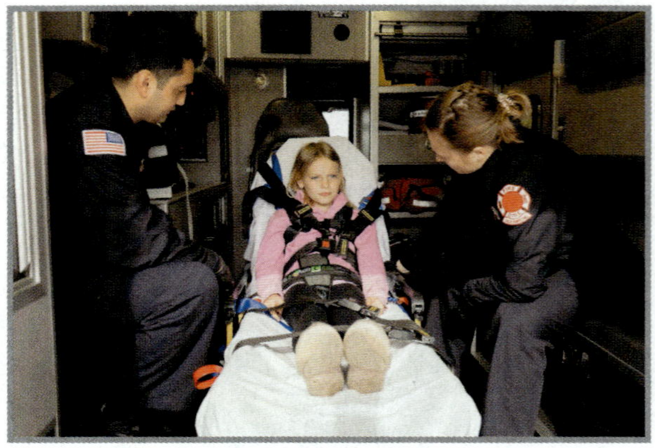

FIGURE 18–5 An ambulance-specific child restraint accommodating children 10 to 40 lbs (4.5-18 kg).

During an ambulance crash, children can slide up the stretcher. The use of shoulder straps can help minimize this movement, but challenges arise because these straps do not fit securely on a child's shoulders, nor do they fully prevent upward movement during a crash. Ideally, the straps should be secured similarly to those in a car seat, adjusted at or below the shoulder level. The straps should enter through the stretcher padding and be secured to the frame of the stretcher at the height of the shoulders. Unfortunately, this setup is rarely available on most currently used stretchers. However, a few ambulance-specific restraint systems are now available that make securing a child to the stretcher safer. These devices must first be secured to the stretcher, and then adjusted to fit the patient (**FIGURE 18–5** and **FIGURE 18–6**). Use of the pediatric restraint devices made for stretcher application helps to properly secure most pediatric patients.

OTHER DANGERS IN TRANSPORTING CHILDREN

Using an appropriate transport device is the first step in ensuring safe transport for the child. It is essential to recognize that crew members, parents/caregivers, and loose equipment can create a significant hazard to the patient during a collision. When transporting a child, all equipment must be secured or stored before leaving the scene. Monitors, portable oxygen tanks, equipment bags, and other loose objects can become projectiles during a collision, posing dangers to both crew members and patients. Crew members and parents/caregivers must wear a seat belt during transport to prevent injury. Ambulance crash tests have shown that unrestrained passengers in the patient compartment can be launched during a

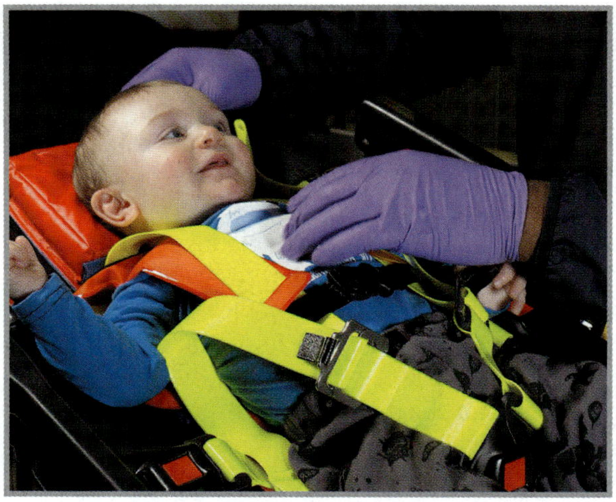

FIGURE 18-6 An ambulance-specific child restraint.

Photo courtesy of EMS Solutions.

collision, potentially landing on the patient, increasing risk to the child.

TIP

Securing all occupants, monitoring devices, and other equipment during transport is extremely important. Even hard braking can cause harm to the patient if objects are unrestrained.

TIP

Crash tests of ambulances have shown that unrestrained passengers in the patient compartment present a risk to the patient during a collision by potentially being launched and landing on the patient. All occupants, including EMS clinicians, must be restrained.

Summary of Child Restraint Systems

Whenever possible, a child who is in stable condition should be transported in a size-appropriate CRS in an upright position. Follow guidelines for proper use of car seats for children of different weights, ensuring the devices are securely fastened to the ambulance to maximize safety. If local EMS policy permits using the child's own car seat in the ambulance, make sure it is not damaged, meets all the NHTSA criteria for reuse after a crash, and is securely fastened. Additionally, if EMS policy allows and the individual can be properly restrained, encourage the presence of the caregiver in the ambulance to provide comfort and solace to the child and to improve ongoing assessment.

Transport Mode

Emotions can run high on pediatric calls, often leading to a strong desire for rapid transport. However, lights-and-sirens transport poses risks to both ambulance occupants and bystanders, and typically shaves only a few minutes off the total transport time. To minimize the dangers, it is essential to decide the mode of transport according to the type of call, the patient's condition, and their degree of instability. The highest priority for lights-and-sirens transport is the critically injured child who needs urgent interventions, such as blood products or surgery.

CONTROVERSY

Lights-and-sirens transport carries significant risks to the ambulance occupants and bystanders. The benefits of faster transport time must be weighed carefully against these dangers.

Transport Destination

The decisions regarding where and how to transport a pediatric patient depend on the child's condition, the cause of the illness or injury, the pediatric readiness of the receiving facility, local EMS policy, weather, and resources. In some cases, air transport may be appropriate, although separation from the caregiver can add stress because not all aircraft can accommodate both the patient and caregiver.

CAUTION

Although air transport can be lifesaving, the inability to bring a caregiver may increase patient and family stress. This should be carefully considered when deciding on the transport method.

Multiple Patients

When there are multiple pediatric patients, additional transport units may be required to ensure that each child is safely secured, as ambulances have limited space for car seats and proper restraint adjustments.

Summary of Transport Mode and Multiple Patients

Choosing the appropriate transport mode should be done before transport begins. Lights and sirens are reserved for extremely time-sensitive cases involving trauma patients in unstable condition or those who are critically ill. When multiple children are involved, additional units should be activated to ensure everyone is safely transported.

CASE STUDY ANSWERS

CASE STUDY 1

This case demonstrates an important dilemma. Although family-centered care is highly desirable, it must take place without placing the patient, family member, accompanying child, or EMS clinician at increased risk. Whenever possible, arrange alternative safe care and/or transportation for the child so that the medical providers can focus their attention on the patient. This includes care by or transportation with a competent adult, ensuring that appropriate child restraints are available and in use. Additional options for transporting the child could include a supervisor's vehicle, an auxiliary vehicle, or a child service's transportation vehicle. Transporting the infant in the front seat of the ambulance or in the rear seat of a police car or other emergency vehicle is dangerous. A vehicle in which the CRS is to be used in the front seat must have an airbag deactivation switch.

Parent and child separation, however, may cause undue distress to the mildly injured parent. In that case, if the system allows the transport of the infant in the ambulance, follow proper procedures to secure the child in the appropriate restraint system and in the correct position. This method of transportation must include enough participants to meet the child's and the patient's needs and to ensure that observation or tending to the immediate needs of either one does not detract from that of the other. This option is often unavailable because of space or personnel resource limitations.

CASE STUDY 2

This case involves the need for appropriate positioning, airway and vascular access, monitoring, and perhaps intervention during the transport process. "Stabilization" in a car seat meets none of these requirements and therefore should not be used. This child should be restrained using an appropriate CRS on the ambulance stretcher, with attention to airway positioning, vascular access, and appropriate observation. Here, accompaniment of the parent can often be advantageous to parent and child. Although the medical team can attend to the physiological needs of the child, they cannot meet the child's emotional needs. Be sensitive to the parent's need to offer support to their child and ability to keep the child calm. The parent may also be able to provide additional history and assist in reassessments. However, the parent cannot be allowed to carry the child during transport, either on their lap while seated or with the parent and child secured together to a stretcher.

Local protocol often dictates where and how this patient should be transported, as well as whether a parent can accompany the child and specific requirements for doing so. These protocols should include a preferred parental seating location and safety instructions for the parent before transport. Parents must be instructed that the primary role of the providers is to care for the sick child, and that precious attention cannot be diverted from that task. Having the parent sit in the front seat is one way to include them in the environment, while allowing some separation for the EMS clinicians.

Providers may express concern that parents will critique their techniques or skills during the transport or that they will be nervous when confronted with this situation. However, parental reports are generally very positive about the experience, and parents mainly comment on the caring nature of the providers, not on their technical capabilities.

CASE STUDY 3

Assessment of infants after a collision is difficult in the best of environments. The significant mechanism of this incident necessitates assessment during the transport process and medical evaluation of the infant at the appropriate emergency department. The question then is how to best transport the child. If a careful inspection of the child yields no physiological or anatomical abnormality requiring further stabilization or intervention, and the child is accessible to completely assess and reassess as needed when secured in the car seat, this method is appropriate. If a detailed inspection of the child's convertible car safety seat does not yield evidence of fracture or abnormality; it is an appropriate seat for the child's weight; it is not damaged and meets NHTSA criteria; and EMS policy allows, then use this seat and secure it in the usual rear-facing position in the emergency vehicle, unless the ambulance has its own CRS. If there is any question as to the appropriateness or structural integrity of the child's car seat, then use another, more appropriate car seat. Remember that a rear-facing-only or infant-only car seat cannot be safely secured to the ambulance stretcher and may only be secured to a forward-facing attendant seat.

Suggested References

ARTICLES

Becker LR, Zaloshnja E, Levick N, Li G, Miller TR. Relative risk of injury and death in ambulances and other emergency vehicles. *Accid Anal Prev*. 2003;35(6):941–948. doi: 10.1016/S0001-4575(02)00102-1

Child safety seats and the emergency responder. *EMS World*. July 2004. Accessed October 6, 2024. https://www.hmpgloballearningnetwork.com/site/emsworld/article/10324627/child-safety-seats-and-emergency-responder#:~:text=Always%20use%20a%20child%20restraint%20device%20when%20transporting,one%20strap%20secures%20the%20child%20to%20the%20stretcher%29

Cochran-Caggiano N, Till S, Holt C, et al. Children and restraints study in emergency ambulance transport: an observational study and analysis of current pediatric ambulance transport practices. *Pediatr Emerg Care*. 2023;39(10):e66–e71. doi: 10.1097/PEC.0000000000002919

Fidacaro GA Jr, Jones CW, Drago LA. Pediatric transport practices among EMS clinicians. *Pediatr Emerg Care*. 2020;36(11):e632–e635. doi: 10.1097/PEC.0000000000001564

Fischer PE, Perina DG, Delbridge TR, et al. Spinal motion restriction in the trauma patient—a joint position statement. *Prehosp Emerg Care*. 2018;22(6):659–661. doi: 10.1080/10903127.2018.1481476

Graham L, Thomas D, Finstad K, Dennert R, Southcott T. Analysis of ground ambulance crash data from 2012 to 2018. National Highway Traffic Safety Administration. July 2023. Accessed December 1, 2024. www.ems.gov/assets/Analysis-of-Ground-Ambulance-Crash-Data-From-2012-to-2018_FINAL.pdf

Leonard JC, Browne LR, Ahmad FA, et al. Cervical spine injury risk factors in children with blunt trauma. *Pediatrics*. 2019;144(1):e20183221. doi: 10.1542/peds.2018-3221

Lerner EB, Studnek JR, Fumo N, et al. Multicenter analysis of transport destinations for pediatric prehospital patients. *Acad Emerg Med*. 2019;26(5):510–516. doi: 10.1111/acem.13641

Nowak T. Mom holding onto baby isn't an acceptable transport option. EMS1. June 3, 2024. Accessed September 27, 2024. https://www.ems1.com/patient-safety/articles/mom-holding-onto-baby-isnt-an-acceptable-transport-option-xRN97ZTMqfvu3iQR/

OTHER RESOURCES

Automotive Safety Program. Indiana University School of Medicine. Accessed October 6, 2024. https://preventinjury.medicine.iu.edu/

The do's and don'ts of transporting children in an ambulance. National Highway Traffic Safety Administration and Health Resources and Services Administration. May 23, 2000. Accessed October 6, 2024. www.cpsboard.org/wp-content/uploads/2014/01/Safe-Transportation-of-Children-in-an-Ambulance_R1010.pdf

National Association of State Emergency Medical Services Officials. Safe Transport of Children Committee. Accessed October 6, 2024. https://nasemso.org/content.aspx?page_id=22&club_id=157064&module_id=683437

National Highway Traffic Safety Administration. Working group best-practice recommendations for the safe transportation of children in emergency ground ambulances. September 2012. Accessed October 6, 2024. https://static.nhtsa.gov/nhtsa/downloads/p2017-documents/811677.pdf

CHAPTER 19

Making a Difference

Aaron Bates, NRP
Michael K. Kim, MD, FAAP

LEARNING OBJECTIVES

1. **Describe emergency medical services (EMS) for children (EMSC) and the EMS-EMSC continuum.**
2. **Discuss how EMS can interface with public health, as well as the role of EMS in injury and illness prevention and promotion.**
3. **Identify primary and secondary prevention strategies involved in injury prevention.**
4. **Outline the 3 components and the 3 phases of an injury event.**
5. **Discuss EMSC partnerships with other injury-prevention agencies and programs.**
6. **Define the role of the child's "medical home" and identify its importance in the EMS-EMSC care continuum.**
7. **Identify unique quality and safety issues for children in prehospital care.**
8. **Discuss the importance of data collection and information management in EMSC.**
9. **Describe the role of EMS in the prevention continuum.**

Introduction

Effective emergency care for children requires seamless collaboration among health care professionals both inside and outside hospitals, public health agencies, and the community. To ensure that care is safe and effective, these entities must develop and implement comprehensive clinical services and oversight mechanisms that are tailored specifically for children with acute illness and injury. Professionals must also recognize the limitations of the traditional emergency care system, which is largely oriented toward treatment after an illness or injury. Prevention is essential to reducing the overall burden of emergencies, particularly pediatric emergencies. For children, community activities focused on prevention of acute injury and illness is by far the most cost-effective way to improve health.

Emergency medical services professionals play a crucial role not only in responding to emergencies but also in advocating for and practicing injury prevention in their communities. This includes understanding and supporting the prevention and safety programs conducted through the federal Emergency Medical Services for Children (EMSC) and local emergency medical services (EMS) systems. Emergency

CASE STUDY 1

You have been called to the scene of a motor vehicle crash between a compact car and a minivan. A 3-year-old girl, who was not properly restrained at the time of the crash, was thrown from the minivan and lies approximately 15 feet from the vehicle. She is unconscious; has no abnormal airway sounds, retractions, or nasal flaring; and is cyanotic. Respiratory rate is 6 breaths/min, heart rate is 40 beats/min, and blood pressure is difficult to palpate. You transport the child to the nearest emergency department (ED), but the child dies shortly after arrival.

1. How could this have been prevented?
2. What could you do to help others avoid this type of tragedy?

medical services systems can make a substantial difference and can foster a robust infrastructure through advocacy and community involvement, working toward the goal of improving pediatric emergency care while minimizing acute illnesses and injuries through effective prevention.

Emergency Medical Services for Children

Although children younger than 18 years account for only 10% of prehospital transports, the evaluation, treatment, triage, and transport of this group can often create significant stress and a variety of challenges for EMS clinicians. Pediatric patients vary in size, developmental stages, and medical needs, requiring providers to adapt their approaches in ways different from how they care for adults. The lower frequency of pediatric encounters, combined with the need for specialized equipment and medication dosing, can add to the pressure. Emergency medical services clinicians must be skilled in both medical management and communication with young patients and their families, which can ease the complexity of care.

Emergency Medical Services for Children (EMSC) is a federal program initiated in 1973 to improve outcomes for children across prehospital and emergency department (ED) settings. The EMSC Innovation and Improvement Center (EIIC) supports and accelerates EMSC program efforts through quality improvement science, education, and collaboration. Each state, territory, and commonwealth is funded to develop specific programs that improve pediatric emergency care in the prehospital, ED, and beyond through partnership grants. As of this book's publication date, recent years have seen significant advances in the outcomes of children in EDs thanks to the the pediatric readiness program. Since 2018, attention has been focused on prehospital care through the National Prehospital Pediatric Readiness Project (PPRP) to empower EMS and fire-based EMS agencies to become "pediatric ready," or prepared to provide high-quality care for children in accordance with national recommendations.

In 2020, a joint policy statement from the American Academy of Pediatrics, the American College of Emergency Physicians, the Emergency Nurses Association, the National Association of Emergency Medical Services Physicians, and the National Association of Emergency Medical Technicians provided a framework for how prehospital pediatric care can be improved to reduce morbidity and mortality. In summer 2024, the first-ever assessment survey was completed with the goal of assessing the pediatric readiness of EMS agencies across the country. In 2023, the EIIC began work on developing a pediatric readiness recognition program to assist EMS agencies in being better prepared to care for children.

The other site targeted for pediatric readiness is the ED. Because there are relatively few specialized pediatric centers (**pediatric critical care centers** and **pediatric trauma centers**), 83% of children receive emergency care in general hospitals. Hence, improving pediatric readiness among community and rural EDs has shown to be critical in reducing morbidity and mortality in children. The National Pediatric Readiness Project has provided guidance and support to EDs since 2017 to reduce morbidity and mortality in ill and injured children. A recent policy statement from the American Academy of Pediatrics, The American College of Emergency Physicians, the Emergency Nurses Association and the American College of Surgeons provides updated recommendations. Furthermore, the American College of Surgeons is requiring EDs to participate in pediatric readiness for trauma verification to include infrastructure, administration and coordination of care, personnel, pediatric-specific policies, equipment, and other resources that ensure each center is prepared to provide care to an injured child.

> **TIP**
>
> Improved pediatric readiness in EDs reduces morbidity and mortality.

The **EMS-EMSC continuum** is the planned and organized interface among the clinical services. The 5 major phases in the overall continuum are as follows:

- Prevention
- Primary care and the child's medical home
- Prehospital care
- In-hospital care
- Rehabilitation

These phases represent a cycle of care for a single event that should bring the child back to prevention and the child's medical home. The prehospital care professional has the responsibility to support children's emergency care throughout all phases of the continuum. An active partnership with public health programs, collaboration with the community, and continued advocacy through prevention and training empower EMS systems to make a difference.

Summary of EMSC

The EMSC program began as a federal grant initiative aimed at enhancing prehospital pediatric care within the community EMS system. Over the past 5 decades, this work has significantly expanded, evolving into a comprehensive model known as the EMSC-EMS continuum. This model integrates multiple clinical services in the community that are tailored to children and focus on the cohesive system of care that spans the key phases: prevention, the medical home, prehospital care, in-hospital care, and rehabilitation. Each phase plays a vital role in ensuring that children receive appropriate, timely, and coordinated care throughout the continuum of emergency services.

TIP

The EMSC program covers a wide range of health care settings, including rural, community, and specialized pediatric hospitals, as well as prehospital emergency services. This comprehensive network ensures that pediatric emergency care is coordinated across various hospital types and EMS agencies, providing essential services to children in both urban and rural areas.

Public Health Interface

Emergency medical services systems have been evolving as an important part of the public health interface. Emergency medical services clinicians can directly affect disease prevention through vaccination and education and through continued screening and care aimed at limiting disease progression. Prehospital care reports act as disease surveillance in helping to identify disease and symptom patterns, identifying outbreaks earlier than otherwise possible through current means. Proper documentation, as well as participation in screenings, health fairs, clinics, and education forums, gives EMS clinicians an opportunity to better prepare their community. In a disaster, an act of terrorism, or another major event, it is critical to be familiar with your partners in public health.

Prevention and Injury Control

Injury and illness prevention play a vital role in public health and are key components of the EMSC continuum. Despite children's receiving the best possible medical care, pediatric mortality resulting from injuries and illnesses remains high. Thus, we must place a greater focus on prevention, which is more effective in saving lives than is optimal medical care. Prevention represents the first phase of the EMSC continuum. Although both injury and illness prevention are important, prehospital services have focused primarily on emergency management after illness or injury occurs. The 10 steps of developing an injury prevention program emphasize an objective and scientific approach (**TABLE 19–1**). For EMS clinicians, injury prevention means understanding the causes of injuries, recognizing environmental risks, and actively engaging with community partners to prevent injuries before they occur.

TABLE 19–1 Ten Steps for Developing an Injury Prevention Program

1. Gather and analyze data
2. Select the target injury and population
3. Determine intervention steps
4. Develop an implementation plan
5. Identify, select, and commit community agencies to implement the program
6. Develop an action plan
7. Orient and train agencies/individuals implementing the intervention plan
8. Implement the program
9. Monitor and support the program
10. Evaluate and revise the program

INJURIES ARE NOT ACCIDENTS

When injury patterns are carefully studied, it is clear that injuries, like illnesses, vary with the seasons, can occur in epidemics, and often have local trends and demographic distributions. Injuries are largely predictable, whether they are unintentional (eg, drowning) or intentional (eg, handgun assaults), and they also are preventable.

True accidents that result in injuries are rare. Even apparently random events, such as lightning strikes or tornadoes, have predictable features and can be anticipated. For example, weather forecasting can predict potentially deadly storms and alert the public in advance. "Injuries are not accidents" has become a common slogan of injury care professionals. The slogan reflects the current scientific understanding of how injuries occur. Experts refer to automobile collisions as "crashes" rather than "accidents," because crashes have predictable and preventable features. For example, crash injuries commonly result from driving while intoxicated or speeding, or from improper use of child restraints. By identifying these predictable factors, we can intervene and prevent the setup for any future injuries.

> **TIP**
> Injuries are not accidents. They are predictable and preventable.

COMPONENTS OF AN INJURY EVENT

Part of understanding how injuries occur involves looking at the 3 components of an injury event: the host, the agent, and the environment (**FIGURE 19–1**).

The **host** is the recipient of the injury. An injury occurs when potentially destructive energy is too much for the host to tolerate. Human hosts have different levels of tolerance. Children, because of their unique **anatomical** and **physiological** features, are particularly vulnerable to high-energy transfers. Their smaller body size means the energy that is transferred to the body during a collision transfers over a larger percentage of body surface, placing the child at higher risk of experiencing serious injuries in a traumatic event.

The **agent** is a form of energy. The major agents of injury are kinetic, thermal, chemical, electrical, and radiation energy. Most injuries are associated with these types of energy. Kinetic energy is the most common injury agent in circumstances that involve EMS clinicians. For example, falls, automobile-passenger injuries, and pedestrian-versus-automobile and bicyclist-versus-automobile events all involve a human as the host and kinetic energy as the agent. Burns, in contrast, involve thermal, chemical, or electrical energy.

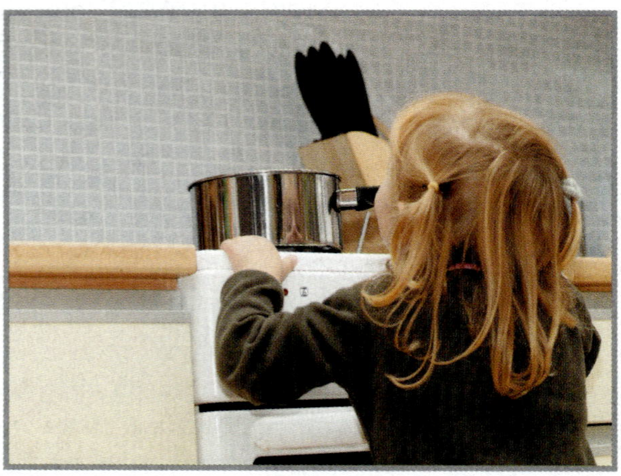

FIGURE 19–1 Components of an injury event: the host, the agent, and the environment. The child is the host, the heat from the boiling water is the agent, and the dangerously placed handle is the environment for a burn injury.

Libortom/iStockphoto.com.

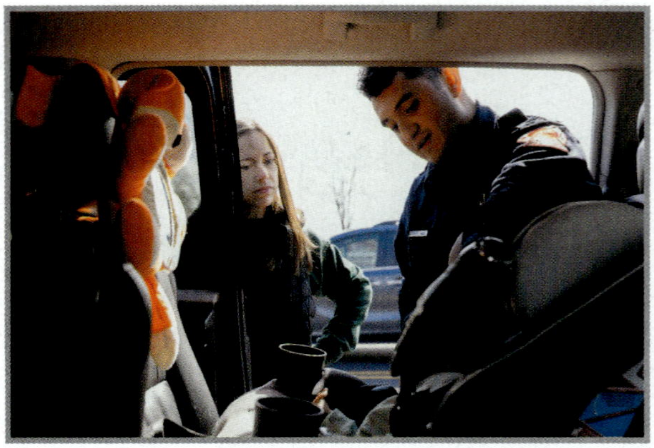

FIGURE 19–2 EMS professionals can become involved directly in injury prevention by attending a child safety seat technician training program and then by providing a child safety seat checkpoint program.

The **environment** is the setting in which the agent interacts with the host, causing or influencing the injury event. Examples include an unsupervised or unfenced swimming pool, a poorly lit road, or an open upper-story window without a protective barrier. Each of these environmental factors creates conditions in which an injury event may occur that involves a child as a host and kinetic energy as an agent. While assessing injury events, the prehospital care professional should identify which components of an injury can be modified to prevent future incidents (**FIGURE 19–2**). Modifying the host's behavior, such as preventing drowning or head injury, might involve education in swimming skills or safe driving practices. Modifying the agent could include providing bicycle helmets (**FIGURE 19–3**) or installing soft surfaces in playgrounds to minimize the effect of kinetic energy on vulnerable brains. Environmental modification to reduce risks of injury may include installing fencing around swimming pools, stair gates, or window bars.

PHASES OF INJURY

There are 3 phases of every injury that need to be considered when devising control strategies: the pre-event period, the event itself, and the postevent period.

Pre-event factors are conditions related to the host, the agent, or the environment that influence the likelihood of an injury's occurring. For example, wearing a helmet while riding a bicycle is a pre-event factor that can significantly reduce the risk of injury.

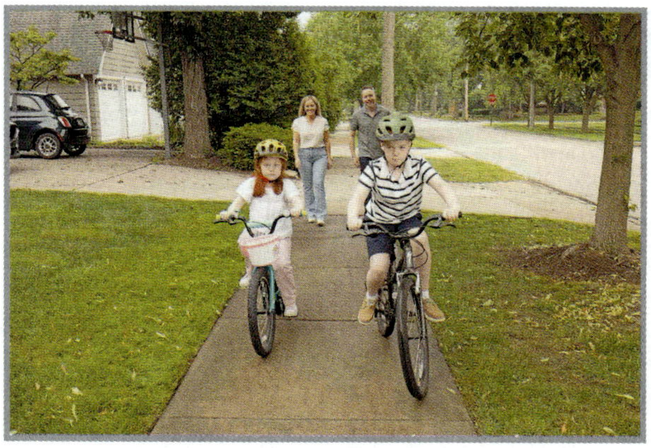

FIGURE 19-3 When worn correctly, bicycle helmets significantly reduce the complications and incidence of death resulting from closed-head injuries. Emergency medical services clinicians have an important community role in teaching simple injury-control strategies.

Event factors refer to conditions that amplify or mitigate the effect of the agent on the host during the injury event. An example of an event factor that decreases the risk of injury in a vehicle crash is the use of seat belts at the time of a crash. Postevent factors involve conditions that affect the outcome for the host after the injury has occurred. For example, effective airway management by a prehospital care provider can significantly impact the prognosis of a child who has severe head injury. Traditionally, prehospital care has focused almost exclusively on the postevent period, providing medical care and transport after the injury has already occurred. However, EMS clinicians should recognize their potential to impact the pre-event and event phases of injury by serving as community educators and advocates. Data collected from patient-care reports help identify patterns and trends that inform prevention programs. Effective prevention is best achieved through collaborative partnerships enhanced by EMSC and other local health care systems and services.

TIP

Prevention is a vital component of all EMS systems and offers EMS clinicians a unique opportunity to significantly improve the health and well-being of all residents, from children to elderly people.

CONTROVERSY

Until recently, injury or illness prevention were not part of the training for EMS clinicians. Although incorporating prevention into their scope of practice presents exciting opportunities, the role of EMS in injury prevention has not yet been fully explored.

Summary of Prevention and Injury Control

Injury and illness prevention are essential components of EMSC and represent the first phase of the EMS-EMSC continuum. Injuries should not be labeled as "accidents"; they are almost always preventable. Emergency medical services clinicians play a vital role in community injury control by responding to the scene, where they can accurately assess the key components in an injury or illness event. This assessment includes evaluating the child (the host), the energy type or agent of injury, and the environment, as along with understanding the pre-event, event, and postevent phases of injury. National and state EMSC resources facilitate collaboration with other programs to enhance available support and resources.

The Medical Home

The second vital link in the EMS-EMSC continuum is the child's primary care provider, or **medical home**. The American Academy of Pediatrics defines a medical home as the child's primary source of medical care. Establishing an effective medical home necessitates ensuring that infants, children, and teenagers have access to continuous, comprehensive, family-centered, coordinated, compassionate, and culturally effective services close to home. The child and family must develop a partnership of mutual trust and responsibility with their primary care provider, particularly children with special needs (see Chapter 12), who often require specialized medical care. Pediatricians and family physicians play an essential role in creating the medical home, managing and facilitating ongoing pediatric primary care while maintaining connections to the EMS system for situations requiring emergency services beyond the office or clinic. Some practices have written protocols and procedures outlining how to identify an emergency, when to alert EMS services, and what emergency care should be provided immediately. Families and primary care providers should reach out to local EMS services and local EDs/hospitals to make collaborative emergency plans. Through this effort, all the players in the medical home have an accurate, up-to-date understanding of the pediatric capabilities of the EMS system and the capacity and resources of the closest hospital for emergency care. Understanding the local EMS system's policies and procedures regarding

CASE STUDY 2

You are dispatched to a local elementary school for a 7-year-old girl with a history of cerebral palsy and seizures. On arrival, the nurse states the patient has been experiencing seizures for 15 minutes, and she has just administered midazolam through the patient's gastrostomy tube. The patient is no longer experiencing seizures; she is sleepy, but responds to voice; she has no increased work of breathing; and her skin is pink. She has respirations of 20 breaths/min, a heart rate of 120 beats/min, a blood pressure of 92/64 mm Hg, and a blood glucose of 86 mg/dL. The child's father arrives and states the patient is demonstrating her usual status after a seizure. He requests transport to the children's hospital 45 minutes away and states he will take her if you cannot go that far, refusing ambulance transport to the local ED. The child is now awake, alert, at her normal developmental level, and deemed medically stable after discussion with medical command.

1. What are your options in the care and transport of this child?
2. How can you assist the parents with safe transportation for this child?

triage, transport, and treatment of children by family and primary care providers is important.

> **TIP**
>
> Communication and teamwork for all members of the medical home are critical components of the EMS-EMSC continuum.

THE EMERGENCY MEDICAL SERVICES CLINICIAN AND THE MEDICAL HOME

Traditionally, EMS clinicians have had little contact with the primary care physicians in the medical home, even though both are integral parts of the EMSC continuum within the community. There are robust opportunities for collaboration between the provider in the child's medical home and the EMS clinicians. With parent's or guardian's consent, the primary care provider can share valuable history and information with the prehospital team. This is especially important when treating children with special health care needs. This information may be communicated in the form of a written care plan or by means of a telephone consultation on scene. This should not delay the care by the EMS clinician or transport, but it can provide critical information when the parent or guardian are not available. In some cases, the primary care physician may be available on scene and assist EMS clinicians or accompany the child to the ED. For this collaboration to be effective, the primary care provider must be familiar with the local scope of practice, including medications, equipment, and supplies available. Emergency medical services clinicians should also have and share a "physician on scene" policy that clearly defines the roles and responsibilities.

Communication is critically important when treating a child with special care needs. An **emergency information form (EIF)**, as described in Chapter 12 (**FIGURE 19–4**), can provide essential details to prehospital care providers during an emergency. Communicating with the family before the emergency can also provide familiarity with the child's baseline health status, thus allowing for a more informed and comfortable emergency response. Effective communication and teamwork are key components in strengthening the connections across all parts of the EMSC continuum.

Occasionally, determining the appropriate destination facility can lead to debate. Choices are typically influenced by patient condition, transport time, available resources, the capabilities of local hospitals, and patient or family preferences. Clearly, the decision should be made according to the above factors; however, several publications have specified criteria that recommend preferential transport to hospitals equipped to provide higher-level pediatric care for seizures, significant soft-tissue injury or complex wounds, altered mental status in children younger than 2 years, shock accompanied by an abnormal Pediatric Assessment Triangle score, or respiratory distress with hypoxia or serious signs and symptoms. Communication within the medical home team can play a valuable role in supporting this often complex decision-making process. The positive impact of these recommendations is reflected in the EIIC's National Pediatric Readiness Program. This program has accelerated the recognition of pediatric-capable facilities across the United States, with more EDs developing pediatric-specific resources. As a result, the challenges of transporting

Emergency Information Form for Children With Special Needs

Last name:

American College of Emergency Physicians®

American Academy of Pediatrics

Date form completed	Revised	Initials
By Whom	Revised	Initials

Name:	**Birth date:** **Nickname:**
Home Address:	**Home/Work Phone:**
Parent/Guardian:	**Emergency Contact Names & Relationship:**
Signature/Consent*:	
Primary Language:	**Phone Number(s):**

Physicians:

Primary care physician:	**Emergency Phone:**
	Fax:
Current Specialty physician:	**Emergency Phone:**
Specialty:	**Fax:**
Current Specialty physician:	**Emergency Phone:**
Specialty:	**Fax:**
Anticipated Primary ED:	**Pharmacy:**
Anticipated Tertiary Care Center:	

Diagnoses/Past Procedures/Physical Exam:

1.	**Baseline physical findings:**
2.	
3.	**Baseline vital signs:**
4.	
Synopsis:	
	Baseline neurological status:

*Consent for release of this form to health care providers

FIGURE 19–4 An emergency information form.

American College of Emergency Physicians and American Academy of Pediatrics.

Last name:

Diagnoses/Past Procedures/Physical Exam continued:

Medications:

1.
2.
3.
4.
5.
6.

Significant baseline ancillary findings (lab, x-ray, ECG):

Prostheses/Appliances/Advanced Technology Devices:

Management Data:

Allergies: Medications/Foods to be avoided **and why:**

1.
2.
3.

Procedures to be avoided **and why:**

1.
2.
3.

Immunizations (mm/yy)

Dates					
DPT					
OPV					
MMR					
HIB					

Dates					
Hep B					
Varicella					
TB status					
Other					

Antibiotic prophylaxis: Indication: Medication and dose:

Common Presenting Problems/Findings With Specific Suggested Managements

Problem	Suggested Diagnostic Studies	Treatment Considerations

Comments on child, family, or other specific medical issues:

Physician/Provider Signature: **Print Name:**

FIGURE 19–4 *(continued)*

pediatric patients to appropriate care facilities should decrease. Furthermore, the integration of pediatric readiness requirements in trauma center verification by the American College of Surgeons to include infrastructure, administration and coordination of care, personnel, pediatric-specific policies, equipment and other resources will ensure that each center is prepared to provide care to an injured child.

Recent advancements in community paramedicine have expanded the scope of how EMS can engage with the community, including making home visits to manage urgent but low-acuity conditions and injuries. Although the long-term effectiveness of these programs is still being evaluated, they show promise in reducing unnecessary hospital visits. In response to the rise in behavioral and mental health incidents, some EMS agencies have introduced specialized programs such as Community Alternative Response Emergency Services (CARES). Personnel in these programs are specially trained to handle mental health crises, providing de-escalation, resources, and appropriate care options for patients. These teams aim to prevent the overuse of EMS and EDs for patients who might need not acute medical care but rather mental health support. By redirecting these patients to appropriate services, these programs reduce strain on traditional EMS systems and EDs, while improving patient outcomes in behavioral health emergencies. As these community paramedicine models evolve, they represent a critical step toward a more integrated, patient-centered approach to care within the medical home.

Summary of the Medical Home

The medical home is the child's primary source of medical care, typically provided by a pediatrician or family physician, sometimes in collaboration with other medical practitioners. It serves as a crucial hub for key information and decision making regarding the child's health. When appropriate, prehospital care providers should leverage the expertise of the primary care provider in decision making about emergency care. For children with special health care needs, always ask if they have an EIF on hand. Currently, emergency information access for EMS agencies is inconsistent. However, efforts are under way to establish a standardized system in the future, aiming to streamline and improve information availability across all EMS services. Primary care physicians should also be knowledgeable about the pediatric capabilities and scope of practice of the local EMS clinicians, as well as those of hospitals and services offered by other components of the EMSC continuum. Alternative EMS services, such as community paramedicine and CARES teams, further highlight innovative EMS services for patients within the medical home.

Quality and Safety in EMSC

Quality improvement (QI) has long been recognized as a method of ensuring efficiency, decreasing waste, and increasing customer satisfaction in industrial settings. In 2001, the Institute of Medicine released *Crossing the Quality Chasm: A New Health System for the 21st Century*. The 6 domains describe essential dimensions of health care quality. These domains provide a framework for improving quality of health care delivery across all sectors, including the prehospital setting. The 6 domains are as follows:

- *Safety*: Health care should avoid causing harm to patients. Safety in health care involves reducing and preventing errors, injuries, accidents, and infections that could harm patients. Care must be delivered in a way that minimizes risks to patients.
- *Effectiveness*: Health care should be based on scientific knowledge and evidence, providing services that are proven to benefit patients. It involves delivering treatments and interventions that have been demonstrated to improve health outcomes, while avoiding underuse of effective treatments or overuse of unnecessary ones.
- *Patient-centeredness*: Health care should be responsive to individual patient preferences, needs, and values. It emphasizes treating patients with dignity, respect, and compassion, as well as ensuring that patient values guide all clinical decisions. This domain encourages patients' active participation in their own care.
- *Timeliness*: Health care should minimize delays and wait times, both for patients seeking care and for those providing care. Timely care reduces harmful delays and ensures that patients receive the right care at the right time.
- *Efficiency*: Health care should avoid waste of resources, including time, equipment, supplies,

and energy. Efficiency in health care means maximizing the value of health care delivery by minimizing unnecessary or duplicative services and making better use of health care resources.

- *Equity*: Health care should not vary in quality because of personal characteristics such as sex, ethnicity, geographic location, or socioeconomic status. Equity in health care ensures that everyone has access to the same standard of care, regardless of their background or circumstances.

Among the 6 domains, safety is of paramount concern, especially for EMS clinicians, who face unique risks in the field. Medical errors and safety in the prehospital environment are issues now receiving increasing attention. Error rates in areas such as medication dosing, performance of critical procedures, and diagnosis are higher in children than in adults. This disparity is likely due to the lower frequency of pediatric calls and of opportunities to reinforce pediatric knowledge and skills in the field. To improve pediatric medication safety, recommended interventions include an improved weight estimation tool, availability of pediatric checklists, and dosage cards. Efforts are needed in implementing competency-based pediatric training modules, use of software to assist in equipment sizing and medication dosing, and development and dissemination of guidelines of care for common or critical pediatric emergencies. Additionally, conducting routine run reviews can help identify factors that contribute to adverse outcomes related to field care. The emerging use of mobile decision support systems (**FIGURE 19–5**) has been shown to reduce acute perceived stress and reduce pediatric care errors. The EMSC initiative has played a crucial role in developing regional prehospital pediatric protocols, pediatric hospital destination agreements, and pediatric care policies. These resources equip EMS clinicians with the tools and guidance they need to effectively and safely manage pediatric calls.

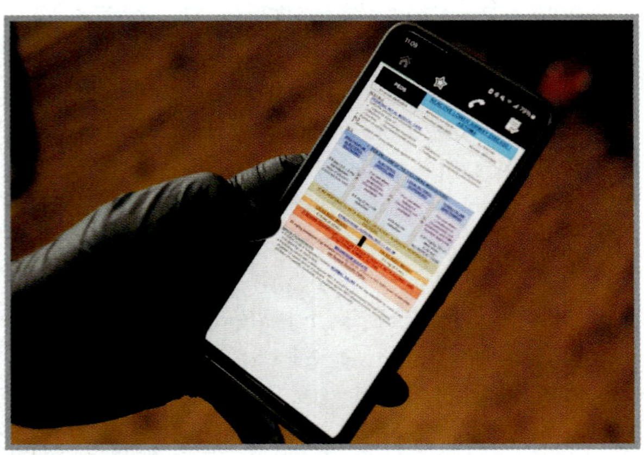

FIGURE 19–5 Pediatric medical decision support software systems are readily available for EMS clinicians on vehicle computers and cell phones.

To emphasize the significance of pediatric QI in emergency care, the National EMS Quality Alliance has identified key measures for EMS agencies to track and enhance, focusing on what is most relevant to their patient populations. Of the 21 measures, one pediatric-specific measure stands out: it tracks the "percentage of EMS responses from 911 requests for patients [younger than] 18 years of age who received weight-based medication and had their weight documented in kilograms or through a length-based estimate." Recognizing the unique challenges in pediatric care, all EMS systems should adopt these quality measures to enhance care at the local level.

Data and Information Management

In the context of QI science, enhancing systems of care requires a thorough understanding of how the system currently operates. This involves collecting baseline data to establish a starting point, as well as postimplementation data to measure the impact of changes. Quality improvement is an active and iterative process that begins with answering the following 3 questions before implementation:

1. **What are we trying to accomplish?** Clearly define the specific goals or outcomes the improvement effort aims to achieve.
2. **What changes can we make that will result in improvement?** Identify measurable indicators that will demonstrate whether the changes made are leading to improvements.
3. **How will we know that change is an improvement?** Determine the specific strategies or interventions that drive meaningful improvements in the system.

These guiding questions help ensure that the QI process is focused, measurable, and evidence-driven.

A PREHOSPITAL QI CASE STUDY

Consider the following hypothetical scenario: An ED physician contacts the manager of your EMS agency with concerns about 2 children who were transported over the past month after on-scene endotracheal intubations following apparent febrile seizures. Both had been treated in the field with intravenous

(IV) lorazepam, resulting in respiratory depression that in turn led to endotracheal intubations, and both underwent extubation shortly after their arrival in the ED. A survey of your agency's electronic database reveals a total of 10 children over the past year with a diagnosis of seizure who were intubated in the field after treatment with IV lorazepam. Knowing that most febrile seizures are brief and self-limited, you are concerned that the potential complications of intubation outweigh the benefits of lorazepam administration. You bring this to the QI committee for review. They ask the following questions:

Question #1: What are we trying to accomplish?

Answer #1: We want to decrease the incidence of children experiencing respiratory depression leading to intubation associated with benzodiazepine treatment for seizures.

Question #2: What changes can we make that will result in improvement?

Answer #2: Possible changes might include education regarding indications for benzodiazepines in children with seizures, adding computer-based decision support software or length-based resuscitation tapes to ensure administration of correct dosing of benzodiazepines, switching from IV to intranasal midazolam administration, and emphasizing/providing training in advanced airway maneuvers such as bag-mask ventilation before intubation.

Question #3: How will we know if a change is an improvement?

Answer #3: Our intubation rate for children with seizures will decrease, without an associated increase of children with respiratory insufficiency on arrival at the ED.

In collaboration with your medical director, you develop a new protocol for assessing and managing pediatric seizures, conduct in-service training, and implement a data sheet to be completed after each seizure call. After 6 months, you discover that your intubation rate for children with febrile seizures has decreased by 75%. This data-driven approach highlights the importance of evaluating current practices and identifying opportunities to improve prehospital care.

IMPORTANCE OF DATA COLLECTION AND INFORMATION MANAGEMENT IN EMERGENCY MEDICAL SERVICES FOR CHILDREN

Injury prevention begins with a comprehensive understanding of the community's injury patterns. Properly collected, integrated, and interpreted data transform into valuable information that can guide prevention efforts. A well-maintained injury database allows EMS clinicians to identify patterns of preventable injury within the community. This information is crucial for generating financial and political support for targeted prevention programs and evaluating programs' effectiveness in reducing injury frequency and severity.

Key elements of an injury database useful for EMS system management include the type, severity, and frequency of both fatal and nonfatal injuries; identification of at-risk populations; geographic locations; time of day and year; and contributing factors such as alcohol use, weather conditions, and improper use of protective devices. Analysis of these data can help prioritize program planning and evaluation. For example, if data indicate there is a high rate of injury among unrestrained young children in car crashes, then an injury prevention program focused on car seat use is needed. The next step is to determine why these children are not properly restrained. Is it lack of education, lack of access to car seats, or perhaps a cultural belief that a baby is safest in a parent's arms? Understanding the root of the problem through data is critical in determining the best intervention strategy.

Summary of Quality, Safety, Data Collection, and Information Management

Quality improvement is now a critical component of EMSC, offering numerous opportunities to evaluate pediatric clinical practice and implement system improvements to reduce errors. Accurate and comprehensive data collection is a key to this process. Although there are many types of EMS data that pertain to children, simply collecting any data is not enough. For data to drive meaningful improvements, they must be accurately collected, systematically reviewed, and analyzed with a focus on identifying and solving a specific problem. When managed effectively, these data become a powerful tool for improving pediatric care. They can guide targeted education and program development, helping to address gaps in practice and reduce errors. By identifying trends and areas for improvement, quality initiatives can enhance the safety and quality of care for children in the prehospital setting, ensuring that the interventions are both evidence based and outcome driven.

TIP

To reduce errors in pediatric emergency care, ensure the availability of pediatric-specific checklists, dosing tools, and competency-based training modules. These resources are critical for improving medication safety and the overall quality of care.

TIP

Collect accurate data on pediatric care to identify gaps in practice and drive improvements. This includes monitoring key quality measures and reviewing case outcomes to reduce errors and enhance patient safety.

Prevention: The Prehospital Professional's Role

Emergency medical services clinicians have a great responsibility to influence and support their communities through illness and injury prevention. *They can have a greater impact on health by reducing illness and injury through prevention than they can through treatment alone*. However, to effectively achieve this role, EMS clinicians require specialized education and training. The first step in developing community intervention programs is understanding how injuries and illnesses can be prevented. This knowledge is essential for designing and implementing effective prevention activities that benefit the entire community.

BEFORE THE CALL

Prevention can begin well before an emergency call through effective and proactive preparedness. Collaborating with your community on programs such as the Community Emergency Response Team initiative, the EIF, CPR and first-aid training, babysitting classes, and car seat safety checks helps to build and strengthen the infrastructure for prevention and management of emergencies. Educational programs and skills training not only enhance community readiness but also improve your response to emergencies. The better prepared your community is to recognize and respond to potential events, the greater the likelihood of successful and effective emergency response.

ROLE ON SCENE

Prevention efforts by the EMS clinician begin during the scene size-up and include ensuring scene safety and performing an **environmental assessment**. Ensuring scene safety involves prevention of injury and illness in everyone present, including prehospital professionals, other medical and law enforcement personnel, and bystanders. This includes identifying potential communicable diseases in the child that can be transmitted to scene personnel without proper precautions. Additionally, ensuring scene safety may help prevent further injury to the child or to the caregiver.

It is crucial that the EMS clinician perform an environmental assessment is to understand the overall picture at the scene. Observation and documentation of the physical and interpersonal environment at the scene provides important information that can guide prevention efforts. These actions may include advising caregivers about safety hazards such as lack of smoke detectors, stair gates, or window bars to prevent potential future injuries and illnesses.

Another type of environmental assessment involves observing signs of possible maltreatment by the caregiver. Communicating any concerns to the ED physician is a preventive action that may save the child's life, as explained in Chapter 13.

CASE STUDY 3

You are called to a recreational complex for an 8-year-old boy who was hit in the chest with a baseball and collapsed. Before your arrival, his coach and teammates started cardiopulmonary resuscitation (CPR) and attached an automated external defibrillator; despite initial defibrillation, he is still in ventricular fibrillation. As you arrive on scene, you are told what happened and what care was administered before your arrival. As you continue resuscitation efforts, you calculate medications and equipment size with a length-based tool and deliver another defibrillation with return of spontaneous circulation before transport. The boy is awake on arrival at the ED and after hospitalization discharged home in 2 days.

1. How did the community prepare for this event? How did EMS?
2. What resources are available in a community?

ROLE IN SAFE TRANSPORT

A crucial aspect of childhood injury prevention for the EMS clinician is ensuring safe transport. *Many serious and fatal vehicular injuries occur to occupants who are improperly restrained.* This pertains to both ambulance and automobile transport. The essential safety steps are simple: Always wear a seat belt, secure all equipment, and secure the pediatric patient in an appropriate child restraint device for the entire transport. These measures also apply to every prehospital professional, reinforcing safety for both providers and patients. For a full description of transportation considerations, see Chapter 18. With regard to safe transport of children in the community, EMS professionals can play a significant role in the community by becoming credentialed car safety seat technicians, assisting parents in obtaining and properly installing car safety seats in their vehicles.

ROLE IN THE COMMUNITY

Detailed and accurate observations made at the scene can initiate or reinforce community-wide strategies for injury and illness control. For instance, in Europe and Australia, EMS clinicians played a key role in recognizing the link between sleep position and **sudden unexplained infant death (SUID)**. Their scene observations contributed to scientific studies that confirmed the increased risk of SUID associated with infants who slept **prone** and assisted in the campaign that has decreased SUID **mortality**. Chapter 15 discusses SUID in more depth.

Emergency medical services clinicians can enhance the understanding of community injury and illness patterns by documenting the mechanism and scene circumstances surrounding acute events in the prehospital record and by assisting in other local data-collection efforts. **TABLE 19–2** lists some specific community injury prevention activities that EMS clinicians might consider in their expanded roles as community advocates, public educators, and trainers.

TABLE 19–2 Examples of Common Injuries and Possible Prevention Strategies

Injury	Prevention
Vehicle trauma	Infant and child restraint seats Seat belts and air bags Pedestrian safety programs Motorcycle helmets Safe driving
Cycling	Bicycle helmets Bicycle paths separate from vehicle traffic Obeying traffic signals and signs
Recreation	Appropriate safety padding and apparel Cyclist/skateboard/skater safety programs Soft, energy-absorbent playground surfaces
Drowning	Four-sided locked pool enclosures Pool alarms Immediate adult supervision Caretaker training in cardiopulmonary resuscitation Swimming lessons Pool/beach safety instruction Personal flotation devices
Poisoning and household items	Proper storage of chemicals and medications Child safety packaging
Burns	Proper maintenance and monitoring of electrical appliances and cords Fire/smoke detectors Proper placement of cookware on stove top Proper supervision of fireworks
Other	Discouragement of infant walker use Gated stairways Babysitter first-aid training Child care worker training in first aid

TIP

Scene observations sparked the scientific studies that confirmed the increased risk of sudden unexplained infant death in babies who slept in prone position.

Summary of Roles in Prevention

The EMS clinician has crucial and ample opportunities to educate and promote prevention both on the job and as a community member (**FIGURE 19–6**). Recognizing scene safety issues, documenting suspicious home circumstances, and recording injury mechanisms are essential responsibilities and duties in an effective EMS system. By ensuring accurate equipment sizing and drug dosing, EMS clinicians can significantly reduce errors and prevent adverse outcomes related to prehospital medical care. Balancing the duties of ensuring child passengers' safety during transport while allowing ongoing monitoring and

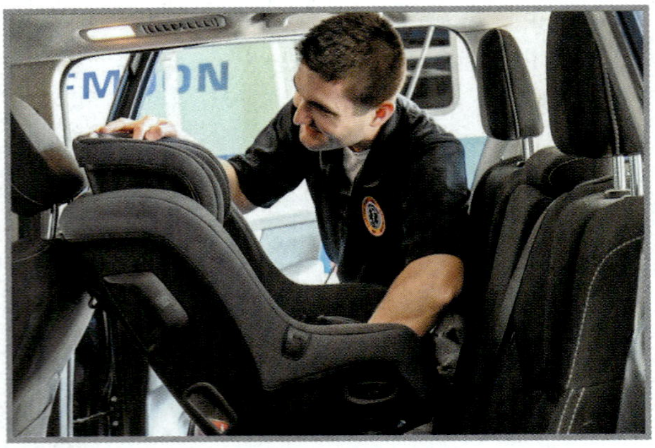

FIGURE 19-6 EMS clinicians have the opportunity to teach prevention.

treatment remains a challenge for EMS professionals. Furthermore, it is a duty of EMS clinicians to advocate for and be an integral part of any community injury and illness prevention programs as a part of the EMSC continuum.

Call to Action: Advocacy for EMSC

EMS clinician advocates play a crucial role in supporting EMSC both on and off the ambulance. They can engage in numerous clinical and operational aspects of EMSC, addressing countless challenges within their community. National and state EMSC programs offer many excellent models and templates for system improvement, often accompanied by funding to support new programs focused on children's care. Numerous funding agencies, both public and private, have resources aimed at bolstering children's services and improving pediatric emergency care in the community. Advocacy for EMSC involves exploring innovative support outside traditional EMS to strengthen pediatric services.

Advancing children's care within EMS may take many forms, including active participation on EMSC committees at the state level and/or daily advocacy for training, equipment, policies, procedures, and protocols specifically designed for children. Other roles may include volunteering as an educator in schools, developing first-aid services for students, serving as a CPR trainer, or engaging in community injury prevention programs and children's health issues. National associations such as the American Academy of Pediatrics, the American College of Emergency Physicians, and the Emergency Nurses Association, as well as local fire departments and prehospital care organizations, sponsor initiatives aimed at pediatric illness and injury prevention. However, the success of these visionary programs requires advocacy and active participation for success.

Partnerships forged within your community can help empower tomorrow's generation through education today. When a child understands that they are not helpless in times of emergency, they become a powerful ally on the scene, which can also reduce psychological trauma. Civic organizations have successfully impacted lives through preparedness initiatives, and EMS has a unique opportunity to further those efforts exponentially. Through this partnership in training and education, we can make a difference.

There is unprecedented potential for transformative improvements in saving lives, alleviating pain and suffering, preventing injury and illness, and facilitating the intricate interface of prehospital pediatric care, community services, and in-hospital care through collaboration with public health. Ensuring the health and safety of children requires ongoing advocacy and vigilance from all EMS clinicians to maintain high-quality pediatric services in EMS systems today and to foster the continued evolution of EMSC in the future.

CASE STUDY ANSWERS

CASE STUDY 1

Several prevention interventions may have prevented or lessened the outcome in this case, including car safety education in schools and communities that emphasizes measures such as the use of seat belts and child restraint seats; proper use of restraints and car seats; reduced vehicle speed; application of advanced automobile safety technology; and improved traffic signage.

For the prehospital professional, the key prevention steps include performing scene size-up, documenting critical scene conditions, providing appropriate care onsite, and rapidly transporting the child to the appropriate medical facility. Noting the mechanism of injury and informing hospital

CASE STUDY ANSWERS—cont'd

professionals of the child's lack of car restraints offers multiple opportunities to formulate prevention strategies. The best medical intervention may have changed this child's outcome; effective prevention programs certainly could have.

Accurate documentation of the circumstances of injury also contributes to data collection, which in turn helps to identify injury patterns within the community. The prehospital professional, as a community advocate, can play a vital role in injury prevention, educating parents and policy makers about known risks and promoting solutions to reduce childhood illnesses and injury. A critical incident response team can be considered for a psychological first-aid debriefing after such incidents, which can be initiated either by EMS clinicians or by hospital staff.

CASE STUDY 2

This child's primary care physician plays a crucial role in managing her chronic illness and is likely best qualified to make care decisions. Given the child's medically stable condition after treatment, contacting the medical control to discuss transport destination is reasonable. Effective prehospital care, as a part of the EMS-EMSC continuum, requires not only appropriate equipment and education of prehospital personnel, but also teamwork, knowledge of community resources, and clear communication. Transport of this child to her "medical home," if allowed by local EMS policies, may offer advantages that must be weighed against potential risks of clinical deterioration. When local protocols restrict transport beyond local facilities, alternative safe transport can be arranged. Additionally, an EIF can provide valuable insight into the patient's baseline status and provide robust clinical information before the parent's arrival. Understanding the pediatric readiness of your local and regional hospitals would also aid in the destination decision.

CASE STUDY 3

The community's rapid response, scene efficiency, and lifesaving interventions prior to EMS arrival significantly impact both the patient and the bystanders. Through education, training, access to necessary equipment, and emergency preparedness, communities enhance their abilities to handle emergencies with optimal outcomes. The ability to respond appropriately ensures a seamless continuum of care. Programs such as CPR and AED training, AED placement, community response teams, pediatric-specific training empowers a community to make a meaningful difference. Use of proper equipment such as a length-based weight estimation tool and a computer-based decision support system can assist the EMS clinician in selecting the appropriately sized equipment and medication dosages. Having well-organized pediatric equipment enhances the professional's ability to locate it quickly and safeguard the care of the child.

Training and education empower communities to take an active role in emergency care and improve patient outcomes. Emergency medical services clinicians play a key role in preparing their communities through EMSC resources and communication efforts, strengthening overall community readiness.

Suggested References

ARTICLES AND BOOKS

Ames SG, Davis BS, Marin JR, et al. Emergency department pediatric readiness and mortality in critically ill children. *Pediatrics*. 2019;144(3):e20190568. doi:10.1542/peds.2019-0568

Anders JF, Fishe JN, Fratta KA, et al. Creating a pediatric prehospital destination decision tool using a modified delphi method. *Children (Basel)*. 2021;8(8):658. doi:10.3390/children8080658

Hoyle JD Jr, Crowe RP, Bentley MA, Beltran G, Fales W. Pediatric prehospital medication dosing errors: a national survey of paramedics. *Prehosp Emerg Care*. 2017;21(2):185–191. doi: 10.1080/10903127.2016.1227001

Hoyle JD Jr, Sleight D, Henry R, Chassee T, Fales B, Mavis B. Pediatric prehospital medication dosing errors: a mixed-methods study. *Prehosp Emerg Care*. 2016;20(1):117–124. doi: 10.3109/10903127.2015.1061625

Institute of Medicine (US) Committee on Quality of Health Care in America. *Crossing the Quality Chasm: A New Health System for the 21st Century*. Washington, DC: National Academies Press; 2001. PMID: 25057539

Lacour M, Bloudeau L, Combescure C, et al; PedAMINES Prehospital Group. Impact of a mobile app on paramedics' perceived and physiologic stress response during simulated prehospital pediatric cardiopulmonary resuscitation: study nested within a multicenter randomized controlled trial. *JMIR Mhealth Uhealth*. 2021;9(10):e31748. doi: 10.2196/31748

Moore B, Shah MI, Owusu-Ansah S, et al; American Academy of Pediatrics, Committee on Pediatric Emergency Medicine and Section on Emergency Medicine EMS Subcommittee; American College of Emergency Physicians, Emergency Medical Services Committee; Emergency Nurses Association, Pediatric Committee; National Association of Emergency Medical Services Physicians, Standards and Clinical Practice Committee; National Association of Emergency Medical Technicians, Emergency Pediatric Care Committee; Pediatric Readiness in Emergency Medical Services Systems; Policy Statement; Organizational Principles to Guide and Define the Child Health Care System and/or Improve the Health of All Children. Pediatric readiness in emergency medical services systems. *Ann Emerg Med*. 2020;75(1):e1–e6. doi: 10.1016/j.annemergmed.2019.09.012

Newgard CD, Lin A, Malveau S, et al; Pediatric Readiness Study Group. Emergency department pediatric readiness and short-term and long-term mortality among children receiving emergency care. *JAMA Netw Open*. 2023;6(1):e2250941. doi: 10.1001/jamanetworkopen.2022.50941

Remick K, Gausche-Hill M, Joseph MM, et al; American Academy of Pediatrics, Committee on Pediatric Emergency Medicine, Section on Surgery; American College of Emergency Physicians, Pediatric Emergency Medicine Committee; Emergency Nurses Association, Pediatric Committee; Pediatric Readiness in the Emergency Department; Policy Statement; Organizational Principles to Guide and Define the Child Health Care System and/or Improve the Health of All Children. Pediatric readiness in the emergency department. *Ann Emerg Med*. 2018;72(6):e123–e136. doi: 10.1016/j.annemergmed.2018.08.431

Remick KE, Foster AA, Jensen AR, et al; American Academy of Pediatrics, AMERICAN COLLGE OF EMERGENCY PHYSICIANS, Pediatric Emergency Committee; EMERGENCY NURSES ASSOCIATION, Pediatric Committee; AMERICAN COLLEGE OF SURGEONS; Committee on Trauma. Pediatric Readiness in the Emergency Department: Policy Statement. Pediatrics. 2026;157(2):e2025075318.

OTHER RESOURCES

The American Association for the Surgery of Trauma. Ten steps for developing an injury prevention program. Accessed April 4, 2025. https://www.aast.org/resources-detail/ten-steps-developing-injury-prevention-program -

American College of Emergency Physicians; American Academy of Pediatrics. Emergency information form. Accessed Febrauary 10, 2026. https://www.acep.org/siteassets/uploads/uploaded-files/acep/clinical-and-practice-management/resources/emergency-medical-services/emergency_information_form_for_children_with_special_needs1.pdf

City of Madison [Wisconsin]. Community Alternative Response Emergency Services (CARES). Accessed February 10, 2026. https://www.cityofmadison.com/fire/emergency-medical-services/community-alternative-response-emergency-services-cares

Health Resources and Services Administration (HRSA) of the US Department of Health and Human Services. EMSC Improvement and Innovation Center. https://emscimprovement.center

Jensen A. Addressing the new pediatric readiness standards at your trauma center. Presented at American College of Surgeons Trauma Quality Improvement Program, January 26, 2022. Accessed February 10, 2026. https://web4.facs.org/TQIPFiles/2022.1ACS_Peds_Readiness.pdf

National EMS Quality Alliance. NEMSQA measures. Accessed April 4, 2025 https://www.nemsqa.org/nemsqa-measures

Procedure 1: Field Reporting

Tabitha Cheng, MD
Maggie Coen Murphy, BS, EMT-P

Introduction

Gathering and organizing pertinent information about pediatric patients to report to other prehospital professionals, medical oversight personnel, and the receiving emergency department (ED) are important pieces of the continuum of care. Clear and concise communication is imperative when describing children and their clinical problems to medical oversight personnel, when informing a receiving ED about an incoming patient, and before transferring patient care. Field reporting should be clear, concise, organized, and pertinent, adhere to confidentiality practices in compliance with HIPAA or similar regulations protecting the privacy of the patient. Do not include the patient's name in the report. The reporting is usually done via a secure radio transmission, a telephone, or another form of secure real-time communication. Different emergency medical services (EMS) regions may have unique requirements for field reporting to medical oversight and to receiving EDs.

In addition to spoken field reports, pediatric-specific documentation is essential for later review and analysis. Emergency medical services agencies typically have their own reporting form or template on which the prehospital professional must record clinical facts, as well as the necessary information for billing and for detailed incident or system analysis.

INDICATION

Use the appropriate field reporting procedure in any radio, telephone, facsimile (fax), or personal/direct communication with medical oversight personnel, a receiving ED, or other prehospital providers regarding on-scene or inbound pediatric emergency patients. Pediatric-specific documentation should be used for all written reports or records concerning pediatric patients.

CONTRAINDICATION

A relative contraindication to appropriate field reporting is the child with a physiological abnormality requiring constant hands-on care. Another is suspected child maltreatment, when the perpetrator may be present. This situation may make it difficult for the prehospital professional to communicate fully with a receiving ED or medical oversight team during transport. When possible, the prehospital professional should have a coworker, such as a partner, assist with notifying pertinent parties that a distressed child is en route. However, complete reporting of patient assessment, treatment, and response to treatment may not be feasible under these circumstances. There are no contraindications to accurate reporting through written documentation.

> **TIP**
> A call to the hospital with an opening line of a specific situation or other disclaimer that shares a "heads up" can notify the hospital that you request assistance from medical control, or that there is a very ill or injured child en route.

EQUIPMENT

Equipment requirements vary depending on the EMS system and may include telecommunications equipment, real-time computerized data transmission, or video. The patient care record is essential, as are other assessment worksheets in some EMS systems.

Rationale

A logical and descriptive format for presentation of key information about ill or injured children is essential for everyday field practice. It promotes the cost-efficient use of communications equipment and personnel time. Proper field reporting also integrates efforts from all emergency care professionals (prehospital professionals, nurses, and doctors) and helps ensure that vital data are transmitted completely and concisely. Pediatric-specific reporting techniques complement appropriate age-related modifications in assessment, treatment, triage, and transport.

Preparation

1. The prehospital professional should prepare for and practice field reporting on pediatric patients.
2. It is helpful to have a field reporting format that is agreed on by the EMS agency, medical oversight personnel, and the transport providers. The desired format can be an actual document or checklist; this may help facilitate the gathering of patient information during situations in which the prehospital professional has multiple tasks and when the environment or equipment makes communication difficult.

Possible Complications

Using incorrect, deceptive, or unclear terminology, or failing to distinguish the pediatric report from the more frequent adult-oriented report, may delay medical oversight and preparation by the receiving ED.

TIP

1. Field reports should be approximately 30 seconds in length, providing enough patient information for the ED and/or medical oversight team to determine the appropriate level of care.
2. Use the Pediatric Assessment Triangle (PAT) to guide assessment reporting. See **TABLE 1-1 in Chapter 1.**

Components of a Prehospital Field Report

1. Unit's identification and level of service (advanced or basic life support)
2. Patient's age, sex, and approximate weight
3. Chief complaint
4. Brief, *pertinent* history of present illness or injury
5. *Pertinent* medical history, medications, and allergies
6. Pertinent physical examination findings (PAT)
7. Abnormalities in airway, breathing, circulation, and level of consciousness (Alert, Verbal, Pain, Unresponsive [AVPU] scale or pediatric Glasgow Coma Scale [GCS])
8. Diagnostic findings (eg, glucose level)
9. Treatments and patient responses
10. Estimated time of arrival (ETA)
11. Request for orders or any additional questions for medical oversight
12. Repetition of medical oversight orders to confirm understanding if given

PROCEDURE 1-1

Field Reporting

1. State the child's age, sex, and estimated body weight.
2. Give the child's chief complaint.
3. Provide, in one sentence, the mechanism of injury or history of illness, and state pertinent medical history, medications, and allergies (usually none or brief).
4. Summarize the assessment and establish the level of severity and urgency for treatment using the PAT. Address all 3 elements of the PAT, using appropriate descriptive words and terms, as listed in **TABLE P1-1**.
5. Report abnormalities in airway, breathing, circulation, or level of consciousness, using AVPU or pediatric GCS without focusing solely on vital signs.
6. Report any diagnostic findings.
7. State treatment and patient's response.
8. State the ETA.
9. Request agreement from medical oversight personnel regarding interventions and request additional orders as per local EMS protocol.

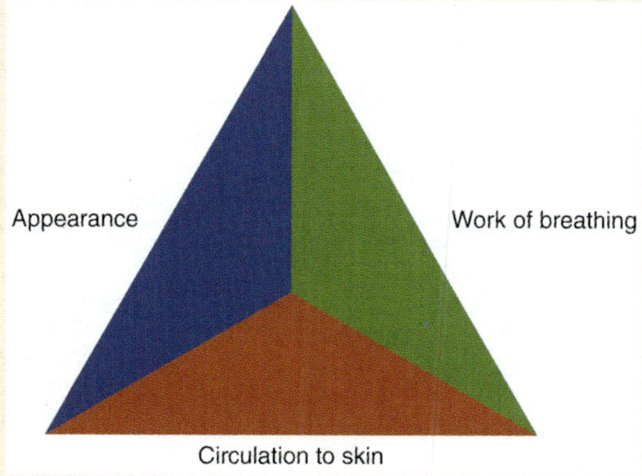

10. Repeat medical oversight orders to confirm understanding.

Refer to **TABLE P1-2** for a sample pediatric reporting template that can serve as a quick reference in high-stress or time-sensitive situations.

TABLE P1-1 Examples of Pediatric-Specific Terminology for the Pediatric Assessment Triangle

Appearance[a]	Work of Breathing	Circulation to Skin
Tone Active, vigorous, good muscle tone Limp, listless, motionless, will not sit or walk	Apneic	Pink, good color
Interactiveness Alert, interactive, attentive, playful Restless, agitated, screaming	Abnormal positioning (sniffing position, tripoding)	Mottled, dusky
Consolability Consolable or distractible by caregiver, comfortable Cannot be consoled	Abnormal airway sounds (snoring, stridor, wheezing, grunting)	Pale
Look/Gaze Fixes gaze, maintains good eye contact Will not engage or make eye contact	Retractions (supraclavicular, intercostal, subxiphoid)	Cyanotic
Speech/Cry Strong cry, normal speech Weak cry, cannot speak	Nasal flaring	Not applicable

[a] Following the TICLS mnemonic to recall individual features: tone, interactiveness, consolability, look/gaze, and speech/cry.

TABLE P1-2 Sample Pediatric Reporting Template

We are [on scene] or [en route to (name of ED)] with a [state age in days, weeks, months, or years as appropriate] [state male or female] patient weighing [state approximate body weight in kilograms].	
CC	The patient's chief complaint is [state chief complaint in 1 or 2 words].
HPI	State brief history of present illness/injury.
PMH	State brief, pertinent medical history, medications, and allergies.
PAT	Appearance: Describe the patient's appearance using descriptive terms.[a] Work of breathing: Describe the work of breathing using descriptive terms. Circulation to skin: Describe the circulation to skin using descriptive terms.
Initial ABCDEs assessment	Summarize key findings from the ABCDEs (see Chapter 1 for more information on the AVPU Scale and Chapter 9 for more information on the pediatric GCS).
Diagnostic findings	Summarize any diagnostic findings.
TX	Report the treatment and the patient's response. Use these elements as the basis for ongoing assessment: the PAT, the ABCDEs, repeating vital signs, and reassessing of positive anatomical findings in distressed children who have received the focused and detailed examinations.
ETA	Our ETA to [state receiving ED] is______minutes. Do you have any advice or questions? [Request additional orders as per local protocol at this point.]

Abbreviations: AVPU, alert, verbal, painful, unresponsive; CC, chief complaint; ED, emergency department; ETA, estimated time of arrival; GCS, Glasgow Coma Scale; HPI, history of present illness; PAT, Pediatric Assessment Triangle; PMH, pertinent medical history; TX, treatment.

[a] See Table P1–1 for examples of pediatric-specific descriptive terminology.

Procedure 2: Length-/Weight-Based Resuscitation Tape

Tabitha Cheng, MD
Maggie Coen Murphy, BS, EMT-P

Introduction

Selecting the appropriately sized equipment or calculating drug dosages is often challenging during encounters with pediatric patients. Using a length-based pediatric emergency resuscitation tape in the prehospital setting reduces medication dosing errors significantly. Several types of length-based systems are available to help determine correct equipment sizes and drug doses. These tapes are simple and effective tools for measuring body lengths and estimating weights.

INDICATION

Pediatric patients weighing 3 to 36 kg requiring appropriate-sized equipment as well as accurate volume and medication dosing based on weight

EQUIPMENT

Length-based resuscitation tape
Pediatric drug dosing tools such as computer or cell phone applications based on length-based resuscitation tape

Rationale

Treatment of infants and children in the prehospital setting is difficult. Equipment size, volume resuscitation, and medication dosages in the pediatric population are all based on the child's weight.

Mistakes are common when selecting appropriate equipment and medications in critically ill pediatric patients without the benefit of an accurate weight. Pediatric resuscitation equipment/methods for such calculations use weight or length as a valid marker of size-specific equipment and medication needs. These devices are portable, easy to use, and applicable to all prehospital equipment and medications. The use of a computer- or cell phone–based application to determine the correct drug dose in milliliters (versus milligrams) is beneficial, but it is important to verify the concentrations of the particular drug to ensure it is the same being used by your agency.

Medication Dosing

Caring for pediatric patients differs from caring for the adult population, because most pediatric emergency interventions are weight based. These interventions include medication doses, intravenous fluid requirements, defibrillation energy doses, and equipment sizes. It is important that pediatric measurement of weight be consistent so as to provide children the right dose of medication, prevent errors, and preserve patient safety and care quality. The kilogram, instead of the pound, is the standard unit of measurement for pediatric patients. Most medications use the metric system, which is compatible with weight measured in kilograms.

There are numerous ways to determine the weight of a pediatric patient in kilograms, which include length-based tapes/systems (eg, Broselow or Handtevy) and age-based weight formulas. For a step-by-step explanation, see **Procedure 2-1**, **Length-Based Resuscitation Tapes**. The original advanced pediatric life support formula tended to underestimate the actual weight, and the margin of error increased with age. There is increasing evidence that methods based on the length of the child are more accurate than are age-based formulas; however, this requires accurate physical measurement. The length-based tapes are accurate for equipment sizing, but with increasing childhood obesity, they may underestimate the child's weight, especially in older children; in some impoverished countries with childhood malnutrition, they may, in fact, overestimate the weight. However, for resuscitation medications, length-based doses should be used. A key factor is to ensure that the concentration of the medication carried is the same as on the tape (eg, atropine and naloxone come in different concentrations). In addition, whereas most of the recent tapes have doses in milliliters, some older tapes had doses in milligrams, except for resuscitation drugs.

As with all patients, the right medication should be administered to the right patient for the right reason via the right route and at the right time. It is also important to check the child's history of allergies and medications already taken to prevent potential negative consequences.

Some drugs may be given according to standing orders, whereas others may be given after consultation with medical control personnel. Verbal orders should always be repeated back to medical control to assure that there is no misunderstanding. Orders that are confusing, unclear, or not within an emergency medical services (EMS) clinician's scope of practice or regional protocols should be questioned to avoid misunderstanding or breaches of standards of care. A medication should be checked carefully to assure it is the correct medication, is not expired, is not contaminated or damaged in any way, and is without particulate matter or discoloration.

Medication administration in children is particularly risky because of the potential for incorrect dosages. Most medications given to children in the prehospital setting are weight based. It is important to remember that weight-based dosing references the amount of drug to be given per kilogram (eg, mg/kg or mL/kg), not per pound. One kilogram equals 2.2 pounds, so if a calculation is inadvertently based on pounds, the dosage will be too high and can lead to an overdose.

In an emergency setting, it is very easy to miscalculate doses, so the use of medication aids is extremely beneficial. There are different types of aids. Some show the calculated dose when figured with a child's known weight in kilograms; these include wheels, cards, or smartphone applications. Others, such as length-based measuring tapes, determine the length of the child and then give the calculated doses based on the average weight of children of that height. Any of these aids help to decrease mathematical errors, especially the misplacement of decimal points in the calculated dose. A misplaced decimal point can cause a calculation 10 times larger or smaller than the dose should be. Some medications are prepackaged in doses specifically for children and adults. An example of this is an epinephrine autoinjector. It is essential that the correct package be selected to administer the correct dose. For example, an adult epinephrine autoinjector is typically 0.3 mg, twice the amount of the usual pediatric epinephrine autoinjector at 0.15 mg.

Because overdoses of medications can occur easily, with potentially serious consequences, it is essential that the EMS clinician do everything possible to safely administer any medications during treatment of the child. It is also important that accurate and complete documentation of any medication doses be done and provided verbally to the ED team during patient report/handoff to prevent potential overdoses due to hospital staff's not knowing what was given in the prehospital setting.

Possible Complications

- Incorrect measurement
- Incorrect drug concentration

TIP

Store the length-based resuscitation tape in an easily accessible location, such as the pediatric equipment kit.

TIP

Arrange your pediatric medication bag to reduce errors. For example, avoid putting "look-alike" drugs in close proximity.

PROCEDURE 2-1

Length-Based Resuscitation Tape

1. Place the patient in a supine position.
2. Extend the patient's legs.
3. Measure the child's length from head to heel with the tape, aligning the red end at the head ("red to head")See Figure 2-1. Note and verbalize the weight in kilograms that corresponds to the child's measured length at the heel. If the child is longer than the tape, use adult equipment and medication doses. From the tape, identify appropriate equipment sizes as well as appropriate medication doses and fluid volumes.

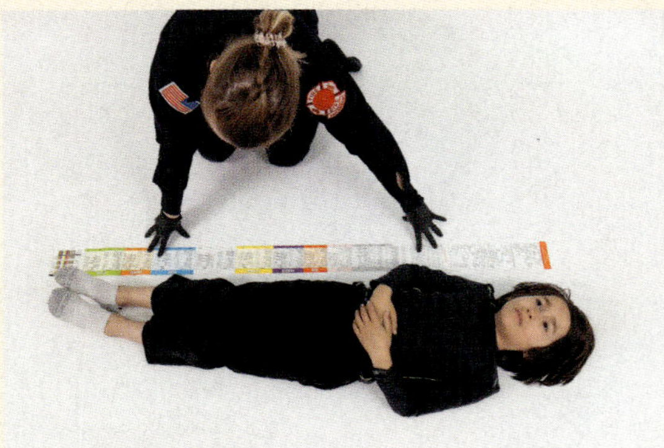

CONTROVERSY

There are several different brands of length-based pediatric resuscitation tapes, which are based on an average-sized US child. Studies have shown these tapes underestimate the weight of obese children, especially toward the longer lengths. However, the equipment sizes are still accurate in terms of length.

CAUTION

Measuring to the child's toes (instead of heel) adds a number of kilograms to the estimated weight and may result in equipment sizes that are too large or excessive drug doses.

CONTROVERSY

Pediatric length-based resuscitation tapes are based on ideal body weight. With the epidemic of obesity in children, there is concern about the accuracy of length-based resuscitation tapes. However, most emergency medications doses are based on what a patient should ideally weigh. Thus, there is rarely a need to increase resuscitation medication doses in obese children.

PROCEDURE 2-2

Pediatric Resuscitation Software

1. Pediatric drug dosage calculators based on length-based resuscitation tapes now exist for a computer or smart phone. It is crucial to use a length-based method to determine the weight of the child. You can then use software to help you determine a drug dose; it is usually in milliliters, rather in milligrams, but look carefully to determine the unit. In addition, it is crucial to verify the concentration of the particular drug to ensure it is the same being used by your agency (eg, atropine and naloxone come in different concentrations).
2. Enter the child's weight into the software program, then select the clinical condition or type of resuscitation. The software will calculate the dose on the basis of the child's weight.

Procedure 3: Oxygen Delivery

Ann Dietrich, MD, FAAP, FACEP
Tyler Diettert, NREMTP, EC

Introduction

Hypoxia in the infant or child causes cardiopulmonary distress and may lead to organ failure. Careful assessment of the child's cardiopulmonary status includes standard physical assessment techniques, pulse oximetry, and end-tidal CO_2 ($EtCO_2$). A normal room air pulse oximetry reading is equal to or greater than 94%. A pulse oximetry value of less than 94% in room air is an indication for supplemental oxygen; a value less than 90% with the child receiving 100% oxygen is also an indication for ventilatory support. Maintain the airway and administer oxygen as appropriate with a target of achieving $>94\%$ SpO_2. Some respiratory problems will improve with simple measures. Rapid intervention may slow or reverse cardiopulmonary distress or failure and prevent the need for additional ventilatory support. The goal is to stop progression from respiratory distress so that the child does not develop respiratory failure, something that can happen quickly in infants and children. Although respiratory disease is usually the cause of hypoxia in children, other conditions, such as hypovolemic shock, severe poisonings, or seizures, may also result in hypoxia.

There are different procedures for giving oxygen to children that vary the amount of actual oxygen supplementation. Use an oxygen delivery technique that matches the child's clinical condition, age, and need for oxygen. When necessary, escalate support methods to maintain normal oxygenation. For the child in no or mild distress who has an open airway, give oxygen via nasal cannula or simple mask; for the child with moderate to severe respiratory distress, give oxygen via a nonrebreathing mask or bag-mask device. For severe respiratory distress or impending respiratory failure, more advanced methods of oxygen delivery may be required, such as continuous positive airway pressure (CPAP), bilevel positive airway pressure (BiPAP), intermittent positive-pressure breathing, humidified high-flow nasal cannula, and/or bilevel nasal CPAP. Use caution with use of positive-pressure delivery methods in children with asthma or bronchospasm; use of such methods can lead to air leaks such as pneumothoraxes and pneumomediastinum.

Rarely, a child in critical condition requires endotracheal intubation or supraglottic airway for assisted and oxygen administration. When supplemental oxygen does not improve the child's condition, consider other possible diagnoses, such as a cardiac disorder (eg, cyanotic congenital heart disease), a circulatory disorder (eg, hypovolemic shock), or, rarely, a toxicologic disorder (eg, methemoglobinemia).

Under some circumstances, giving blow-by oxygen may avoid agitating the child and increasing their distress. In a newborn, be careful about oxygen delivery; it is unnecessary if the newborn is vigorous and pink, and a high concentration of supplemental oxygen may be harmful to the immature brain.

TIP

The appropriate oxygen delivery technique is based on the child's condition, age, and need for oxygen.

INDICATIONS

- Cardiac arrest
- Respiratory distress
- Pulse oximetry reading of less than 94% in room air
- Respiratory failure
- Partial upper airway obstruction
- Partial lower airway obstruction
- Worsening of chronic lung disease
- Status epilepticus
- Overdose
- Shock resulting from any cause
- Multiple trauma
- Any condition possibly causing decreased oxygen delivery to tissues
- Smoke inhalation
- Carbon monoxide poisoning

CONTRAINDICATIONS

There are few absolute contraindications to oxygen delivery to a child who may have hypoxia. A relative contraindication is a child with known cyanotic heart disease. It is important to ask the parent or caregiver what the child's normal pulse oximeter reading should be. You can then provide oxygen to meet this oxygen saturation. Oxygen has proper doses and routes of administration for maximum benefit, minimum toxicity, optimal feasibility, and reasonable cost.

Rationale

A child's immature anatomy and physiology make respiratory distress and failure common pediatric emergencies. When apnea or hypoventilation occurs, hypoxia develops quickly. Therefore, give oxygen to any child who has clinical signs of cardiopulmonary distress or failure, or who has a history suggesting possible abnormalities in gas exchange. *Children out of the newborn period seldom have a condition in which excess oxygen suppresses their respiratory drive, so it is better to overtreat with oxygen than to undertreat.*

Preparation

1. Connect the pressure regulator and flow meter to the oxygen source. Turn on the tank.
2. Match the correct oxygen delivery device with the patient assessment (child's condition, age, and need for oxygen) (**TABLE P3–1**).

Equipment

- Infant and pediatric nasal cannula
- Pediatric mask sizes
- Pediatric nonrebreathing mask
- Oxygen connecting tubing
- Oxygen source
- Pulse oximeter and probes

Possible Complications

There is the potential for injury, if the pressurized tank is punctured or a valve breaks off, and for fire, because oxygen supports combustion.

In preterm newborns, there is a risk of brain injury owing to unnecessary high concentrations of supplemental oxygen.

TIP

An oxygen mask may frighten a child.

TIP

For nasal cannula: The percentage of oxygen delivered is affected by respiratory rate, tidal volume, and extent of mouth breathing. An infant may receive a higher FiO_2 concentration than older patients (eg, 30%–35% with 1 L/min oxygen, 26%–32% with 0.5 L/min oxygen).

CAUTION

Do not give oxygen to a newborn who does not have hypoxia. It is also important to realize that the normal preductal SpO_2 is 85% to 95% at 10 minutes after birth.

CAUTION

Do not force the child to lie down, because it may increase the child's anxiety and agitation.

TIP

Add humidification to nasal cannula flow to avoid nasal irritation and bleeding and to loosen secretions.

TABLE P3-1 Oxygen Delivery Technique and Patient Assessment

Device	Flow Rate	Concentration Delivered	Considerations
Nasal cannula	1–6 L/min	24%–44%	▪ Low-flow system ▪ Least restrictive ▪ Slowly start flow of oxygen after cannula is secured to avoid frightening child ▪ May help to tape cannula to child's cheeks ▪ Use in infants who are obligatory nose breathers or if there is difficulty in obtaining a correctly sized mask
Simple mask	5–12 L/min	35%–50%	▪ Low-flow system ▪ Infant-, pediatric-, and adult-sized masks are available ▪ At least 6 L/min flow rate is needed to prevent rebreathing of exhaled CO_2
Nonrebreathing mask (Face mask and reservoir bag with a valve on the exhalation mask port and a valve between the mask and the reservoir bag)	10–15 L/min	60%–90%	▪ High-flow system ▪ Use in spontaneously breathing patients who require highest concentration of oxygen available (children with respiratory distress and shock) ▪ Make sure the flow rate keeps the reservoir bag inflated ▪ With a snug fit, delivers highest oxygen concentration available by mask ▪ Pediatric and adult masks are available ▪ Partial rebreathing masks are indicated in neonates and infants who cannot overcome valve resistance
Blow-by	10 L/min	Approximately 30%–40%; dependent on proximity to face	▪ Indicated for infant or young child requiring oxygen who will not tolerate mask on the face ▪ Start oxygen flow through simple mask, corrugated tubing, or oxygen tubing threaded through the bottom of a cup ▪ Hold the delivery device as close to the child's nose and mouth as tolerated

PROCEDURE 3-1

Oxygen Delivery

1. Explain to the child and family why oxygen is needed and how the device works. Use developmentally appropriate language. **TABLE P3–2** suggests methods to ease anxiety in the child who does not want to cooperate with oxygen delivery. For blow-by oxygen using a paper cup, punch a hole in the bottom of the cup and insert the tubing through the hole. Placing stickers or drawing smiley faces on the cup may decrease the child's anxiety. Also consider attaching the oxygen tubing to a favorite toy and encouraging the child to hold the toy near their face.

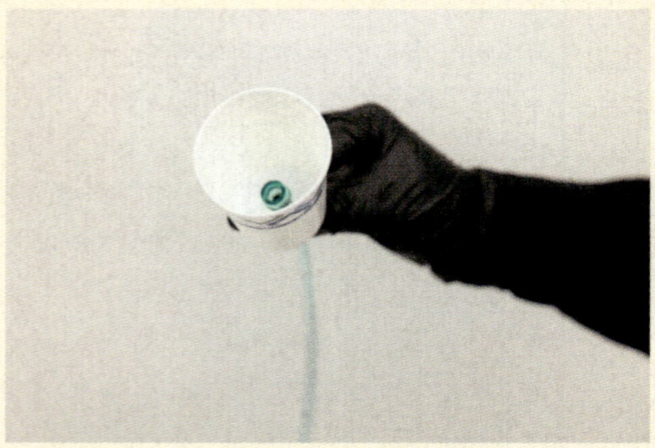

2. **For blow-by oxygen, instruct the caregiver to hold the tubing, paper cup, or favorite toy close to the child's face to maximize oxygen delivery.**

3. Allow the child to remain in a position of comfort, which may be sitting on the caregiver's lap. In the ambulance, the child must be safely restrained.

4a. To apply a mask, select the correct size. The mask should extend from the bridge of the nose to the cleft of the chin. Avoid placing pressure on the eyes.

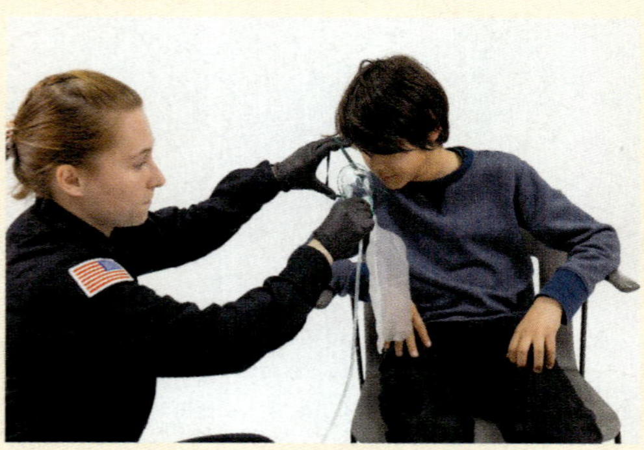

4b. Place the mask over the child's head, starting from the nose downward. Squeeze the nose clip and adjust the head strap.

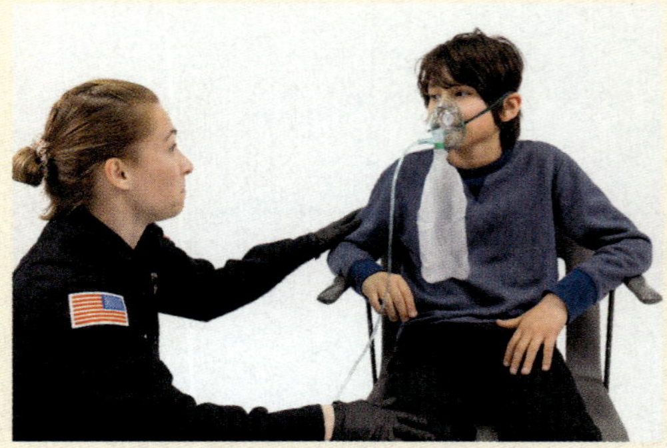

5. To apply a nasal cannula, curve the plastic prongs back into the nostrils. Loop the tubing around the ears.

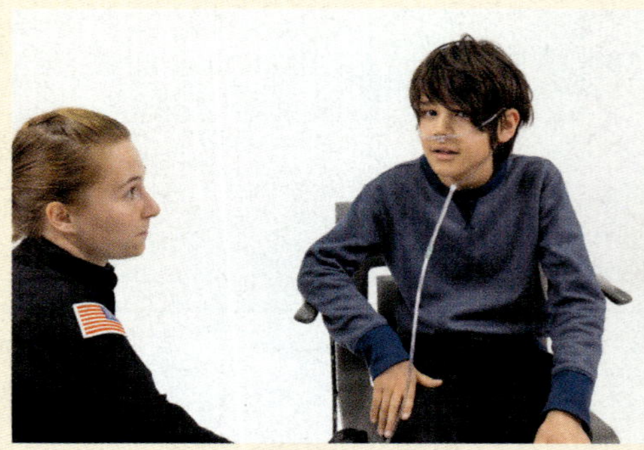

6. For blow-by oxygen, instruct the caregiver to hold the tubing, paper cup, or favorite toy close to the child's face to maximize oxygen delivery.

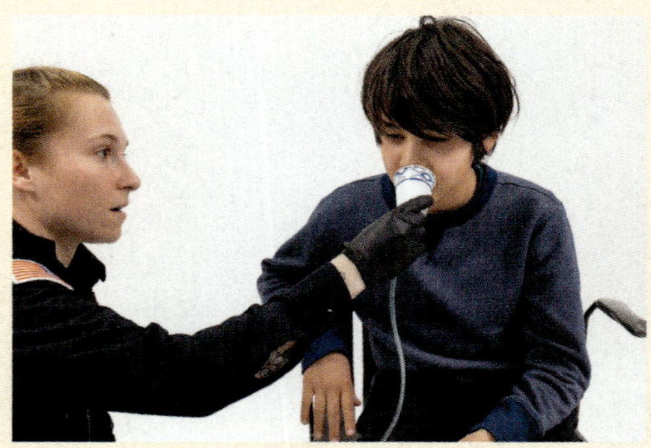

TABLE P3–2 Methods to Gain Child's Cooperation With Oxygen Delivery

Allow the child to hold the mask before placing it on their face.
Allow the child to feel the flow of oxygen before placing the mask on their face.
Describe the mask in appealing terms, such as a space mask or superhero mask.
If the child struggles, consider using the blow-by technique to avoid agitation and increasing the oxygen demands. Placing stickers or drawing smiley faces on the cup may decrease the child's anxiety. Also consider attaching the oxygen tubing to a favorite toy and encouraging the child to hold the toy near their face.

CONTROVERSY

The amount of oxygen to give to children with chronic lung disease is unknown and probably differs for each individual. In some children, oxygen delivery may have the unexpected effect of worsening hypoxia. That said, administration of oxygen to patients with chronic lung disease who retain carbon dioxide at baseline rarely results in hypoventilation in pediatric patients. If the child has a history and assessment suggesting acute hypoxia and increased work of breathing, give oxygen but be ready to assist ventilation with a bag-mask device.

Suggested References

National Association of State EMS Officials. *National Model EMS Clinical Guidelines, Version 3.0*. National Association of State EMS Officials; 2022

Topjian AA, Raymond TT, Atkins D, et al; Pediatric Basic and Advanced Life Support Collaborators. Part 4: Pediatric basic and advanced life support: 2020 American Heart Association guidelines for cardiopulmonary resuscitation and emergency cardiovascular care. *Circulation*. 2020;142(16 suppl 2):S469–S523

Procedure 4: Suctioning

Ann Dietrich, MD, FAAP, FACEP
Tyler Diettert, NREMTP, EC

Introduction

Children of all ages are prone to airway obstruction caused by secretions, vomitus, pus, blood, or edema. In newborns, airway obstruction caused by amniotic fluid, meconium, and blood is a common and potentially critical problem that is usually treatable with suction alone. In infancy and childhood, conditions such as closed head injury or status epilepticus may cause the loss of airway protective reflexes and put the child at risk of losing airway patency because of aspiration or airway obstruction. Children needing endotracheal intubation often have diseases or trauma associated with fluid in the endotracheal tube and airway sacs; this fluid must be removed to ensure adequate oxygenation and ventilation. Children with tracheostomy tubes may accumulate secretions or mucus in the tubes, which must be suctioned and possibly removed.

INDICATIONS

- Some newborns
- Infants or children with mucus or secretions in the nasopharynx or oropharynx
- Intubated patients with fluids or secretions in the endotracheal tubes
- Patients who have tracheostomy tubes with secretions or mucus in the tubes

CONTRAINDICATIONS

- Children with severe airway obstruction and suspected airway foreign body
- Children with suspected croup or epiglottitis
- Children with basilar skull fractures
- Minimize suctioning in intubated children with increased intracranial pressure and at risk of experiencing herniation

EQUIPMENT

- Bulb syringes, 1- and 2-piece types
- Endotracheal tube suction catheters, sizes 8 to 14 French (Fr)
- Suction catheters 5/6Fr (premature newborn), 8Fr (newborn-6 months), 10Fr (1–8 years), 10-14Fr (> 8 years) or approximately ½ the size of the tip of the nostril
- Large-bore rigid suction catheter

Rationale

Suctioning is a basic technique for maintaining an open airway. Children have small airways that are easily obstructed. The type of suction device and suctioning procedure depend on the child's age and clinical issue (**TABLE P4–1**). Bulb syringes remove thin secretions from newborns or infants but do not permit deep suctioning. When suctioning newborns, avoid suctioning vigorously or deeply. Deep suctioning can cause vagal stimulation, bradycardia, and laryngospasm in the newborn, particularly in the first hours during initial transition to extrauterine life. Brief, gentle suctioning with a bulb syringe (mouth, then nose) is usually adequate to remove secretions. Suction catheters remove thin secretions

TABLE P4–1 Suction Techniques, According to Patient's Age and Type of Obstructing Material

Age and Obstruction	Technique
Newborns	Bulb syringe or suction catheter
Infants and children with thin secretions	Bulb syringe or suction catheter
Newborns, infants, and children with endotracheal tube	Suction catheter
Infants and children with thick secretions or particulate matter	Large-bore suction catheter

from the mouth, nose, or throat and are useful in all age groups. Suction catheters are also necessary for endotracheal tube suctioning. Large-bore rigid suction catheters are useful in infants and children (not newborns) to remove thick secretions, vomitus, pus, blood, or particulate matter from the mouth.

Preparation

1. Use personal protective equipment.
2. Select an appropriate suction device according to clinical condition or type of obstruction and age. If there is no functioning negative-pressure or suction source (vacuum outlet, battery- powered or electric portable suction, or hand-powered portable suction), use a bulb syringe for thin secretions.
3. Make sure the suction device is operational.
4. Determine the correct catheter size with the pediatric length-based resuscitation tape. The suction catheter should be smaller than the nostril. For a child with a tracheostomy, most uncuffed tubes are 39 to 46 mm in length. A cuffed tube is 50 to 56 mm in length.
5. Open the catheter package.
6. Connect the suction tubing or rigid suction catheter to connecting tubing and the suction source.
7. Set suction vacuum (newborn–1 month, 60–80 mm Hg; infants, 80–100 mm Hg; children and adolescents, 100–120 mm Hg), being careful to avoid injuring sensitive tissues.

Possible Complications

- Injury to the mouth, nose, airway, or lung
- Gagging, vomiting
- Aspiration of stomach contents
- Hypoxia resulting from prolonged suctioning
- Pushing foreign body into trachea with suction device
- Increased intracranial pressure

PROCEDURE 4-1

Oropharyngeal / Nasopharyngeal Suctioning With Bulb Syringe

1. Squeeze the bulb away from the infant to remove air. Suction the mouth, then the nose.

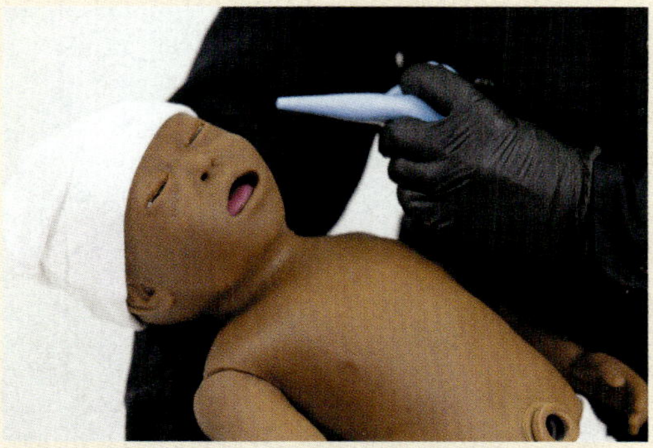

2. Open the mouth and insert the syringe tip at the side of the mouth, then advance the syringe to remove thin secretions. Avoid inserting the syringe tip into the deeper soft tissues at the back of the mouth. Do not use a 2-piece bulb syringe in the mouth because it may come apart.

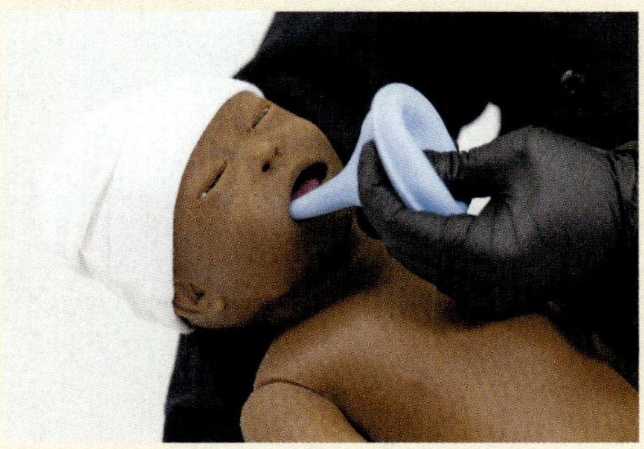

3. Lift the nostril slightly and suction the nose. Insert the syringe tip straight back into the nostril or at a right angle to the face.

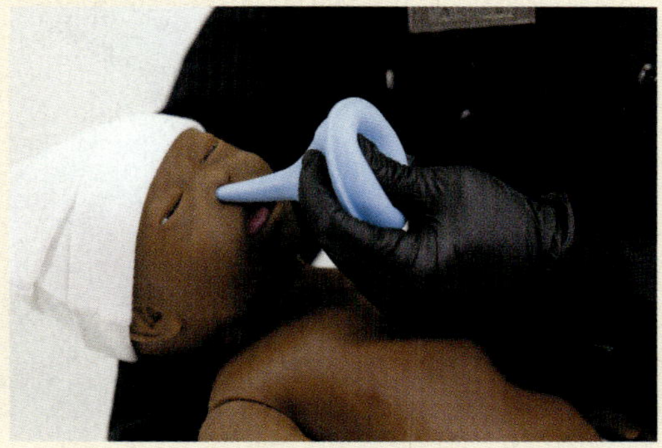

PROCEDURE 4-2

Oropharyngeal / Nasopharyngeal Suctioning With Suction Catheter

1. Suction the mouth, then the nose. Open the mouth and advance the catheter until the tip touches secretions.

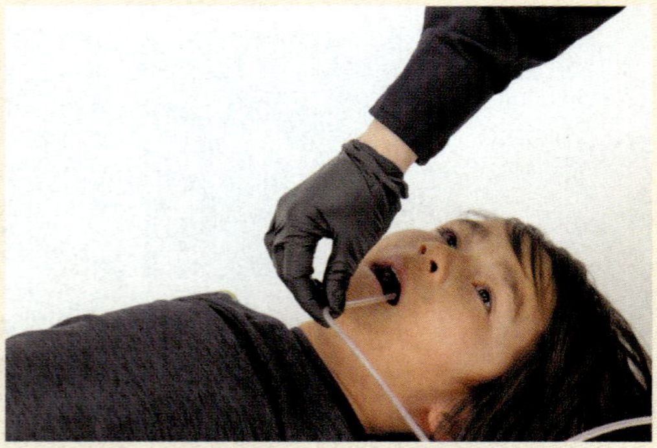

2. Block the side port and begin suctioning. Do not do deep suctioning beyond what is in direct vision. Remove the catheter with a twisting motion.
3. Put a small amount of lubricant on the side of the tip of the catheter (do not occlude the tip). Insert the catheter into the nostril, after measuring from the tip of the nose to the bottom of the ear lobe.

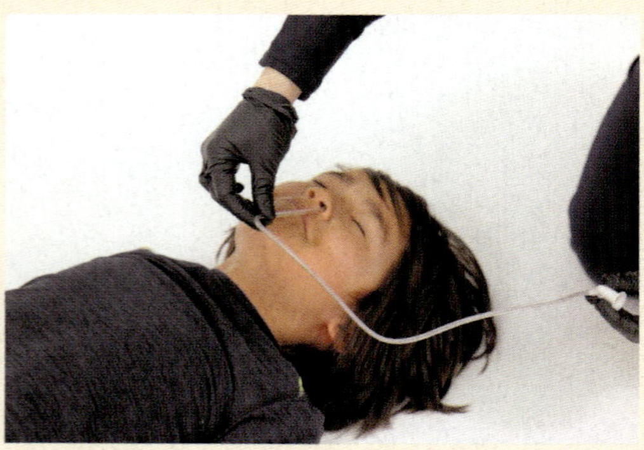

4. Block the side port to begin suctioning when the tip touches secretions. Remove the catheter with a twisting motion. Never suction longer than 5 seconds.

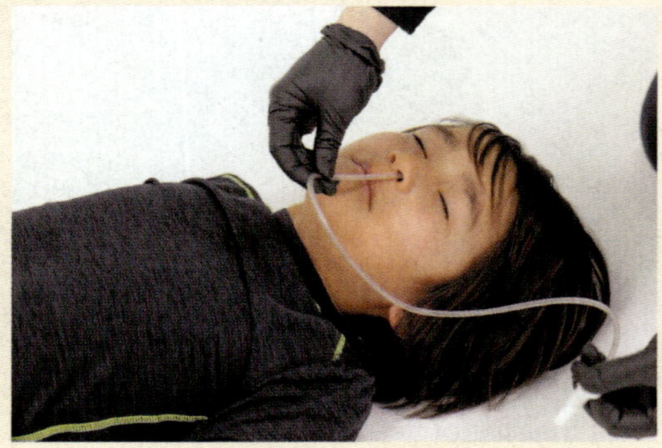

TIP

In suspected foreign body aspiration, look into the airway before suctioning.

TIP

Suction for less than 5 seconds, but use enough time to remove secretions.

PROCEDURE 4-3

Tracheal Tube Suctioning With Suction Catheter

1. Ask your partner to preoxygenate the patient with 5 to 6 breaths from a bag-mask device using 100% oxygen.

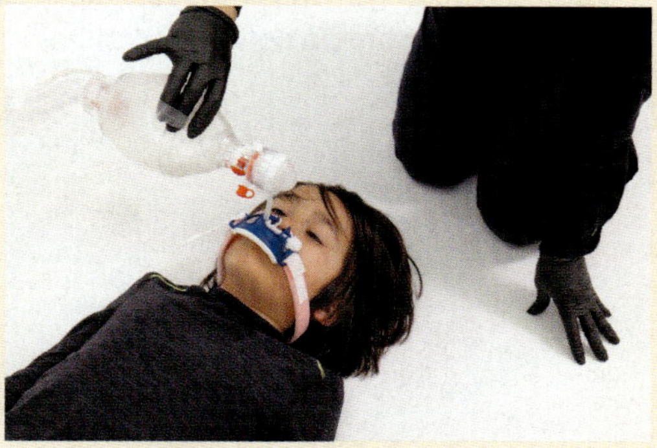

2. With thumb off the side port, insert suction catheter through the endotracheal tube and down the trachea until resistance is met.

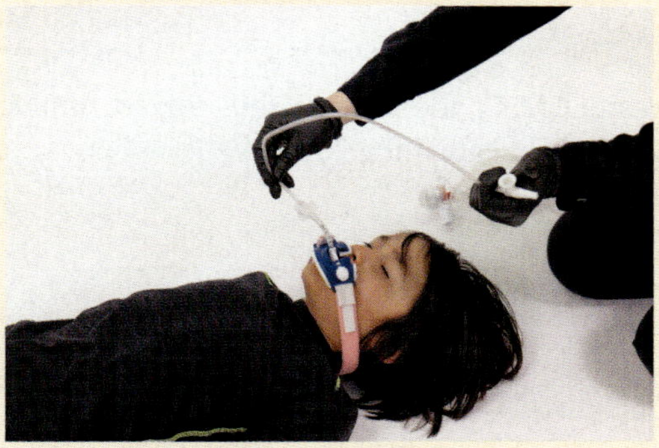

3. Apply suction off and on by placing thumb over the side port while withdrawing and twisting the catheter (maximum, 5 seconds).

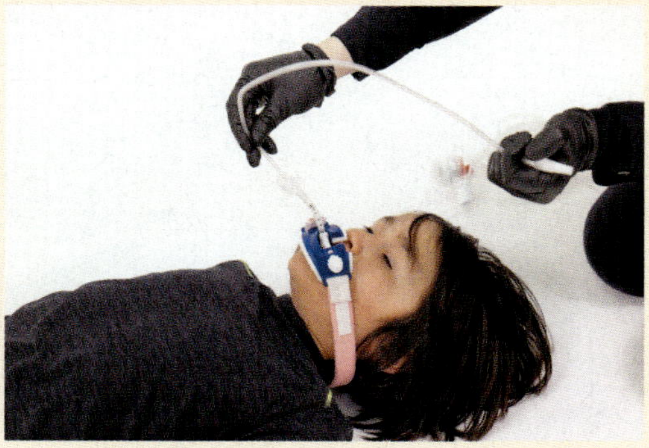

4. Irrigate catheter with normal saline.

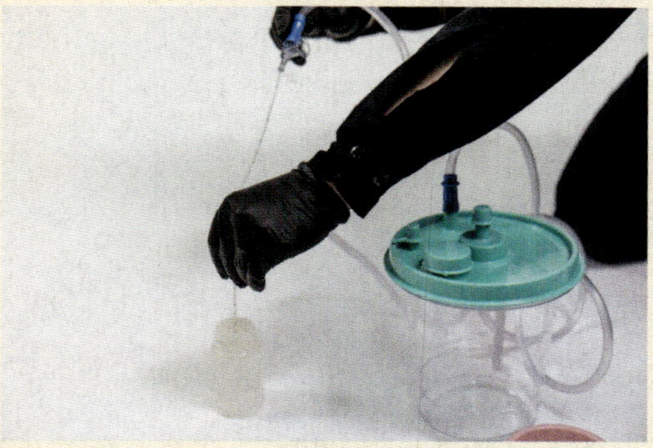

5. Ask your partner to oxygenate 5 to 6 times. Repeat as necessary.

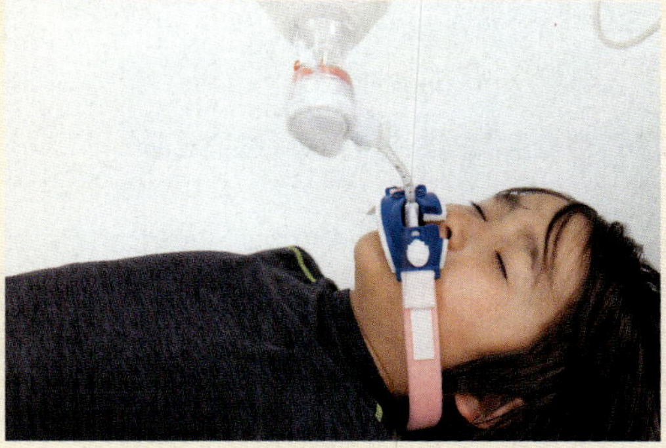

PROCEDURE 4-4

Oropharyngeal Suctioning With Large-Bore Rigid Suction Catheter

1. Open the mouth and advance the catheter until it touches secretions.

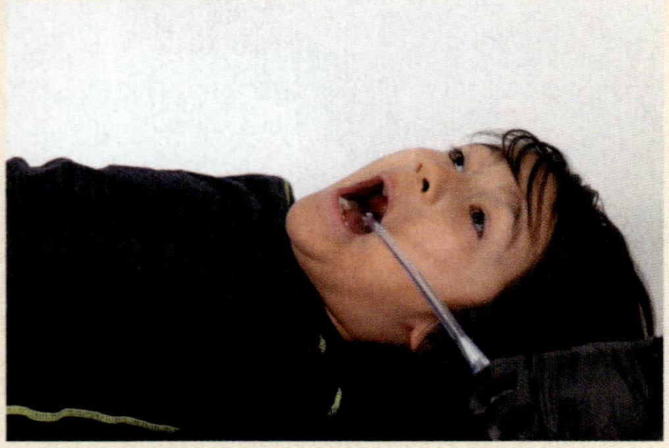

2. Close the side port or turn on suction to begin suctioning. Remove the catheter with a twisting motion. Do not suction more than 5 seconds.

Suggested Reference

American Academy of Pediatrics, American Heart Association. *Textbook of Neonatal Resuscitation.* Weiner GM, Cooper C, Lee H, eds. 9th ed. American Academy of Pediatrics; 2025

Procedure 5: Airway Adjuncts

Theresa Censoplano, MS, RN, NRP
Alexandra Cheetham, MD, MEd, FAAP

Introduction

An oropharyngeal (OP) or nasopharyngeal (NP) airway adjunct is often helpful to maintain an open airway for optimal ventilation. Sizing is important, because improperly sized OP or NP airways may press on structures in the posterior pharynx or upper airway and cause further obstruction. The prehospital professional must know when to use an OP or NP airway adjunct, how to determine the proper size, and how to insert the adjunct safely and effectively.

INDICATIONS

- Respiratory insufficiency
- Airway obstruction, NP or OP
- Seizures, including postictal state (NP airway)

CONTRAINDICATIONS

Oropharyngeal airway:

- Intact gag reflex (including conscious or semi-conscious patients)
- Ingestion of a caustic or petroleum product

Nasopharyngeal airway:

- Complete nasal obstruction
- Possible basilar skull fracture
- Major trauma to the face or head

EQUIPMENT

- Nasopharyngeal airways
- Oropharyngeal airways

Rationale

Opening the airway of a small infant or child by positioning alone, with head-tilt/chin-lift maneuvers or jaw thrust, may not keep the tongue from obstructing the airway. Adequate ventilation often requires placement of airway adjuncts. They are easy to insert and may markedly improve airway patency. Adjuncts may immediately improve the efficacy of the child's spontaneous ventilation. In addition, they may allow more effective bag-mask ventilation, reduce gastric inflation, and avert the need for endotracheal intubation.

Preparation

1. Position patient's airway:
   Medical patient
   - Perform the head-tilt/chin-lift maneuver to open the airway. Avoid hyperextension of the neck, because it may cause airway obstruction.
   - Use padding such as a folded sheet or towel under the shoulders of an infant or small child to achieve neutral airway position. Neutral airway position is accomplished when the external auditory meatus (opening to the ear canal) and sternal notch are horizontally aligned.

CAUTION
Never attempt to insert an oropharyngeal airway in a conscious child.

CAUTION
Do not insert an oropharyngeal airway that is too small, because it will push the tongue back and obstruct the airway.

Trauma patient

- Use the modified jaw thrust maneuver with in-line spinal stabilization to open the airway.

2. Select the properly sized adjunct:

Oropharyngeal airway

- Use length-based resuscitation tape (see **Procedure 2, Length-/Weight-Based Resuscitation Tape**) OR
- Measure the device on the patient:
  - Place OP airway next to face with the flange at the level of the maxillary central incisors (top front teeth) and the bite block segment parallel to the hard palate.
  - The tip of the appropriately sized OP airway should reach the angle of the jaw.

Nasopharyngeal airway

- Use length-based resuscitation tape (see **Procedure 2, Length-/Weight-Based Resuscitation Tape**) OR
- Measure the device on the patient:
  - The outside diameter of the NP airway should be less than the diameter of the nostril.
  - Place the NP airway next to the face with the flange positioned at the tip of the nose. The tip of the appropriately sized NP airway should reach the tragus of the ear.
  - Adjust movable flange (if present) up or down to achieve the appropriate length.

TIP

An NP airway is useful in maintaining an open airway during an active seizure.

PROCEDURE 5-1

Oropharyngeal Airway Insertion

1. Open the mouth to check for foreign material. Suction blood, vomit, or secretions if they block the airway.
2. Depress the tongue with a tongue blade (if available). Next, insert the oral airway with the tip down (to avoid injury to the palate) until the flange rests against the lips.
3. If a tongue blade is not available, insert the airway sideways, with the tip to the side, then rotate it down over the base of the tongue.
4. Insert the OP airway until the flange is resting against the lips.

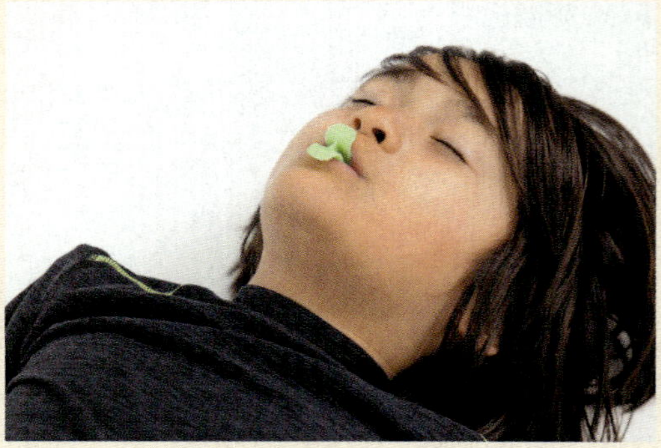

PROCEDURE 5-2

Nasopharyngeal Airway Insertion

1. Lubricate NP airway.

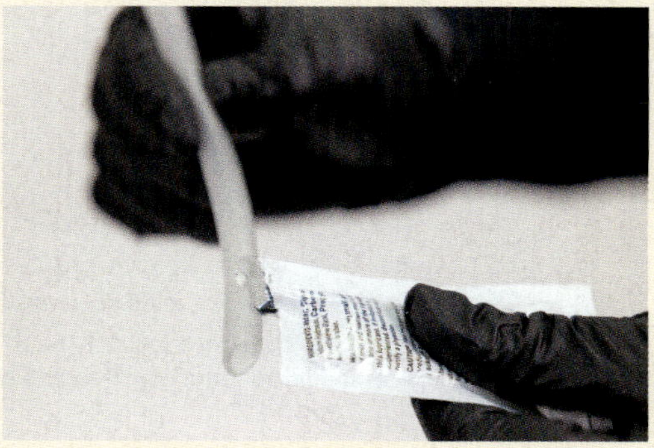

2. Insert with the bevel toward the septum (center of the nose).

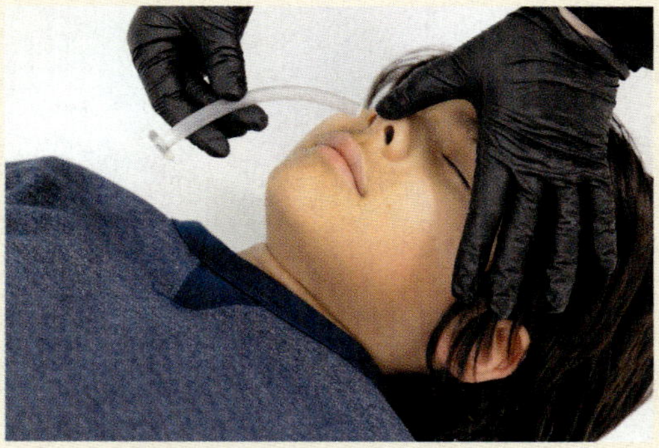

3. Advance the tip along the floor of the nasal cavity.

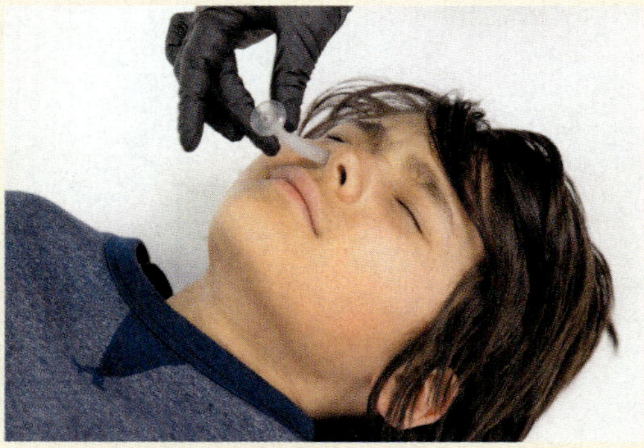

4. If using the right nostril, advance the airway until the flange is seated against the outside of the nostril.

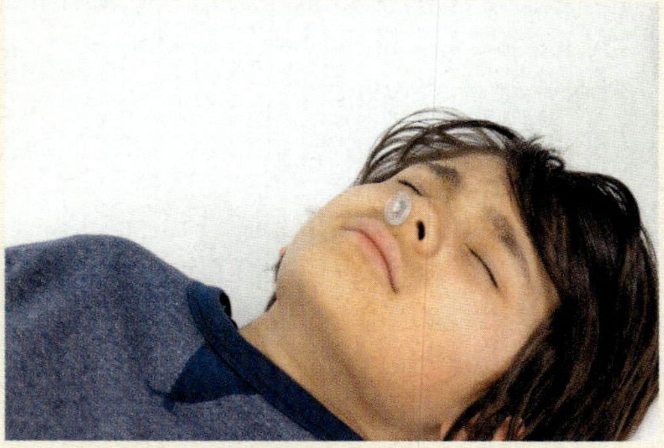

5. If using the left nostril, begin inserting the airway with the curvature upward until resistance is felt, and then rotate the device 180° and advance it until the flange is against the outside of the nostril.

Possible Complications

OROPHARYNGEAL AIRWAY

- If the OP airway is too small, the tongue may be pushed back into the pharynx, obstructing the airway
- If the OP airway is too large, it may obstruct the larynx
- Pharyngeal bleeding
- Laryngospasm
- Vomiting

NASOPHARYNGEAL AIRWAY

- Damage to adenoidal tissue
- Nasal or pharyngeal bleeding
- Obstruction of tube with fluids or soft tissues, causing airway obstruction
- If an NP airway is too long, vagal stimulation or esophageal entry with gastric distension may occur
- Laryngospasm
- Vomiting

CONTROVERSY

The use of airway adjuncts in facial trauma is controversial. If the child has an open fracture of the craniofacial bones, the device could penetrate into the brain and cause further brain injury or hemorrhage. These devices should not be used in the setting of major facial or head injury.

Procedure 6: Foreign Body Obstruction

Theresa Censoplano, MS, RN, NRP
Alexandra Cheetham, MD, MEd, FAAP

Introduction

Foreign body obstruction of the airway is common in toddlers and preschool children, who place objects in their mouths as part of the exploratory behavior normal for children in these age groups. Fortunately, hypoxic brain injury and death are uncommon outcomes.

Liquids are the most common cause of choking in infants, whereas balloons, small objects, and food (eg, hot dogs, round candies, nuts, grapes) are the most common causes of foreign body airway obstruction.

INDICATIONS

- Severe airway obstruction: inability to speak or cry; weak, ineffective cough or no cough
- Severe partial airway obstruction and respiratory failure

CONTRAINDICATION

- Partial/mild airway obstruction with maintenance of the airway

EQUIPMENT

- Laryngoscope and straight blades (Miller sizes 1 and 2)
- Curved blades (MacIntosh sizes 1 and 2)
- Pediatric Magill forceps
- Bag-mask ventilation devices (infant and pediatric)

Rationale

In the setting of severe airway obstruction, prehospital professionals can make the difference between life and death. Immediate removal of an airway foreign body can often be achieved using basic life support (BLS) procedures, yet every year many children suffer serious injury and death because of clinicians' failure to use basic clearance maneuvers. Sometimes, the foreign body is deeper in the airway or embedded in tissue, so that basic maneuvers are unsuccessful. In such cases, using Magill forceps and direct laryngoscopy may be the best option for removal.

CAUTION
Do not perform blind finger sweeps, which may push the foreign body further into the airway.

Preparation

1. Attempt BLS maneuvers first (see **Procedure 6-1**).
2. Move to advanced life support (ALS) maneuvers if BLS maneuvers fail.
3. Attach appropriately sized laryngoscope blade to laryngoscope handle. Use length-based resuscitation tape to determine appropriate blade size (see **Procedure 6-2**).
4. Ensure light on laryngoscope blade is working.

Possible Complications

- Hypoxia
- Foreign body is pushed farther into airway
- Laryngeal and tracheal injury
- Teeth and mouth injury

PROCEDURE 6-1

BLS Maneuvers

1. If foreign body airway obstruction (FBAO) is mild, do not interfere. Allow the victim to clear the airway by coughing while you observe for signs of severe FBAO.
2. If the FBAO is severe (ie, the victim is unable to make a sound), you must act to relieve the obstruction.
3. For a child, perform cycles of 5 back blows followed by 5 abdominal thrusts until the object is expelled or the victim becomes unresponsive.

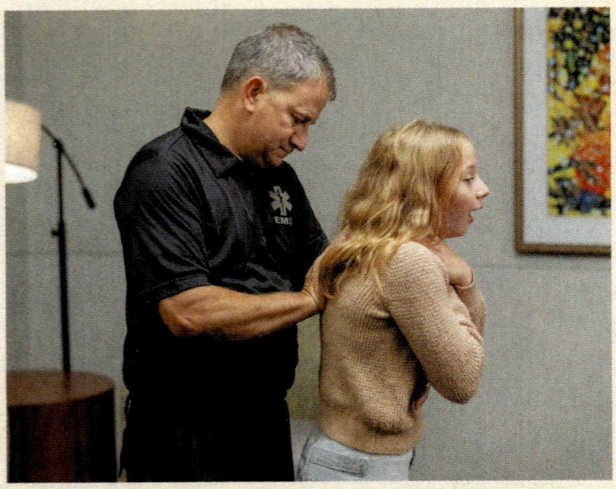

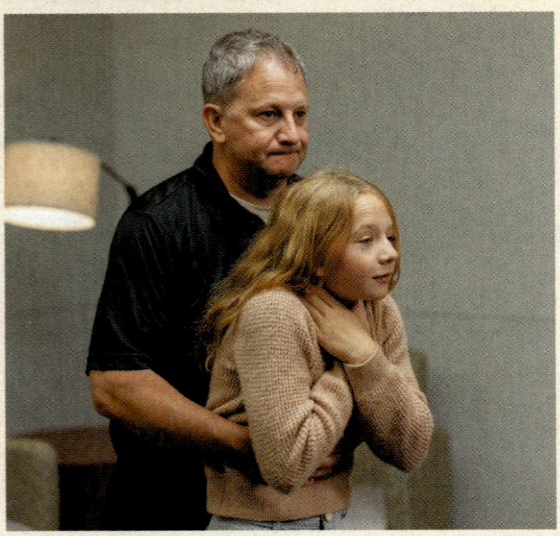

4. For an infant, deliver repeated cycles of 5 back blows followed by 5 chest thrusts until the object is expelled or the victim becomes unresponsive.

For back blows, position the infant face down with their head lower than their body and support their head. Deliver 5 back blows by placing the heel of your hand between the shoulder blades and firmly striking with the heel of your hand. For chest thrusts, use heel of one hand against the sternum.

Abdominal thrusts are not recommended for infants because they may damage the infant's relatively large and unprotected liver.

For chest thrusts, use the heel of one hand.

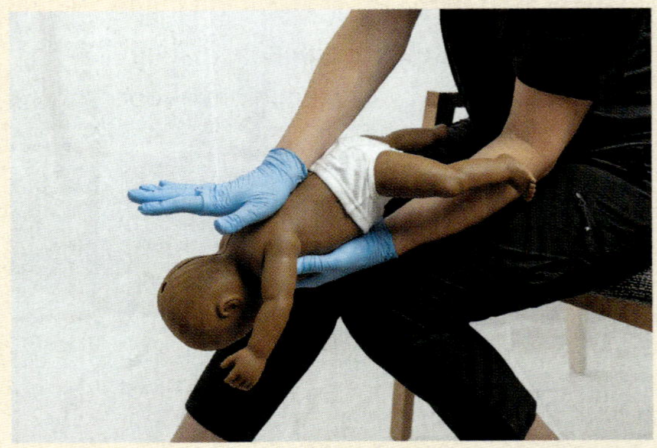

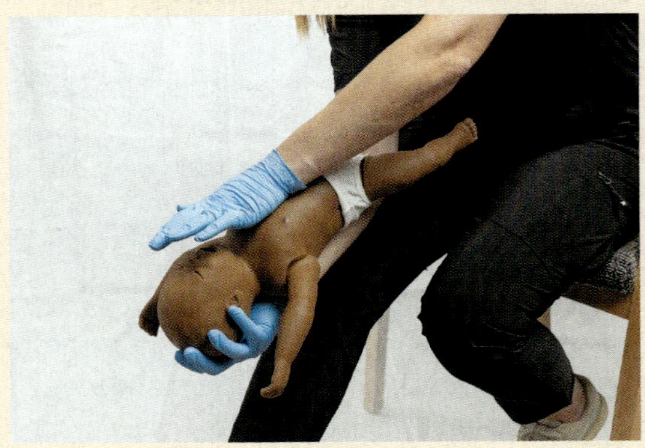

5. If the victim becomes unresponsive, start cardiopulmonary resuscitation (CPR) with chest compressions (do not perform a pulse check).

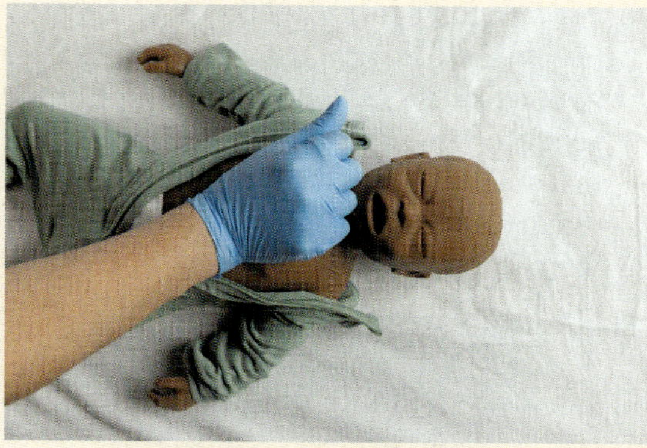

6. If alone after 30 chest compressions, open the airway. If you see a foreign body, remove it; however, do not perform blind finger sweeps, because that may push the object farther into the pharynx. Attempt to give 2 breaths and continue with cycles of chest compressions and ventilations until the object is expelled.

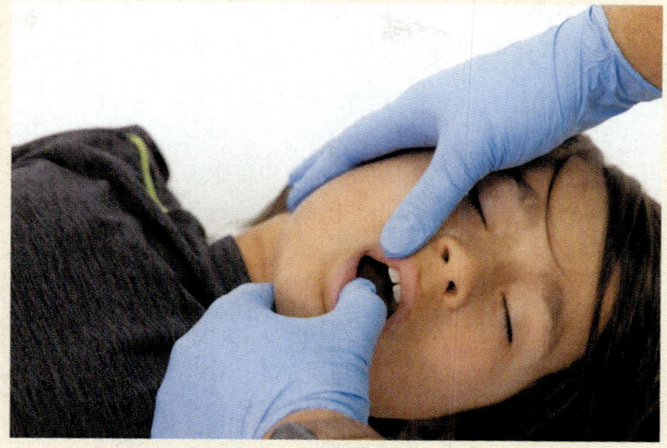

7. If multiple clinicians and at least 1 ALS clinician are available, continue CPR and attempt the following procedure (**Procedure 6-2**).

PROCEDURE 6-2

Laryngoscopy and Magill Forceps (ALS Procedure)

TIP

Attempt BLS maneuvers before using Magill forceps.

1. Grasp the laryngoscope handle in the left hand.

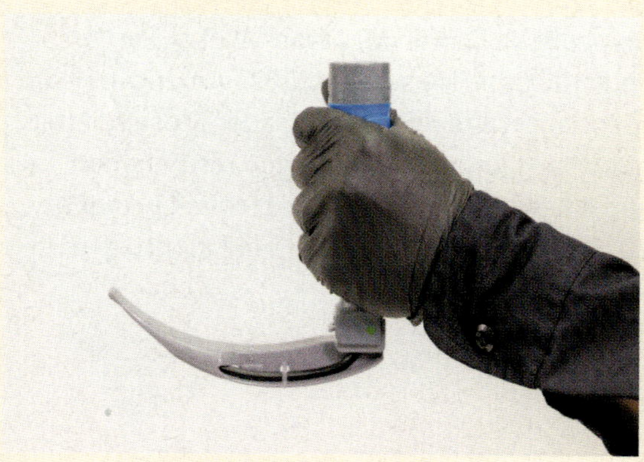

2. Open the mouth by using thumb pressure on the chin or by scissoring open the teeth/gums by using the thumb and middle finger of the left hand. Push the lower teeth/gum down with the thumb and the upper teeth/gum up with the middle finger.

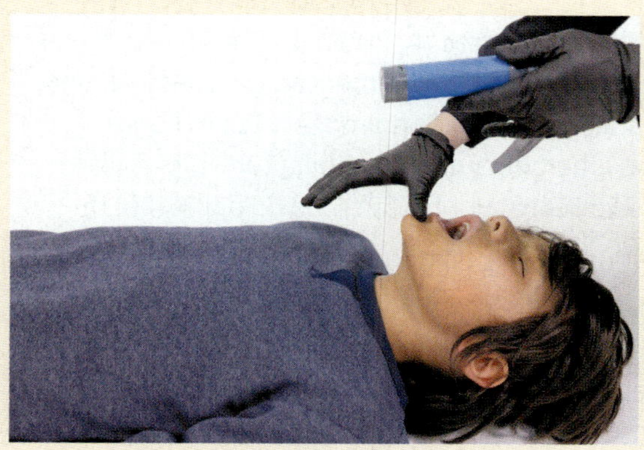

3. Insert the appropriately sized laryngoscope blade into the mouth.

4. Lift the tongue with the blade. Exert gentle traction upward along the axis of the laryngoscope handle at a 45° angle. Do not use teeth or gums for leverage. Advance the blade slowly. Watch the laryngoscope blade tip until the foreign body is visible. Do not go past the vocal cords. Use suction to improve visibility and maintain the airway, if needed.

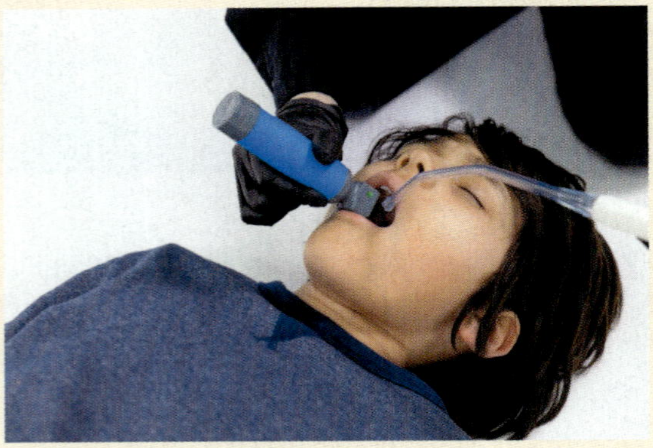

5. Grasp closed Magill forceps in the right hand, palm down. Insert the Magill forceps into the mouth, tips closed. Open the forceps and move the tips around the foreign body. Grasp the foreign body and remove it while looking directly at it. Avoid grasping any part of the airway or soft tissue to avoid damage to the airway. Inspect the airway and make sure it is clear of foreign bodies or debris. Remove the laryngoscope blade. After removing the foreign body, reassess the patient's respiratory status. Use suction if needed. Attempt to ventilate if the child does not breathe spontaneously. If there is no pulse, begin CPR and return to BLS maneuvers if no foreign body is seen via direct laryngoscopy.

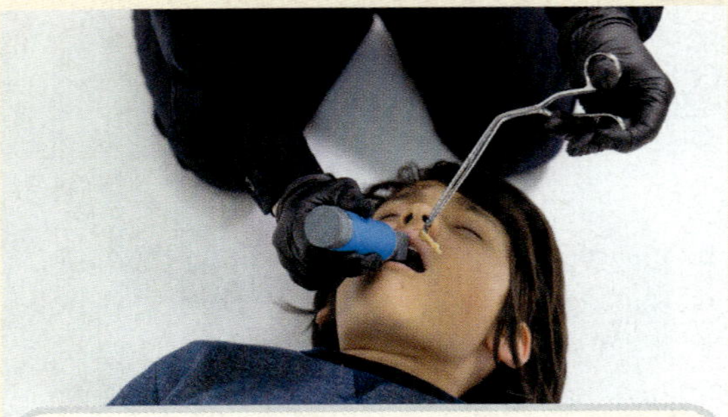

TIP

Repeat BLS procedures if no foreign body is seen via direct laryngoscopy.

CAUTION

Suctioning may push the foreign body farther into the airway, so inspect the airway before suctioning.

Suggested References

Del Rios M, Bartos JA, Panchal AR, et al. Part 1: executive summary: 2025 American Heart Association guidelines for cardiopulmonary resuscitation and emergency cardiovascular care. *Circulation.* 2025;152(16 suppl 2):S284–S312. doi:10.1161/CIR.0000000000001372

Ichikawa M, Oishi S, Mochizuki K, Nitta K, Okamoto K, Imamura H. Influence of body position during Heimlich maneuver to relieve supralaryngeal obstruction: a manikin study. *Acute Med Surg.* 2017;4(4):418–425. PMID: 29123902 doi: 10.1002/ams2.297

Joyner BL Jr, Dewan M, Bavare A, et al. Part 6: Pediatric basic life support: 2025 American Heart Association and American Academy of Pediatrics guidelines for cardiopulmonary resuscitation and emergency cardiovascular care. *Circulation.* 2025;152(16_suppl_2):S424-S447. doi:10.1161/CIR.0000000000001370

Procedure 7: Bronchodilator Therapy

H. Joel Dishroon, PM, IC
Shea Duerring, MD, NRP, FAAP, FACEP, FAEMS

Introduction

Wheezing caused by bronchospasm is one of the most common prehospital pediatric issues. Children who are wheezing are usually in acute respiratory distress and are often anxious, agitated, and uncooperative. The prehospital professional must use a developmentally appropriate approach with the child and the caregiver when providing general noninvasive respiratory care and using β-agonists with or without anticholinergic medications. The caregiver can help by holding, soothing, and supporting a scared child. One method of administering aerosolized β-agonist and anticholinergic medication is using an oxygen-powered nebulizer. Another method is using a metered-dose inhaler (MDI) with a spacer. If the child is uncooperative or unable to use inhaled β-agonist therapy, intramuscular (IM) drug delivery is another possibility.

INDICATION

Wheezing

CONTRAINDICATION

Known sensitivity to bronchodilator drugs

EQUIPMENT

INHALATION THERAPY (NEBULIZER)

- An oxygen-powered nebulizer that aerosolizes the liquid bronchodilator to small particle size that can reach the bronchioles
- Oxygen source set to 6 L/min minimum
- Mask or mouthpiece with liquid reservoir

β-agonist

- Albuterol solution (1.25 mg/3 mL, 2.5 mg/3 mL, prediluted solutions for nebulization; 5 mg/mL solution for nebulization [dilution required])

Anticholinergic

- Ipratropium solution 0.02% (500 µg/2.5 mL or 500 µg/2.5mL)

INHALATION THERAPY (MDI)

- MDI
- Spacer with mask or mouthpiece

β-agonist

- Albuterol MDI (90 µg/puff)

Anticholinergic

- Ipratropium (MDI) (17 µg/puff)

INTRAMUSCULAR THERAPY

Intramuscular therapy

- Tuberculin 1-mL or 3-mL syringe with a 22- to 27-gauge needle

Bronchodilator

- Epinephrine 1 mg/mL concentration

Rationale

For asthma, early bronchodilator therapy, performed on scene and en route to the emergency department (ED), helps immediately open airways, relieve respiratory distress, and improve oxygen delivery. Early bronchodilator therapy may reduce the need for more aggressive hospital therapy, shorten ED and hospital stays, and decrease chances of complications or death. The addition of anticholinergic medication is beneficial; it has been shown to improve pulmonary function tests and decrease the need for hospitalization in children versus β-agonist administration alone. Inhalation treatment with a nebulized β-agonist with or without anticholinergic medication is the best initial approach with severe wheezing and respiratory distress. See **Table P7-1** for nebulized medication side effects.

TABLE P7–1 Possible Complications of Albuterol and/or Ipratropium

Anxiety	Nausea
Chest pain	Nasal stuffiness
Cough	Palpitations
Dizziness	Restlessness
Dry mouth	Tachycardia
Dysrhythmias	Tremors
Headache	Vomiting
Hypertension	

Preparation

INHALATION THERAPY

1. Have the caregiver hold the child on their lap. An older child can sit alone.
2. Place the child in an upright position of comfort.
3. Explain what is happening. Most children need only inhalation bronchodilator therapy by oxygen-powered nebulizer or with an MDI and spacer.

INTRAMUSCULAR THERAPY (EPINEPHRINE)

1. Position the child on the caregiver's lap or straddling the caregiver's leg.
2. Expose the thigh or deltoid area for injection (see **Procedure 14, Intramuscular Injections**).

PROCEDURE 7-1

Inhalation Therapy

1. If the child can cooperate, deliver nebulized β-agonist with or without anticholinergic medication through a mouthpiece or mask. The caregiver can hold the mask to the child's face, if necessary.

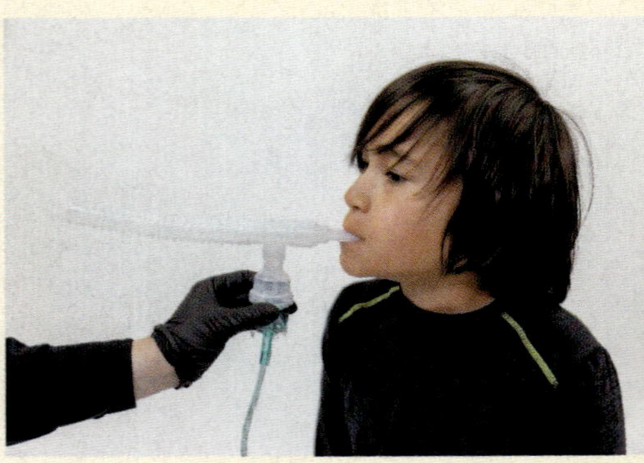

2. If an MDI is used, attach the spacer and mask when the child is too young or unable to trigger aerosol effectively.

3. Monitor respiratory rate, heart rate, pulse oximetry readings, and waveform capnography readings during therapy.

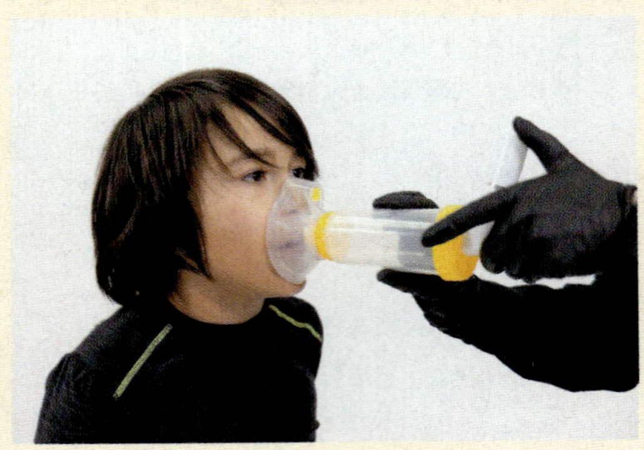

CONTROVERSY

The role of the MDI in prehospital β-agonist therapy is not known. Although ED studies have shown that the MDI is as effective as inhaled drugs for most children, it has not been studied adequately in the prehospital setting. An MDI with mask and spacer can probably deliver an adequate β-agonist dose to most children older than 2 years.

TIP

Use β-agonists for children who are wheezing because of asthma (reactive airway disease).

In children unable to cooperate with a nebulized treatment and/or patients who are unable to properly use an MDI, the emergency medical services clinician can remove the bag from a nonrebreathing mask and insert the medication reservoir into the opening. This allows passive administration of the nebulized medication via mask. Oxygen settings remain the same as when a nebulizer is used in the normal manner.

The nebulizer may also be placed in-line on a bag-mask device when ventilating a patient with wheezing who needs assistance with ventilation.

PROCEDURE 7-2

Intramuscular Therapy

1. If the child is in significant respiratory distress or if the child cannot cooperate with inhalation therapy, give epinephrine via intramuscular injection (**Procedure 14, Intramuscular Injections**). Use 1 of 2 anatomical locations: the lateral aspect of the deltoid in the upper arms (older child) or the anterolateral thigh.
2. Inject the medication intramuscularly.

TIP

Avoid using injectable drugs in cooperative, wheezing patients. The procedure is painful and no more effective than is using an inhaled β-agonist.

Procedure 8: Bag-Mask Ventilation

Kory Lane, MEd, NRP, FP-C, CCP-C, NCEE
Franscesca Miquel-Verges, MD

Introduction

Bag-mask ventilation is a highly effective way to deliver assisted ventilation to a child in respiratory failure. For the newborn, ventilation of the lungs is the single most important and effective step in resuscitation.

INDICATIONS

- Apnea or respiratory arrest
- Respiratory failure
- Cyanosis despite supplemental oxygen*
- Pulse oximetry (SpO_2) reading of less than 90% despite administration of 100% oxygen by nonrebreather mask*

EQUIPMENT

- Transparent masks with soft rim, sizes neonate through adult
- Self-inflating resuscitator bag

*Children with uncorrected cyanotic heart disease may have cyanosis or low oxygen saturations at baseline and despite receiving supplemental oxygen.

Rationale

Assisted ventilation is a method of oxygenating and ventilating a child who is unable to breathe adequately on their own. Although the technique does not provide the definitive airway control that endotracheal intubation does, in many cases bag-mask ventilation will be the best technique for assisting ventilation during resuscitation and transport. Effective bag-mask ventilation is one of the prehospital professional's most useful skills in pediatric prehospital care.

Preparation

1. Measure the mask on the patient. The mask should extend from the bridge of the nose to the cleft of the chin, avoiding compression of the eyes. Transparency allows the rescuer to observe the child for cyanosis of the lips and for emesis. If the mask has an inflatable rim, this should be filled with air before use to ensure an adequate seal.
2. Select an appropriately sized resuscitator bag. Although a small child can be safely and effectively ventilated by using an adult bag, a pediatric bag will not work for a large child, an adolescent, or an adult. Pediatric tidal volume is approximately 8 mL/kg, so the pediatric bag should have a volume of 450 to 750 mL. An adult bag (1,200 mL) is acceptable for larger children or adolescents.
3. If a pop-off valve is present, it may need to be disabled to permit higher inflation pressures and achieve chest rise in certain patients. The pop-off valve is a safety mechanism to prevent excessive inflation pressure, and caution should be exercised when disabling the pop-off valve.
4. Connect one end of oxygen tubing to the resuscitator bag and the other end to the flow meter, set to 15 L/min.

Possible Complications

- Hypoxia
- Barotrauma
- Gastric distension
- Emesis and aspiration

PROCEDURE 8-1

Airway Preparation for Bag-Mask Ventilation

1. Open airway. *Medical patient*: Use head-tilt/chin-lift maneuver. *Trauma patient*: Use jaw thrust with in-line manual cervical spine stabilization.

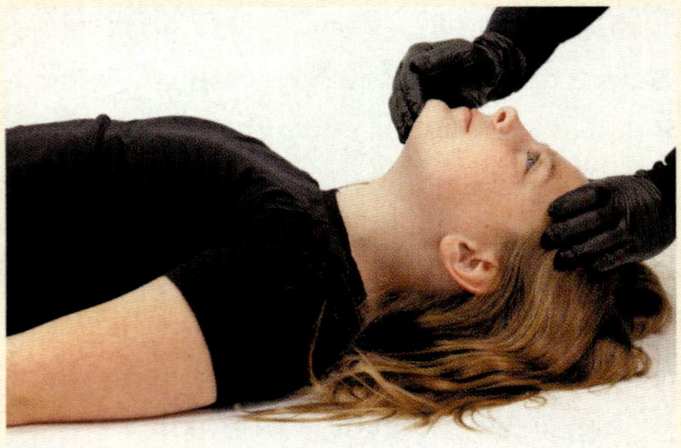

2. Ensure neutral positioning (the sniffing position). Because infants and toddlers have large heads, place a small roll under the shoulders to achieve the sniffing position. Avoid hyperextension of the neck, because this may cause airway obstruction or spinal injury.

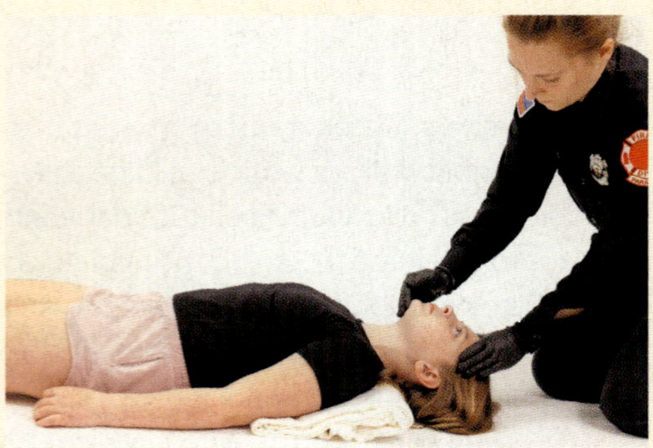

3. Insert an appropriate airway adjunct if airway patency cannot be maintained with the head-tilt/chin-lift or jaw thrust maneuvers (see **Procedure 5, Airway Adjuncts**). Use an oropharyngeal (OP) airway if the patient does not have a gag reflex; use a nasopharyngeal (NP) airway if the patient has an active gag reflex.

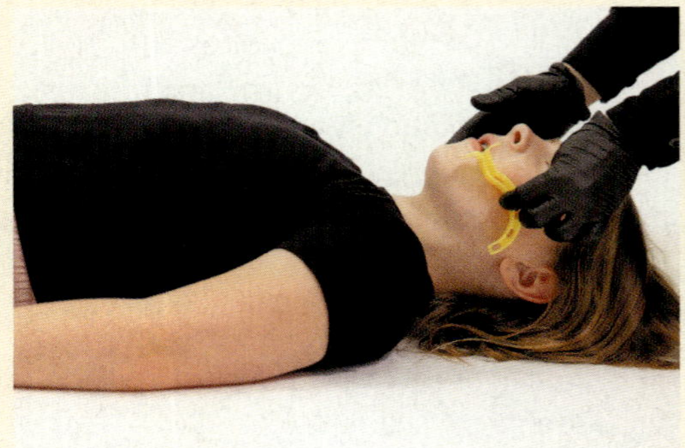

CAUTION

Avoid hyperextension of the neck, which may cause airway obstruction or spinal injury.

TIP

In children with pending respiratory failure due to an obstructive process (ie, status asthmaticus), listening for the end of expiration before delivering the next breath may minimize risk of barotrauma.

TIP

Use an OP or NP airway with the bag-mask device if airway patency cannot be maintained with the head-tilt/chin-lift or jaw-thrust maneuvers.

PROCEDURE 8-2

Bag-Mask Ventilation Using 1-Rescuer Technique

1. Apply the mask to the face (over the nose and mouth) and ensure an airtight seal by placing the thumb and index finger on the mask and the third, fourth, and fifth fingers on the bony portion of the jaw (mandible). This is called the E-C clamp technique.

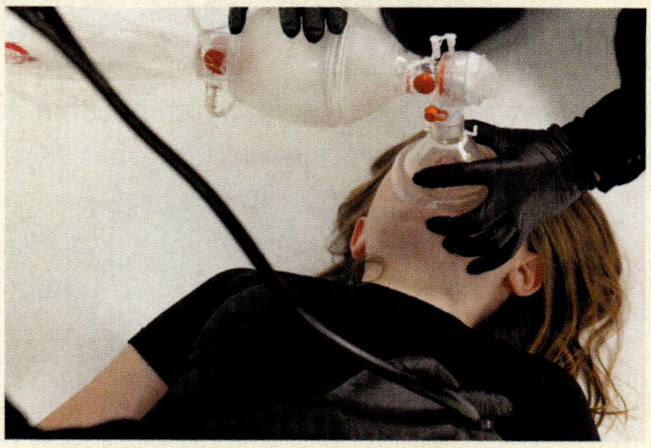

2. Using the third, fourth, and fifth fingers, pull the child's jaw into the mask to establish a seal; avoid pushing the mask into the face. Failure to provide a tight seal may result in delivery of lower oxygen concentrations or an inadequate volume of air. Avoid placing pressure on soft tissues under the chin, because this may compress the airway. Squeeze the bag with the dominant hand, watching for chest rise. Squeeze the bag only until the chest rise is visible, then release. Say, "squeeze, release, release" during ventilation to achieve the correct inflation time and to allow for expiration.
   - Newborn rate: 40 squeezes/minute
   - Child rate: 20-30 squeezes/minute
   - Adult rate: 12 to 16 squeezes/minute.
3. Assess effectiveness of ventilation. Look for adequate bilateral rise and fall of chest. Auscultate for lung sounds at the midaxillary line bilaterally. Monitor oxygen saturation and end-tidal carbon dioxide ($EtCO_2$), if available.

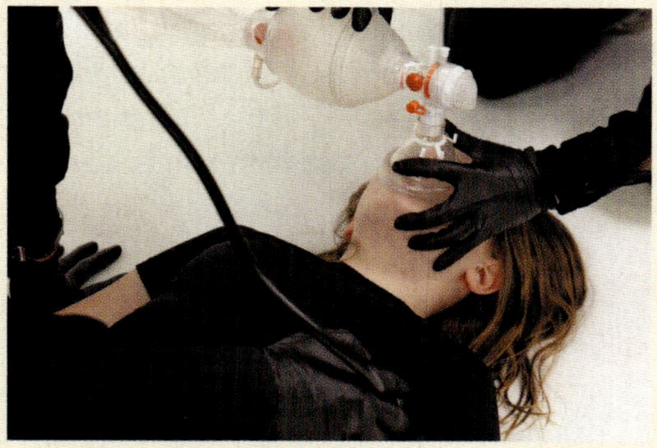

4. If ventilation is not effective, return to the airway opening and troubleshoot. Reposition the head and the mask, consider airway suction or use of airway adjuncts, check mask size and seal, and increase pressure if needed. If additional rescuers are available, consider using the 2-rescuer bag-mask ventilation technique described below.

TIP

Pull the jaw into the mask, instead of pushing the mask into the face.

TIP

Seeing the chest rise is the best indicator of adequate tidal volume.

CONTROVERSY

Small research studies suggest that bag-mask ventilation is as good as endotracheal tube ventilation in the prehospital setting for children with respiratory failure caused by illness or trauma. Large national studies are still in process in 2026.

PROCEDURE 8-3

Bag-Mask Ventilation Using 2-Rescuer Technique

The 2-rescuer technique is preferable, particularly if the 1-rescuer technique does not create an effective seal.

1. One rescuer applies the mask to the face (over the nose and mouth) and achieves an airtight seal. *Medical patient*: Hold the mask to the face with the thumb and index fingers of both hands; use the other fingers to perform a chin lift (bilateral E-C clamp technique). *Trauma patient*: Perform a jaw-thrust maneuver, lifting the jaw into the mask with both hands, while maintaining in-line cervical spine manual stabilization.

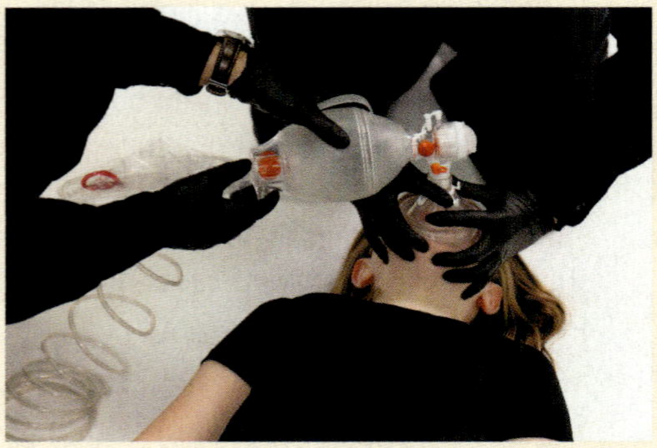

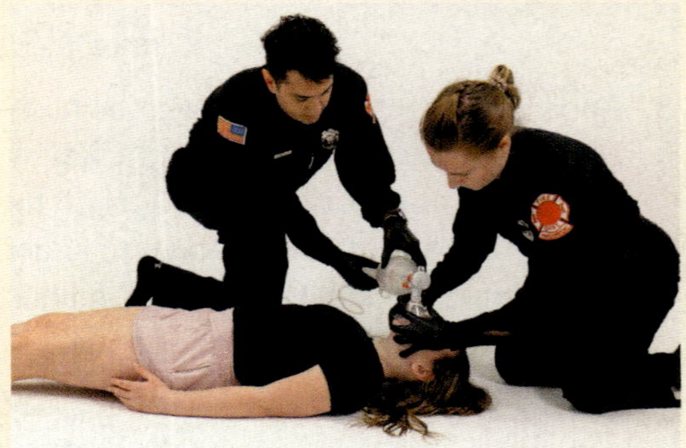

2. Pull the child's jaw into the mask, instead of pushing the mask into the face, to establish a seal. Avoid placing pressure on soft tissues under the chin, because this may compress the airway.

3. The second rescuer ventilates by squeezing the bag only until the chest starts to rise. Squeeze the bag only until the chest rise is visible, then release. Say, "squeeze, release, release" during ventilation to achieve the correct inflation time and to allow for expiration.

- Newborn rate: 40 squeezes/minute
- Child rate: 20-30 squeezes/minute
- Adult rate: 12 to 16 squeezes/minute

4. Avoid gastric distension; watch the abdomen for signs of enlargement during ventilation. If this happens, reposition the airway and observe the chest rise carefully. If bag-mask ventilation continues, consider placement of an orogastric or nasogastric tube for gastric decompression (see **Procedure 10, Orogastric and Nasogastric Tube Insertion**).

5. Assess effectiveness of ventilation. Look for adequate bilateral rise and fall of chest. Auscultate for lung sounds at the midaxillary line bilaterally. Monitor oxygen saturation and $EtCO_2$, if available.

6. If ventilation is not effective, return to the airway opening and troubleshoot. Reposition head and mask, consider airway suction or use of airway adjuncts, check the mask size and seal, and increase pressure if needed.

TIP

The 2-rescuer technique for bag-mask ventilation is preferable to the 1-rescuer technique. Establishing a good seal of the mask on the face is the key to delivering effective ventilations.

CAUTION

A bag less than 450 mL will not generate enough inspiratory pressure to ventilate a large child, adolescent, or adult.

Procedure 9: Pulse Oximetry

Hoi See Tsao, MD, MPH
Evelyn Wilson, EdD, NRP, NCEE

Introduction

Pulse oximetry, which measures oxygenation and pulse rate, can be a useful adjunct in the care of the ill or injured child. Use of the pulse oximeter does not replace clinical assessment of the child. Pulse oximetry measurement is a standard part of the complete respiratory assessment by emergency medical services (EMS) clinicians. Continuous monitoring for changes in pulse oximetry readings may help EMS clinicians determine a patient's response to treatment and guide additional interventions.

Although pulse oximetry is a useful clinical tool, it has limitations. If the child is in shock, inadequate perfusion may make it difficult for the pulse oximeter probe to sense flow, resulting in an inability to obtain a reading or waveform. Pulse oximetry may overestimate true oxygen saturation in patients with darker skin pigmentation. When carbon monoxide (CO) poisoning is suspected, pulse oximetry may also be falsely high. A child with CO poisoning may have a pulse oximetry reading of 100% and still have functional hypoxia. Oximetry detects gaseous saturation of the hemoglobin molecule and cannot discriminate between oxygen and CO. A specialized oximeter is needed to measure CO in the blood.

INDICATIONS

- Medical or trauma condition with the potential for hypoxia
- Respiratory distress
- Hypoxia
- Need for oxygen therapy

EQUIPMENT

- Pulse oximeter probes in sizes for newborns, infants, and children
- Monitoring cable and pulse oximetry monitoring device

Preparing the Child for the Procedure

1. Prepare the child for application of the pulse oximeter probe. This may be explained as being similar to putting on an adhesive bandage or a sticker. Use age-appropriate, child-friendly language and explain that the light can make the child's finger look red. A child's sock can be used to cover the hand or foot where the sensor is located to distract the child from the pulse oximeter probe.
2. Select location for probe placement. In infants, an adhesive pulse oximeter probe can be wrapped completely around the palm of the hand or the whole foot. In older children, you can use any finger or toe. Placement of the pulse oximeter probe on a young child's toe covered by a sock or blanket may be easier to distract children from probe placement compared with placement on fingers and also prevent it from being pulled or kicked off as easily. In poor perfusion states, the earlobe may have more circulation than distal extremities.

CAUTION

Carbon monoxide poisoning will cause falsely high readings on pulse oximetry; do not rely on pulse oximetry when treating a patient with suspected CO poisoning.

Possible Complications

- Incorrect probe placement
- Poor perfusion with poor tracing or waveform
- Inability to obtain an SpO_2 reading

Causes of Inability to Obtain a Reading or Waveform

- Incorrect probe placement
- Poor perfusion
- Poor tracing or waveform

PROCEDURE 9-1

Pulse Oximetry

1. Obtain equipment in the appropriate size. Place probe on a fingertip, a toe, an earlobe, or a wrist as indicated in the manufacturer's instructions.

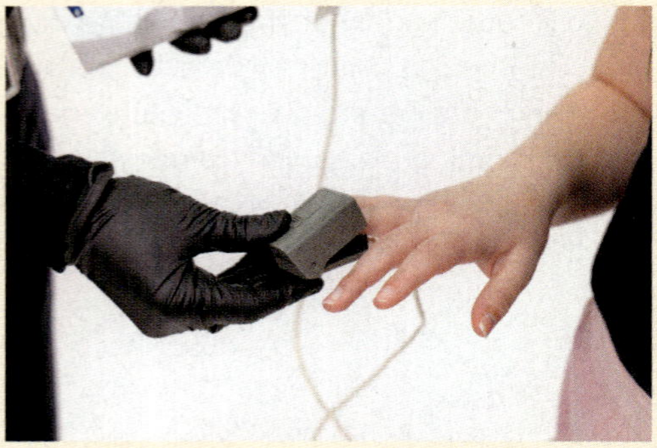

2. Connect the probe to the monitoring cable. Some portable monitoring devices have a reusable probe that has a spring-loaded clip for use only on a fingertip or toe. Note and document oxygen saturation (SpO_2). If the monitoring device being used shows a waveform, observe for correlation with heart rate.

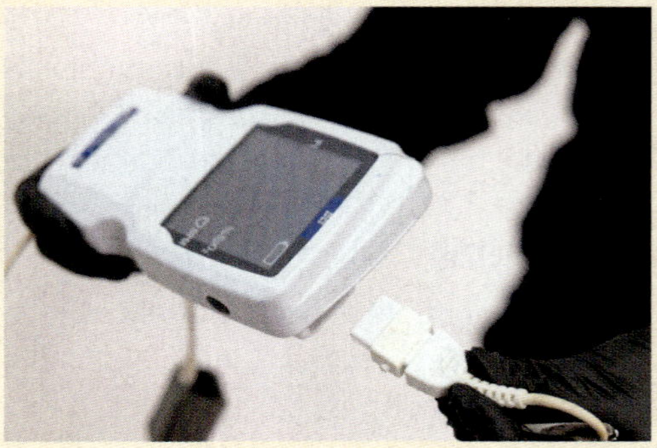

TIP
Use pulse oximetry in the primary assessment of every acutely ill or injured child.

CAUTION
Even when the pulse oximetry reading is normal, if there is increased work of breathing or significantly increased respiratory rate, the child may need therapy, including oxygen.

CAUTION
Pulse oximetry is a very useful tool for measuring oxygen saturation; however, it should not replace a thorough assessment, which includes respiratory rate, auscultation of lung sounds, and palpation of a pulse.

Procedure 10: Orogastric and Nasogastric Tube Insertion

Hoi See Tsao, MD, MPH
Evelyn Wilson, EdD, NRP, NCEE

Introduction

Gastric tubes have multiple purposes, such as gastric decompression in cases of bowel obstruction or distension secondary to assisted ventilation or to provide enteral nutrition, medications, or fluids. The tube may be placed into the stomach through the nose (nasogastric [NG] insertion) or through the mouth (orogastric [OG] insertion). In the prehospital setting, the procedure of gastric tube insertion is indicated primarily for decompression of the stomach during assisted ventilation.

INDICATIONS

Gastric distension that impedes ventilation

CONTRAINDICATIONS

- Nasogastric and orogastric insertion is contraindicated in children with caustic ingestions owing to risk of esophageal damage with passage of the tube.
- Nasogastric insertion is contraindicated for children with severe head or facial trauma, especially with midface injury or if blood or clear fluid is draining from the nose. Use OG tubes in these patients instead.
- Nasogastric insertion is not advised for infants younger than 6 months, because the nostrils are usually too small to accommodate the tube. Use OG tubes in these patients instead.
- Orogastric insertion is not advised in conscious children owing to risk of aspiration. Use NG tubes in these patients instead.

EQUIPMENT

- Gastric tube
- 30- to 60-mL syringe with funnel-tipped adapter for manual removal of stomach contents through tube
- Mechanical suction
- Adhesive tape
- Nonpetroleum lubricant

Rationale

During assisted ventilation or in a child with significant respiratory distress, it is common for air to inflate the stomach as well as the lungs. Gastric distension slows downward movement of the diaphragm and decreases tidal volume, making ventilation more difficult and necessitating higher inspiratory pressures. In the spontaneously breathing child, gastric inflation decreases tidal volume and significantly increases the work of breathing. In addition, inflation of the stomach with air increases the risk that the patient will vomit and aspirate. Gastric tube insertion with an NG or OG tube decompresses the stomach and makes assisted ventilation or spontaneous breathing easier.

Preparing the Child for the Procedure

Unconscious child: Lie the child down supine for the procedure. In an unconscious child, NG or OG tube placement should not take precedence over other emergent airway, breathing, or circulation interventions.

Uncooperative child: Consider wrapping young children in a sheet to help keep their arms and legs down. Alternatively, a family member can hold the child against their chest, wrap their legs around the child's legs, or put one arm across the child's arms and put their other hand on the child's forehead and hold the child's head against the family member's chest.

Awake child: Sit the child up, reclined against the back of the stretcher. Explain to the child what will happen—for example, "I need to put this tube into your nose to help with your breathing. It will be uncomfortable for a few seconds, but it will help if you try to relax as much as you can. You can play a game/watch a video on mom or dad's phone/hug your stuffed toy if you want while I do this."

Preparation

1. Select the proper size tube. Sizing techniques are outlined in **TABLE P10-1**.
2. Measure the tube on the patient. The length of the tube should be the same as the distance from the lips or tip of the nose (depending on if the OG or NG route is used) to the left ear PLUS the distance from the left ear to the left upper quadrant of the abdomen, below the costal margin and about halfway between the xiphoid process and the navel (**FIGURE P10-1**).
3. Mark this length on the tube with a piece of tape. When the tip of the tube is in the stomach, the tape should be at the lips or nostrils.
4. Place the patient in a supine or reclined position.

TABLE P10-1 Methods for Determining Nasogastric/Orogastric Tube Size

1. Refer to a length-based resuscitation tape or resuscitation software (see **Procedure 2, Length/Weight-Based Resuscitation Tape**).
2. Select a tube size that is the same as the size of the patient's nostril, through which it should pass with minimal resistance.
3. Use a tube size twice the endotracheal (ET) tube size (a child who needs a 5.0-mm ET tube needs a 10.0 French nasogastric or orogastric tube).

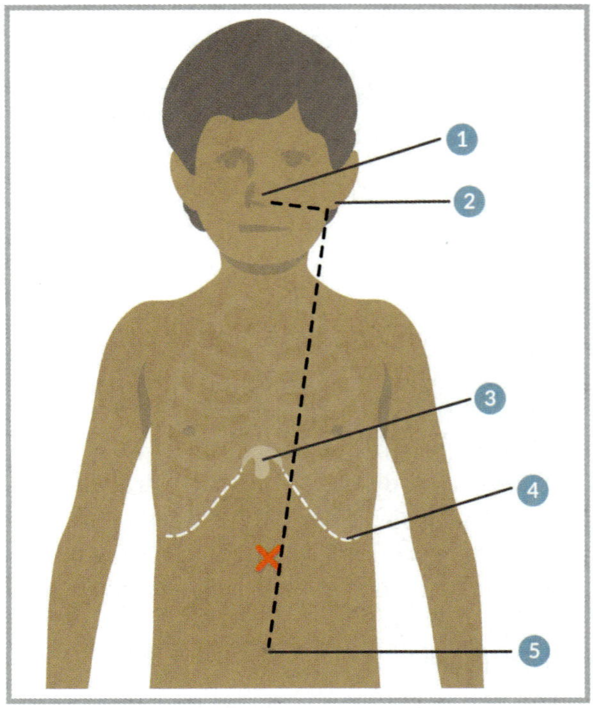

FIGURE P10-1 Technique for measuring the distance to insert a nasogastric or orogastric tube. 1. Tip of nose. 2. Earlobe. 3. Xiphoid process. 4. Costal margin. 5. Navel.

5. Assess the gag reflex. If the patient is unconscious and has a poor or no gag reflex, consider endotracheal intubation before gastric tube insertion.
6. In a trauma patient:
   - Maintain in-line stabilization of the cervical spine if a neck injury is suspected.
   - Choose the orotracheal route if the patient has severe head or facial trauma or has serious midfacial injuries.
7. Lubricate the end of the tube.

Possible Complications

- Placement of the tube into the trachea
- Vomiting and aspiration of stomach contents
- Airway bleeding or obstruction
- Passage of tube into brain when head/facial trauma is present

CONTROVERSY

The value of nasogastric and orogastric tube insertion is unproven. Although these procedures are routine in emergency departments, no studies have tested the benefit of easier ventilation against the potential complications of hypoxia resulting from endotracheal intubation or aspiration of stomach contents.

CAUTION
Never use force to pass an nasogastric or orogastric tube. If the tube is having difficulty passing, consider attempting insertion in the other nostril.

CAUTION
Do not perform orogastric tube insertion on a conscious patient because he or she is at risk of experiencing aspiration.

CAUTION
Insert the nasogastric tube by angling/pointing the tube directly toward the back of the head. Do not angle the tube superiorly.

PROCEDURE 10-1

Nasogastric Insertion

1. Pass the tube gently through the nostril, directing the tube straight back to the posterior pharynx. Do not angle the tube superiorly.
2. If the tube does not pass easily, try the opposite nostril or a smaller tube. Never force the tube. If NG passage is unsuccessful, use the OG approach.

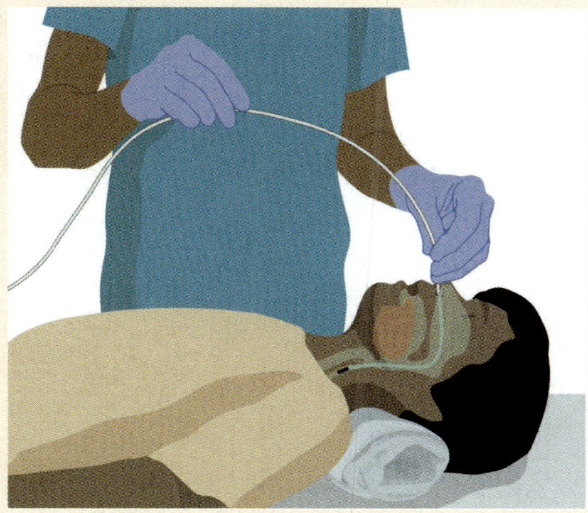

PROCEDURE 10-2

Orogastric Insertion

1. Insert the tube over the tongue, using a tongue blade if necessary to help insertion.
2. Advance the tube into the hypopharynx, then insert it rapidly into the stomach. If coughing, choking, or a change in voice occurs, immediately remove the tube, because it may be in the trachea.

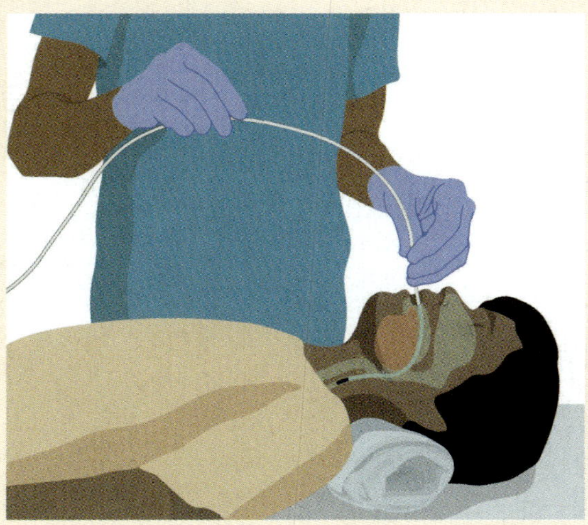

PROCEDURE 10-3

Check Placement of Nasogastric or Orogastric Tube

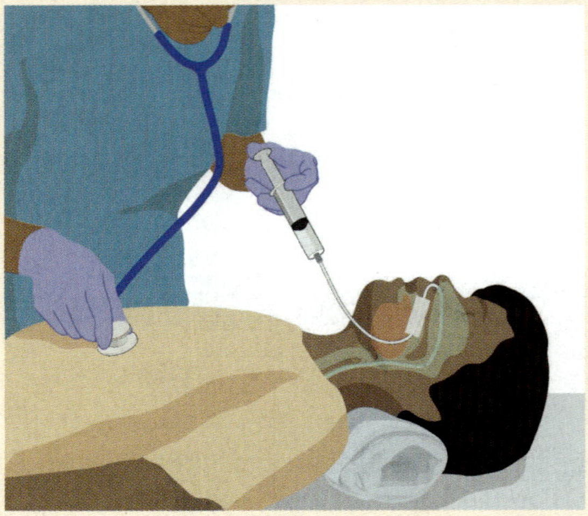

1. Check tube placement by aspirating stomach contents. If pH paper is available, placement can be verified by low pH. An additional method of checking tube placement is to use a syringe with the appropriate adaptor to quickly instill 10 to 20 mL of air through the tube while auscultating over the left upper quadrant. If there is a rush of air over the stomach region, the placement is correct. If correct placement cannot be verified, remove the tube.
2. Secure the tube to the bridge of the nose or to the cheek using adhesive tape. Aspirate air from the stomach, using a 30- to 60-mL catheter-tipped syringe, or connect to mechanical suction at a low, continuous, or intermittent setting.

TIP

Perform orogastric rather than nasogastric insertion in infants younger than 6 months.

TIP

Talking or crying during the procedure is an indication that the gastric tube is not in the trachea.

Procedure 11: Endotracheal Intubation

Tyler Molleur, MSN, RN, CEN, TCRN, CPEN, CTRN, CFRN, AEMT
Karen O'Connell, MD, MEd, FAAP

Introduction

The airway of a neonate, infant, or child should be managed in the least invasive way possible. Advanced airway measures should be used only if bag-mask ventilation fails. Performing endotracheal intubation (ETI) quickly and safely can be difficult. Unsuccessful attempts and malpositioning of endotracheal tubes (ETTs) occur at far higher rates in children than in adults. Inappropriate or unsuccessful intubation attempts may result in hypoxia, aspiration, airway injury, or worsening of cervical spine injury, and in worst-case scenarios they can lead to cardiac arrest. Endotracheal intubation of children in the prehospital setting is an infrequently performed skill that carries potentially significant risk, and it has not shown improvements in outcomes. Basic airway management and ventilation are the key interventions for survival in most respiratory failure or arrest situations.

Several anatomical differences make the pediatric airway more challenging than the adult airway:

- The child's vocal cords/glottic opening are more anterior and superior.
- The tongue is proportionally larger.
- The mandible and oral cavity are smaller.
- The diameter and length of the trachea are narrower and shorter.
- The soft tissues are more fragile.
- The narrowest area of the airway for children 5 years of age or younger is the cricoid cartilage.
- The airway is more pliable, and hyperextension or hyperflexion could cause complete occlusion of the airway.
- The epiglottis is larger and omega-shaped (U-shaped) and can be more difficult to position on intubation.
- The larger occiput and shorter neck make positioning the airway for optimal glottic visualization challenging. The goal is to align the airway axes (oral, pharyngeal, and laryngeal) by positioning the head and neck in a "sniffing" position. Helpful tips include the following:
  - Elevate the patient's head by placing a towel roll under the shoulders in patients younger than 8 years and under the head in patients aged 8 years or older.
  - Align the external ears horizontally with the sternal notch, while avoiding hyperflexion and hyperextension of the neck.

INDICATIONS

- When less invasive methods (eg, bag-mask ventilation; supraglottic airway [SGA], or extraglottic airway placement; positive pressure [continuous, bilevel]) are ineffective in oxygenation and/or ventilation
- Obstruction of ventilation by airway anatomy
- Severe facial or oropharyngeal burns or injuries
- Altered mental status in patient resulting in compromise of ongoing airway patency or loss of airway protective reflexes
- Respiratory failure or cardiopulmonary arrest
- Need for controlled ventilation (eg, traumatic brain injury)
- Severe shock (to decrease myocardial oxygen demand)

CONTRAINDICATIONS

- Effective oxygenation and ventilation achieved by using less invasive methods, such as bag-mask ventilations, and short transport time (relative)
- Clinicians who are inexperienced in or uncomfortable with intubating infants or children
- Patients with tracheostomy tube in place (may or may not be ventilator dependent) (relative)
- Newly born infants
- Difficult airway anatomy (large tongue, hematoma, massive facial injuries) (relative)

EQUIPMENT

- Length-based resuscitation tape *or* a reference material that provides appropriate guidance for equipment sizing based on length/age
- Pediatric laryngoscope handle with extra batteries and bulbs
- Pediatric laryngoscope blades, curved (Macintosh) sizes 2 to 4, and straight (Miller) sizes 0 through 4
- Video laryngoscopy (if available)
- Endotracheal tubes sizes 2.5 through 8.0 mm cuffed (preferred) or 2.5 through 5.5 uncuffed (option)
- 10-mL non-Luer-lock syringes
- Stylets for endotracheal tubes, pediatric and adult sizes
- Bougie for endotracheal tubes, pediatric and adult sizes
- Magill forceps, pediatric and adult sizes
- End-tidal carbon dioxide ($EtCO_2$) detection capability, with continuous waveform capnography preferred
- Pulse oximeter, with continuous pulse oximetry preferred
- Rescue airway device such as a supraglottic airway device (SGA)
- Portable and fixed suction apparatus with a regulator, per federal specifications
- Wide-bore tubing with rigid pharyngeal curved suction apparatus or flexible suction catheters, 6Fr through 16Fr
- Water-soluble lubricant
- Oropharyngeal airways sizes 0 through 5; infant, child, and adult
- Self-inflating resuscitator bag with oxygen reservoir/accumulator and valve: adult (> 1,000 mL) and child (450–750 mL) sizes
- Transparent masks with soft rim, sizes neonate through adult
- Adhesive tape and skin adhesive
- Commercial ETT securing devices if available
- Oxygen source, capable of metered flow with adequate tubing

Rationale

Successful ETI allows optimal oxygenation and ventilation, provides an alternative means for resuscitation medication delivery, and assists with ensuring ongoing airway patency. Properly securing an endotracheal tube is a life-saving intervention when caring for critically ill or injured patients. This procedure requires specialized training and skills and can be associated with significant and serious complications. The decision to intubate should be made after careful risk/benefit consideration.

Endotracheal Intubation

PREPARATION

1. Make sure oxygen delivery equipment is connected to an oxygen source.
2. Select an appropriately sized ETT (**TABLE P11–1**) for oral ETI.
3. For a cuffed ETT: Check cuff for leaks as follows:
   - Inflate the cuff with appropriate volume of air and ensure the cuff stays inflated.
   - Feel the cuff for integrity.

TABLE P11–1 Suggested Endotracheal Tube (ETT) and Suction Catheter Sizes[a]

Age	ETT Size (mm) Uncuffed	ETT Size (mm) Cuffed	Suction Catheter Size (French)
Premature newborn	2.0–2.5	2.0	5
Newborn to 3 months	3.0	2.5	6–8
6 months	3.5	3.0	8
12–18 months	4.0	3.0	8
3 years	4.5	4.0	8
5 years	5.0	4.5	10
6 years	5.5	5.0	10
8 years	Not applicable	6.0	10
12 years	Not applicable	6.5	12
16 years	Not applicable	7.0–8.0	14

[a]Formulas to estimate ETT size in mm: uncuffed ETT 4 + age/4 cuffed ETT 3.5 + age/4

- Deflate the cuff and remove the syringe before insertion.

4. Attach the blade to the laryngoscope handle and make sure the light source is secure and works.
5. Ensure functioning suction equipment is available.
6. Insert the stylet into the ETT, stopping the stylet at least 1 cm from the end of the ETT.
7. Bend the ETT into a gentle upward curve. In some cases, you may need to bend the tube into the shape of a hockey stick. This helps with guiding the ETT to the anteriorly positioned glottic opening in young children.
8. Lubricate the tube with a water-soluble lubricant (optional).
9. Prepare the device for confirmation of ETT placement (continuous capnography waveform monitoring is the reference standard).
10. To predict correct ETT tube position at the gum line, do one of the following:
    - Check color-coded length-based tape or other resuscitation guides.
    - Calculate ETT position with formula: gum line position (in cm) = ~3 × tube size (diameter).
11. Have partner prepare for the following:
    - Performing ongoing patient assessment
    - Providing time counts for ventilation rates
    - Watching monitors (heart rate, pulse oximetry, $EtCO_2$ capnography tracing)
    - Handling suction devices
    - Assisting with ETT handling, stabilization, and securing
    - Applying external laryngeal manipulation assistance, as necessary
    - Ensuring in-line cervical spine immobilization if the child has possible spinal trauma
12. Position patient (avoid hyperextension or hyperflexion of neck).
    - Medical patient: Place the child in the "sniffing" position following the detailed tips provided previously.
    - If spinal trauma is a possibility, place the child in a neutral position with in-line manual cervical spine stabilization.

TIP

Make sure proper equipment is available and functioning before attempting intubation.

CONTROVERSY

The value of performing ETI in children in the prehospital setting is controversial. The airway of a neonate, infant, or child should be managed in the least invasive way possible. The optimal strategy for prehospital pediatric airway management (outcomes comparison of BMV, ETT, SGA) remains unknown; ongoing studies are directly addressing this question. Performing the procedure quickly and safely in the field can be difficult. Malposition of the ETT or aspiration can be nearly 3 times as common in children as in adults. Inappropriate or unsuccessful intubation attempts may result in hypoxia, aspiration, oral trauma or injury to the child's airway, worsening of cervical spine injury, malposition of the ETT (right mainstem intubation, esophageal intubation), and, in the worst cases, hypoxia leading to severe bradycardia and/or cardiac arrest. This is especially important when considering intubation in children, because it is infrequently performed in this age group and has not been shown to significantly improve outcomes.

TIP

Video laryngoscopy offers shared visualization of the intubation process and may enhance intubation success rates. Video-assisted intubation should be used when available.

CAUTION

Because pediatric intubation is an infrequently used skill for many prehospital providers, ongoing education and hands-on practice are essential.

PROCEDURE 11-1

Endotracheal Tube Insertion

1. Oxygenate and ventilate the patient for 1 to 2 minutes with BMV device and 100% oxygen, at a rate of 1 ventilation every 2 to 3 seconds. Say "squeeze, release" or "squeeze, release, release" to reinforce proper rate.

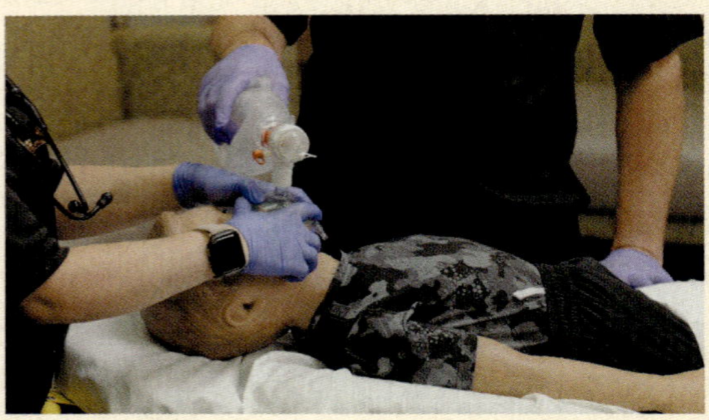

2. There is insufficient evidence to recommend routine cricoid pressure application to prevent aspiration.
3. Grasp the laryngoscope in the left hand. Stop ventilating and begin timing, giving 20- to 30-second counts.

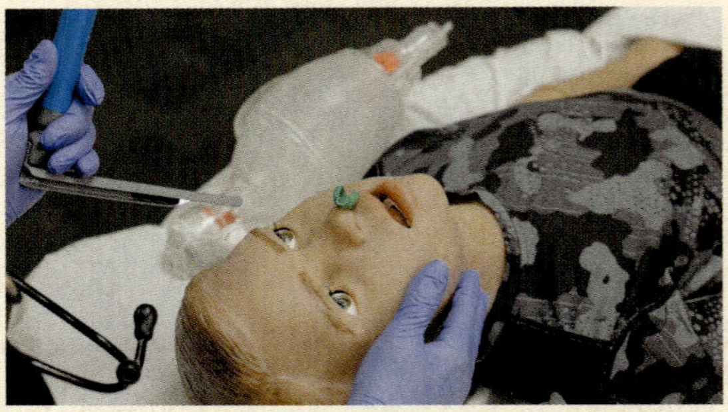

4. Open the mouth by applying thumb pressure on the chin; check the mouth for foreign bodies or loose teeth; remove the oropharyngeal airway if present.

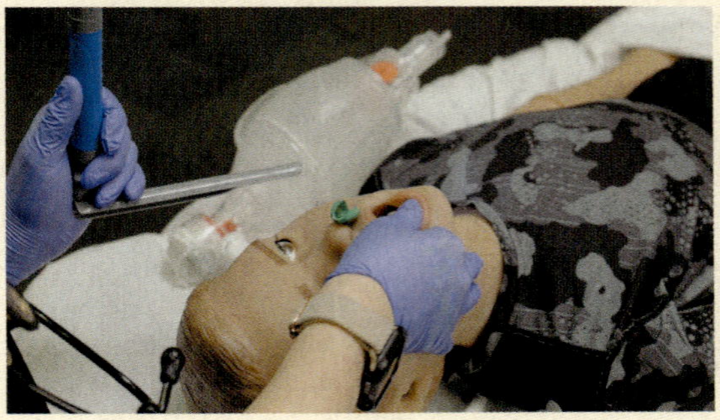

5. Insert the laryngoscope blade into the right side of the mouth and lift the tongue with a sweeping motion to the left for a direct line of sight to the glottic opening/vocal cords.

6. Exert gentle traction upward along the axis of the laryngoscope handle at a 45° angle.

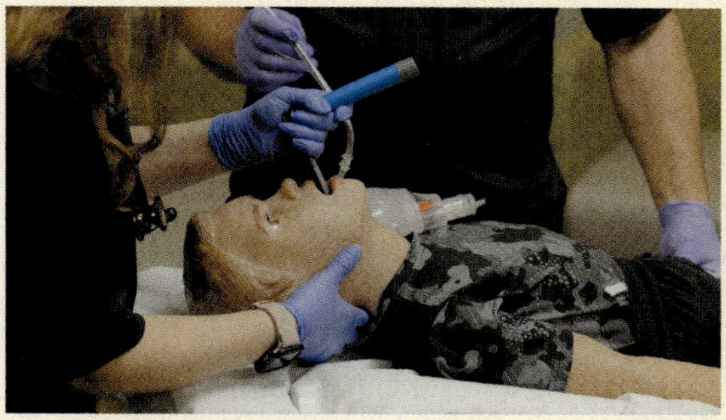

7. Minimize the risk of trauma to the teeth or gums by *not* coming in contact with them. *Do not* bend or rock your wrist backward toward you, which steeply changes the angle of the blade in the oropharynx.

8. Advance the blade straight along the tongue. Continue looking at the blade tip, until the tip is just beyond the epiglottis. Do not take your eyes off the vocal cords. Your partner should hand the ETT to you while you maintain view of the cords.

9. If there is difficulty seeing the vocal cords, consider the following:

(1) remove secretions or particulate matter with rigid, large-bore suction device (or Magill forceps if large solid debris is present)

(2) advance or retract the laryngoscope blade to bring the epiglottis into view, then reposition the tip of the blade to bring the vocal cords into view

(3) have your partner apply the backward-upward-rightward pressure (BURP) maneuver to bring the glottic opening into alignment; or

(4) reposition the head to help with alignment of axes

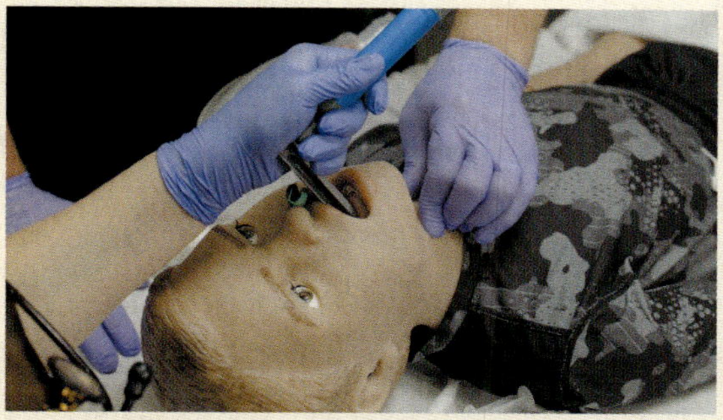

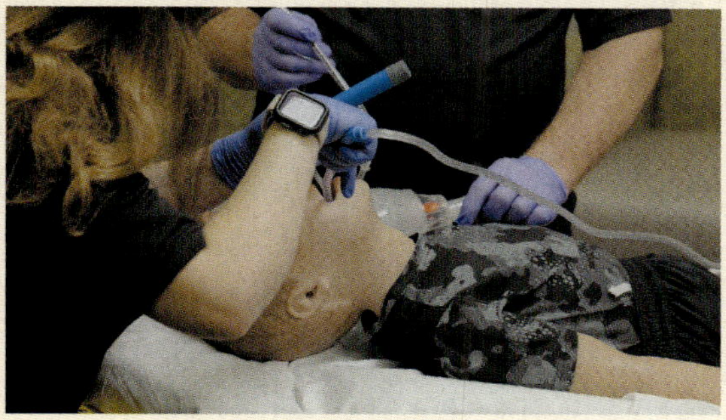

10. Insert the ETT while maintaining constant visualization of the ETT's passage through the vocal cords. Hold the tube like a dart with right hand and insert the tip of the tube from the right corner of the mouth down between the vocal cords. Do not insert the tube in the channel of the laryngoscope blade, because this blocks the view of the vocal cords. Advance a cuffed tube until the balloon passes through the vocal cords. Advance an uncuffed tube until the black-striped marker on the ETT is situated beyond the vocal cords. Look for the centimeter marking on the ETT in relation to the gum line.

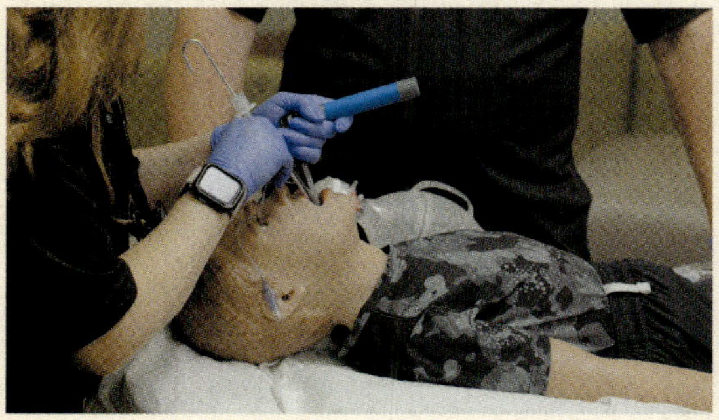

11. Remove the laryngoscope blade while holding the ETT securely in place. Continuously secure the tube manually until it is secured with tape, twill, or a commercial tube holder.
14. Remove the stylet from the ETT.

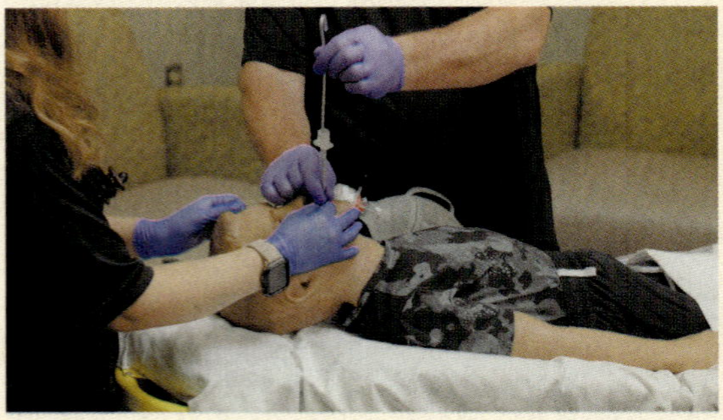

15. If using an ETT with a cuffed end, inflate the cuff with a pilot balloon. Maintain the tube's position by holding the ETT against the upper lip or the hard palate.
16. If a large amount of fluid is evident in the ETT, use a suction catheter to clear the airway. Your partner should maintain the ETT's position and ventilate the patient with a BMV device.
17. Confirm the correct endotracheal position of the tube by using waveform capnography (reference standard), capnometry or colorimetric CO_2 device. Listen for bilateral breath sounds and observe for symmetrical, bilateral chest wall rise. Assess appearance, heart rate, pulse oximetry, and perfusion for recovery after intubation.

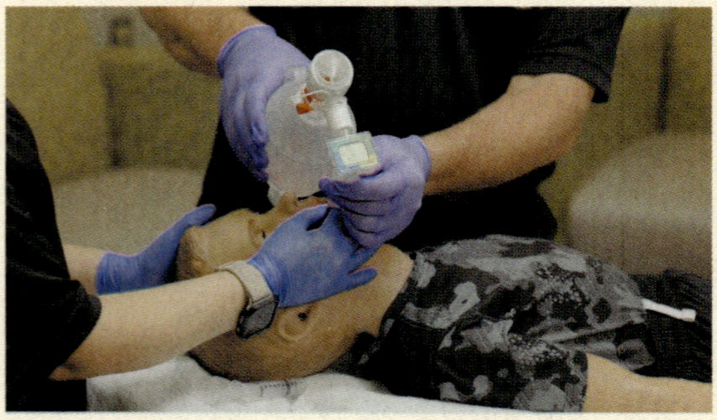

18. Auscultate for bilateral lung sounds at the midaxillary line, third intercostal space (check for 2 breaths on the right and then 2 breaths on the left). If breath sounds are heard only on 1 side (usually the right), pull the ETT back slightly until breath sounds are heard on both sides. The absence of gastric sounds with ventilation is not adequate to verify proper placement; instead, placement can be assessed by ensuring the absence of bubbling or gurgling sounds in the epigastric area, indicating air-water interface (check for 2 breaths).
19. Document tube position using the centimeter mark at teeth or gum line. Mark it on the ETT with indelible pen and monitor frequently for tube movement/displacement.

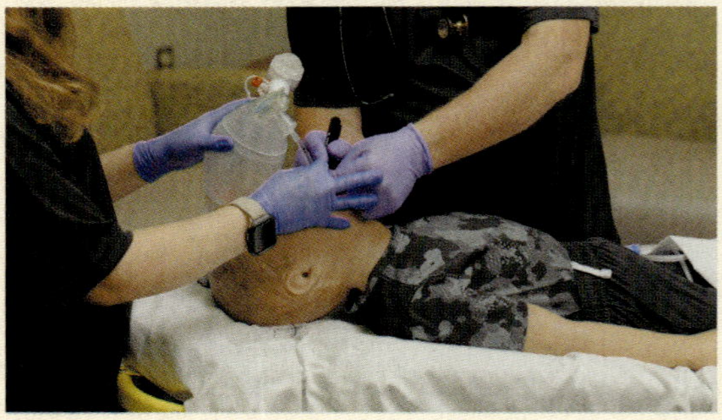

20. Secure the tube with tape or a commercially available ETT securing device. Reassess the proper location of the tube via continuous capnography monitoring.
21. Reapply the cervical collar and/or cervical stabilization device if indicated.
22. Ventilate intentionally for minimal chest wall rise. Pediatric tidal volumes are approximately 6 to 8 mL/kg ideal body weight. Avoid hyperventilation and excessive tidal volumes. Ventilate at the recommended rates: adult, 10 to 12 breaths/min; child, 20 to 30 breaths/min; neonate, 40 breaths/min.
23. Continuously monitor $EtCO_2$ to maintain a level of 35 to 40 mm Hg.
24. Consider sedation with sedative or opioid medications if the patient is agitated.
25. Consider gastric decompression if there is gastric distension to improve oxygenation and ventilation (see **Procedure 10, Orogastric and Nasogastric Tube Insertion**).
26. Transport to the closest appropriate hospital for airway stabilization when respiratory failure cannot be successfully managed.

Indications for Tube Removal

IMMEDIATE TUBE REMOVAL

- No chest rise with ventilation.
- Failure to confirm endotracheal placement with measurement of $EtCO_2$; patients in cardiac arrest may not have measurable $EtCO_2$, and endotracheal placement should be ensured by confirmation of direct visualization of the ETT positioned through the vocal cords.

CAUTION

Ensure ongoing manual in-line stabilization during intubation attempts in trauma patients.

CAUTION

Never assume the ETT is in the trachea unless you see the tube passing through the vocal cords. Misting in the tube or absence of gastric bubbling are not reliable indicators of placement.

TIP

Use continuous waveform capnography to detect $EtCO_2$; this is the reference standard for confirming endotracheal tube placement.

TIP

In addition to preoxygenation, apneic oxygenation (high-flow oxygen via nasal cannula) may prolong the period before hypoxia during an intubation attempt.

TIP

Once an ETT is secure and appropriate placement confirmed, selective resuscitation medications can be delivered via the ETT. Preferred resuscitation medication delivery is by intraosseous (IO) or intravenous (IV) route; however, endotracheal delivery provides a potentially life-saving option. Reminder: only lidocaine, epinephrine, atropine, and naloxone (medications in the mnemonic LEAN) can be given through the ETT route. Medication doses need to be adjusted for this route of administration (refer to a medication formulary).

Drug-Assisted Intubation (DAI)/ Rapid-Sequence Intubation (RSI)

Drug-assisted intubation (also known as rapid-sequence intubation) is a technique for optimizing intubation conditions and minimizing complications. The medications available can be divided into neuromuscular blockers (eg, succinylcholine, vecuronium, and rocuronium) and analgesics/sedatives/anxiolytics (eg, midazolam, diazepam, fentanyl, ketamine). See **TABLE P11–2**. Local protocols define medication availability and recommendations. It is important to realize that each drug or combination of drugs is associated with a risk/benefit profile. The premedication atropine has been used in infants with the intentions of blunting the vagal response associated with laryngoscopy, but its benefits remain unclear. American Heart Association guidelines recommend against routine use of prophylactic atropine. However, it may be reasonable in specific situations at high risk of inducing bradycardia, such as when succinylcholine is used for paralysis. The use of neuromuscular blocking medications before endotracheal tube insertion has been associated with improved success and decreased complications in emergency intubations. It is extremely important to note that inducing paralysis in a patient causes apnea. Assisted ventilation is required during this phase to prevent hypoxia and its associated complications.

CAUTION

Pediatric DAI/RSI should not be performed without prior training, and clinicians who do not routinely use medications for DAI/RSI should not perform DAI/RSI on children. The use of DAI/RSI should be reserved for clinicians under a comprehensive program with ongoing training and quality assurance measures.

TABLE P11–2 Drug-Assisted Intubation Medications

Drug	Type	Dose
Atropine (infants)	Anticholinergic	0.02 mg/kg IV/IO; use only if HR < 100
Diazepam	Anxiolysis/sedative	0.1 mg/kg IV/IO/IM
Fentanyl	Analgesia	1 μg/kg IV/IO 1–2 μg/kg Intranasal
Ketamine	Analgesic/anesthetic	1–2 mg/kg IV/IO 3–4 mg/kg IM
Lorazepam	Anxiolysis/sedative	0.1 mg/kg IV/IO/IM
Midazolam	Anxiolysis/sedative	0.1 mg/kg IV/IO/IM 0.2 mg/kg Intranasal
Rocuronium	Paralytic/neuromuscular blockade	1 mg/kg IV/IO
Succinylcholine	Paralytic/neuromuscular blockade	1–2 mg/kg IV/IO/IM
Vecuronium	Paralytic/neuromuscular blockade	0.2 mg/kg IV/IO

IM, intramuscular; IO, intraosseous; IV, intravenous.

INDICATIONS

- Respiratory failure in pediatric patients who are not in cardiac arrest
- Severe head trauma accompanied by need for airway protection or hyperventilation

CONTRAINDICATIONS

- Abnormal airway anatomy that poses increased risks of intubation failure and in which removal of a patient's own respiratory drive may cause critical complications
- Upper airway obstruction, severe facial or neck trauma, or suspected laryngeal fracture in which cricothyrotomy may be indicated

EQUIPMENT

- Endotracheal intubation equipment
- Medications for DAI/RSI

PREPARATION

1. Prepare the child for ETI.
2. Review the SOAP-ME preintubation safety checklist: **s**uction, **o**xygen source, **a**irway and **p**ositioning plan for optimal visualization, **m**edications, **e**quipment ready with **E**tCO_2 detection and monitor.
3. Ensure the presence of a working IV or IO line (if available).
4. Double-check medications with appropriate mg/kg dosing on length-based resuscitation tapes (see **Procedure 2, Length/Weight-Based Resuscitation Tape**).

PROCEDURE 11-2

Drug Assisted Intubation/ Rapid-Sequence Intubation

1. Prepare equipment and medications; ensure the team shares an understanding of the plan.
2. Preoxygenate with a 100% nonrebreather face mask or bag-mask device if ventilation is compromised.
3. Premedicate with atropine (as needed).
4. Administer sedation/analgesia/anxiolysis.
5. Administer a neuromuscular blocking agent.
6. Perform ETI with visualization of the ETT passing through the vocal cords. Use external laryngeal manipulation and ask a colleague to assist with direct pressure on the trachea as needed to achieve adequate visualization of glottic opening.
7. Confirm ETT placement ($EtCO_2$ detection is reference standard; bilateral breath sounds detected; adequate chest wall rise).
8. Tape ETT in place (or use commercial device if available).

TIP

The induced muscular paralysis resulting from DAI/RSI allows the EMS clinician to insert an ETT through relaxed vocal cords with little resistance. This improves success and decreases complications arising from forced insertion attempts.

CAUTION

If RSI fails, BMV use should be resumed immediately to provide adequate oxygenation and ventilation.

PROCEDURE 11-3

Reconfirm Endotracheal Tube Placement

CAUTION

Ongoing assessment is critical when an airway device is in place. Acute worsening of respiratory status or evidence of hypoxemia can be secondary to displacement or obstruction of the airway device, pneumothorax, or equipment failure.

TIP

Always reassess tube location after patient movement or when there is a change in patient status.

1. Verify presence of CO_2 with waveform capnography, capnometry, or colorimetric CO_2 detector.
2. Reassess breath sounds bilaterally at the midaxillary line, third intercostal space (2 breaths on the right and then 2 breaths on the left). Take extra care handling an ETT in a pediatric patient because it can be easily dislodged. Reassess after the patient is in the ambulance (and after change of position or change in patient status). Report and record findings.

Possible Complications

- Aspiration of stomach contents
- Tracheal tube malposition (esophageal intubation) and/or dislodgement of ETT from trachea
- Hypoxemia/hypoxia
- Tube obstruction
- Barotrauma resulting from excessive ventilation and large tidal volumes
- Adverse reactions to sedative or paralytic medications (see the **Appendix, Medication Formulary**)
- Injury to laryngeal, tracheal, pharyngeal, esophageal structures; teeth or mouth trauma
- Partial or complete vocal cord avulsion

PROCEDURE 11-4

Extubation

Postresuscitation extubation is rarely indicated in the field. All 3 of the following situations must be present: (1) spontaneous breathing with adequate rate and tidal volume, (2) conscious patient, and (3) coughing or gagging causing distress.

1. Ensure rigid large-bore suction device is functioning.
2. Suction the oropharynx.
3. Turn the patient on their left side.
4. Deflate the cuff completely (if the cuff is inflated).
5. Remove the ETT quickly at the end-inspiratory phase, while suctioning.

Suggested References

ARTICLES

Harris M, Lyng JW, Mandt M, et al. Prehospital pediatric respiratory distress and airway management interventions: an NAEMSP position statement and resource document. *Prehosp Emerg Care*. 2022;26(suppl 1):118–128. doi: 10.1080/10903127.2021.1994675

Lasa JJ, Dhillon GS, Duff JP, et al. Part 8: Pediatric Advanced Life Support: 2025 American Heart Association and American Academy of Pediatrics Guidelines for Cardiopulmonary Resuscitation and Emergency Cardiovascular Care. *Pediatrics*. 2026;157(1):e2025074351. doi:10.1542/peds.2025-074351

Lyng J, Adelgais K, Alter R, et al. Recommended essential equipment for basic life support and advanced life support ground ambulances 2020: a joint position statement. *Prehosp Emerg Care*. 2021;25(3):451–459. PMID: 33557659 doi: 10.1080/10903127.2021.1886382

OTHER RESOURCES

American Heart Association. *Highlights of the 2020 American Heart Association Guidelines for CPR and ECC*. American Heart Association; 2020. Accessed October 20, 2024. https://cpr.heart.org/en/resuscitation-science/cpr-and-ecc-guidelines

National Association of State EMS Officials. *National Model EMS Clinical Guidelines, Version 3.0*. National Association of State EMS Officials; 2022. https://nasemso.org/docs.ashx?id=1444322

Procedure 12: Confirmation of Endotracheal Intubation and Use of End-Tidal Capnography

Karen O'Connell, MD, MEd, FAAP
Tyler Molleur, MSN, RN, CEN, TCRN, CPEN, CTRN, CFRN, AEMT

Introduction

Performing pediatric airway management in the prehospital setting may be difficult or impossible even for experienced prehospital professionals. Accurate confirmation of proper position of the endotracheal tube (ETT) in the trachea after intubation is essential. Inadvertent esophageal intubation and ETT dislodgement are common and potentially lethal complications that must be detected immediately. Adequate measurement of end-tidal carbon dioxide ($EtCO_2$) can also assist with verifying proper supraglottic airway placement and guide successful ventilation by using bag-mask ventilation or advanced airways.

There are several methods of primary confirmation of ETT placement:

- Continuous waveform capnography (reference standard; both graphical waveform and numerical values)
- Use of exhaled CO_2 detection device (colorimetric CO_2 detector)
- Use of digital capnometry (quantitative $EtCO_2$ with numerical value)

INDICATIONS

- Endotracheal intubation
- Insertion of a supraglottic device
- Ventilation with a bag-mask device

CONTRAINDICATION

- An adult CO_2 detector cannot be left in place in a child weighing less than 15 kg.

EQUIPMENT

- Stethoscope
- End-tidal CO_2 waveform capnography *or* colorimetric $EtCO_2$ detector device *or* quantitative $EtCO_2$ capnometry

Rationale

Properly positioned endotracheal tubes (ETTs) and supraglottic devices make it possible to effectively oxygenate and ventilate critically ill or injured children. Esophageal placement of an ETT, however, is usually harmful or lethal. Inadvertent esophageal placement or dislodgement of an ETT has potentially life-threatening consequences. Relying on clinical assessment of placement of the ETT alone can be inaccurate, especially in the prehospital environment where ambient noise (traffic, family members) can make it difficult to hear breath sounds. It is challenging to discern actual lung breath sounds from sounds that are transmitted from the esophagus or stomach throughout a child's chest.

Fortunately, several mechanical adjuncts are available to supplement clinical assessment, help confirm correct tracheal placement of the ETT, and allow the emergency medical services (EMS) clinician to continuously monitor adequate ventilation. These devices work primarily by measuring or verifying the presence of CO_2 on exhalation, which will be present if an advanced airway is allowing for appropriate ventilation.

Preparation

1. Determine the patient's weight.
2. Intubate the infant or child with a correctly sized ETT (see **Procedure 11, Endotracheal Intubation**) or insert the correctly sized supraglottic device (see **Procedure 13, Supraglottic Airway Insertion and Pediatric Difficult Airway**), or initiate bag-mask ventilation with the proper size device and good mask-to-face seal.
3. Suction any fluid from the ETT or supraglottic airway.

END-TIDAL CARBON DIOXIDE WAVEFORM CAPNOGRAPHY

1. Connect the capnography device to monitoring equipment. Ensure the monitoring equipment has calibrated the capnography device and the waveform is displayed on the monitoring equipment before proceeding.
2. Connect the device to the end of the ETT.
3. Observe for a waveform and a numerical value.
4. A flat waveform or value of 0 means the ETT is in the esophagus.

DIGITAL CAPNOMETRY

1. Place the sensor as indicated by the manufacturer.
2. Attach the sensor probe to the monitoring cable.
3. Observe for the presence of a numerical value that indicates detection of exhaled CO_2 and proper ETT placement.
4. Absence of a numerical value indicates the ETT is improperly placed.

COLORIMETRIC EXHALED CARBON DIOXIDE DETECTOR

1. Determine correct size of the CO_2 detector.
   - Use a pediatric device if the child weighs less than 15 kg.
   - Use an adult device if the child weighs 15 kg or more.
   - If an adult device is used on a small child, remove it after 6 breaths (initial confirmation of placement).
2. Check the expiration date on the CO_2 detector package.
3. Remove the CO_2 detector from its packaging and inspect it before use. The detector should be dry and be a bright purple or dark blue color.

PROCEDURE 12-1

Clinical Assessment

1. Look for bilateral rise and fall of the chest. Listen for breath sounds in the right midaxillary line, then in the left midaxillary line. If breath sounds are equal, secure the tube. If breath sounds are greater on the right side than on the left side, then the tube may be in the right mainstem bronchus. Slowly pull back the ETT until breath sounds are equal.

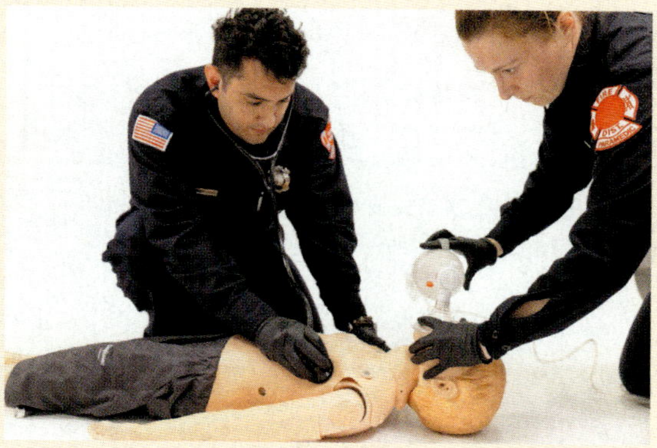

2. Secondary assessment can include listening for breath sounds over the stomach. If gurgling is present (sounding like a straw in milk), the ETT may be in the esophagus. If there is an absence of an $EtCO_2$ waveform or numerical value, desaturations, or bradycardia, remove the ETT immediately. If the patient is hemodynamically stable (blood pressure, heart rate, and oxygen saturation are adequate), then provide 6 breaths and monitor for color change of the device. If there is continued concern regarding proper ETT placement in a stable patient, direct visualization via laryngoscopy for tube placement through the vocal cords can be performed.

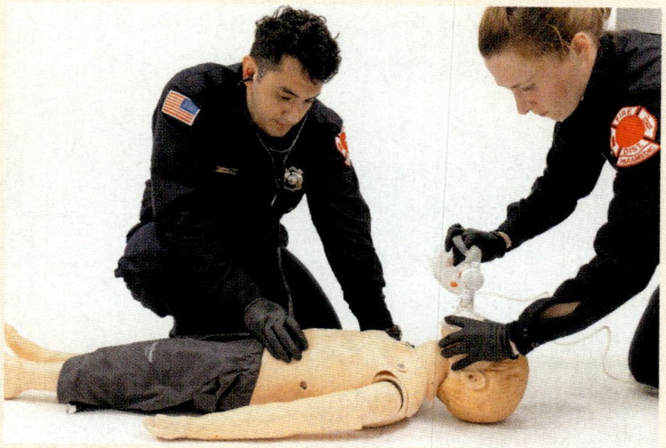

CAUTION

Do not remove the ETT just because breath sounds are heard in the stomach, because they may be transmitted sounds from the lungs. If the patient has continued desaturations or bradycardia, perform a direct laryngoscopy to ensure the ETT is through the vocal cords. If it is not, or you are unsure, and the patient has continued desaturations despite giving effective breaths with positive end-expiratory pressure, then remove the ETT and deliver oxygen with bag-mask ventilation.

PROCEDURE 12-2

End-Tidal Carbon Dioxide Waveform Capnography and Capnometry

Waveform capnography is the best diagnostic study and the reference standard in determining exhaled CO_2, because it provides both a continuous waveform and a number. This may be used as a standalone methodology, or it may be built into a cardiac monitor used by EMS clinicians. In patients who require assisted ventilation, an adapter can be attached between the band and the mask, ETT, or supraglottic airway.

The capnograph is the waveform that shows how much CO_2 is present at each phase of the respiratory cycle, and it normally has a square peak-and-trough shape (**FIGURE P12-2A**). Capnography also measures and displays the respiratory rate. The shape of the waveform (amplitude and width) provides clues about respiratory effort and causes of respiratory distress and gives real-time feedback about how management is working (**FIGURE P12–1**). For example, a shark-fin waveform can indicate bronchoconstriction (**FIGURE P12–2B**). Capnography can also detect poor perfusion states such as shock or cardiac arrest, and it can assist with determining the effectiveness of cardiopulmonary resuscitation (CPR) (**FIGURE P12–3**).

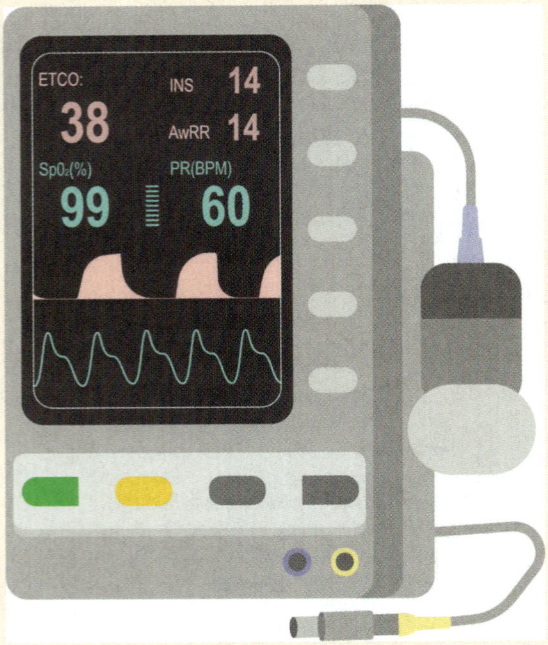

FIGURE P12–1 Capnography monitor.

Once the waveform capnography is connected, it is important that a waveform and a number are observed on the monitor. A flat wave indicates that the ETT is not in the airway and is likely in the esophagus. If there is an initial waveform that then flattens, this is an indication that the ETT has become misplaced, obstructed, or dislodged. **TABLE P12–1** describes several patterns of waveform shape and/or numerical $EtCO_2$ measurement that may be useful to the EMS clinician.

The number is capnometry, which is the partial pressure of CO_2 detected at the end of exhalation. This is $EtCO_2$, which is normally 35 to 45 mm Hg. An above-normal $EtCO_2$ is likely an indication of hypoventilation, causing CO_2 levels to increase in the bloodstream.

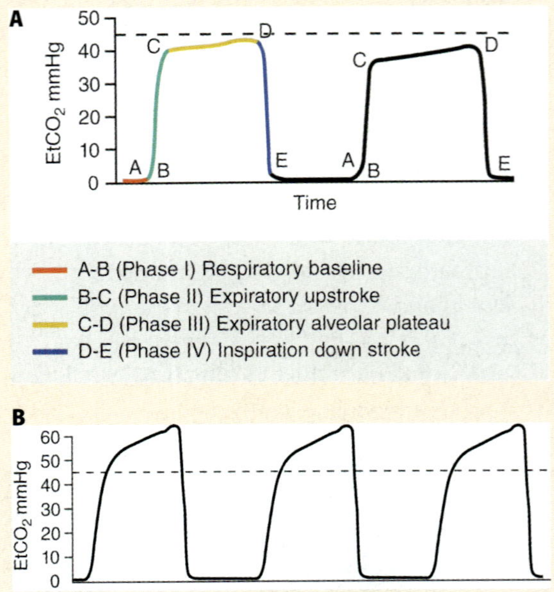

FIGURE P12–2 **A.** A normal waveform. **B.** A shark-fin waveform can indicate constriction.

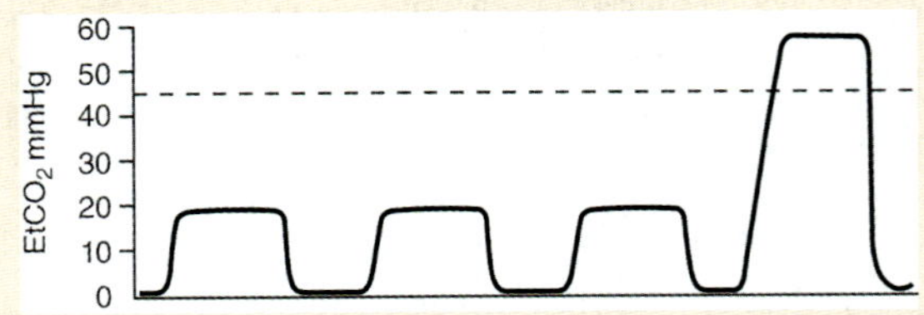

FIGURE P12–3 Capnography can also aid in determining the effectiveness of CPR.

A below-normal $EtCO_2$ could be the result of hyperventilation or poor perfusion. Poor perfusion does not allow for CO_2 to exit the bloodstream via the lungs in adequate amounts and may indicate shock. End-tidal CO_2 as a measurement of perfusion can also be used to assess CPR adequacy (**FIGURE P12–3**) and return of spontaneous circulation.

TIP

Capnography and capnometry can be used to assess adequacy of ventilations, placement of advanced airway, and the patient's overall perfusion.

Continuous $EtCO_2$ monitoring will show real-time changes within seconds and is a more timely indicator of inadequate ventilation than is waiting for changes in oxygen saturation, which lag minutes behind.

CAUTION

Discerning and interpreting measurable $EtCO_2$ is tricky in patients in cardiac arrest, with pulmonary edema or pulmonary hemorrhage caused by low amounts of exhaled CO_2.

If the child is pulseless and inadequate chest compressions are being performed, there will be a very low (or zero) reading on quantitative capnometry. Assess the quality of CPR (depth, rate, recoil).

TABLE P12–1 Use of Waveform Capnography in the Patient With Assisted Ventilations

Waveform Pattern	Significance	Clinician Actions
Decreasing over time	Ventilation: Patient may be hyperventilated	Verify rate of ventilation is appropriate for patient's age/clinical situation; adjust as necessary
	Perfusion: Patient's cardiac output is decreasing	Assess patient's capillary refill, skin color, blood pressure, and other signs of perfusion; correct as necessary with hemorrhage control, fluids, and vasopressors; if performing cardiopulmonary resuscitation (CPR), verify adequacy of rate, depth, and recoil of chest compressions
Sudden drop in end-tidal carbon dioxide ($EtCO_2$) to zero	Ventilation: Endotracheal tube has become dislodged, disconnected, or obstructed	Verify connections attached and not kinked Look at vocal cords with laryngoscope If tube is incorrectly placed: • Extubate • Ventilate with bag-mask device • Reintubate
	Perfusion: Patient is in cardiac arrest	Reassess patient condition, including presence of a pulse; begin CPR if patient is pulseless or has pulse $<$ 60 beats/min despite appropriate ventilation delivery
Shark-fin waveform	Ventilation: Bronchoconstriction	Use in-line nebulization kit with bag-mask device, if available, to provide bronchodilators while ventilating Pay attention to ensure that ventilation rates and volumes are appropriate to reduce the risk of pneumothorax
Triangular pattern and/or decreasing $EtCO_2$ with each breath	Ventilation: Air leak around endotracheal tube	Troubleshoot: Add air to cuff; visualize placement to see if repositioning endotracheal tube is needed (deflating cuff, advancing tube, and re-inflating cuff); add three-way stopcock to pilot balloon valve if valve is leaking Otherwise, extubate, ventilate with bag-mask device, and reintubate
$EtCO_2$ increasing over time	Ventilation: Patient may be hypoventilated	Verify rate of ventilation is appropriate for patient's age/clinical situation; adjust as necessary
	Perfusion: Patient's cardiac output is increasing	Assess patient's capillary refill, skin color, blood pressure and other signs of perfusion
Sudden increase in $EtCO_2$	Ventilation: Ventilations resumed and/or sampling occurring from respiratory tract	Continue ventilations and perform clinical assessment to verify tube placement and ventilation adequacy
	Perfusion: Return of spontaneous circulation	Reassess patient for a pulse and ventilatory effort; maintain adequate cardiac output and ventilations

PROCEDURE 12-3

Colorimetric Carbon Dioxide Detector Device

1. Attach the device to the end of the ETT and attach the other end to the bag-mask device.

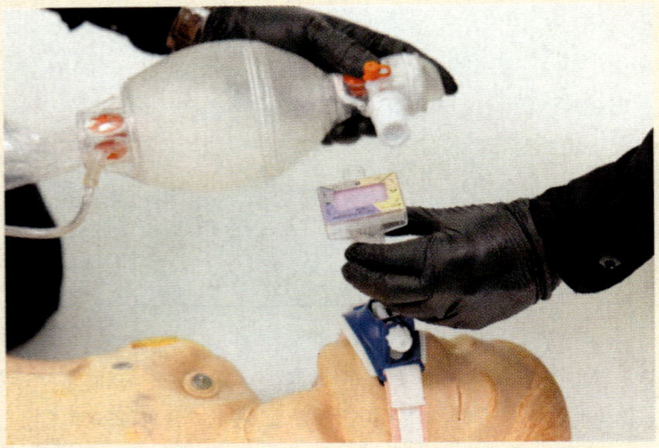

2. Begin ventilation.

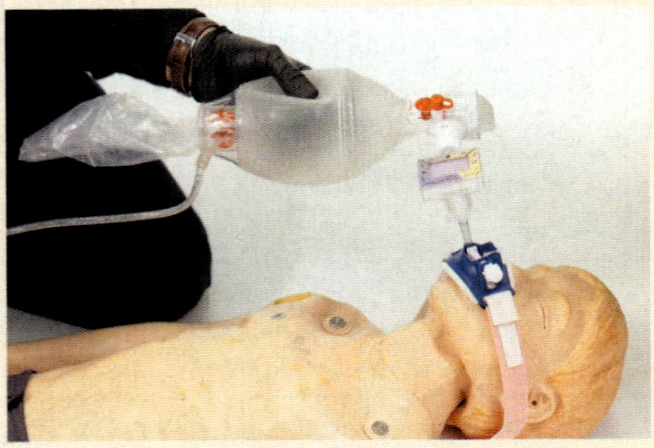

3. Observe the CO_2 detector for color change during exhalation. Read only after a total of 6 breaths. Check the color and act accordingly (**TABLE P12–2**). Regardless of whether the ETT is in the trachea, the CO_2 detector will change to a purple or dark blue color when 100% oxygen is squeezed through the bag device and ETT into the lungs. The color on exhalation is the one to note, because a yellow color in the expiratory phase of breathing reflects CO_2 detection. Document observations and changes with interventions.

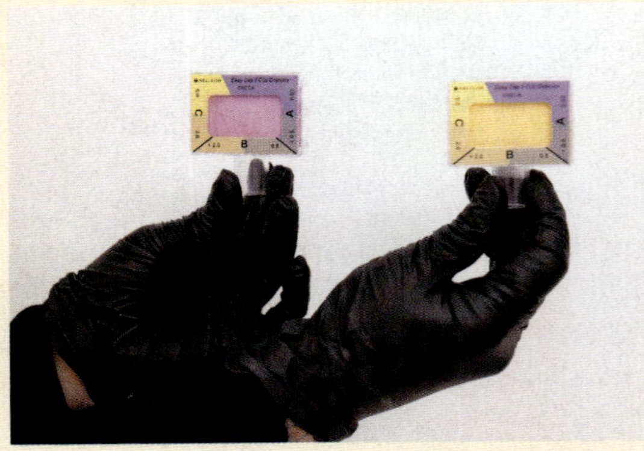

4. However, do not leave an adult CO_2 detector in place after initial confirmation of tube position on a patient weighing less than 15 kg. The adult device has too much dead space, and an infant can rebreathe CO_2 if it is left in line.

CAUTION

Remove the colorimetric CO_2 detector from the ETT if endotracheal drugs are given, because a wet detector may not show a correct color change from purple to yellow.

TIP

If the child weighs less than 15 kg, use a pediatric colorimetric exhaled CO_2 detector.

CAUTION

If the child is in cardiac arrest and not receiving chest compressions, color change may not occur, even if placement is correct, because CO_2 in the blood is not being pumped to the lungs.

TABLE P12–2 Interpretation of Colorimetric Exhaled Carbon Dioxide (CO_2) Detector for Endotracheal Tube (ETT) Placement

<table>
<tr><th>CO_2 Detector Color & Significance</th><th colspan="2">Clinician Actions</th></tr>
<tr><td>Yellow
Confirmed placement</td><td colspan="2">Carbon dioxide detected (tube is correctly placed)
Leave tube in place and secure it</td></tr>
<tr><td>Tan
Inconclusive placement</td><td colspan="2">Some carbon dioxide detected (needs further assessment)
Ventilate 6 more times (while reassessing tube placement)
Reassess detector for color change; if still tan, leave tube in place and secure it
Attempt to correct any possible cause of low perfusion or low CO_2
Consider direct laryngoscopy to visualize ETT placement</td></tr>
<tr><td rowspan="2">Purple or dark blue
Problem with placement</td><td colspan="2">No carbon dioxide detected (tube incorrectly placed or lack of perfusion)</td></tr>
<tr><td>WITH A PULSE
Assume ventilation problem: Tube incorrectly placed
Extubate
Ventilate with bag-mask device
Reintubate</td><td>WITHOUT A PULSE
Direct laryngoscopy to visualize vocal cords and tube; if tube is not going between cords, proceed with ventilation steps
If tube is between vocal cords on direct visualization and vocal cord marker is below vocal cords, it is likely a perfusion problem
Leave tube in place
Check adequacy of cardiopulmonary resuscitation
Proceed with advanced life support protocol</td></tr>
</table>

Other Resources

Lasa JJ, Dhillon GS, Duff DP, et al. Part 8: Pediatric Advanced Life Support: 2025 American Heart Association and American Academy of Pediatrics Guidelines for Cardiopulmonary Resuscitation and Emergency Cardiovascular Care. *Pediatrics*. 2026;157(1):e2025074351. doi:peds.2025-074351

National Association of State EMS Officials. *National Model EMS Clinical Guidelines, Version 3.0.* National Association of State EMS Officials; 2022. Accessed October 20, 2024. https://nasemso.org/projects/model-ems-clinical-guidelines

Nickson C. Endotracheal tube cuff leak. Life in the Fast Lane. Published July 5, 2024. Reviewed and revised September 8, 2024. Accessed April 14, 2025. https://litfl.com/endotracheal-tube-cuff-leak/

Nowicki T, Jamal Z, London S. Carbon dioxide detector. In: *StatPearls*. [Internet] StatPearls Publishing; 2023. Accessed April 14, 2025. https://www.ncbi.nlm.nih.gov/books/NBK482169/

Procedure 13: Supraglottic Airway Insertion and Difficult Airway Management

Kory Lane, MEd, NRP, FP-C, CCP-C, NCEE
Vishal Naik, MD, MEd, FAAP

Introduction

Many emergency medical services (EMS) systems allow EMS clinicians to perform supraglottic airway (SGA) insertion for assisted ventilation. Currently, there is not enough evidence to show whether these devices are superior to endotracheal intubation or bag-mask ventilation. Research into use as a primary airway modality is ongoing. However, SGA devices are well recognized as a rescue airway for the child with a difficult airway when bag-mask ventilation has failed or endotracheal intubation cannot be achieved.

The EMS clinician should always assess for an anticipated difficult airway when performing airway management. Generally speaking, pediatric airway management is always "difficult" compared with adult airway management, and children with congenital syndromes frequently have very difficult airway anatomy. Two methods discussed here (SGA and gum elastic bougie) are commonly performed in EMS management of the difficult airway.

Difficult airway situations in children include the following:

- Massive head trauma and airway edema
- Hematomas of the mouth or upper airway
- Multisystem injuries
- Infants with significant congenital or acquired airway abnormalities

DIFFICULT AIRWAY

Characteristics of children that are red flags for possible problems in managing the airway include the following history or physical findings:

History

1. History of difficult intubation or problems with ventilation
2. Children with congenital anomalies affecting facial bones and oropharyngeal structures (including the tongue), such as Down syndrome and Pierre-Robin sequence
3. History of recurrent stridor or upper-airway obstruction

Physical Findings

1. Inability to open the mouth widely
2. Difficulty in fully extending the neck
3. Presence of a large tongue or dysmorphic facial features
4. Inability to visualize the entire uvula when depressing the tongue with a tongue blade
5. Trauma to the face, mouth, tongue, or neck

TABLE P13–1 LEMON Mnemonic for Predicting a Difficult Airway

L	Look for external signs of difficult airway such as trauma or large tongue.
E	Evaluate using the 3–3-2–1 rule. The mouth should open at least 3 fingers wide (use size of the patient's finger), the hyoid/mental distance should be at least 3 fingers wide, and the thyroid to hyoid at least 2 fingers wide. The jaw should not subluxate more than 1 cm.
M	Mallampati score should be at least III (3) (**FIGURE P13–1**).
O	Obstruction: Check airway for obstructions such as tumors or hemangiomas and/or trauma.
N	Neck mobility: Assess limitations such as cervical collar, high muscle tone.

A good mnemonic for predicting a difficult airway is LEMON (look, evaluate, Mallampati score [assessment of the relative size of the base of the tongue compared to the oropharyngeal opening in hopes of predicting the difficult airway], obstruction, neck mobility) (**TABLE P13–1**).

Supraglottic Airway Devices

Supraglottic airway devices are widely used in hospitals, primarily for children undergoing short episodes of anesthesia. They are also available as a rescue airway when intubation is difficult. Supraglottic airways have been widely adopted for EMS use over the past decade owing to the relative ease of insertion compared with endotracheal tubes. The SGA is designed for blind insertion (without direct laryngoscopy) and consists of a tube with a mask that sits just above the epiglottis and allows ventilation through the vocal cords and relative blockage of the air down the esophagus. This airway is less secure than an endotracheal intubation, but more so than in bag-mask ventilation.

Many different types of SGA are available from a wide range of manufacturers. Currently, the devices most commonly used by EMS include the soft gel mask and the laryngeal mask. These devices share indications and contraindications, but the insertion procedures differ significantly and will be addressed separately.

INDICATIONS

- Child who requires assisted ventilation
- As a rescue device when bag-mask ventilation has failed
- As a rescue device when endotracheal intubation has failed

CONTRAINDICATIONS

- Responsive patients with intact gag reflex
- Severe upper-airway obstruction or limited mouth opening
- Known esophageal disease
- Caustic ingestion (eg, drain cleaner)

EQUIPMENT

- Appropriately sized SGA
- Water-soluble lubricant
- Syringe (for laryngeal mask; not needed for soft gel mask)
- Oxygen source

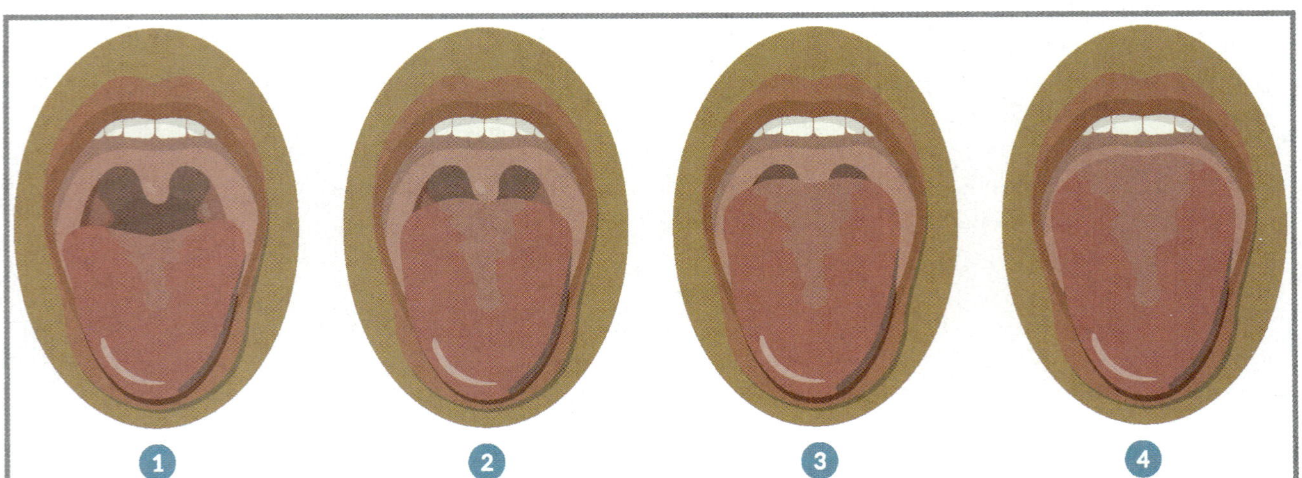

FIGURE P13–1 The Mallampati classifications. 1. Class I: Entire posterior pharynx is fully exposed. 2. Class II: Posterior pharynx is partially exposed. 3. Class III: Posterior pharynx cannot be seen; base of uvula is exposed. 4. Class IV: No posterior pharynx structures can be seen.

- Suction
- Ventilation bag
- Monitors (pulse oximeter, capnograph)

SOFT GEL MASK SUPRAGLOTTIC AIRWAY

The soft gel mask is a SGA device with a soft, gel-like, noninflatable cuff that is designed to fit and adhere over the laryngeal inlet. The soft gel mask was designed for ease and speed of insertion and is the device most widely studied in prehospital use. This device is unique in that it has no cuff to inflate; instead, the gel-like cuff softens at body temperatures and molds to create a seal over the laryngeal inlet. As with other SGAs, it can be used for assisted ventilation or spontaneously breathing patients. As with all SGAs, the soft gel mask may not fully protect against regurgitation and aspiration. The soft gel mask has a built-in bite block, and most sizes have a gastric access port through which a gastric tube can pass for decompression of the stomach.

CAUTION

Do not allow peak airway pressures during ventilation to exceed 40 cm water.

EQUIPMENT

- Appropriately sized soft gel mask

PREPARATION

1. Choose the correct size based on the patient's weight (see **TABLE P13–2** for sizing) or use length-based tape (**Procedure 2, Length/Weight-Based Resuscitation Tape**) to select correct size.
2. Inspect the packaging to ensure there is no damage.
3. Apply water-soluble lubricant to the integral bite block, back, sides, and front of the device.
4. Inspect the device to ensure the airway is patent and there are no foreign bodies or lubricant obstructing the opening of the airway or gastric port.
5. Check that the 15-mm connector fits the patient connection.
6. Place the patient in the sniffing position.

TABLE P13–2 Soft Gel Mask Sizing and Information

Soft Gel Mask	Neonate	Infant	Small Pediatric	Large Pediatric	Small Adult	Regular Adult	Large Adult
Size	1	1.5	2	2.5	3	4	5
Connector color	Pink	Blue	Gray	Clear	Yellow	Green	Orange
Recommended patient weight	2–5 kg	5–12 kg	10–25 kg	25–35 kg	30–60 kg	60–90 kg	90+ kg

Source: https://www.intersurgical.com/info/igel

PROCEDURE 13-1

Soft Gel Mask Insertion

1. Grasp the lubricated soft gel mask firmly at the integral bite block and position the device so the soft cuff outlet is facing toward the chin (soft gel toward the tongue and the hard tip toward the roof of the mouth).

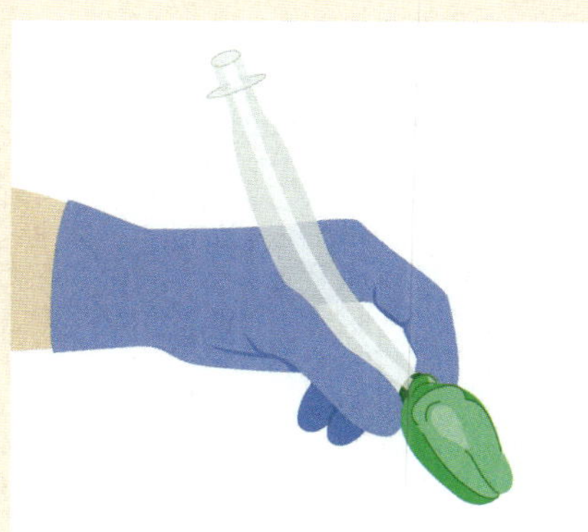

2. With the patient in the sniffing position and with the head extended, open the mouth by pressing the chin down.

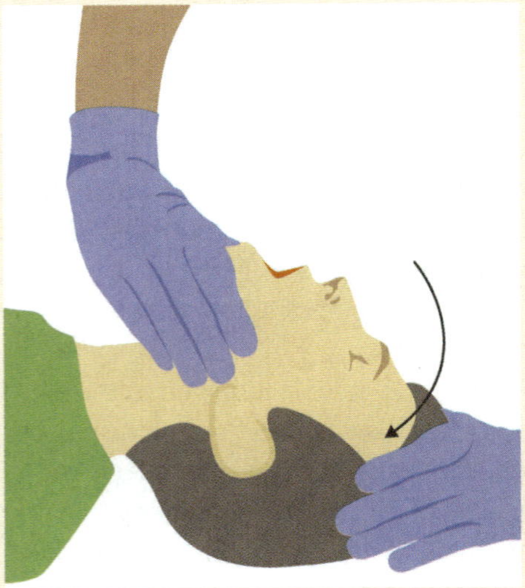

3. Introduce the device into the mouth with the open side toward the tongue and advance the tip toward the hard palate.

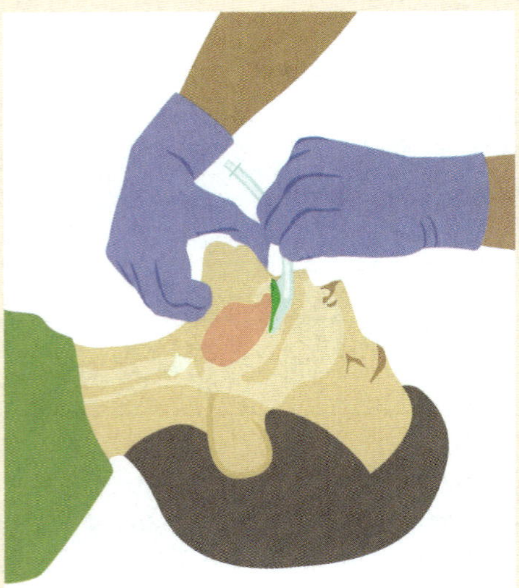

CAUTION

Sometimes a sensation of "giving way" is felt before the end resistance is met owing to the passage of the bowl of the soft gel mask through the faucial pillars (pharyngoepiglottic folds).

4. Glide the device down and back along the hard palate with a gentle continuous push until resistance is felt.

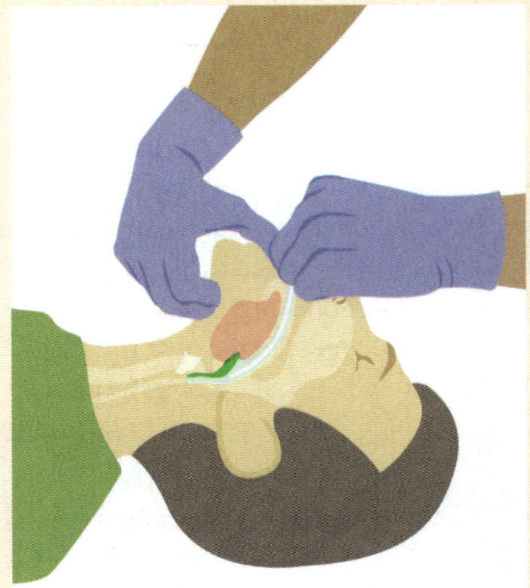

5. Hold the soft gel mask in correct position while the device is being secured with tape or a commercially available device and begin ventilations.

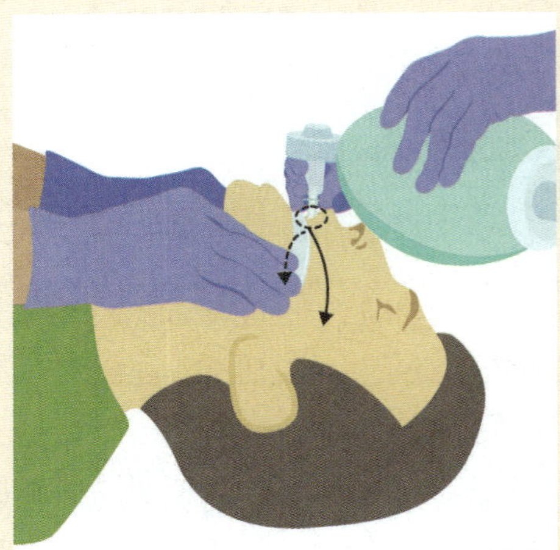

TIP

If the chin-lift method does not open the mouth sufficiently to allow easy advancement of the tube, a laryngoscope or tongue depressor can be directly applied to lift the tongue anteriorly.

LARYNGEAL MASK

The laryngeal mask is a device used frequently in hospitals to ventilate children. It consists of a tube with a distal mask that is inserted into the mouth. When the mask is properly placed, a seal is created over the laryngeal inlet and directs air from the tube into the trachea. A self-inflating bag can be connected to the tube to provide rescue breathing. There are multiple types of laryngeal masks available in pediatric sizes, including a gastric decompression port and/or the ability to intubate through the laryngeal mask. The laryngeal mask has classically been the alternative airway of choice for in-hospital pediatric difficult airway situations, but there is little experience with laryngeal masks in prehospital settings. However, the procedure is simple and fast, and its success rates in hospitals are excellent. The mask is quite flexible before inflation; the tip of the mask can fold backward, or the epiglottis may flip over and prevent good positioning of the laryngeal mask device. In either case, a large air leak would be seen by EMS and inadequate ventilation achieved.

EQUIPMENT

- Appropriately sized laryngeal mask

Preparation

1. Select the correct size based on the patient's weight (see **TABLE P13–3**). Use a length-based tape to estimate weight (**Procedure 2, Length/Weight-Based Resuscitation Tape**).

TABLE P13–3 Laryngeal Mask Size/Cuff Volume According to Patient Weight

Laryngeal Mask Size	Cuff Volume	Weight of Patient
1	4 mL	< 5 kg
1.5	7 mL	5–10 kg
2	10 mL	10–20 kg
2.5	14 mL	20–30 kg
3	20 mL	30–50 kg
4	30 mL	50–70 kg
5	40 mL	> 70 kg
6	50 mL	> 100 kg

2. Select an appropriate resuscitator bag; although a small child can be safely and effectively ventilated using an adult bag, a pediatric bag will not work for a large child. Pediatric tidal volume is approximately 6 to 8 mL/kg. The bag should have a volume of 450 to 750 mL. An adult bag (1,200 mL) is acceptable for larger children or adolescents.

CONTROVERSY

The laryngeal mask has not been studied in children in the prehospital setting, and risks and benefits of its use there are unknown.

3. Connect the oxygen tubing.
4. Once inserted, connect the bag device to the end of the laryngeal mask.

PROCEDURE 13-2

Laryngeal Mask Insertion Methods: Classic

1. Deflate the cuff of the mask if needed.

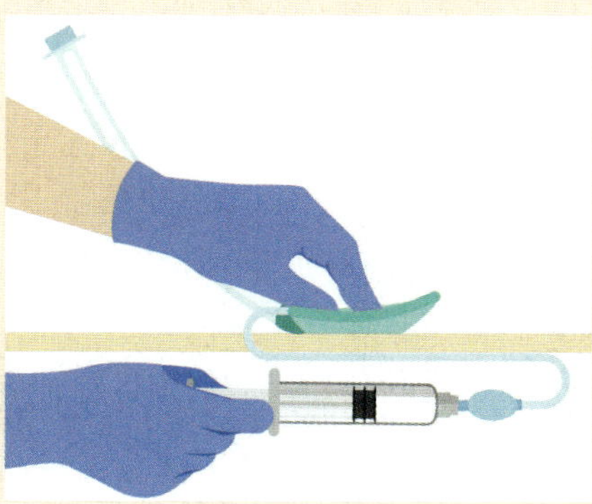

2. Hold the laryngeal mask like a pen, with the index finger of the dominant hand at the junction of the mask and the tube.

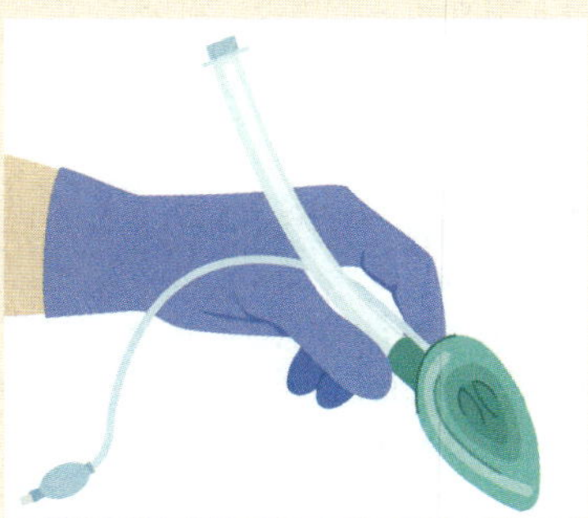

3. Slide the laryngeal mask along the hard palate, pushing it back against the palate as it is advanced toward the hypopharynx. This prevents the tip from folding over on itself and reduces interference from the tongue.

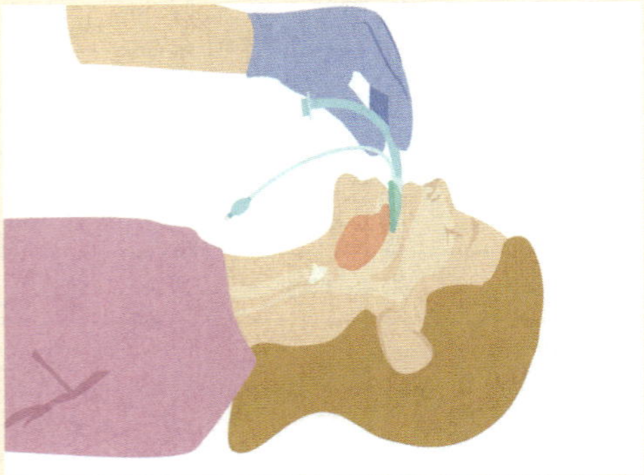

4. Advance with gentle pressure until resistance is met.
5. If necessary, continue pressure on the tube with the nondominant hand to fully advance the laryngeal mask to its proper position.

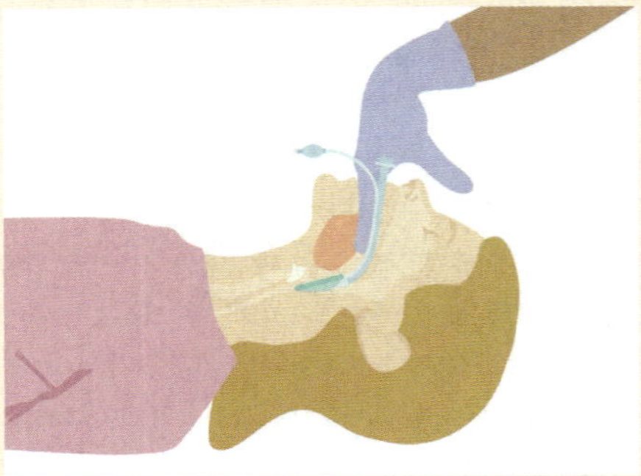

6. Once the laryngeal mask is in place, loosen your grip. Then inflate the cuff, allowing it to acquire its natural position.
7. Attach the laryngeal mask to a bag device.

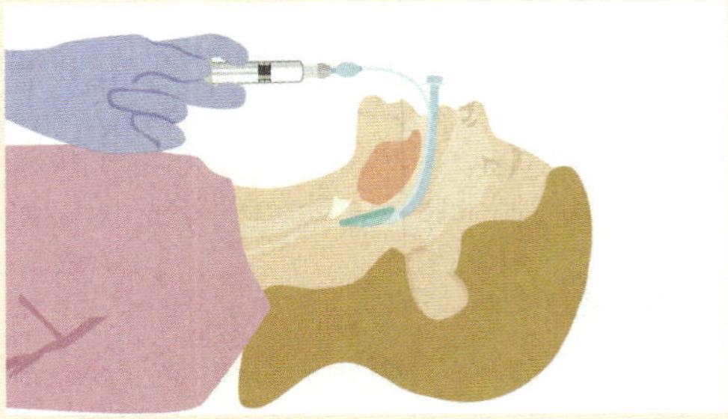

PROCEDURE 13-3

Laryngeal Mask Insertion Methods: 180° Rotation

1. Invert the deflated mask inside out.
2. Insert the laryngeal mask into the mouth in a 180° rotated position, with the mask's orifice facing the palate.
3. Push the laryngeal mask toward the hypopharynx until it enters the pharynx (detected by a sudden loss of resistance). In contrast to the classic method, do not use the index finger as a guide.
4. Turn the laryngeal mask 180° back to its normal position.
5. Inflate the cuff. Apply a water-soluble lubricant to the posterior surface. Rub the lubricant over the anterior hard palate.
6. Attach the laryngeal mask to a bag device.

Gum Elastic Bougie

The gum elastic bougie or ETT introducer is a long, flexible stylet that facilitates insertion of an ETT with limited visualization of the vocal cords. There are several versions of the gum elastic bougie. The classic bougie has a 5-mm diameter and a 38° bend in the distal end. It will work with ETTs larger than 5.0. If the child is old enough, usually $>$8 years, the trachea will have formed cartilaginous rings that allows the operator to feel the ridges when passing the gum elastic bougie to the correct location. The bent end of the semi-rigid bougie can be angled between the cords and advanced into the trachea. As the device brushes against the tracheal rings, the user will receive tactile feedback that the bougie is in the trachea. Once in place, the device serves as a guide for placement of the ETT. For small children needing ETTs 5.0 mm and smaller, there is a 10 French (3.3-mm) bougie that will work with ETTs as small as 3.5 mm. The pediatric version does not have the 38° distal bend, and the trachea of a young child will not provide the same tactile feedback to verify placement. The bougie should be advanced slowly to reduce risk of airway injury.

TIP

A gum elastic bougie is particularly helpful when a very anteriorly placed larynx makes visualization of the cords difficult.

CAUTION

The immature airway (in children <8 years of age) does not contain full cartilaginous rings; therefore, the bougie will not produce the same "click" or tactile feedback to verify tracheal placement. Use in young children requires specialized training and airway experience.

INDICATIONS

- An adjunct for the difficult airway when direct visualization of the vocal cords is impossible because of secretions or blood obstructing the view

CONTRAINDICATIONS

- Major facial trauma
- Laryngeal fracture
- Severe upper airway obstruction
- Endotracheal tube is too small to pass over the bougie

EQUIPMENT

- Gum elastic bougie device in pediatric and adult sizes
- All equipment described under endotracheal tube insertion (ETI) (**Procedure 11, Endotracheal Intubation**)

Preparation

1. Prepare the child for ETI (see **Procedure 11, Endotracheal Intubation**).
2. If using adult size, ensure the distal end of the gum elastic bougie points upward in a J-shape configuration.

PROCEDURE 13-4

Gum Elastic Bougie Device

1. Place the lubricated ETT over the straight end of the gum elastic bougie.
2. Visualize the cords via laryngoscopy.
3. Insert the distal end of the gum elastic bougie through the cords, advancing the device until clicks are palpated, indicating the presence of tracheal rings (if the child is >8 years old).
4. Slide the ETT over the gum elastic bougie into the trachea.
5. Remove the laryngoscope, then the gum elastic bougie.
6. Ensure the ETT is in the trachea by means of end-tidal carbon dioxide detection or an esophageal detector device and that the tube has a correct position at the lips.
7. Attach the ETT to the bag-mask device.
8. Secure the ETT.

Suggested References

ARTICLES

Harris M, Lyng JW, Mandt M, et al. Prehospital pediatric respiratory distress and airway management interventions: an NAEMSP position statement and resource document. *Prehosp Emerg Care*. 2022;26(suppl 1):118–128. doi: 10.1080/10903127.2021.1994675

Procedure 14: Intramuscular Injections

Sean Davis, MSEd, CIC, NRP, FESI-2
Michael J. Stoner, MD, FAAP

Introduction

The intramuscular (IM) route is the preferred route for several lifesaving medications. For others, it is an alternative when vascular access is not available. Some common emergent medications administered IM include epinephrine, midazolam, morphine, and ketamine. Noted benefits of the IM route include quick delivery and availability when inhalation, intravenous (IV), or intraosseous (IO) delivery of the medication is not possible. Intramuscular administration does have limitations, including slower absorption of medication and discomfort or agitation caused by the injection, which is especially important in children.

INDICATION

- Rapid administration of medications when vascular access or other routes are not available or practical

CONTRAINDICATIONS

- Poor perfusion
- Alternative routes are available: oral, inhalation, IV, intranasal, or IO (relative)

EQUIPMENT

- Tuberculin or 3-mL syringe, 22- or 25-gauge needle (⅝- to 1½-inch for IM injection)

Rationale

Intramuscular administration allows the medication to absorb slowly but steadily. The effects of IM medications may take 10 to 20 minutes to materialize but are often quicker. The advantage of the IM technique is ease in delivery. The disadvantages are poor patient acceptance and delayed effect. Avoid IM medication administration in patients with low perfusion, because their absorption is unpredictable. Sometimes, in situations involving a child with low venous pressures, such as in anaphylaxis, IM is an excellent first choice for delivery while vascular access is being attempted.

Preparation

1. Prepare the child to ease stress and anxiety. Explain the procedure using developmentally appropriate terminology. Avoid using the word "shot" or "stick" because the child may associate this with being shot by a gun or being hurt with a stick. Describe the needle stick as a pinch or a poke. Be honest and tell the child it will hurt but be over quickly.
2. Select the medication, noting that some IV and IM medications have different concentrations and/or dosing. Double check for any medication allergies the child may have.
3. Select the appropriate syringe and needle, keeping needles out of the child's sight.

   Needle Length for IM Injection
   - For the ventrogluteal or dorsogluteal sites, use a needle slightly longer than ½ of the distance between the thumb and finger when the skin at the injection site is grasped.
   - For the deltoid and vastus lateralis sites, use a 1-inch needle if the skin is grasped. If the muscle is stretched, use a ⅝-inch needle.
4. Cleanse the top of the medication vial with an alcohol wipe or open the ampule.

5. Withdraw the appropriate volume of medication according to the child's weight-based (milligram per kilogram) dose. Calculate the dose or obtain it from a length-based resuscitation tape or resuscitation software (see **Procedure 2, Length/Weight-Based Resuscitation Tape**).
   - Administer the maximum-volume IM injection at a single site as follows:
     - 2 mL in older children
     - 1 mL in small children and older infants
     - 0.5 mL in small infants
6. Select the appropriate injection site (**TABLE P14–1**).
   Consider the following factors:
   - The volume of medication
   - The condition of the muscle
   - The level of muscle development
   - The type of medication
   - The condition of overlying skin (avoid injecting through infected or damaged skin)
   - The child's ability to be properly positioned
7. Position and secure the child. For an anxious small child, consider letting the caregiver hold the child in one of these ways:
   - Have the child sit on the caregiver's lap, facing to the side. Put one of the child's arms around the caregiver's waist and have the caregiver hold the child close to their chest. The caregiver can hold the child's arms or legs.
   - Position the child straddling the caregiver's lap, sitting chest to chest. Tell the caregiver to hug the child. The caregiver can help to hold an arm or leg.

Possible Complications

- Abscess
- Cellulitis
- Injury to blood vessel, nerve, or tendon
- Redness or swelling at the site
- Adverse reaction to the medication
- Pain at injection site
- Injection into the joint space

TABLE P14–1 Appropriate Sites for IM Injections

Sites	Indications	Landmarks	Considerations	Disadvantages
Deltoid (upper arm)	Use for small volumes of medication; do not exceed volume of 1 mL This is the preferred site for ages > 3 years to adult	Palpate the acromion process and go 2 fingerbreadths (3–5 cm) below it Administer the injection in the upper third of the muscle	Faster absorption rate than gluteal site Fewer side effects from the injection and less painful site	May damage the radial nerve in young children Because of the limited muscle mass, only small volumes of medication can be injected
Dorsogluteal site (buttocks)	Generally discouraged owing to sciatic nerve injury risks but sometimes used for large-volume, oil-based, or thick injections in children older than 3 years and adults	Have the child lie on their stomach and rotate the legs and toes inward Palpate greater trochanter and posterior iliac spine; draw an imaginary line between these 2 points Inject lateral to and above the imaginary line	In an older child, larger volumes of medication (2 mL) can be injected because the muscle mass is larger	Contraindicated in children younger than 2-3 years and those who have not been walking for at least 1 year Medication may inadvertently be injected into fat in an older child with a large fat mass May damage the sciatic nerve, which tracks out from the lower lumbar spine and goes underneath the gluteal muscles

TABLE P14-1 Appropriate Sites for IM Injections—cont'd

Sites	Indications	Landmarks	Considerations	Disadvantages
Vastus lateralis muscle: largest muscle group in children younger than 3 years (thigh)	Use in infants and small children Preferred site for children younger than 3 years	Palpate the greater trochanter and the knee joint; divide the distance into thirds Use middle third for injection site	Can be used for IM injections in young children	Possible thrombosis of the femoral artery More painful than deltoid or gluteal sites
Ventrogluteal muscle: large muscle with few nerves and blood vessels (lateral upper thigh/buttocks)	Use in children of all ages, especially for thick or irritating medications	Have the child lie on their side and bend the upper leg forward in front of the lower leg Palpate greater trochanter and anterior and posterior iliac crests Place palm over greater trochanter with fingers open in a V shape pointing toward iliac crests Inject into center of the V shape	Use well-defined landmarks to identify the site	None

Abbreviations: IM, intramuscular.

PROCEDURE 14-1

Intramuscular Injections

1. The vastus lateralis site (lateral thigh) is the preferred location for infants and small children. The deltoid is preferred for older children. Use the ventrogluteal or dorsogluteal sites if the thigh muscle is not accessible in children older than 3 years.
2. Stretch the skin and insert the needle at a 90° angle.
3. If the patient's muscle mass is small, grasp the body of the muscle between the thumb and forefingers.

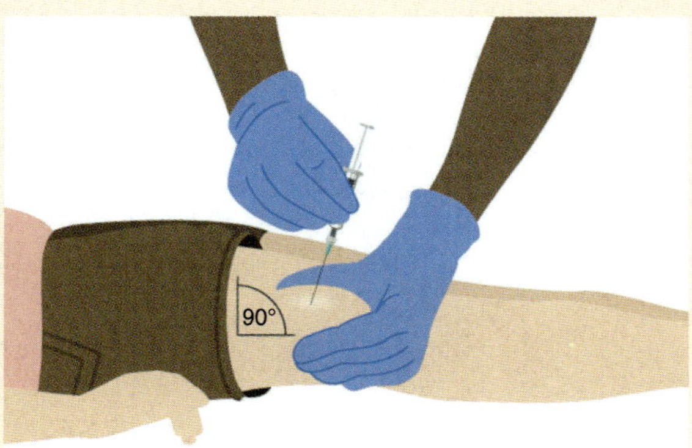

4. Apply gentle pressure to the site with a gauze pad. Do not massage the site.

TIP

Select the injection site according to age, anatomical considerations, muscle development, and volume of medication to be given.

CAUTION

Injection in the dorsogluteal site carries a higher risk of injury to nerve (sciatic nerve) and vasculature (gluteal artery). Avoid this site in children who have not been walking for at least 1 year (those aged < 2-3 years).

PROCEDURE 14-2

After the Injection

1. Activate the safety device over the needle, if applicable.
2. Dispose of the syringe and needle in a sharps container.
3. Praise the child. Apply an adhesive bandage to the site.
4. Write down the name of the medication, dosage, route, time, location of the injection, and any effects.

TIP

The anterolateral thigh (vastus lateralis) is the preferred location for IM injections in children younger than 3 years old.

Suggested References

Rishovd A. Pediatric intramuscular injections. *Am J Maternal/Child Nurs*. 2014;39(2):107–112

Silbergleit R, Durkalski V, Lowenstein D, et al; NETT Investigators. Intramuscular versus intravenous therapy for prehospital status epilepticus. *N Engl J Med*. 2012;366(7):591–600. PMID: 22335736 doi: 10.1056/NEJMoa1107494

Procedure 15: Intranasal Medication Administration

Ann Dietrich, MD, FAAP, FACEP
Robert Sharkey, EMT-P, IC

Introduction

Intranasal medication administration has become a popular route for delivering certain medications in the prehospital setting. It is particularly beneficial when there is no intravenous (IV) access established and urgent medication administration is necessary. Such instances include medications that are needed for pain control, anxiolysis, seizures, and opioid reversal. The highly vascular nasal mucosa allows certain medications to rapidly achieve therapeutic drug concentrations. Delivery of intranasal medication is also relatively painless and easy and can be administered via the droplet or atomized method.

INDICATIONS

- Pain control
- Anxiolysis
- Sedation
- Seizure control
- Opioid reversal

CONTRAINDICATIONS

- Secure IV/intraosseous access (relative)
- Cardiac arrest
- Head trauma with altered level of consciousness
- Facial trauma
- Nasal septal deformity, obstruction, or recent surgery
- Epistaxis
- Recent use of nasally administered vasoconstrictors (eg, cocaine, oxymetazoline, phenylephrine) may limit absorption of medications administered intranasally (relative)

EQUIPMENT

- 1-mL Luer-lock syringe
- Blunt filtered needle (if drawing from a glass ampule)
- Mucosal atomization device (MAD)
- Gloves

Rationale

The rich vascular plexus of the nasal cavity provides a direct route into the bloodstream for small, simple, lipophilic-molecule medications to easily cross mucous membranes. The direct absorption into the bloodstream of many intranasal medications bypasses the first-pass metabolism of enteric medications and allows for plasma concentrations to be comparable with those of IV medications and typically better than those of medications administered via subcutaneous or intramuscular routes. Intranasal drug administration is essentially painless and is often an easier route by which to administer certain medications than is IV when an IV line has not already been established.

Limitations

A limited list of medications have data to support intranasal administration. Common examples include midazolam, fentanyl, ketamine, naloxone, hydromorphone, haloperidol, and glucagon.

Studies suggest the ideal volume per nostril is 0.2 to 0.3 mL. In practice, the maximum volume for a single administration into one nostril is 0.5 mL in pediatric patients and 0.1 mL in neonates. Larger volumes should be divided equally, with half the dose in each nostril. Therefore, the available concentration of the medication and resulting total volume can be a limitation.

The molecular size and composition of the medication also play a role. Medications that are lipophilic and have a small molecule size have the best absorption. The physiologic pH of the nasal mucosa is 5.0 to 7.0. Medications outside this pH range may cause irritation and affect absorption.

Intranasal delivery will be less effective if there is obstruction resulting from a nasal foreign body or secretions, or if the mucosa is swollen (as seen with allergies or an upper respiratory infection). The clinician should remove any devices such as a nasopharyngeal airway or a nasogastric tube before attempting to use the nostril.

Preparation

1. Perform hand hygiene and don gloves.
2. Ensure the medication can be administered via the intranasal route.
3. Determine the volume of medication to be administered. If the volume of medication is greater than 0.5 mL, then divide the volume equally between each nostril. If the volume per nostril exceeds 0.5 mL, the dose should be administered in 2 separate applications 5 to 10 minutes apart. Spacing between doses allows the previous dose to be absorbed.
4. Draw the prescribed amount of medication into a 1-mL Luer-lock syringe. If using a MAD, draw an additional 0.1 mL of medication to account for dead space in the syringe and MAD.
5. Remove the needle from the syringe and dispose of it properly, in a sharps container.
6. Position the patient supine or held by caregiver with head tilted back.
7. If the child is awake, explain what you are going to do in age-appropriate terms.

PROCEDURE 15-1

Intranasal Administration Using a Mucosal Atomization Device

1. Connect the MAD to the syringe by twisting it in place.

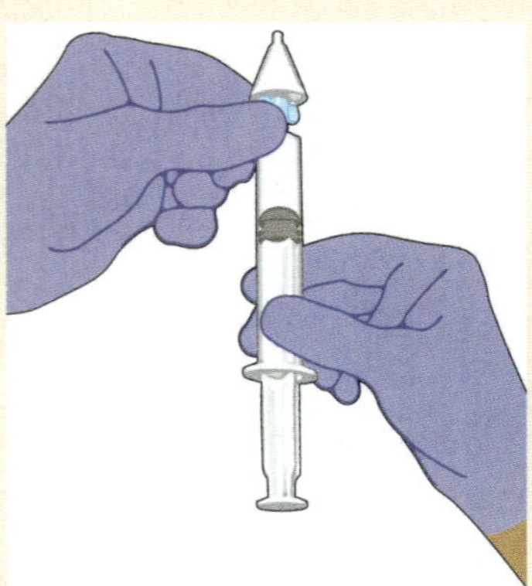

2. Inspect the nostril for anything that might impair the absorption of the medication.

3. Use your free hand to hold the crown of the head stable.

4. Place the tip of the MAD into the nostril, aiming it up and slightly outward (toward the top of the ear).

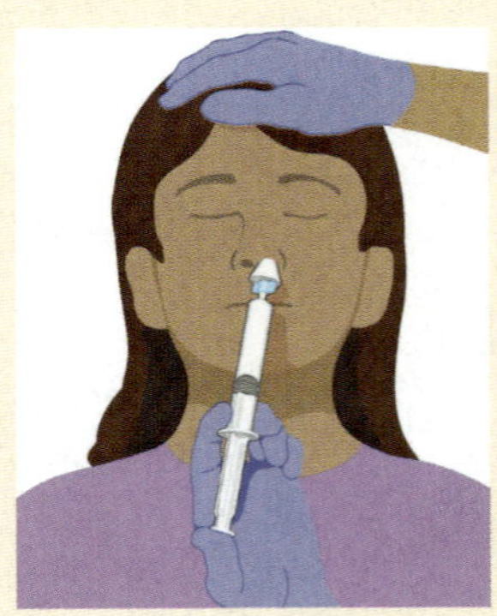

5. Briskly compress the syringe plunger to deliver medication.
6. Remove the syringe from the patient's nostril.

TIP
Ensure the atomizer is firmly attached to the tip of the syringe.

TIP
In neonates or small children, removal of the foam tip may provide a better fit.

PROCEDURE 15-2

Intranasal Administration Using the Drip Method

1. Inspect the nostril for anything that might impair the absorption of the medication.
2. Use your free hand to hold the crown of the head stable and place the patient's head in a sniffing position.
3. Slowly depress the syringe plunger to drip the medication into the patient's nostril and administer a few drops at a time.

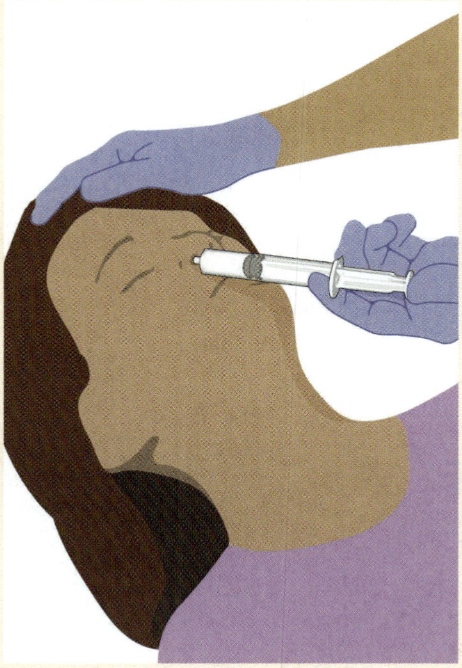

Suggested References

Emergency Nurses Association. Clinical practice guideline: intranasal medication administration. Accessed April 15, 2025. https://media.emscimprovement.center/documents/Intranasal_Medication_Administration.pdf

Wolfe T. Therapeutic intranasal drug delivery. Accessed April 15, 2025. http://www.intranasal.net

Procedure 16: Intravenous Access

Elizabeth Blizzard, BA, NRP, FP-C, CCP-C
Theresa A. Walls, MD, MPH, FAAP

Introduction

Establishing intravenous (IV) access is a time-honored method of fluid and drug administration. However, unlike in an adult, securing IV access in a pediatric patient is often difficult or impossible in the prehospital setting. Fortunately, most pediatric patients do not require IV access before emergency department (ED) arrival, and many prehospital medications do not require an IV route for administration.

INDICATIONS

- Cardiopulmonary arrest
- Shock
- Trauma
- Cardiac dysrhythmia
- Illness or injury possibly requiring immediate IV drug or fluid administration
- Consider vascular access on the way to the ED when there is multisystem injury

CONTRAINDICATIONS

- Availability of another reliable administration route
- Brief transport time
- Limited available vasculature (available vessels of substantial quality to access)
- Consider intraosseous access as initial modality for time-sensitive, critical illness

EQUIPMENT

- Intravenous catheters, 14- to 24-gauge
- Intravenous tubing (macrodrip or microdrip)
- Extension connector
- Intravenous solution
- Rubber band or elastic band tourniquet
- Adhesive tape or adhesive transparent dressing
- Gauze pad
- Alcohol pad
- Pediatric arm board

Rationale

Intravenous access makes it easier to administer medications and provides a route for fluid therapy in illness or injuries in which there is possible blood or fluid loss. Intravenous delivery is the reference standard for delivering medications because it permits predictable delivery and more rapid onset of action for most important drugs. The indications for IV access must be carefully weighed against common complications and possible risks associated with the procedure. These include distraction from airway and breathing management, possible delays in ED care, and causing excessive pain to the child. Also, there is a risk for the prehospital professional involving exposure to bloodborne pathogens. However, in certain children, such as the critically ill child experiencing shock, IV therapy in the field can be lifesaving.

Preparation

1. Assemble the equipment. Select the appropriate IV solution and tubing.
   - Inspect the solution for cloudiness, expiration date, leakage, or contamination. Verify the solution name.

- Use microdrip IV tubing or a saline lock for administering medications. For fluid administration, use a macrodrip in older children; small children may require a pump, a controlled infusion device, or a push-pull system to prevent administration of excessive amounts of fluid.
- For medication administration, consider a saline lock: a male Luer-lock device with an injection port and a sterile normal saline flush.
- Spike the fluid bag with the tubing, clamp the tubing, squeeze the drip chamber until it is half full, open the clamp, and flush the tubing.
- Select the appropriate catheter, depending on the need for fluid volume. Use a smaller catheter when only medications are indicated.

2. Prepare the child and family for the procedure. Use developmentally appropriate language to explain the procedure.
   - Allowing a parent or caregiver to hold the child during the procedure, if feasible, may reduce distress. Distracting the child during the procedure is also often helpful.
   - If time allows, explain the procedure to the child first (using terminology they can understand) and consider demonstrating it on a stuffed animal or another toy.
   - Do not lie to the child about the procedure; be realistic, but emphasize the short duration of pain and the importance of the procedure. For example, say, "You will feel a quick pinch, but the pain won't last long, and afterward I can give you medicine to make you feel better."
   - Do not ask the child if they want an IV unless their refusing it is a legitimate choice. Instead, offer a neutral choice such as "Do you want the IV here or there?" This allows the child to have some control over the situation without placing the clinician in a position of having to overrule the answer the child gave.
   - A possible script for explaining an IV to a child would be as follows: "I need to place a small straw into your arm so I can give you medicine to help you get better. This needle helps me get the straw in, but it won't be in your arm for long." As with describing the pain of the procedure, do not lie to the child about the presence of a needle, but do emphasize the need for it and that it will not be there for long.
3. Select the site.
   - The best IV sites in the infant are the hands, the antecubital fossa, and the saphenous vein at the ankle or feet. The dorsum (back) of the hand is a good site in chubby infants. To access the back of the hand, grasp the child's hand with the fingers closed and flex the wrist downward (**FIGURE P16-1**).
   - In toddlers and older children, potential IV sites are the hands and antecubital areas. Use the child's nondominant extremity if possible. When feasible, allowing the child to choose where they want the IV can help them feel in control.
   - Ideally, avoid inserting the catheter over a joint.
   - Consider the antecubital fossa when fluid boluses are required because veins that are more distal in the forearm or hand are usually smaller.
   - Hand veins are often mobile under the skin and may move with contact with the catheter. Maintain firm tension on the skin during the initial puncture to keep the vein in place.
4. Position the patient supine, or in the caregiver's lap if the child is younger than school age. Secure

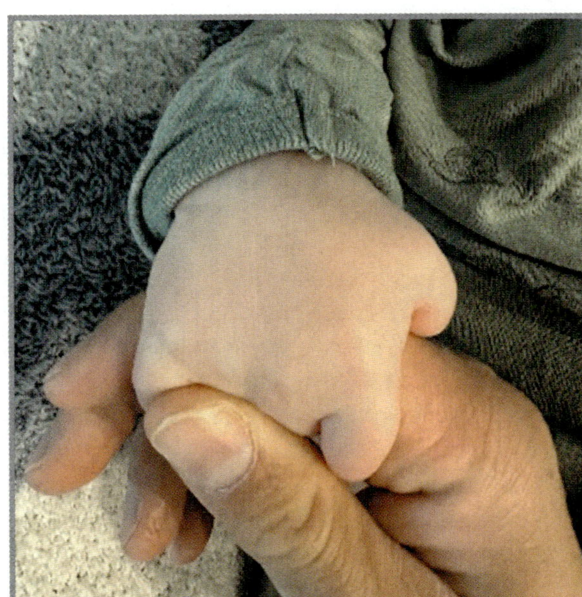

FIGURE P16-1 Accessing the back of the infant hand for an IV site.

John Creagh, MD

the child's legs and arms to avoid flailing. The caregiver can help hold the child and immobilize the insertion site.

5. Apply the rubber band or tourniquet proximal to the entry site. Do not make it too tight. The tourniquet should not block arterial flow. If it is necessary to make the vein more visible, do the following:
   - Place the extremity in a dependent position.
   - Tap or massage the site.
   - Ask an older child to clench and unclench their fist.
6. Consider using a local anesthetic spray, if permitted by local medical protocols, to decrease patient pain. This is sometimes described as "magic spray" and can help make the child less frightened.
7. Cleanse the site with antiseptic solution such as chlorhexidine gluconate with alcohol, isopropyl alcohol, or povidone-iodine.

TIP

When describing the procedure to a child, be honest about what will happen while explaining it in simple terms appropriate to the child's age—for example, "You will feel a quick pinch" and "The IV is like a straw to help give you medicine."

TIP

If IV access is solely for administering medication, use microdrip tubing or a saline lock. For administering fluid, use macrodrip tubing.

CAUTION

Never delay transport in any critically injured infant or child; consider attempting IV access while en route to the hospital.

TIP

Position the child and secure the site before beginning the procedure.

PROCEDURE 16-1

Intravenous Access

1. Insert the needle. Stabilize the vein by pulling the skin taut distally from the insertion site. Insert the catheter through the skin with the bevel up, at a 30° angle. Insert the catheter slowly; blood return may be delayed for a few seconds. When there is visible blood in the hub of the catheter, advance the needle slightly, fully advance the catheter into the vein, and then remove the needle. Never pull the catheter back over the needle, because this may cause shearing of the catheter tip. Release the tourniquet. Compress the vein proximal to the site to prevent blood loss through the catheter (if it is not self-occluding) while connecting the tubing. It is also helpful to position a gauze pad under the catheter at this point. Connect the tubing or male Luer lock to the catheter. If a saline lock (a male Luer lock with an injection port) is used, a 2- to 5-mL saline flush should be used to maintain patency.
2. Stabilize the catheter with tape or transparent adhesive dressing. Avoid placing an excess amount of tape or gauze over the site, because it obstructs the view of the site. Use a clear medicine cup or other device to protect the site while allowing access and visualization.

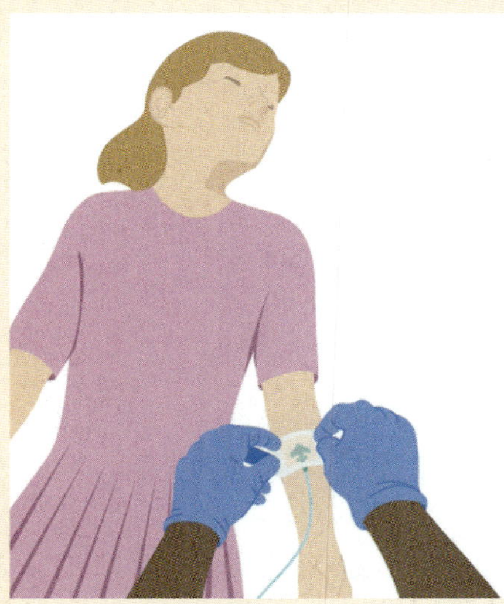

3. Immobilize the extremity. Be careful not to apply the tape too tightly, because this blocks the flow of blood through the vein.
4. Monitor the solution drip rate to avoid administering too much or too little fluid.
5. Dispose of the needle properly.

Troubleshooting

1. If the fluid is not infusing properly, take the following steps:
   - Make sure the tourniquet has been released.
   - Make sure the child's arm is not bent.
   - Make sure the tape is not too tight.
   - Make sure the tubing is not kinked.
   - Make sure the clamp is open.
   - Lower the fluid bag below the extremity and assess for a backflow of blood into the tubing.
   - Raise the fluid bag higher, if possible.
2. If none of the above measures is effective, discontinue the IV and restart it in another site.

Possible Complications

- Pain
- Infiltration (observe for pain or edema at the site, inability to infuse fluids, or lack of blood return; discontinue IV and insert it at another site)
- Hypothermia resulting from administering too much room-temperature fluid to an infant
- Skin or bloodstream infection
- Extravasation (leaking of vesicant drugs into surrounding tissue)
- Thrombophlebitis
- Inadvertent fluid overload
- Catheter shear
- Inadvertent arterial puncture

CONTROVERSY

Few children require IV access in the field or on the way to the ED. Most injured children should be transported before IV access is attempted. For ill children, especially if there is a short transport time, the determination of which ones need IV access and whether IV access is beneficial to the patient or causes undue anxiety or stress to the child is controversial. It is important to carefully weigh the benefits against the risks before inserting an IV in a child in the prehospital setting.

CAUTION

Be careful not to secure the tape too tightly to immobilize the extremity, because this blocks blood flow in the vein.

TIP

Reward and comfort the child after the procedure.

Procedure 17: Intraosseous Needle Insertion

Archana Reddy Bongurala, MD, FAAP
Dawn Poetter, Oregon Paramedic

Introduction

Establishing vascular access is often difficult or impossible during life-threatening emergencies in infants and young children. The intraosseous (IO) route for the delivery of resuscitation fluids and medications has been used since the early to mid-1900s, and many studies have confirmed that the IO space is an excellent route for administering medications and fluids in children and adults. The primary technical problem is successfully piercing the bony cortex (the outer layer of the bone) in older children. The bones of neonates and infants are usually soft and the intramedullary space is relatively large, so needle insertion is easier in younger children. Good equipment, preparation, and effective technique are especially important for success.

INDICATION

Severe illness or injury requiring immediate administration of drugs or fluids in cases in which intravenous (IV) access is unsuccessful or unlikely to be possible

CONTRAINDICATIONS

- Available secure IV line
- Fracture or deformity in same bone as insertion site
- Previous attempt in same bone
- Skin or soft-tissue infection over insertion site
- Osteogenesis imperfecta

EQUIPMENT

- Intraosseous needle/insertion device
- Skin cleansing solution
- Normal saline and IV tubing
- 10-mL syringe
- Extension connector and 3-way stopcock (optional)

Rationale

Using an IO needle to give drugs or fluids is an excellent alternative to cannulating peripheral veins in critically ill or injured children. The IO space is highly vascular and functions as a temporary, noncollapsible access. Needle insertion into this space is quick, simple, effective, and usually quite safe. Several sites can be used for intraosseous access, including the sternum, clavicle, humeral head, iliac crest, distal femur, proximal tibia, distal tibia, and calcaneus. The distal femur, proximal tibia, and distal tibia are generally preferred for infants and neonates owing to their ease of access and reduced risk of complications in these age groups. The IO space is suitable for infusion of all parenteral medications, crystalloid fluids, or blood products, which are quickly absorbed from small veins of the bone into the central circulation. Complications are usually minor and infrequent.

Preparation

TIBIA AND FEMUR SITES

1. Place the patient in the supine position.
2. Put a small towel roll under the knee.
3. Clean the skin over the insertion site with an antiseptic solution.

Possible Complications

- Compartment syndrome
- Failed infusion
- Growth plate injury (especially in young children)
- Bone infection (osteomyelitis)
- Skin infection
- Bone fracture

PROCEDURE 17-1

Traditional Intraosseous Insertion

1. Pierce the bony cortex with a firm, twisting motion. Use a back-and-forth twisting motion to enter the marrow space. Do not push hard on the needle. A "pop" may be felt as the needle passes through the bony cortex and into the marrow cavity.

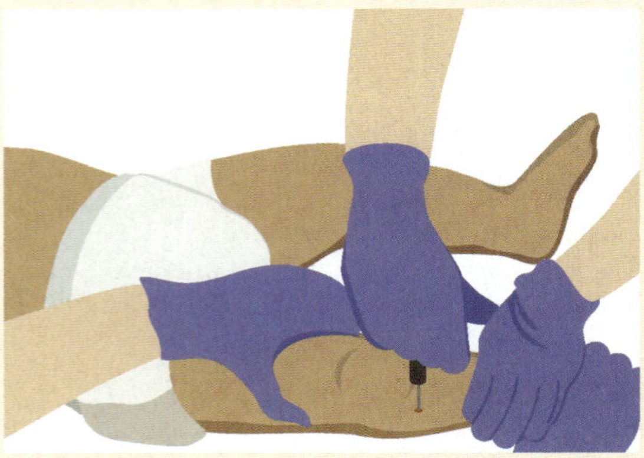

2. Remove the stylet and aspirate the marrow contents. Keep any bone marrow aspirate for glucose check or for other tests in the emergency department. Sometimes, marrow cannot be aspirated. Confirm correct placement by infusing 10 mL of normal saline without resistance or swelling in the soft tissue adjacent to or behind the needle.

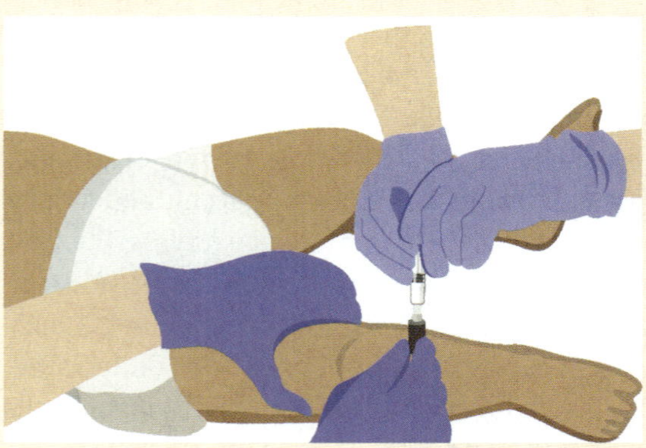

3. Attach IV line to the hub, or to an extension connector and stopcock, and infuse fluids or drugs directly into the IO space.

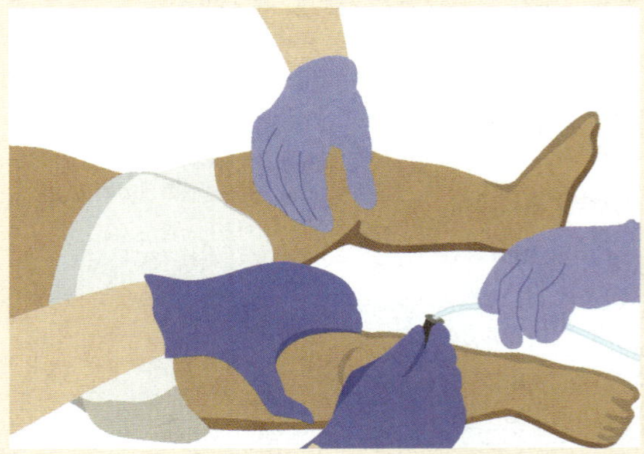

4. Secure the needle to the overlying skin with tape. Monitor the surrounding soft tissue to ensure that there is no swelling to indicate leakage of fluid.

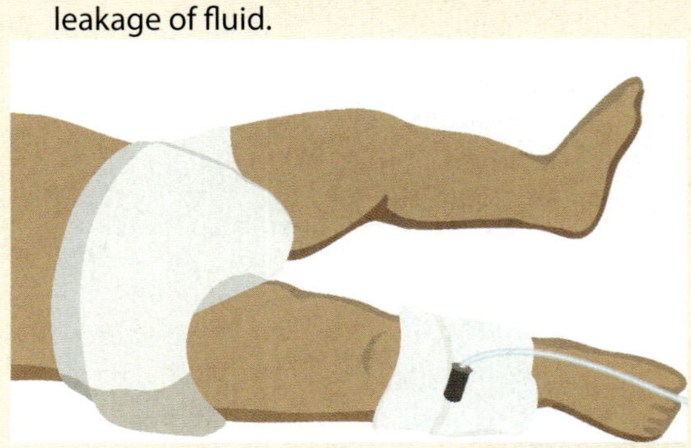

5. Continuously infuse fluids to maintain the patency of the IO line.

6. Do not use an infusion pump to deliver fluids; use the "push-pull" method by using a 3-way stopcock, or use a pressure bag.

TIP

When placing a traditional IO needle, use firm pressure and a twisting motion.

CAUTION
Insert the IO needle gently. Too much force may push the needle all the way through the bone and into the soft tissues.

CAUTION
Avoid placing your hand behind the insertion site to prevent possible injury resulting from through-and-through IO needle penetration.

PROCEDURE 17-2

Mechanical IO Insertion

An alternate to the traditional manual IO is the mechanical IO (**FIGURE P17-2-1**). Some devices are FDA cleared for IO access only in children weighing 3 kg or more in the proximal humerus, distal femur, proximal tibia, and distal tibia. Review the manufacturer's specifications to become familiar with approved weight ranges for your device.

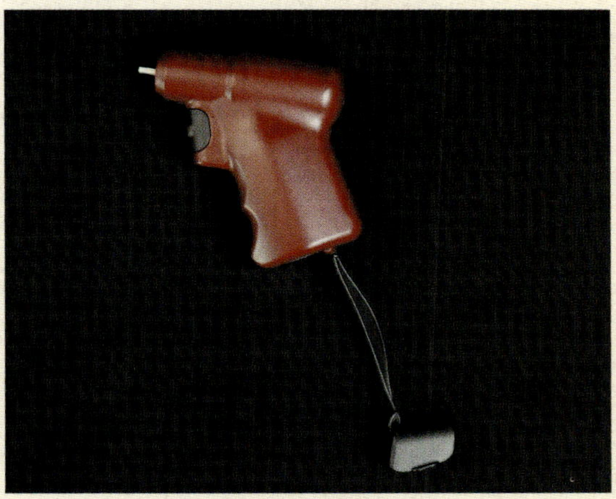

FIGURE P17-2-1 A mechanical IO drill.

1. After palpating the insertion site, select the appropriate needle for the patient according to the patient's weight and anatomy and to the clinician's judgment. The mechanical IO 45-mm needle set (yellow hub) should be considered for proximal humerus insertion in patients weighing 40 kg or more, and for patients who have excessive tissue over any insertion site. The mechanical IO 25-mm needle set (blue hub) should be considered for patients weighing 3 kg or more.
2. Attach the needle to the mechanical IO drill.
3. Position the needle and mechanical IO drill at 90° to the bone for all sites except the proximal humerus, for which the needle and drill should be at a 45° angle to the anterior plane and posteromedial. With the tip of the needle set touching bone, the 5-mm marker must be visible above the skin for confirmation of adequate length before drilling. Press the trigger on the drill handle and apply gentle pressure, while letting the drill do the work for you. When you feel the "pop," you have gained access; immediately release the trigger, avoiding recoil. Do *not* pull back on the driver when releasing the trigger. As with traditional IO insertion, refrain from placing your other hand behind the insertion site to prevent possible palm penetration resulting from excessive force.

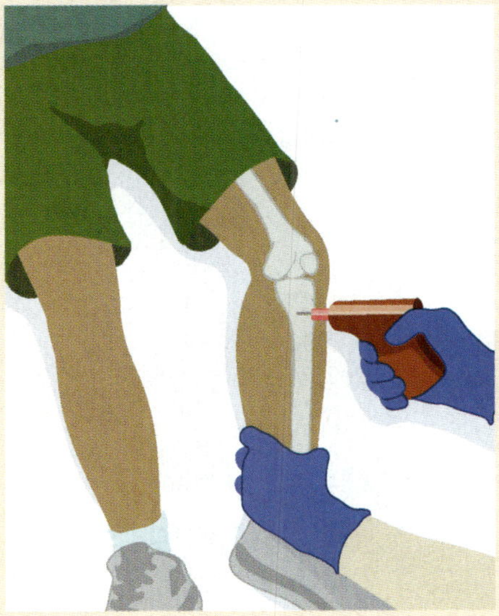

4. Disconnect the mechanical IO drill while stabilizing the needle set to avoid dislodgement from the medullary space.

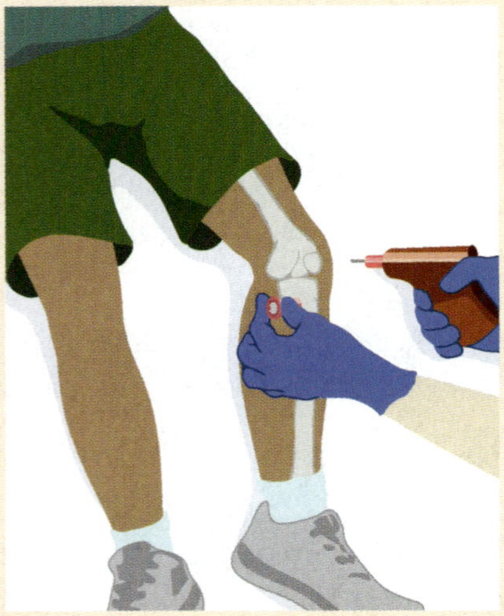

CAUTION
If the drill stops, you are pushing too hard.

5. Withdraw the needle stylet and confirm placement by aspirating blood with the syringe; however, the inability to aspirate blood does not necessarily indicate improper placement. Confirm correct placement by infusing 10 mL of normal saline without resistance or swelling in the soft tissue adjacent to or behind the needle.

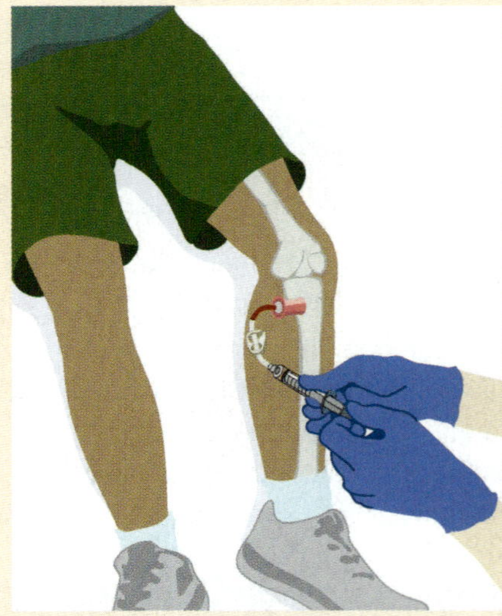

PROCEDURE 17-3

Proximal Tibia Site

1. Use the flat surface of the proximal medial tibia, just below and medial to the tibial tuberosity on the flat side of the bone.

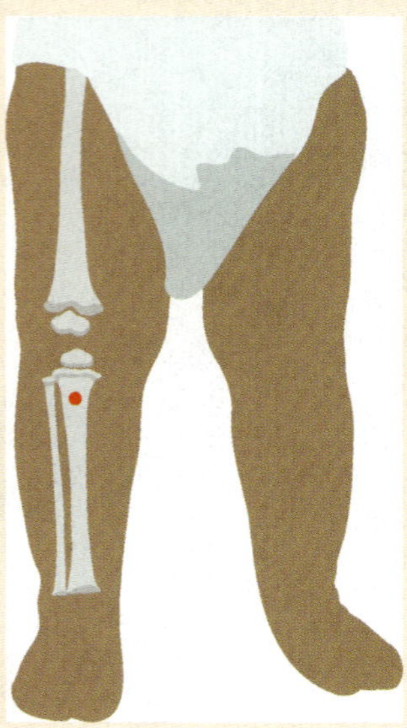

2. Introduce the traditional IO needle in the skin directed away from the growth plate or pointing toward the foot until the tip touches the bone. The mechanical IO is inserted at a 90° angle, but avoid the growth plate, and follow the previously detailed steps for insertion into the intramedullary space.

PROCEDURE 17-4

Distal Tibia Site

1. Use the flat surface of the medial distal tibia above the medial malleolus.

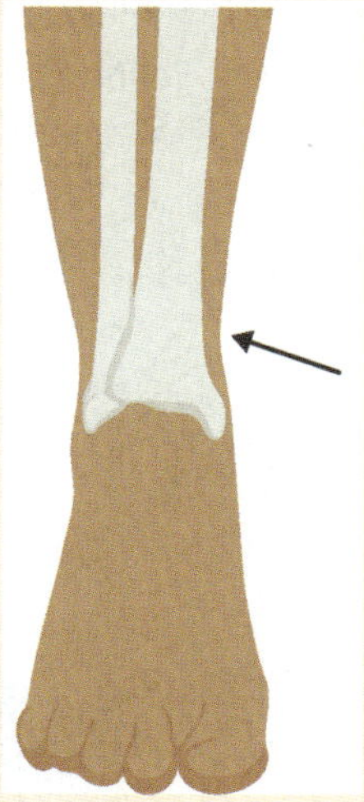

2. Introduce the traditional IO needle in the skin directed away from the growth plate or toward the knee until the tip touches the bone. Insert the mechanical IO at a 90° angle, but avoid the growth plate. Follow the previously detailed steps for insertion into the intramedullary space.

PROCEDURE 17-5

Distal Femur Site

1. Use the distal third of the femur, estimate the distance through soft tissue to reach the bony surface of the femur, and ensure that the correct length of needle is chosen or that the needle has been adjusted to a length that allows bony penetration.

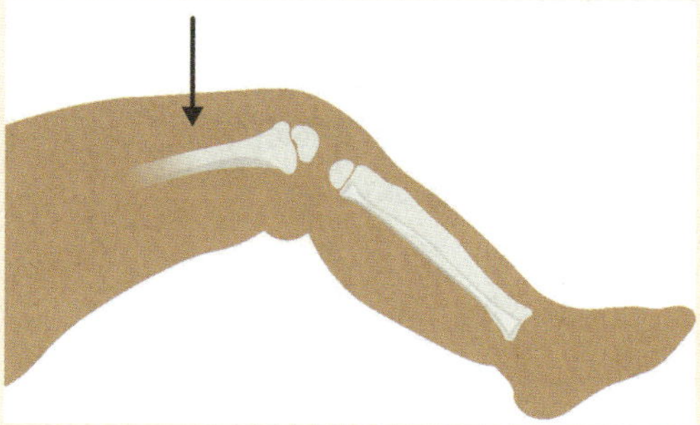

2. Introduce the traditional IO needle in the skin, directed away from the growth plate or pointing toward the trunk until the tip touches the bone. The mechanical IO is inserted at a 90° angle, but avoid the growth plate. Follow the previously detailed steps for insertion into the intramedullary space.

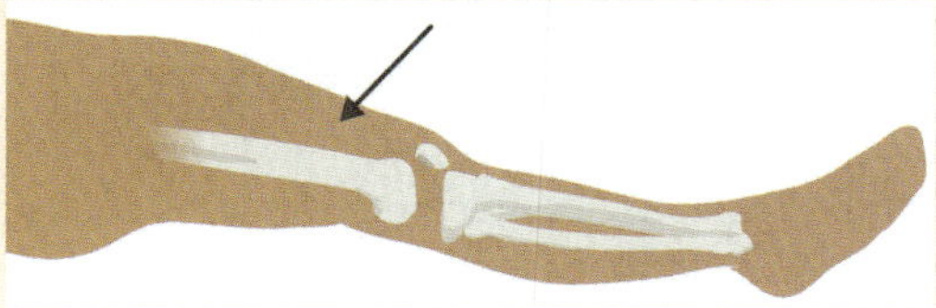

PROCEDURE 17-6

Proximal Humerus Site

1. With the child's hand resting on their abdomen and their elbow held close to their body (**FIGURE PR17–6–1**), place the palm of your hand on the child's shoulder. This area, which feels like a "ball," is the proximal humerus. Place one hand vertically in the axilla, with your fifth digit against the skin. Then take your other hand and place it vertically in the midline of the upper arm, with your fifth digit against the skin. Cradle the humerus so your thumbs meet in the middle. This is the vertical line of insertion. Use 1 thumb to climb up the humerus until a "notch" or "groove" is felt; this is the surgical neck.

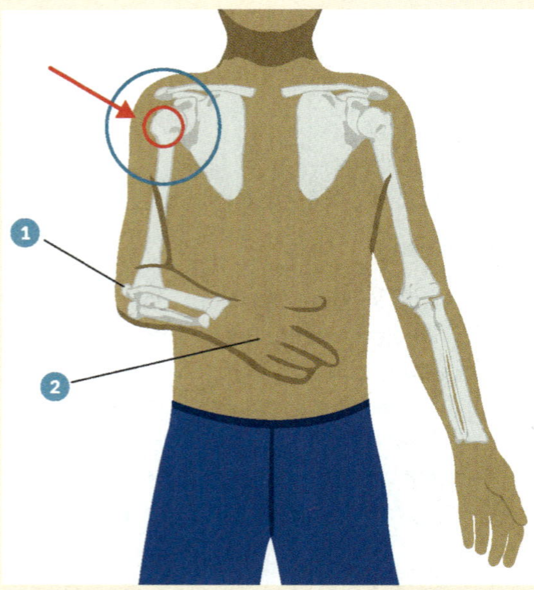

FIGURE PR17–6–1 1. Elbow should remain adducted and posteriorly located. 2. Place the hand over the umbilicus for humeral positioning and safety.

2. The insertion point for the IO needle is located approximately 1 cm above the surgical neck until the tip touches the bone (**FIGURE PR17–6–2**). Follow the steps below for insertion into the intramedullary space.
3. Secure the arm in place to prevent accidental dislodgement of the IO catheter.

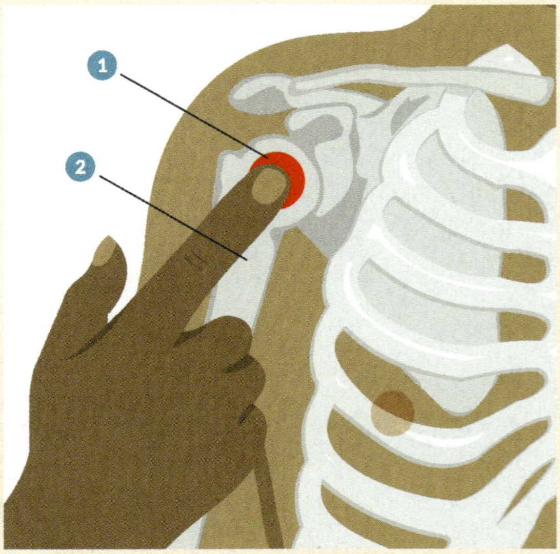

FIGURE PR17–6–2 1. Insertion point. 2. Surgical neck.

CAUTION

The proximal humerus should be used for IO insertions only in children whose appropriate anatomical landmarks can be identified. Humeral IOs often dislodge during patient care and movement.

Procedure 18: Cardiopulmonary Resuscitation

T.J. Bishop, AS, NRP, NCEE
Kayla Long, DO, MS, MAPP, FACEP, FAEMS

Introduction

Cardiopulmonary arrest (CPA) occurs when a patient's heart and lungs stop functioning. In children, CPA usually begins as a primary respiratory arrest. This contrasts with adults, in whom CPA or "sudden death" is almost always a primary cardiac event that occurs with onset of ventricular fibrillation (VF) and an abrupt change in the heart's electrical activity. Because cessation of effective breathing is often the precipitating factor in pediatric CPA, airway management and ventilation are to children in CPA what defibrillation is to adults.

Cardiopulmonary resuscitation (CPR) refers to chest compressions, airway management, and breathing via ventilations (circulation, airway, breathing [CAB]) to provide oxygen and circulation to core organs: the heart, brain, and lungs. In children, CPR has been shown to improve survival of drowning, and it may also benefit patients in CPA resulting from other causes. Asphyxial cardiac arrest is more common than VF cardiac arrest in infants and children; thus, ventilation is extremely important in pediatric resuscitation.

INDICATIONS

- Newborn, neonate, infant, or child of any age who is apneic and pulseless
- Newborn, infant, or child with a heart rate less than 60 beats/min whose condition does not improve after ventilation
- Neonates, infants, and children with a heart rate less than 60 beats/min and poor perfusion

CONTRAINDICATION

- Newborn, neonate, infant, or child with sustained, effective perfusion

EQUIPMENT

- Mouth-to-mask device
- Neonate, infant, child bag-valve-mask devices with appropriately sized masks
- Airway adjuncts

Rationale

Cardiopulmonary resuscitation encompasses the basic procedures recommended by the American Heart Association for sustaining critical oxygenation, ventilation, and perfusion. The pediatric techniques are modified from the adult techniques to reflect the known differences in CPA between age groups. Furthermore, there are specific differences between newborns/neonates, infants, and children, including number of rescuers required, placement of hands, rates of ventilation, and rates and depth of chest compressions.

Preparation

- Position the child on a hard surface.

Pediatric Assessment

1. Perform airway, breathing, circulation (ABC) assessment if patient is awake and moving.
2. If the patient is unresponsive and not adequately breathing (gasps do not count as breathing), perform the CAB assessment, beginning with checking the pulse.
3. If no pulse is centrally palpated in 10 seconds, or if the heart rate is less than 60 beats/min, start chest compressions (see ratios in **TABLE P18–1**).
4. If the heart rate is less than 60 beats/min, ventilate with a bag valve mask device for 30 to 60 seconds. If the heart rate does not increase to 60 beats/min, start chest compressions.
   - Newborn/Neonate basic life support (BLS) guidelines apply from birth to hospital discharge.
   - Infant BLS guidelines apply to infants younger than 1 year.
   - Child BLS guidelines apply to children aged 1 year to puberty. Puberty is defined as breast development in girls and the presence of axillary hair in boys.
   - Adult BLS guidelines apply at and beyond puberty.

HIGH-QUALITY CPR

High-quality CPR is defined by the following:

1. Chest compressions are of appropriate rate and depth.
2. Push fast: Push at a rate of 100 to 120 compressions per minute. Use of a metronome or other audio/visual prompting device is highly recommended.
3. Push hard: Push with sufficient force to depress at least one-third the anteroposterior (AP) diameter of the chest, or approximately 1.5 inches (4 cm) in infants and 2 inches (5 cm) in children.
4. Allow complete chest recoil after each compression to allow the heart to refill with blood. Incomplete recoil during CPR is associated with higher intrathoracic pressures and significantly decreased venous return, coronary perfusion, blood flow, and cerebral perfusion.
5. Minimize interruptions of chest compressions to a hands-off time of 10 seconds or less.
6. Avoid excessive ventilation. Consider placing an orogastric or a nasogastric tube to eliminate gastric inflation.
7. See ratios in **TABLE P18–1** for ratio of chest compressions to ventilation.
8. Rescuers should rotate the compressor role every 2 minutes to avoid fatigue.

TABLE P18–1 Chest Compressions to Ventilation Ratios

Age	Compressions (min)/Ratios	Depth (inches)	Hand Placement
Newborn/Neonate	120 compressions/min, 3:1 ratio of compressions to ventilations (90 compressions to 30 breaths every minute)	Compress approximately one-third of AP chest diameter	Two thumbs encircling the chest and supporting the back or heel of one hand
Infant	100–120/min; 30:2 ratio of compressions to breaths for 1 rescuer and 15:2 if 2 rescuers	Compress at least one-third the depth of the chest or about 4 cm (1.5 inches)	One rescuer (whether lay rescuers or health care professionals) should compress the sternum with 2 thumbs encircling the chest or heel of 1 hand placed just below the intermammary line; do not compress over the xiphoid or ribs
Child	100–120/min; 30:2 ratio of compressions to breaths for 1 rescuer and 15:2 if 2 rescuers	Compress at least one-third of the AP dimension of the chest or approximately 5 cm (2 inches)	One rescuer (whether lay rescuers or health care professionals) should compress the lower half of sternum with heel of 1 or 2 hands
Adolescent	100–120/min; 30:2 ratio of compressions to breaths	Compress at least one-third of the AP dimension of the chest or approximately 5 cm (2 inches)	Place the heel of 1 or 2 hands on the center of the chest (lower half of the sternum); place the heel of the other hand over the first hand

Abbreviation: AP, anteroposterior.

9. When the patient is intubated (has an advanced airway), it is reasonable to provide ventilations at a rate of 1 breath every 2 to 3 seconds (20 to 30 breaths/min) while providing continuous chest compressions.

TIP

Manipulation of the head to keep the airway in a neutral position, aligning the ear canal to the sternum, is essential for effective ventilation. A towel roll under the shoulders of the infant or small child may help maintain neutral head position.

PROCEDURE 18-1

Performing Cardiopulmonary Resuscitation on an Infant

1. Position the infant on a firm surface. Place heel of one hand or encircle chest with both hands and place 2 thumbs in the middle of the sternum just below a line between the nipples. Use 2 thumbs or heel of hand to compress the chest at least one-third the AP diameter of the chest or about 4 cm (1.5 inches) at a rate of 100 to 120 per minute. Allow the sternum to return to its normal position between compressions.

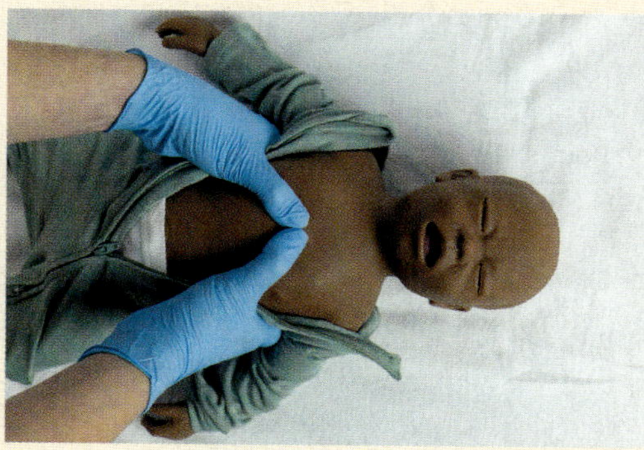

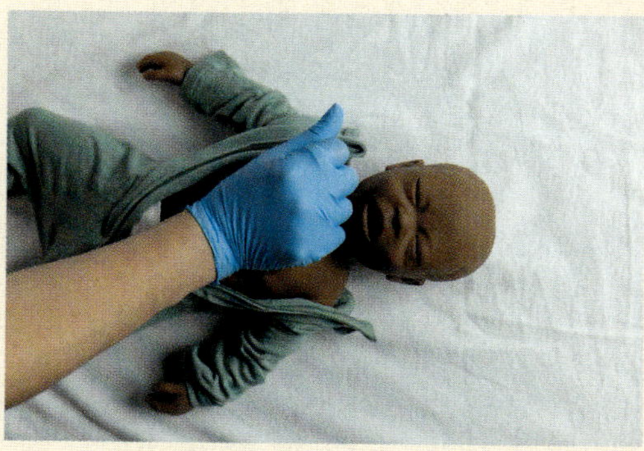

2. Coordinate compressions with ventilations in a 30:2 ratio (1 rescuer) or 15:2 (2 rescuers), pausing for 2 ventilations at the end of each cycle. Continue cycles of compressions and ventilations until a defibrillator becomes available or the infant shows signs of spontaneous breathing. Perform bag mask ventilation with 100% oxygen. Give 2 breaths of 1 second each.

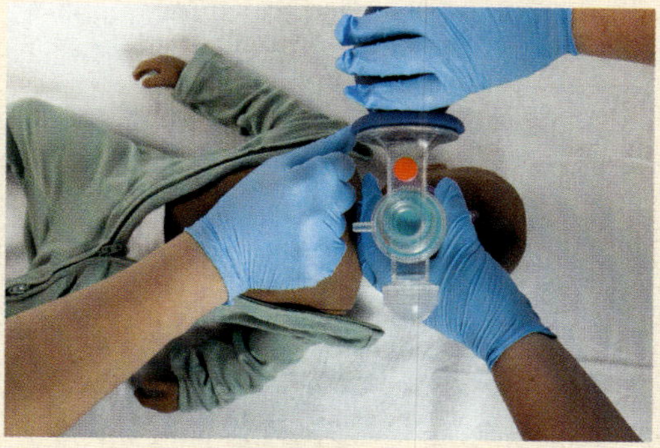

3. If 2 rescuers are present, compressions can also be performed at a ratio of 15 compressions to 2 breaths using the 2-thumbs-encircling-hands technique or heel of 1 hand.

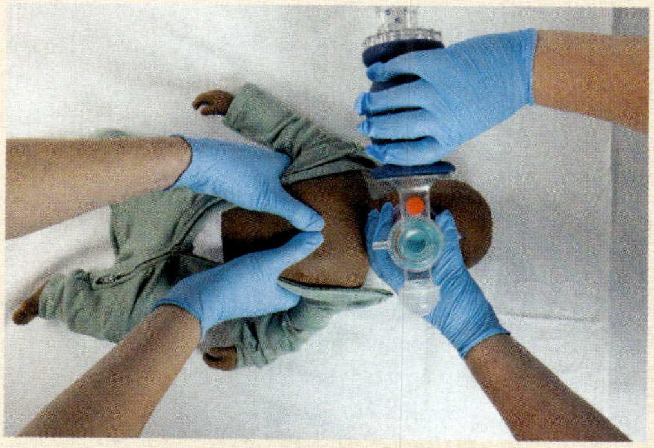

4. Newborn/Neonate CPR is performed at 120 compressions per minute with a 3:1 compression-versus-ventilation ratio.

PROCEDURE 18-2

Performing CPR on a Child

1. Place the child on a firm surface. Prepare to place the heel of 1 or 2 hands in the center of the chest, in between the nipples, avoiding the xiphoid process.

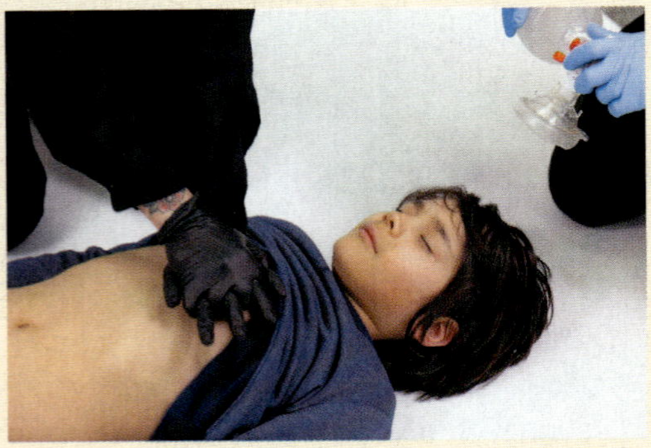

2. Compress the chest at least one-third the AP diameter of the chest or approximately 5 cm (2 inches) at a rate of 100 to 120 per minute.

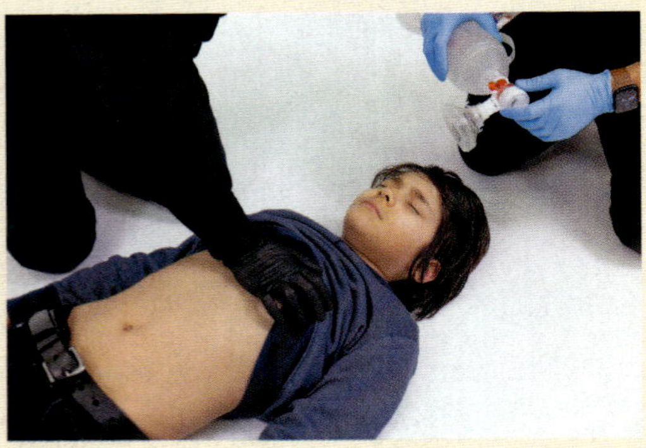

3. Coordinate compressions with ventilations in a 30:2 ratio (1 rescuer) or 15:2 (2 rescuers). At the end of each cycle, pause for 2 ventilations. Perform bag mask ventilation with 100% oxygen. Give 2 breaths of 1 second each.

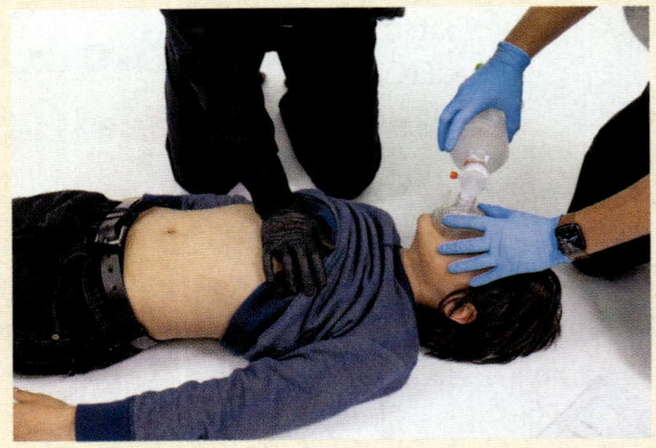

4. Continue cycles of compressions and ventilations until a defibrillator becomes available or the patient shows signs of spontaneous breathing. If the child resumes effective circulation and breathing, place them in the recovery position.

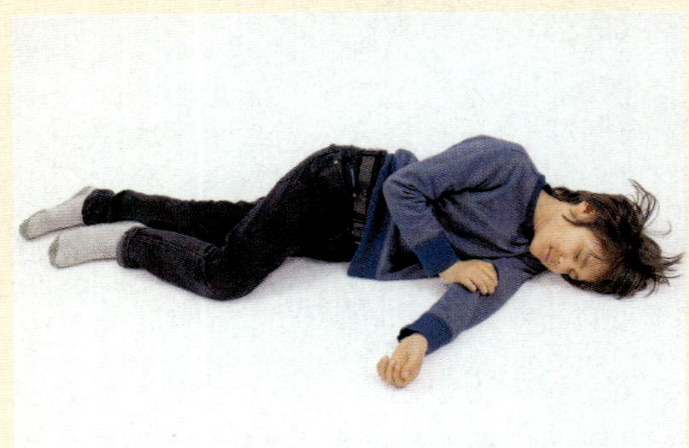

CAUTION

A common problem in the transition from 1-rescuer to 2-rescuer child CPR is the lack of coordination between ventilations and compressions.

Possible Complications

- Coronary vessel injury
- Diaphragm injury
- Hemopericardium
- Hemothorax
- Interference with ventilation
- Liver injury
- Myocardial injury
- Pneumothorax
- Rib fractures
- Spleen injury

Use of End-Tidal Carbon Dioxide to Monitor Quality of Compressions

1. Exhaled carbon dioxide (CO_2) is reflective of cardiac output during a cardiac arrest, because pulmonary blood flow must exist for end-tidal carbon dioxide ($EtCO_2$) to register, and measurement of $EtCO_2$ is recommended for CPR in intubated patients.
2. Quantitative $EtCO_2$ may be used to monitor quality of CPR. Normal $EtCO_2$ with a good mask seal or if the patient is intubated is approximately 35 to 45 mm Hg. During a cardiac arrest, the $EtCO_2$ value will be much lower and can theoretically reach zero if the patient has no pulse and is not receiving chest compressions.
3. End-tidal CO_2 levels $<$10 mm Hg indicate chest compressions need improvement. End-tidal CO_2 levels above 20 mm Hg indicate high-quality chest compressions.

Procedure 19: Automated External Defibrillators and Defibrillation

Kathleen Adelgais, MD, MPH, FAAP, FAEMS
John A. Erbayri, MS, NRP, CHSE

Introduction

Synchronized cardioversion for tachydysrhythmias has long been part of adult emergency care. However, ventricular dysrhythmias are rare in children, especially in infants, and pediatric supraventricular tachycardia (SVT) is usually treatable with medical therapy. All prehospital professionals should be prepared to provide synchronized cardioversion or defibrillation in appropriate situations. Ventricular fibrillation (VF) is observed in 5% to 15% of pediatric and adolescent arrests. However, when a child develops VF or pulseless ventricular tachycardia, defibrillation (unsynchronized cardioversion) may be lifesaving. Synchronized cardioversion may resuscitate a child in shock who has SVT. Synchronized cardioversion provides a shock that is timed (synchronized) with the QRS complex, avoiding delivery during the refractory period of the cardiac cycle, when a shock could produce VF. Clinicians should use the synchronized mode for selected cases of SVT or ventricular tachycardia with a pulse, and the unsynchronized (defibrillation) mode for VF or ventricular tachycardia without a pulse.

INDICATIONS

- Ventricular fibrillation
- Pulseless ventricular tachycardia
- Supraventricular tachycardia with shock and no vascular access rapidly available (synchronized)
- Ventricular tachycardia with shock and unresponsiveness with pulse (synchronized)
- Atrial fibrillation or atrial flutter with shock (synchronized)

CONTRAINDICATION

- Conscious patient with good perfusion

EQUIPMENT

- Automatic external defibrillator with pads appropriate for age*
- Standard defibrillator with paddles or pads appropriate for age*

*If pediatric pads are not available, use adult pads.

Rationale

When a child's heart rhythm deteriorates into ventricular tachycardia or ventricular fibrillation, there is usually a severe systemic insult, such as profound hypoxia, ischemia, electrolyte abnormalities, electrocution, or myocarditis. Death may result if treatment is delayed. Supraventricular tachycardia, in contrast, is usually a more stable cardiac rhythm. When the child is pulseless and has VF or ventricular tachycardia, perform defibrillation as quickly as possible with the appropriate technique. If a child has ventricular tachycardia with a pulse or SVT with poor perfusion, use synchronized cardioversion. *Do not attempt to perform synchronized cardioversion on a child with SVT who is well perfused;* medical therapy is indicated in such a case.

Preparation

1. Open airway and ventilate the patient with a bag-mask ventilation (BMV) device with 100% oxygen if indicated, while assembling equipment for cardioversion or defibrillation.
2. If child is pulseless, begin chest compressions until an automated external defibrillator (AED) or conventional defibrillator is available.

CAUTION

Do not deliver synchronized cardioversion to a conscious child with SVT or ventricular tachycardia unless the child is in shock and has no intravenous or intraosseous access rapidly available for medical treatment.

TIP

For a child with ventricular fibrillation or pulseless ventricular tachycardia, use the unsynchronized (defibrillation) mode.

CONVENTIONAL DEFIBRILLATOR USE

1. Select the proper paddle or pad size. Use the 8-cm adult paddles if these will fit on the chest wall and be separated by 2 cm of each other; otherwise, use the 4.5-cm pediatric paddles.

TABLE P19–1 Paddle Size

▪ 8-cm adult paddles (use in children older than 12 months or weighing more than 10 kg) on anterior chest wall *or* in anterior-posterior position if paddles touch when positioned on anterior chest
▪ 4.5-cm pediatric paddles (use in infants up to 12 months of age or weighing less than 10 kg) on the anterior chest wall

Ensure pediatric pads are compatible with your monitor or defibrillator (**TABLE P19–1**).

2. Prepare paddles or skin electrodes with electrode jelly, paste, or saline-soaked gauze pads, or use self-adhesive defibrillator pads. Do not let jelly or paste from one site touch the other and form an "electrical bridge" between sites, which could result in ineffective defibrillation or skin burns.
3. Establish appropriate electrical charge (**TABLE P19–2**).
4. Select synchronized or unsynchronized mode as indicated. Synchronize for SVT or any rhythm with a pulse; use the unsynchronized mode for ventricular tachycardia or ventricular fibrillation.

TIP

Maintain high-quality chest compressions until defibrillator is charged when you are analyzing rhythm *or* as long as possible when using AED mode. Immediately resume compressions once rhythm is analyzed and does not suggest a shock *or* immediately after a shock is delivered.

CAUTION

Failure to firmly apply paddles to the chest wall decreases the effective delivery of charge.

TABLE P19–2 Appropriate Electrical Charge for Countershock

Dysrhythmia	Mode	Charge
Ventricular fibrillation Ventricular tachycardia without a pulse	Defibrillation (unsynchronized)	2 J/kg, then 4 J/kg Subsequent shocks 4 J/kg after CPR and each dose of medication Do not deliver more than 10 J/kg or adult dose
Ventricular tachycardia with pulse, SVT	Synchronized cardioversion	0.5–1.0 J/kg Can increase to 2 J/kg if needed
Atrial fibrillation and atrial flutter with shock	Synchronized cardioversion	If no result with 0.5–1.0 J/kg, may use up to 2 J/kg

Abbreviations: CPR, cardiopulmonary resuscitation; SVT, supraventricular tachycardia.

PROCEDURE 19-1

Conventional Defibrillator Use

1. Apply the paddles or pads directly to the skin. Place one paddle or pad on the anterior chest wall on the right side of the sternum inferior to the clavicle and the other paddle or pad on the left midclavicular line at the level of the xiphoid process. The pads should not touch; if they do, use the anterior-posterior position.

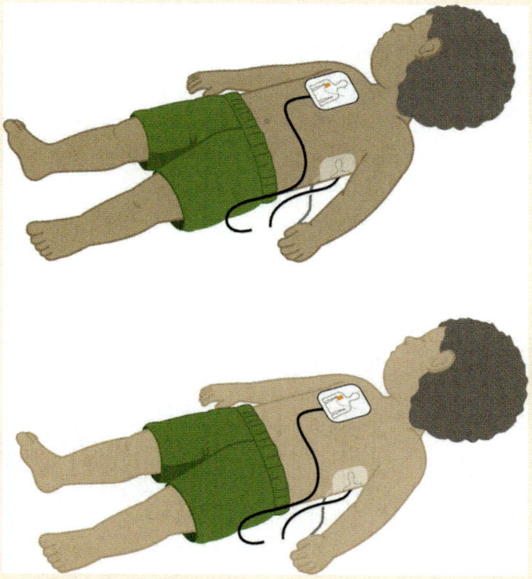

2. Press the charge button and clear the nearby area to avoid shocking someone. Announce, "I am going to shock on three. One, I am clear. Two, you are clear. Three, everybody is clear."
3. Begin recording the rhythm. Paddles are no longer used.
4. If CPR was being performed before shock was induced, resume CPR for 2 minutes. Then check the monitor for a change in rhythm and check the pulse.
5. If the first electrical shock is unsuccessful, resume CPR, then reanalyze the rhythm after another 2 minutes of CPR. Give specific dysrhythmia treatment with epinephrine or other drugs, as per protocol. Treat bradycardia or other dysrhythmias.

CONTROVERSY

The preferred paddle location in children is controversial, and no study in humans has involved comparison of the 2 techniques. Anterior chest wall placement has the advantage of a supine position for the child and easier airway management. Anterior-posterior placement may allow larger paddles and more effective delivery of electricity.

TIP

Consider giving a benzodiazepine before synchronized cardioversion if the patient is awake.

PROCEDURE 19-2

One Rescuer With an Automated External Defibrillator

For children younger than 8 years, use a child-pad cable system if available.

1. Verify unresponsiveness.
2. Look for an absence of breathing or only gasping and check the pulse.
3. If the patient is not breathing but has a pulse, begin BMV.
4. If the patient has no pulse, begin CPR with 30 compressions and 2 breaths.

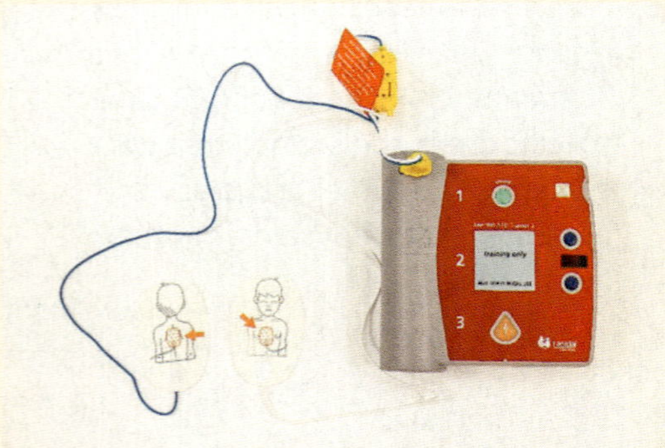

5. Apply the AED as soon as available.
6. Power on the AED and follow the voice prompts. Some devices will turn on when the AED lid or carrying case is opened.
7. Attach the AED. Select the correct pads for the patient's size and age (adult versus child). Peel the backing from the pads. Attach the adhesive pads to the patient as shown on the pads. (If only adult pads are available, and they overlap when placed on the chest, use an anterior [chest] and posterior [back] placement.) Attach the electrode cable to the AED (if not preconnected).
8. Allow the AED to analyze the victim's rhythm ("clear" the patient during analysis). Deliver a shock if needed ("clear" the patient before delivering the shock). Reasonable variations in this sequence are acceptable.

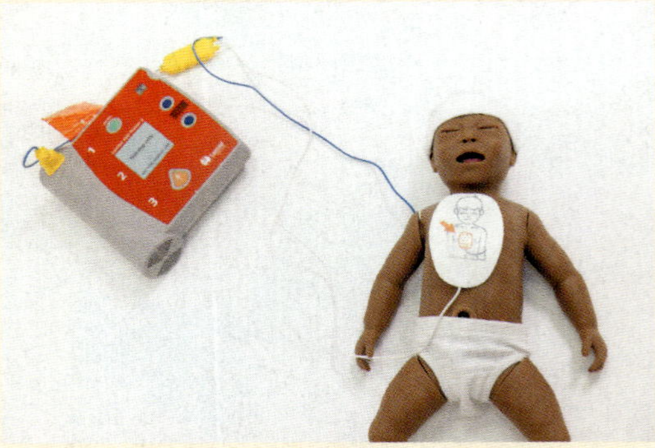

9. Resume CPR.

Possible Complications

- Ineffective delivery of cardioversion because of failure to charge, improper positioning on the chest, incorrect paddle size, pads incompatible with monitor or defibrillator, or improper conduction medium
- Burns on the chest wall
- Failure to "clear" before voltage discharge, leading to electrical shock of a team member or bystander
- Tachydysrhythmia
- Bradycardia
- Myocardial damage or necrosis
- Cardiogenic shock
- Embolic phenomena

PROCEDURE 19-3

Two-Rescuer Automated External Defibrillator Sequence of Action

1. Verify unresponsiveness. Have your partner get the AED.
2. Look for an absence of breathing or only gasping and check the patient's pulse.

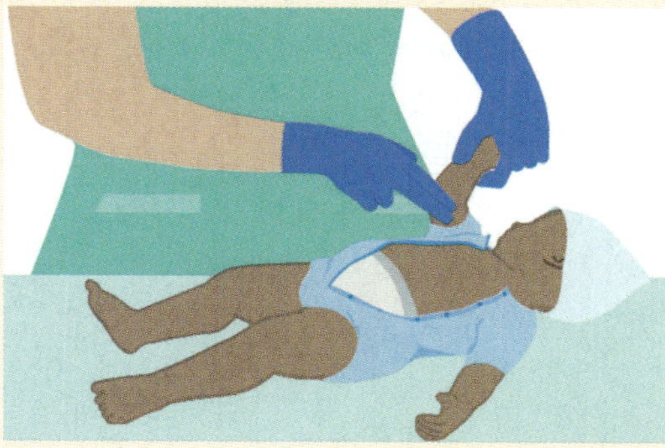

3. If the patient has no pulse, start CPR. If the patient is not breathing but has a pulse, begin bag mask ventilation.

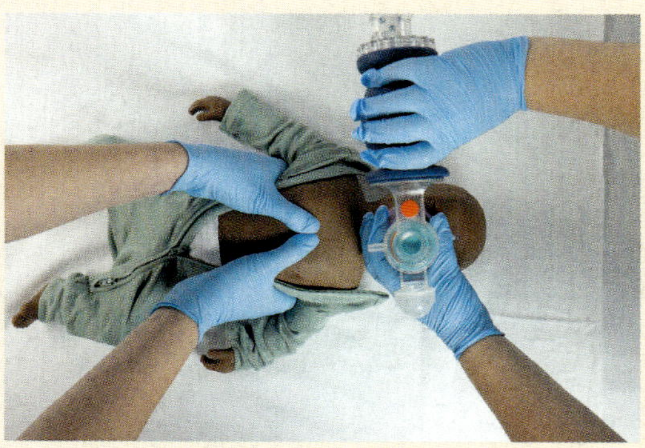

4. Apply AED as soon as it is available.
5. Attempt defibrillation with the AED if no signs of circulation are present. Place the AED near the rescuer who will be operating it. The AED is usually placed on the side of the patient opposite the rescuer who is performing CPR. The rescuer begins performing CPR while the rescuer who was performing CPR prepares to operate the AED. (It is acceptable to reverse these roles.)

The AED operator takes the following actions:

6. Power on the AED first (some devices will turn on automatically when the AED lid or carrying case is opened).
7. Attach the AED to the patient. Select correct pads for the patient's size and age. Peel the backing from the pads. Ask the rescuer performing CPR to stop chest compressions. Attach the adhesive pads to the patient as shown on the pads. (If only adult pads are available, and they overlap when placed on the chest, use an anterior [chest] and posterior [back] placement.) Attach the AED connecting cables to the AED (if not preconnected).

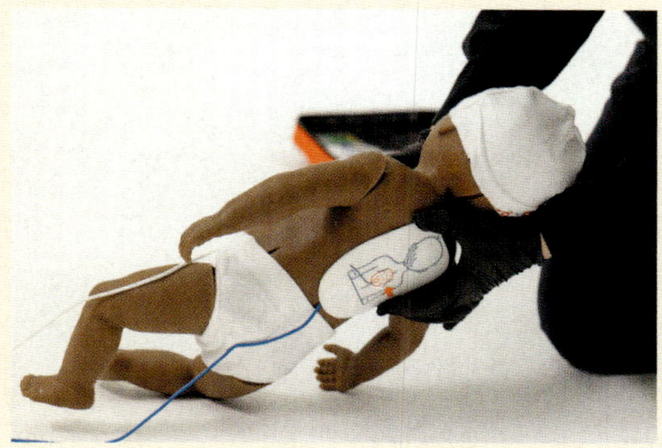

8. Analyze the rhythm. Clear the patient before and during analysis. Check that no one is touching the patient. Press the "analyze" button to start rhythm analysis (some brands of AEDs do not require this step).

   If the "Shock Indicated" message appears, resume CPR until AED is charged and ready to deliver shock. Clear the patient once more before pushing the "shock" button ("I'm clear, you're clear, everybody's clear"). Check that no one is touching the patient. Press the "shock" button (patient may display muscle contractions).

   If the "No Shock Indicated" message appears, resume CPR immediately.
9. After 2 minutes of CPR (or when prompted by the AED), analyze rhythm, then follow the "shock indicated" or "no shock indicated" steps detailed above as appropriate.

Procedure 20: Endotracheal Tube Drug Instillation

Jonathan P. Carolla, BSc, NRP, FPC
Shea Duerring, MD, NRP, FAAP, FACEP, FAEMS

Introduction

The ability of the airways of the lungs to absorb medicines has been recognized for more than a century. Administering medication through an endotracheal (ET) tube is an alternative to intravenous (IV) or intraosseous (IO) drug delivery in a cardiopulmonary resuscitation, when necessary. The airways are well vascularized and can absorb certain emergency medications. Drug dosages and dilutions in ET delivery are different than in IV or IO administration. Endotracheal drug delivery has been deemphasized; although this route of administration is better than no drug delivery, it is less effective than IV or IO. Once vascular access has been achieved, consideration should be given to repeating drug administration if there has been no response to the ET drug delivery.

INDICATIONS

- Cardiopulmonary resuscitation
- Lack of IV or IO access

CONTRAINDICATION

- Functioning IV or IO access

EQUIPMENT

- Endotracheal tube
- Long catheter (feeding tube, suction catheter, nasogastric tube, or umbilical catheter)
- Catheter size (in French units): approximately 2 times ET tube size (in mm) (**TABLE P20–1**)
- Desired drug/diluent mixture
- Normal saline
- Self-inflating ventilation device
- Diluent: 1 to 3 mL in infants and 5 to 10 mL maximum in older children

Rationale

If neither IV nor IO access is available for administering drugs during cardiopulmonary resuscitation, the ET route is a good alternative for pediatric drugs (lidocaine, **epinephrine**, atropine, and naloxone [LEAN]). The absorption, blood levels, onset, and duration of action are different with each drug. Endotracheal doses are unique for each agent and are higher than IV or IO doses because absorption is not as good. Although ET drugs are probably not as effective as IV or IO drugs, they can help improve the chances of successful resuscitation while IV or IO access is established.

TABLE P20–1 Suggested Catheter Size per Tracheal Tube

Endotracheal Tube Size (mm)	Catheter Size (French)
2.5	5
3.0	6
3.5–4.5	8
5.0–6.5	10
7.0	12

Preparation

1. Intubate the patient.
2. Stabilize and secure the ET tube.
3. Preoxygenate and ventilate.

TIP

Endotracheal drug administration is a potential route for medications during early phases of resuscitation.

Possible Complications

- Hypoxia
- Hypercarbia
- Pneumonitis
- Tracheal injury
- Adverse effects of the drug itself

TIP

The IV and IO routes of drug administration are better than the ET route.

PROCEDURE 20-1

Endotracheal Drug Delivery

1. Draw the calculated drug dose into a syringe (doses must be increased 2 to 3 times for lidocaine, atropine, and naloxone, and increased 10 times for epinephrine).
2. Dilute the medication with normal saline.
3. Insert the tip of a small feeding tube or catheter past the distal tip of the ET tube.
4. Instill solution directly into the trachea.
5. Follow with positive-pressure breaths.
6. Ventilate 3 times with bag ventilation device to disperse the solution into the entire lung. Repeat medications if indicated.

CAUTION

Never give sodium bicarbonate or dextrose via the ET route; they pose substantial risk of injury to lung tissue.

TIP

Doses via the ET route must be increased 2 to 3 times for lidocaine, atropine, and naloxone and increased 10 times for epinephrine.

TIP

These drugs are approved by the US Food and Drug Administration for ET instillation: lidocaine, epinephrine, atropine, and naloxone.

Procedure 21: Rectal Administration of Benzodiazepines

Rehman Chowdhry, MD, FAAP
Aaron Bates, NRP

Introduction

Rectal drug administration is a well-known delivery technique in children and is useful for many medications, including antipyretics and anticonvulsants. The only rectal medication approved in most emergency medical services (EMS) systems is diazepam for pediatric status epilepticus. Status epilepticus is a pediatric medical emergency that requires prompt treatment. Although the priority is airway and breathing, additional therapy may include medication to terminate the seizure. There remains significant controversy, from a safety and effectiveness stance, regarding the administration of rectal drugs. Rectal administration of diazepam is an effective route with few added complications when other routes of administration are not immediately available. It is important to ask if the caregivers have administered a rectal gel form of diazepam before EMS arrival.

TIP

Many patients with a known seizure disorder will receive prescriptions for diazepam for rectal and intranasal administration in emergency situations. It is important to ask caregivers if any medication was administered before EMS arrival on scene.

INDICATION

Status epilepticus

CONTRAINDICATIONS

- Newborn age (1 month or less) (relative)
- Recent rectal surgery (eg, for Hirschsprung disease, imperforate anus) (relative)

EQUIPMENT

- Lubricant
- Tuberculin syringe, or 14- to 20-gauge over-the-needle catheter with 3- to 5-mL syringe
- Intravenous (IV) solution of diazepam
- Tape (optional)

Rationale

The rectum is an effective alternative route for emergency drug administration. The rectum is highly vascularized, and certain drugs are quickly absorbed through its mucosa. Diazepam is a lipid-soluble benzodiazepine that is reliably absorbed through the rectum and terminates most seizures without further treatment. It takes a few minutes longer to stop the seizure after rectal administration of diazepam as compared with IV administration. Occasionally, as with the IV diazepam preparation, more than 1 dose of rectal diazepam is necessary owing to the drug's short duration of action.

Rectal lorazepam also has been used in the treatment of status epilepticus. This is less frequently encountered in the prehospital setting because of the manufacturer's recommendations to keep this drug refrigerated. If used in the prehospital setting, lorazepam may be stored for up to 30 days unrefrigerated at room temperature.

TIP

A rare but potentially serious complication of rectal diazepam is respiratory depression, which is usually caused by the drug, but may be a result of the prolonged seizure or the underlying cause of the seizure.

Preparation

1. Use a length-based resuscitation tape or software to determine the child's weight (see **Procedure 2, Length/Weight-Based Resuscitation Tape**) or establish the patient's weight from information provided by the caregiver. Note: You may have to convert the given weight in pounds to kilograms.
2. Draw up the calculated dose of IV medication into a disposable tuberculin syringe or a 3- to 5-mL syringe.
3. Lubricate the syringe or catheter:
   - If using the tuberculin syringe as the administration device, *remove the needle* and apply lubricant to the tip of the syringe.
   - If using a 3- to 5-mL syringe (or tuberculin syringe, to draw up medication only), *remove the needle*, attach an over-the-needle catheter (plastic portion only), and lubricate the catheter.

Possible Complications

- Respiratory depression
- Rectal trauma

PROCEDURE 21-1

Rectal Administration of Benzodiazepines

1. Position the patient in the decubitus position, knee-chest position, or supine position with a second prehospital professional or the caregiver holding the legs apart.

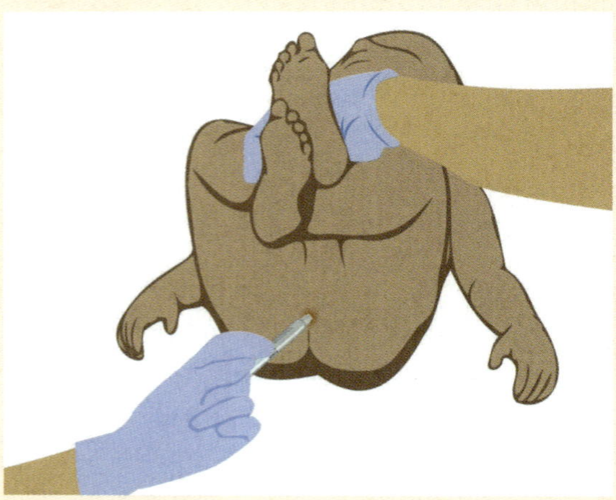

2. Carefully introduce the lubricated syringe or over-the-needle catheter approximately 5 cm (2 in) into the rectum. Inject the solution into the rectum. Remove the syringe. Hold buttocks closed for 10 seconds. Tape buttocks closed (optional) (**FIGURE PR21-1-1**).

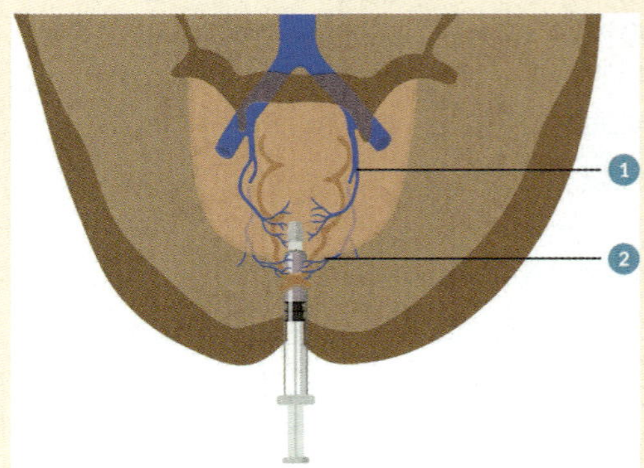

FIGURE PR21-1-1 1. Middle rectal vein. 2. Rectal vein.

TIP

The rectal dose of diazepam for infants, children, and adolescents is 0.5 mg/kg, to a maximum dose of 20 mg. The onset of action for rectal diazepam is slower than the IV dose but quicker than the oral dose.

CAUTION

Administration of diazepam too high into the rectum may decrease its anticonvulsant effect, because the drug may be absorbed differently and broken down more quickly in the liver.

Procedure 22: Spinal Motion Restriction

Claire Gahm, MD, MPH, FAAP
Debra L. Bell, MS, CCEMTP, EMT-T, NJ-CEM

Introduction

Spinal motion restriction (SMR) in pediatric patients is a practice used to prevent further injury during transport in cases of suspected spinal cord injury. It entails the use of a cervical collar (C-collar) and transport stretcher to maintain neutral alignment of the spine and reduce excessive movement that may worsen existing spinal trauma and neurological deficits. Spinal motion restriction has been standard practice in emergency medical services (EMS) for decades—supporting restriction whenever there is a clinical suspicion of spine injury, including high-risk mechanism of injury, pain or tenderness of the spine, or signs and symptoms of weakness or loss of sensation. Since the 1980s, studies have demonstrated the potential for harm with total spinal immobilization (C-collars and backboards), including aspiration risk, respiratory distress, agitation and pain, pressure ulcers, and exaggerated flexion or extension of the natural curvature of the spine that leads to further spinal injury. Practice has therefore shifted toward the judicious use of restriction techniques, limiting the use of backboards to extrication and specific clinical scenarios.

Spinal injuries may be subtle and difficult to recognize owing to altered mental status, distracting injuries, or, in infants and young children, the inability to communicate neck or back pain. Similarly, an injured and anxious child may express pain throughout an examination because of fear and anxiety, making it difficult to localize injuries. These nuances can provide specific challenges for EMS professionals in cases of pediatric trauma. It is thus especially important to rely on updated agency protocols to direct care. Failure to recognize and treat potential spinal injury can lead to permanent disability or death.

HOW IS SPINAL MOTION RESTRICTION ACHIEVED?

- Application of a cervical collar
- Securing the patient to a stretcher with appropriately sized pediatric restraint devices
- When the patient is not ambulatory, use of a long spine board, scoop stretcher, or flexible stretcher to move the patient to the ambulance stretcher

INDICATIONS FOR USE OF A RIGID COLLAR IN PEDIATRIC PATIENTS

- Neck or spine pain
- Deformity of the neck or spine
- Unexplained numbness or paresthesia in extremities
- Muscle spasm of the neck (torticollis)
- Altered mental status
- High-risk trauma (eg, high-energy motor vehicle accident, hyperextension neck injury, and significant upper-body injury)

CONTRAINDICATIONS TO USE OF RIGID IMMOBILIZATION DEVICES

- Penetrating trauma
- Fixed neck deformity
- Massive cervical swelling for which collar placement may impinge the airway or prohibit circulatory stabilization (hemorrhage control)

SPECIAL CONSIDERATIONS

- Perform in-line stabilization for any airway procedure that necessitates removal of a C-collar (intubation, cricothyrotomy).
- If the risks of agitation and increased spinal movement resulting from spinal motion restriction are greater than the benefits, consider more acceptable but less definitive stabilization options (eg, towel rolls).
- Alternate methods of stabilization may also be needed if the C-collars or other devices do not fit the patient appropriately (eg, infants). Clearly document the rationale.

EQUIPMENT

- Long spine board, scoop stretcher, flexible stretcher, or approved EMS stretcher
- Padding materials (blankets, towels)
- Rigid cervical collars in pediatric sizes
- Straps with fastening device
- Wide tape (2 or 3 in)
- Optional equipment: Head cushions from a cervical immobilization device (CID)

Rationale

The spinal column is made of 33 articulating bones, and its structure changes significantly during childhood. The age of the child and the physical state of spinal growth are important factors in the incidence and types of pediatric spinal injuries. Children younger than 8 years have relatively large heads, weak cervical muscles, short necks, and a predominance of cartilage (because the spinal bones ossify over the first 1 to 3 years after birth), which makes them particularly prone to axial cervical spine injury. Whenever the mechanism of injury, signs, or symptoms suggest possible spinal injury, the entire spine should be stabilized. The neck is placed in a cervical collar while the body is placed in the supine position in a neutral, in-line position. As discussed, placing the patient on a backboard for transport is not usually indicated; however, the proper mechanism for spinal immobilization in pediatric patients is detailed in this section. When the scene or situation makes these techniques difficult, maintain the anatomical stability of the entire spinal column as carefully as possible using age-specific considerations to minimize spinal movement. Padding voids and areas with potential for movement can help maintain the head and neck in a neutral position.

Unconscious or critically unstable patients should be immobilized on a spinal immobilization device such as a long backboard.

PROCEDURE 22-1

Spinal Motion Restriction

1. Prepare the child and caregiver for the procedure by explaining your actions.
2. While one rescuer holds the child's head in a neutral position, a second rescuer measures and applies an appropriately sized cervical collar.

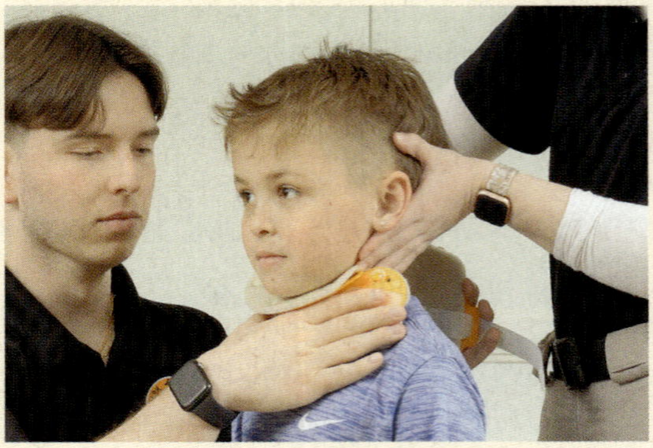

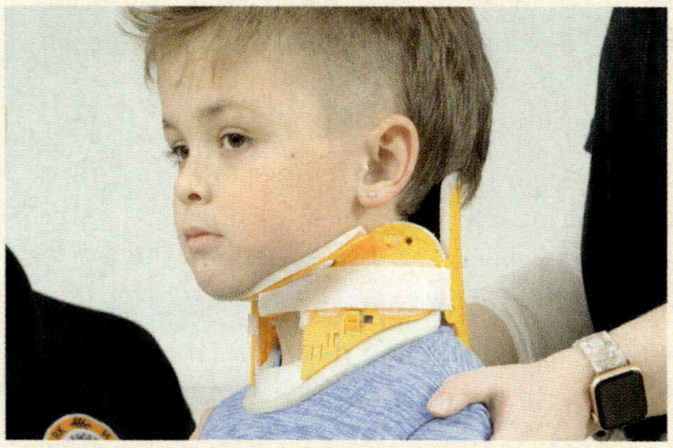

A properly placed cervical collar.

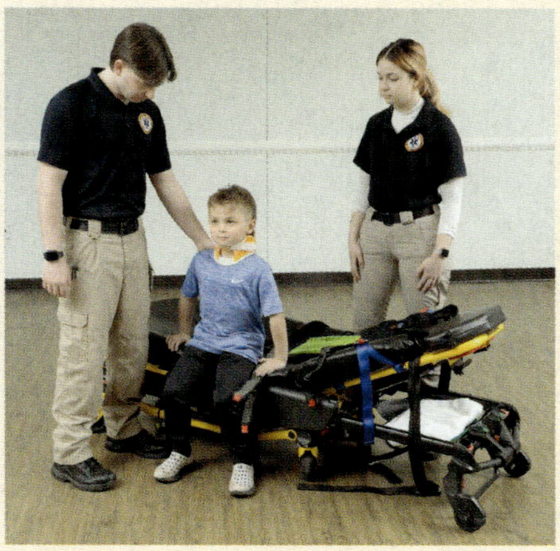

3. The rescuers accompany the child to the ambulance stretcher. Instruct the child to sit on the stretcher.

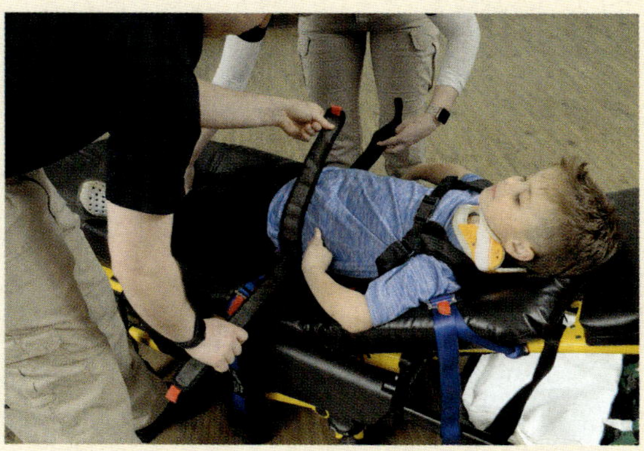

4. Rescuers position and secure the patient on the stretcher with an appropriate child restraint system.

5. Once properly secured, the patient can be transferred to the ambulance. The head of the stretcher can be elevated for comfort but no more than 30 degrees to avoid compressing the spinal column.

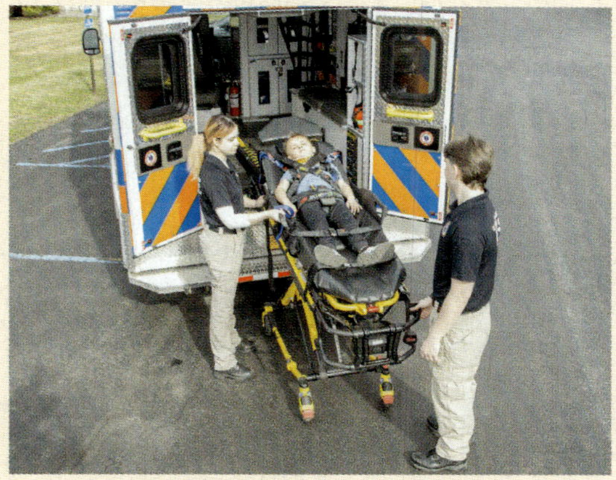

TIP

Reassure nervous children that the spinal motion restriction is only temporary, but it is necessary. Try distraction.

TIP

Assign 1 rescuer to in-line neck stabilization of a combative child.

CAUTION

Verify sizes for cervical collars ("pediatric" or "infant") by measuring each patient individually. One size does not fit all.

Possible Complications

- Airway obstruction
- Anxiety and combativeness
- Impairment of ventilation
- Obscured hemorrhage or other neck injuries
- Spinal injury resulting from improper technique
- Back pain
- Pressure ulcer

PROCEDURE 22-2

Securing an Unstable Patient to a Spinal Immobilization Device

1. After applying an appropriately sized cervical collar, secure the patient to a rigid carrying device such as a scoop stretcher or backboard.

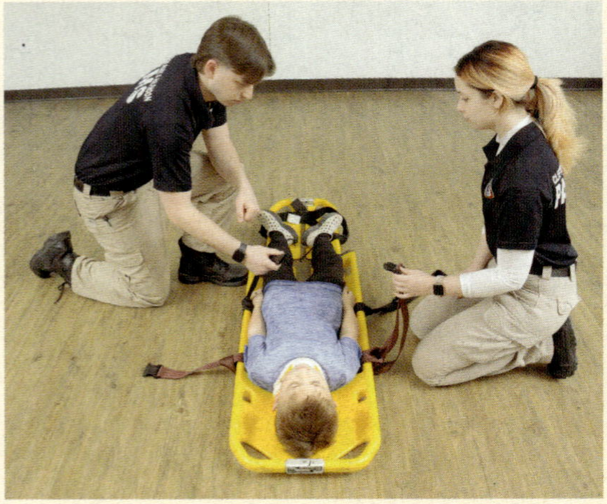

2. Transfer the patient to an ambulance stretcher with a previously placed child restraint system.

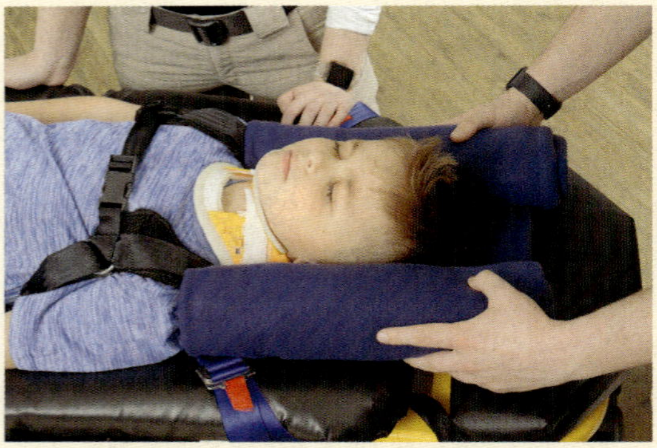

3. The patient's head can be secured with a commercial device or a rolled blanket. Avoid chin straps that may complicate airway maintenance.

4. Reassess airway, breathing, and circulation for any changes after spinal immobilization.

5. If a parent will be accompanying the child in the patient compartment, assure the parent is properly belted.

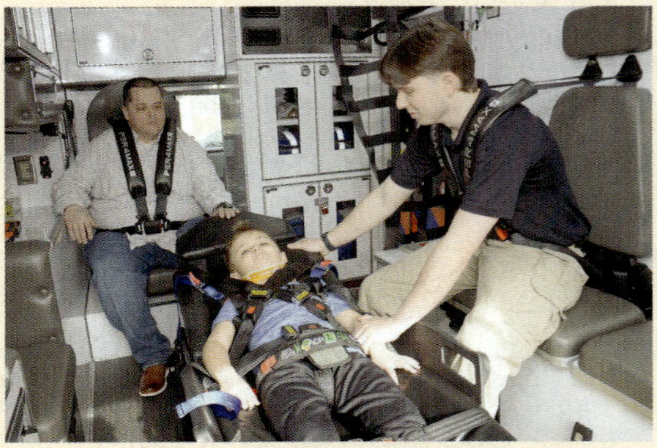

CAUTION

Do not use sandbags or weighted material because of the risk of injury in the event of movement.

CAUTION

There is no role for spinal immobilization in penetrating chest or abdominal trauma.

TIP

When using tape, use the longest strips possible to maximize adhesive surface and security.

Tools

PECARN cervical spine injury prediction rule. MDCalc. Accessed April 18, 2025. https://www.mdcalc.com/calc/10552/pecarn-cervical-spine-injury-prediction-rule

Pediatric Emergency Care Applied Research Network (PECARN). Clinical decision rule for cervical spine injury in children. Accessed April 18, 2025. https://pecarn.org/wp-content/uploads/2024/06/EMS240529_CSpineGraphics_Full240605.pdf

Procedure 23: Needle Thoracostomy

Chris Coughlin, PhD, NRP
Rudy Kink, MD, FAAP

Introduction

A pneumothorax occurs when air accumulates between the 2 pleural membranes of the lung, a space that is normally empty during regular breathing conditions.

Tension pneumothorax develops when the air trapped in the pleural space exerts pressure, causing shifting of the internal contents and impairing the function of the lungs, heart, and major vessels. This reduces venous return to the heart and diminishes cardiopulmonary function, which can lead to shock and cardiopulmonary arrest if left untreated. Tension pneumothorax in children is often a consequence of assisted ventilation in the field, leading to increased work of breathing and hypoxia. Although pneumothoraces can occur spontaneously in diseases such as asthma or cystic fibrosis, tension pneumothorax in these cases is rare. Classical signs seen in adults, such as a deviated trachea or diminished breath sounds on the affected side, may not be as evident in infants or children. If the tension pneumothorax severely impairs cardiac output, the child may also experience shock.

INDICATIONS

- Penetrating chest wall injury in a child with poor perfusion, respiratory distress, and hypoxia
- Blunt chest wall injury in a child with respiratory distress and hypoxia, especially if symptoms worsen with assisted ventilation

CONTRAINDICATION

- History of a severe bleeding disorder, such as hemophilia (relative contraindication)

EQUIPMENT

- 14- or 16-gauge 5-cm (2-in) over-the-needle catheter
- 30-mL syringe
- Skin cleansing solution

CAUTION

In a 2019 study, a standard 5-cm (2-in) 14- to 16-gauge needle for chest decompression was more than twice as long as needed for children younger than 13 years according to chest wall thickness as shown on computerized tomography.

Rationale

When the mechanism of injury, signs, and symptoms suggest a tension pneumothorax, it is crucial to relieve the elevated intrapleural pressure by creating an opening between the pleural space and the external environment. This intervention re-expands the lung, improves venous return, and restores cardiopulmonary function. The simplest method for achieving this is creating an open pneumothorax by using a large-bore needle to relieve pressure.

CONTROVERSY

The frequency of tension pneumothorax after blunt chest wall injury is not known, and the indications for needle thoracostomy in this prehospital situation are controversial.

Preparation

1. Position the child supine.
2. Raise the arm above the head on the affected side and have the caregiver or second rescuer hold it.
3. Select the site:
   - Second intercostal space (over the top of the child's third rib) at the midclavicular line *or*
   - Fourth intercostal space (the nipple is usually at the fourth intercostal space) at the anterior axillary line
4. Double-check rib count to ensure correct site location.
5. Prepare the site with skin-cleansing solution.

Possible Complications

- Open pneumothorax
- Hemothorax
- Diaphragm penetration
- Bowel penetration
- Hemopericardium
- Intercostal nerve or vessel or other intrathoracic vessel injury

CAUTION

Do not insert the needle under the rib margin, because the vessels and nerves there are easily injured. Instead, insert above the rib.

PROCEDURE 23-1

Needle Thoracostomy

1. Attach the needle (with catheter in place) to the syringe.
2. Insert the needle through the skin at 90° through the skin and advance until the tip contacts a rib (**FIGURE PR23–1–1**).

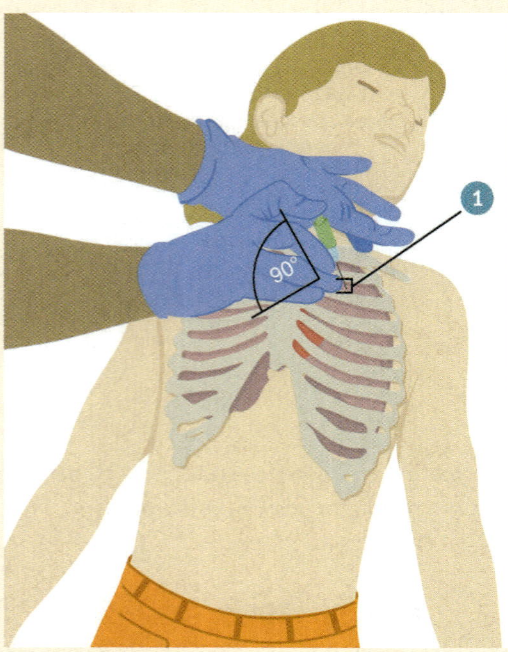

FIGURE PR23–1–1 1. Second intercostal space.

3. Move the needle over the top of the rib to avoid damaging the intercostal nerve and blood vessels located along the lower edge of each rib.
4. Advance the needle tip into the pleural space. You will often feel a slight "pop" when the needle pierces the pleural membrane (parietal pleura).
5. Aspirate air by pulling back the syringe plunger to confirm you are in the pleural space.
6. Remove the syringe and needle, leaving the catheter in the pleural space. Anchor the catheter securely to the chest wall to prevent displacement.
7. Monitor the child's clinical status, including work of breathing, skin, circulation, heart rate, respiratory rate, and blood pressure. If the child's condition does not improve, consider performing needle thoracostomy on the opposite side (contralateral needle thoracostomy).

CAUTION
A shifted trachea or diminished breath sounds may not be detectable in an infant or young child with a tension pneumothorax.

TIP
Suspect a tension pneumothorax when a child with chest injury worsens with assisted ventilation.

Suggested Reference

Mandt MJ, Hayes K, Severyn F, Adelgais K. Appropriate needle length for emergent pediatric needle thoracostomy utilizing computed tomography. *Prehosp Emerg Care*. 2019;23(5):663–671. PMID: 30624127 10.1080/10903127.2019.1566422

Procedure 24: Removing and Replacing a Tracheostomy Tube

Aaron Bates, NRP
Michael K. Kim, MD, FAAP

Introduction

With the advent of advanced technology and emphasis on home care, an increasing number of children living in the community have tracheostomy tubes. Most have parents and caregivers who are trained in emergency tracheostomy tube care, but 911 calls for emergencies in these patients do occur, and prehospital professionals must know how to evaluate and manage acute tracheostomy tube problems.

INDICATIONS OR ISSUES

The most common issues with tracheostomy tubes are decannulation and obstruction. However, bleeding, infection, subcutaneous air or pneumothorax, tube malfunction ,or aspiration may result in a call for emergency help.

CONTRAINDICATIONS OR BARRIERS

Occasionally, the stoma may be too small for the insertion of a new tracheostomy tube. In this case, the clinician should insert a smaller tracheostomy tube, if available, or an endotracheal tube. If no replacement tracheostomy tube is available, an endotracheal tube can be inserted in the stoma.

EQUIPMENT

- Suction equipment
- Sterile suction catheters
- Oxygen
- Bag-mask ventilation device with a mask that is appropriately sized for the patient
- Tracheostomy cannulas, appropriately sized for the patient and 1 size smaller, if available
- Endotracheal tubes, standard pediatric and adult sizes
- Laryngoscope handle with blades
- Tape or tracheostomy ties
- Gauze pads
- 5- or 10-mL syringe
- Water-soluble lubricant
- Scissors
- Sterile saline
- Stethoscope

TIP

When a tracheostomy tube is dislodged or removed, the stoma can shrink rapidly, making reinsertion difficult. Do not hesitate to consider a smaller device if you encounter difficulty in attempting to reinsert the tracheostomy tube.

Rationale

The tracheostomy complications most likely to be encountered by emergency medical services (EMS) personnel include obstruction (resulting from mucus plugging) and displacement. Although obstruction often responds to suctioning, in severe cases the mucus may be so thick that suctioning is ineffective, thus necessitating removal of the original tube and insertion of a new tube. The decision to change a tracheostomy tube should be made quickly and decisively. When a tracheostomy tube is displaced, the stoma will begin to close, and significant respiratory distress can develop. This requires immediate placement of a new tracheostomy tube or alternative airway by prehospital personnel to maintain or stabilize the airway and save the child's life.

Preparation

1. Ask the caregiver if there are any special problems with the child's trachea or special requirements involving the child's tracheostomy.
2. Confirm the age of the tracheostomy, because a new tracheostomy (7–10 days after placement) presents additional potential complications such as bleeding, soft-tissue injury, and false tract creation.
3. Ask the caregiver if a replacement tracheostomy tube is available.
4. Speak directly to the child about what to expect and attempt to enlist their cooperation.
5. Place a pulse oximeter on the child.

Possible Complications

- Creation of a false tract
- Subcutaneous air
- Pneumomediastinum
- Pneumothorax
- Bleeding at insertion site
- Bleeding through tube
- Mainstem intubation with endotracheal tube (usually the right mainstem)
- Failed cannulation

PROCEDURE 24-1

Preparing the New Tracheostomy Tube

1. Prepare a clean surface for equipment: new tracheostomy tube, syringe, lubricant, water, and gauze.
2. Open the new tracheostomy tube and check the integrity of the balloon (if present): inflate the balloon slowly to confirm it is intact. Remove all air.
3. Apply lubricant to the new tracheostomy tube.
4. Insert the obturator, if present, into the tracheostomy tube. If the tube has an inner and outer cannula, use the outer cannula and obturator for insertion.

PROCEDURE 24-2

Removing an Old Tracheostomy Tube

1. Position the child with the head and neck slightly hyperextended to expose the tracheostomy site.
2. Apply oxygen over the mouth and nose.
3. If the existing tube has a cuff, deflate it by connecting a 5- to 10-mL syringe to the valve on the pilot balloon and draw air out until the balloon collapses. Cutting the balloon will not deflate the cuff.
4. Cut or untie the ties that hold the tracheostomy tube in place.
5. Apply the new tie around the neck.
6. Ask patient to take a deep breath in. Withdraw the tracheostomy tube during exhalation, using slow, steady outward and downward motion.
7. Visually inspect the stoma for any evidence of foreign body, inflammation, or bleeding.
8. Assess the airway for patency and adequate ventilation.
9. Proceed with the insertion of the new tube.

PROCEDURE 24-3

Replacing the Tracheostomy Tube

Whenever possible, insert a tracheostomy tube of the same size and model. If this is not available, use a smaller tube or an endotracheal tube of the same inner diameter as the tracheostomy tube.

1. Hold the device by the flange (wings) or hold the actual tube like a pencil.
2. Position the head in a neutral or slightly extended position.
3. Gently insert the tube with an arching motion (follow the curvature of the tube) posteriorly and then downward. Slight traction on the skin above or below the stoma may help. *Do not use force, because this may create a false tract.* If resistance is encountered, reduce the degree of neck extension.

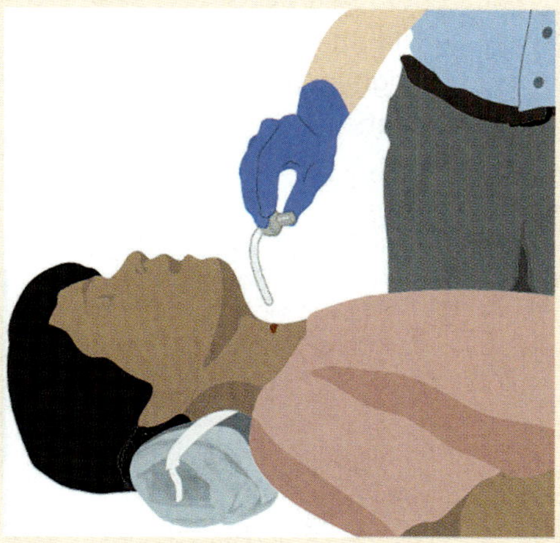

4. Once the tube is completely inserted, remove the obturator, attach the bag-mask device, and ventilate. If the tube uses an inner cannula, insert it to allow mechanical ventilation with a bag-mask device.

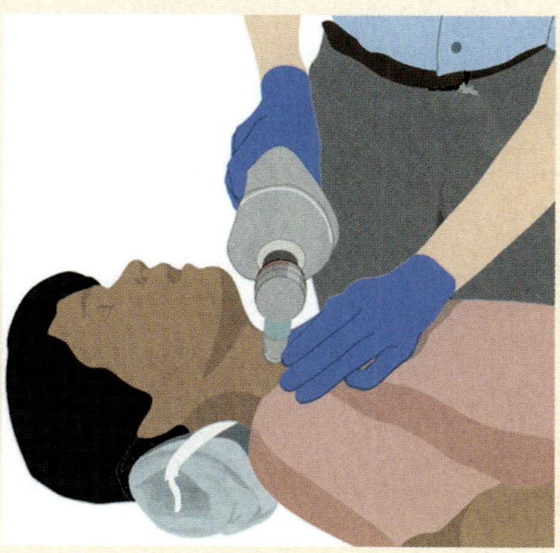

5. Confirm proper placement by watching for bilateral chest rise, listening for equal breath sounds, monitoring for an increase in the pulse oximeter reading, and observing the patient. If waveform capnography is available, it should be used to confirm ventilation. Signs of improper placement include lack of chest rise or air entry on auscultation, resistance to assisted ventilation, air in the surrounding tissues, no increase in the pulse oximeter reading, lack of patient improvement, and an absent or unclear capnography waveform.
6. If you notice difficulty in insertion, remove the tube, administer oxygen, and ventilate as needed.
7. Use a smaller tracheostomy tube for the second attempt. If it is still unsuccessful, insert an uncuffed endotracheal tube through the stoma. Check the length of the original tracheostomy tube, note the markings on the endotracheal tube, and advance it to the same depth as the original tube. The inserted portion of the endotracheal tube will be approximately one-half the distance needed for oral insertion. Do not advance the tube too far, or it may enter a mainstem bronchus.
8. If tube replacement is still unsuccessful, use a suction catheter as a guide. Insert a small, sterile suction catheter through the tracheostomy tube. Without applying suction, insert the suction catheter into the stoma. Slide the tracheostomy tube along the suction catheter and into the stoma until it is in the proper position. Remove the suction catheter. Assess ventilation through the tracheostomy tube.
9. If still unsuccessful, consider orotracheal intubation or transport the patient with ventilation through the stoma using a stoma mask or neonatal mask, or by placing a bag-mask device over the nose and mouth while covering the stoma with a sterile gauze.

After proper tube placement, cut the ends of the tracheostomy ties or tapes diagonally (to allow for easy insertion), pass them through the eyelets (openings) on the flanges, and tie them around the patient's neck so that only a little finger can pass snugly between the ties and the neck.

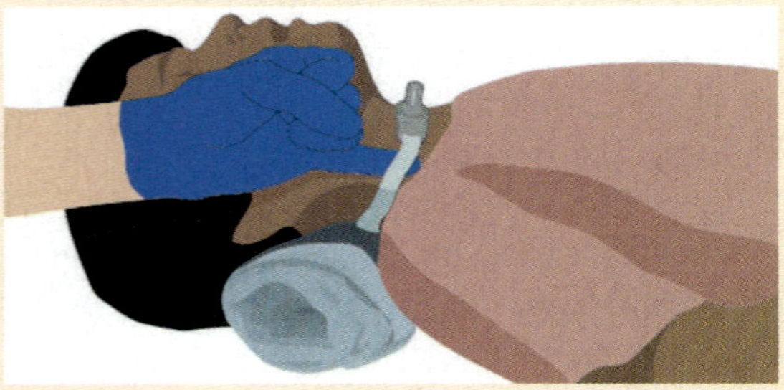

TIP
If the patient is in respiratory distress, it may be possible to assist their ventilations using a standard bag-mask technique over the mouth and nose while occluding the stoma with a gauze.

TIP
Before performing any tracheostomy tube replacement, confirm its necessity and the availability of assistance.

CAUTION
If a patient has a newly created tracheostomy stoma, the clinician must exercise extreme caution, because the stoma is not mature and there are risks of airway collapse, bleeding, and false tract creation. Do not force a tracheostomy tube, especially through a new stoma site. Consider inserting a smaller tracheostomy or endotracheal tube.

Procedure 25: Tourniquet Application

Aaron Bates, NRP
Michael K. Kim, MD, FAAP

Introduction

The "Stop the Bleed" campaign was launched by the White House in 2015 as a national initiative spearheaded by the Department of Homeland Security in collaboration with the American College of Surgeons and other medical organizations. This campaign underscores the urgent need for timely assessment and intervention in life-threatening bleeding through widespread civilian education. Uncontrolled hemorrhage resulting in hypovolemia is the leading cause of shock in victims of all ages, resulting in rapid death or disability once shock sets in.

Advances in trauma care have shown that hemorrhage control in the prehospital setting is achievable, and the use of tourniquets for this purpose is both safe and effective. The likelihood of modern emergency medical services (EMS) professionals encountering pediatric patients with uncontrolled bleeding is increasing, highlighting the importance of hemorrhage control as an essential skill for prehospital professionals as well as civilians. Concerns about limb ischemia resulting from tourniquet use have been reduced, with both combat and civilian research demonstrating tourniquets' effectiveness in saving lives.

Establishing hemorrhage control as quickly as possible to prevent blood loss and subsequent shock remains the highest priority when caring for a victim of trauma, sometimes even before airway and breathing interventions. Timely placement of a tourniquet when direct pressure fails to control bleeding is often the single most important intervention prehospital professionals can take to increase a patient's chance of survival. There are limited data regarding use of tourniquets among children; however, it is supported by the Pediatric Trauma Society in the prehospital setting and during resuscitation of children who are experiencing exsanguination hemorrhage caused by severe trauma to extremities.

> **TIP**
> It is important to prioritize hemorrhage control, sometimes even before airway and breathing interventions.

INDICATION

Uncontrolled hemorrhage refractory to direct pressure

CONTRAINDICATIONS

Embedded or impaled foreign object at the site of intended application

Fracture at the site of intended application

Over joints

EQUIPMENT

Tourniquet (commercial device or improvised)

Rationale

Tourniquet use is intended to stop arterial blood flow to a hemorrhaging extremity. There are very few absolute contraindications to tourniquet application, and most can be addressed. If an embedded object or fracture is present at the site of intended application, the prehospital clinician should attempt to place the tourniquet more proximally if possible. When proximal placement is not feasible, the clinician should prioritize controlling hemorrhage through direct pressure. Junctional hemorrhage can occur at or around the site where an extremity joins the torso, including the base of the neck, areas high in the groin region (proximal to the inguinal ligament), the gluteal region, the perineum, and the axillary region. These sites are not amenable to tourniquet application; however, junctional hemorrhage is compressible. Effective control can typically be achieved by applying significant pressure to deep vessels proximal to the injury.

Numerous styles of commercial tourniquets are available, and the type and style used by prehospital personnel depends on the specific agency's selection for their service. Given this variability, EMS professionals must practice often with the specific tourniquet they have to maintain proficiency with that device.

Commercially available tourniquets employ 2 tightening methods.

1) A windlass mechanism: This consists of a stiff rod that is inserted between the skin and the tourniquet or installed as part of a commercially available device. Twisting the windlass takes up the slack and applies compression to the affected extremity. A windlass-type mechanism can be used with an improvised tourniquet as well.

2) A ratcheting device: This lever-style mechanism advances a ridged belt incrementally, locking it into position with each advancement. As the belt is advanced, it takes up slack and applies greater pressure. This style of mechanism cannot be improvised and is available only on commercial devices.

When a commercially available tourniquet is not accessible, such as when the patient is too small for proper application, an improvised tourniquet is a viable option. This can be made from common items, such as a piece of clothing at least 2 inches wide, combined with a windlass-style device to apply sufficient pressure. Additionally, a tightly inflated blood pressure cuff can serve as an improvised tourniquet; it is essential to check the cuff periodically to ensure there is no leak and it remains inflated.

TIP

There is limited information available regarding commercially available tourniquets for children. A study suggested that the Combat Application Tourniquet was effective in children as young as 2 years of age.

CONTROVERSY

Not too long ago, the use of tourniquets fell out of favor owing to concern that they cause ischemic injury, mainly due to incorrect application, and may lead to a higher incidence of limb loss when applied in the prehospital setting. There is now substantial evidence that refutes these claims. Multiple studies have concluded that *tourniquet use does not increase ischemic injury or limb loss* when used to control massive hemorrhage. It has also been established that the benefit of hemorrhage control and improved chances of survival far outweigh any minimal risk of limb ischemia and loss. The overwhelming consensus is that prehospital use of tourniquets for hemorrhage control saves lives, and that tourniquets should be applied as soon as possible for patients with uncontrolled hemorrhage.

Preparation

1. Place the patient in a position that protects the airway when possible (generally supine or recumbent).
2. If possible, expose the wounded area and confirm that there is no foreign body between the tourniquet and the skin (do not delay treatment for this).
3. Select and prepare an appropriate commercial tourniquet device or fashion an improvised tourniquet if a suitable commercial device is unavailable.

Possible Complication

- Limb ischemia (remote)

PROCEDURE 25-1

Tourniquet Application

1. Have a partner or the patient apply direct pressure to the site of bleeding if possible. If bleeding persists and there is concern regarding significant hemorrhage, proceed to tourniquet application.
2. Place the tourniquet on the affected limb and position it 2 to 3 inches above the site of the bleeding. Do not place the tourniquet on a joint; go above the joint and make sure there is no foreign body beneath the tourniquet. Wrap and secure the tourniquet device around the limb per the manufacturer's directions.

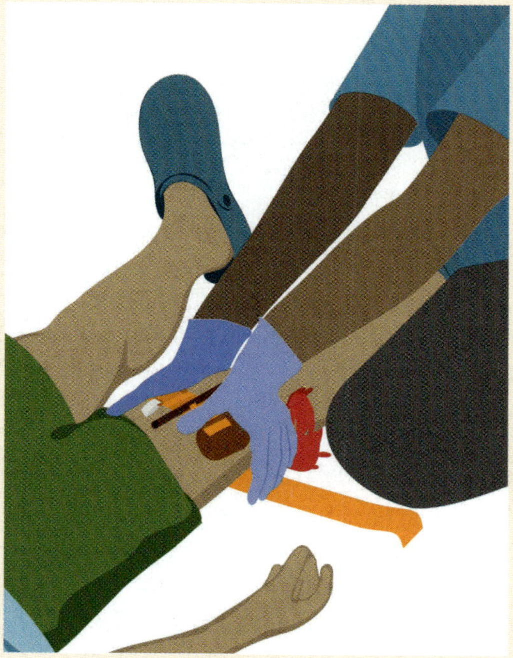

3. Pull the strap through the buckle device to draw the tourniquet down as tightly as possible before using the ratchet or windlass to apply compression. If more than 2 or 3 fingertips can be inserted between the tourniquet and the limb, it should be tightened further before compression is applied.

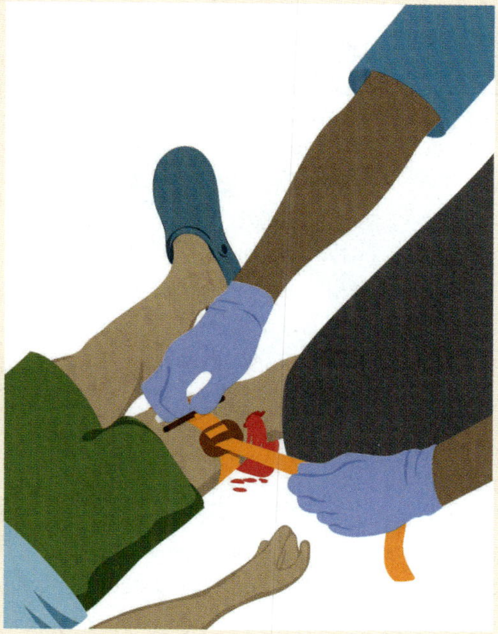

4. Turn the windlass rod or advance the ratcheting device until bleeding has stopped.

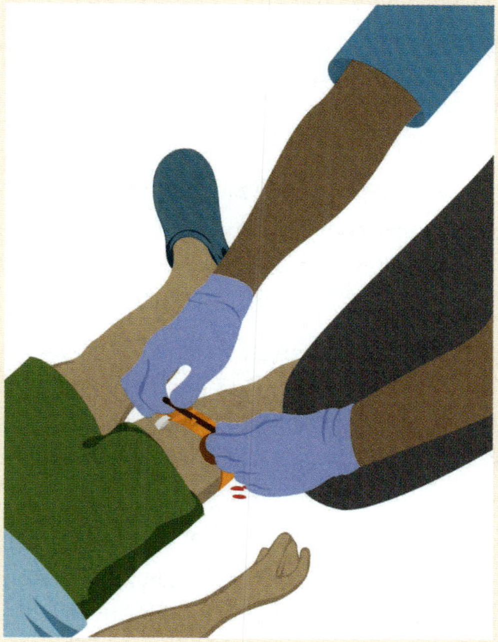

5. Secure the windlass rod or ratcheting device in place. Check again that bleeding has been stopped. If bleeding does not stop or a distal pulse is still palpable, consider using an additional tourniquet if available and/or reinstitute direct pressure in addition to tourniquet(s).

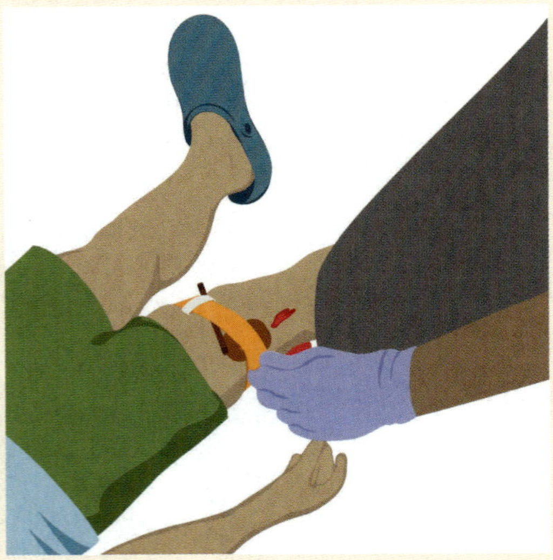

6. Secure any remaining tourniquet band or material so that it does not catch or snag when the patient is moved.
7. Always document the time the tourniquet was applied by writing it directly on the device once it is secured.
8. Continue to check periodically that bleeding remains controlled. Routinely assess distal pulses in the affected extremity to ensure they are absent and assess whether the tourniquet has been tightened sufficiently.

Generally, once a tourniquet is applied, you should not loosen or remove it unless you are directed to do so by medical control personnel. In situations in which transport may be significantly delayed, a physician may request that you either reposition the tourniquet to a location that is 2 to 3 inches proximal to the wound or apply a second tourniquet 2 to 3 inches proximal to the wound and then release the original tourniquet. This will allow for blood flow to as much of the injured extremity as possible without sacrificing hemorrhage control.

Suggested References

Cunningham A, Auerbach M, Cicero M, Jafri M. Tourniquet usage in prehospital care and resuscitation of pediatric trauma patients: Pediatric Trauma Society position statement. *J Trauma Acute Care Surg*. 2018;85(4):665–667. doi: 10.1097/TA.0000000000001839

Kelly JR, Levy MJ, Reyes J, Anders J. Effectiveness of the combat application tourniquet for arterial occlusion in young children. *J Trauma Acute Care Surg*. 2020;88(5): 644–647. doi: 10.1097/TA.0000000000002594

Joarder M, Noureddine El Moussaoui H, Das A, Williamson F, Wullschleger M. Impact of time and distance on outcomes following tourniquet use in civilian and military settings: a scoping review. *Injury*. 2023;54(5):1236–1245. doi: 10.1016/j.injury.2023.01.031

Kragh JF Jr, Littrel ML, Jones JA, et al. Battle casualty survival with emergency tourniquet use to stop limb bleeding. *J Emerg Med*. 2011;41(6):590–597. doi: 10.1016/j.jemermed.2009.07.022

Kragh JF Jr, Nam JJ, Berry KA, et al. Transfusion for shock in US military war casualties with and without tourniquet use. *Ann Emerg Med*. 2015;65(3):290–296. doi: 10.1016/j.annemergmed.2014.10.021

Kragh JF Jr, Walters TJ, Baer DG, et al. Survival with emergency tourniquet use to stop bleeding in major limb trauma. *Ann Surg*. 2009;249(1):1–7. doi: 10.1097/SLA.0b013e31818842ba

Sokol KK, Black GE, Azarow KS, Long W, Martin MJ, Eckert MJ. Prehospital interventions in severely injured pediatric patients: rethinking the ABCs. *J Trauma Acute Care Surg*. 2015;79(6):983–989

OTHER RESOURCES

Stop the Bleed. American College of Surgeons. Accessed April, 25, 2025. https://www.stopthebleed.org/

Procedure 26: Push-Pull Fluid Administration

Susan Fuchs, MD, FAAP, FACEP

Introduction

For a child in shock, rapid fluid administration is important. However, for a small child, a 20-mL/kg bolus is hard to administer via a pressure bag or by squeezing the intravenous (IV) fluid bag, because it is unclear how much fluid is actually delivered. By using the push-pull method, aliquots of 20 mL/kg can be delivered rapidly and accurately via IV or intraosseous administration.

INDICATIONS

Rapid and precise fluid delivery

CONTRAINDICATIONS

Lack of proper equipment
Cardiogenic shock

EQUIPMENT

Intravenous catheters, 14- to 24-gauge
Intravenous tubing
Extension connector
Intravenous solution
20-mL syringe
Three-way stopcock

Rationale

When a child is in shock, rapid delivery of crystalloid fluid is the treatment of choice. Because a bolus of 20 mL/kg is used, it is important to know how much fluid is being administered to a small child. Using the push-pull method, this fluid can be delivered rapidly and accurately.

Preparation

1. Assemble the equipment.
2. Attach the IV tubing to the fluid bag, then the 3-way stopcock to the end of the tubing. Make sure the closed arrow is pointing to the tubing.

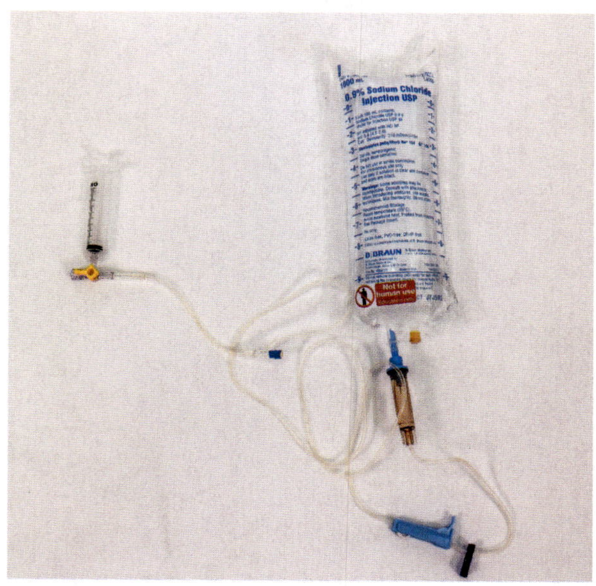

PROCEDURE 26-1

Push-Pull Fluid Administration

1. When the IV is established and secured, attach the extension tubing to the IV catheter hub.
2. Attach the 20-mL syringe to 1 hub of the 3-way stopcock.
3. Attach the last hub of the 3-way stopcock to the extension tubing.
4. Turn the 3-way stopcock so the closed arrow is pointing to the extension tubing. Fill the 20-mL syringe with fluid.

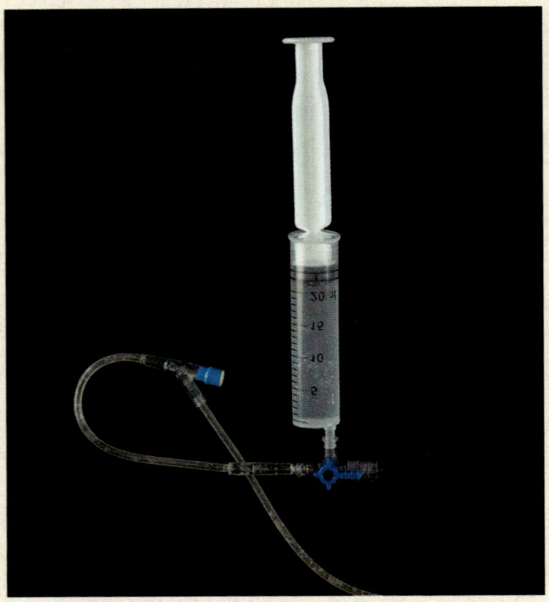

5. Turn the closed arrow of the 3-way stopcock toward the fluid bag and tubing, then administer the 20 mL of fluid to the patient.

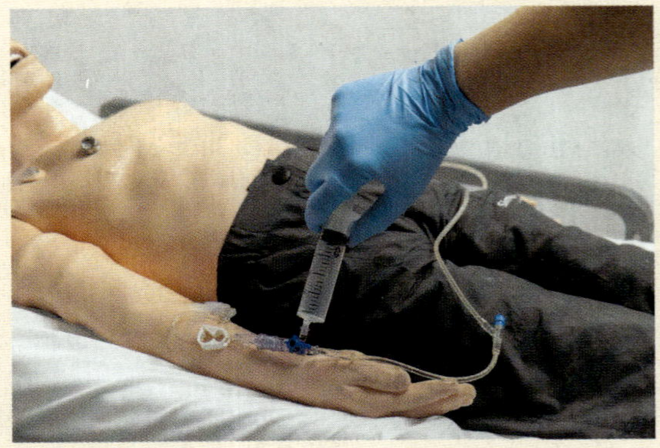

6. Turn the closed arrow of the 3-way stopcock toward the patient and refill the 20-mL syringe.
7. Turn the closed arrow toward the IV tubing and bag and administer 20 mL of fluid to the patient.
8. Repeat this process until you have given the same number of syringes as the patient's weight in kilograms, at which point they have then received a 20-mL/kg fluid bolus.

TIP

This process can be repeated if the child needs additional 20-mL/kg fluid boluses.

CAUTION

If the IV catheter is small (eg, 24-gauge), you can still infuse fluid rapidly; however, monitor the site for infiltration.

Medication Formulary

Chris Coughlin, PhD, NRP
Rudy Kink, MD, FAAP
Amy Mitchell-Van Steele, PharmD, FPPA

Note: The following drugs may be used for pediatric prehospital care. Certain drugs may not be available in some emergency medical services systems per local policy.

Acetaminophen, APAP

Use: Analgesic, antipyretic	**Recommended Dose** PO/G-tube: 15 mg/kg Rectal: 15–20 mg/kg) **Maximum Dose** 1 g	**Precautions:** Ensure proper concentration. Use with caution in patients with liver disease. **Adverse Reactions:** Nausea, vomiting

Activated Charcoal

Use: Gastric decontamination for certain ingestions such as aspirin, tricyclic antidepressants, barbiturates	**Recommended Dose** Initial dose, according to age: • $<$1 year, 10–25 g PO/NG • 1–12 years, 25–50 g PO/NG • $>$12 years, 25–100 g PO/NG **Maximum Dose** 100 g	**Precautions:** According to local emergency medical services policy, the prehospital professional should consult medical oversight or poison control (1-800-222-1222). Iron, lithium, alcohols, ethylene glycol, alkalis, fluoride, mineral acids, and potassium do not bind to activated charcoal. Administer as soon as possible after ingestion. Avoid aspiration. If airway reflexes are impaired, the risk of administering activated charcoal may outweigh the benefits. Commercially available preparations include charcoal with sorbitol (used to produce catharsis) and charcoal in water. Fatal hypernatremic dehydration has been reported after repeated doses of charcoal with sorbitol. With preparations containing propylene glycol, potentially fatal toxicities seen in neonates, such as seizures, lactic acidosis, and respiratory depression. **Adverse Reactions:** Vomiting, constipation, obstruction, development of intestinal bezoar, diarrhea, dehydration, pulmonary aspiration, mouth discoloration

Adenosine

Use	Dose	Precautions
Use: Supraventricular tachycardia (SVT), regular monomorphic wide-complex tachycardia	**Recommended Dose** Initial dose: 0.1 mg/kg rapid IV or IO bolus over 1–2 seconds (maximum, 6 mg); follow with saline flush Second dose: 0.2 mg/kg (maximum, 12 mg; follow with saline flush **Maximum Dose** First dose: 6 mg Second dose: 12 mg	**Precautions:** Use continuous cardiac monitoring. Avoid use in second- or third-degree AV block, sick sinus syndrome. Administer at IV site closest to patient's heart; follow with a rapid saline flush (5–10 mL). **Adverse Reactions:** Nausea, hypotension, dyspnea, bronchospasm, chest pain/pressure, tingling, heart block, dysrhythmias, facial flushing, metallic taste; in those with asthma, bronchoconstriction may occur

Albuterol

Use	Dose	Precautions
Use: Prevention and acute relief of bronchospasm, prophylaxis for exercise-induced bronchospasm	**Recommended Dose** Nebulizer solution (1.25 mg/3 mL, 2.5 mg/3 mL, 5 mg/mL): 2.5 mg every 15–20 minutes for 3 doses; repeat up to 10–20 mg every 1–4 hours as needed; dilute in minimum of 2–3 mL of saline if needed for adequate nebulization; may use continuously for status asthmaticus MDI: 4–8 puffs (90 µg/puff) every 15–20 minutes for 3 doses; repeat every 1–4 hours as needed **Maximum Dose** Not established for status asthmaticus	**Precaution:** Tremors and tachycardia are common. **Adverse Reactions:** Nausea, palpitations, headache, dizziness, tremor, tachycardia

Amiodarone

Use	Dose	Precautions
Use: Life-threatening ventricular arrhythmias: VF or VT	**Recommended Dose** 5 mg/kg IV or IO push for VF or pulseless VT 5 mg/kg IV or IO infusion over 20–60 minutes for wide complex tachycardia May repeat initial loading dose twice for acute treatment **Maximum Dose** 300 mg/dose 15 mg/kg (maximum total dose)	**Precautions:** Must dilute with 20 mL of 5% dextrose before administration to avoid thrombophlebitis and hypotension. May be given undiluted in pulseless VT or VF. May cause hypotension and prolonged Q-T interval; slow rate of infusion if hypotension or bradycardia develop. Should not use in combination with procainamide. Contraindicated in severe sinus node dysfunction, marked sinus bradycardia, second- and third-degree AV block. **Adverse Reactions:** Hypotension, bradycardia, dysrhythmias, vomiting

Aspirin

Use	Dose	Precautions
Use: Analgesic, antipyretic	**Recommended Dose** 10–15 mg/kg **Maximum Dose** 1 g/dose	**Precautions:** Avoid use in patients aged <18 years with chickenpox or influenza due to association with Reye syndrome. Not routinely used in pediatrics. **Adverse Reactions:** Nausea, vomiting, abdominal pain, ulcers, rash, urticaria, bronchospasm

Atropine

Use	Recommended Dose	Precautions
Use: Sinus bradycardia, chemical nerve gas and organophosphate pesticide poisoning, rapid-sequence intubation of infants	**Recommended Dose** IV or IO: 0.02 mg/kg ET tube: 0.04–0.06 mg/kg/dose May repeat dose every 5 minutes to maximum total dose of 1 mg for a child and 2 mg for an adolescent Organophosphate/carbamate/nerve agent poisoning: 0.05–0.1 mg/kg IM, IV, or IO; repeat every 3–5 minutes as needed, with doubling doses titrated to pulmonary status **Maximum Dose** Single dose: 0.5 mg for a child, 1 mg for an adolescent for sinus bradycardia	**Precautions:** Atropine sulfate comes in different concentrations; calculate dosage accordingly. Avoid in tachydysrhythmias. Use caution in children with brain damage or spastic paralysis. Anticholinesterase poisonings may require large doses, so maximum dose does not apply (will also need pralidoxime). Slow IV injection may result in paradoxical bradycardia. **Adverse Reactions:** Dry mouth, blurred vision, tachycardia, constipation, urinary retention

Calcium Chloride

Use	Recommended Dose	Precautions
Use: Hypocalcemia, hyperkalemia, hypermagnesemia, calcium channel blocker toxicity Recommended for cardiac resuscitation only in cases of documented hyperkalemia, hypocalcemia, or calcium channel blocker toxicity	**Recommended Dose** 20 mg/kg IV or IO slowly (if using 10% calcium chloride, dose is 0.2 mL/kg); inject slowly while monitoring HR; repeat dose in 10 minutes as necessary for desired clinical effects **Maximum Dose** 2,000 mg in cardiac arrest when hyperkalemia, hypocalcemia, or calcium channel blocker toxicity is present/suspected; 1,000 mg for all other indications	**Precautions:** Stop injection if symptomatic bradycardia occurs. Calcium chloride administration results in a more rapid increase in ionized calcium concentrations than calcium gluconate and is preferred for the critically ill child. Infuse at a maximum rate of 50–100 mg/min. During cardiac arrest, may administer over 20 seconds. Extravascular administration can result in severe skin injury. Highly irritating to tissues. Avoid scalp vein and small hand or foot veins for IV administration. **Adverse Reactions:** Tissue extravasation and necrosis; may exacerbate metabolic acidosis; hypotension, bradycardia, arrhythmias, VF

Calcium Gluconate (Preferred in Neonates)

Use: Ionized hypocalcemia, hyperkalemia, hypermagnesemia, calcium channel blocker toxicity Recommended for cardiac resuscitation only in cases of documented hyperkalemia, hypocalcemia, or calcium channel blocker toxicity	**Recommended Dose** 60 mg/kg IV or IO slowly (if using 10% calcium gluconate, dose is 0.6 mL/kg); inject slowly while monitoring HR; repeat dose in 10 minutes as necessary for desired clinical effects **Maximum Dose** 3,000 mg in cardiac arrest	**Precautions:** Stop injection if symptomatic bradycardia occurs. Calcium chloride administration results in a more rapid increase in ionized calcium concentrations than calcium gluconate and is preferred for the critically ill child. Infuse at maximum rate of 100 mg/min. Extravascular administration can result in severe skin injury. Highly irritating to tissues. Avoid scalp vein and small hand or foot veins for IV administration. **Adverse Reactions:** Tissue extravasation and necrosis, hypotension, bradycardia, arrhythmias, VF

Dexamethasone

Use: Croup, asthma	**Recommended Dose** Asthma: 0.6–1.0 mg/kg IV, IM, or PO Croup: 0.15–0.6 mg/kg IV, IM, or PO **Maximum Dose** 16 mg/dose	**Precautions:** Long-acting glucocorticoid, so actions and side effects are prolonged. Parenteral dexamethasone may be mixed with a flavored oral solution and given PO. Rapid IV administration is associated with perineal burning and tingling; infuse over 1–4 minutes to decrease perineal discomfort. Oral liquid products may contain alcohol. **Adverse Reactions:** Sodium and fluid retention, hyperglycemia

Diazepam

Use: Seizures, agitation, rapid-sequence intubation	**Recommended Dose** IV: 0.1 mg/kg every 5–10 minutes; administer over approximately 2 minutes to avoid pain at intravenous site PR, according to age: • 2–5 years, 0.5 mg/kg • 6–11 years, 0.3 mg/kg • ≥12 years, 0.2 mg/kg **Maximum Dose** IV: 10 mg/dose PR: 20 mg	**Precautions:** There is an increased incidence of apnea when combined with other sedative agents or when given rapidly. Be prepared to provide respiratory support. Monitor oxygen saturation. Avoid extravasation to prevent venous thrombosis or phlebitis. Avoid prolonged use of parenteral diazepam because it contains 40% propylene glycol as a diluent. To prevent hypotension or respiratory arrest, do not exceed 1–2 mg/min administration time. **Adverse Reactions:** Respiratory depression, drowsiness, bradycardia, hypotension, apnea, pain at injection site

Diphenhydramine

Use: Anaphylaxis, antihistamine	**Recommended Dose** IV or PO: 1 mg/kg **Maximum Dose** IV or PO: 50 mg	**Precautions:** May cause sedation and respiratory suppression, especially if using other sedative agents. May cause hypotension. Overdose may cause hallucinations and seizures. Rapid IV administration may precipitate seizures. Administer undiluted at a rate of ≤25 mg/min. All doses may cause paradoxical excitement or agitation. **Adverse Reactions:** Drowsiness, dry mouth, constipation, urinary retention

Dopamine

Use	Dose	Precautions
Use: Hypotension, shock	**Recommended Dose** Neonates: IV or IO infusion, 2–20 µg/kg/min Children: IV or IO infusion, 2–20 µg/kg/min Titrate up to desired effect by 5–10 µg/kg/min increments: • 5 µg/kg/min = low dose (renal blood flow and urine output) • 10 µg/kg/min = moderate dose (β activity—increases HR, contractility, and blood pressure) • 20 µg/kg/min = high dose (α activity—vasoconstriction and increasing blood pressure) **Maximum Dose** 20 µg/kg/min	**Precautions:** Infusion rates greater than 20 µg/kg/min may produce extreme peripheral vasoconstriction and ischemia. Mix with great caution. Extravascular administration can result in severe skin injury. Avoid small veins; central line preferred. Dopamine is inactivated in an alkaline solution. Correct hypovolemia before use. Do not abruptly stop the infusion; instead, gradually titrate down before discontinuing. **Adverse Reactions:** Ectopic beats, tachycardia, palpitations, vasoconstriction, dyspnea, vomiting

Droperidol

Use	Dose	Precautions
Use: Severe agitation	**Recommended Dose** ≥7 years, according to weight, IM or IV: • <34 kg, 0.625 mg • 34–57 kg, 1.25 mg • 57–68 kg, 1.875 mg • >68 kg, 2.5 mg **Maximum Dose** 2.5 mg	**Precaution:** Avoid use with other drugs that prolong QT interval. **Adverse Reactions:** Dystonic reaction, QT prolongation, black box warning for suicidality

Epinephrine

Use	Recommended Dose	Precautions / Adverse Reactions
Use: Croup, anaphylaxis, acute asthma, cardiac arrest, shock	**Recommended Dose** Anaphylaxis: IM, 0.01 mg/kg/dose = 0.01 mL/kg/dose of 1-mg/mL concentration (maximum, 0.3 mg = 0.3 mL); repeat dose every 5–15 minutes Intranasal: • For children aged ≥4 years and who weigh 15-<30 kg, use 1 mg in 1 nostril • For children ≥30 kg, use 2 mg spray in 1 nostril • Can repeat dose in same nostril if no improvement after 5 minutes Anaphylactic shock: IV, 0.01 mg/kg of **0.1-mg/mL concentration** (maximum, 0.5 mg) Cardiac arrest: • Newborn: IV/IO, 0.01–0.03 mg/kg of 0.1-mg/mL concentration ET: 0.05–0.1 mg/kg of 0.1-mg/ML concentration • Infant and children: IV/IO, 0.01 mg/kg of 0.1-mg/mL concentration ET: 0.1 mg/kg of 1 mg/mL concentration Shock: 0.1–1 µg/kg/min of **0.1-mg/mL concentration** "Push dose": 1 µg/kg (0.1 mL/kg) up to 10 µg/kg (1 mL) of **0.1-mg/mL concentration** Croup: 0.25–0.5 mL/kg of 1-mg/mL concentration in 3 mL of NS by inhalation (maximum, 5 mL/dose) Racemic epinephrine (2.25%) for croup: 0.1 mL/kg by inhalation (maximum, 0.5 mL) in 3 mL of NS; may repeat every 20 minutes	**Precautions:** Use length-based resuscitation tape or computer software to verify correct dose. Read concentration on label carefully. Incompatible with alkaline solutions. Extravascular administration can result in severe skin injury. • Anaphylaxis: Preferred location is IM, in the anterolateral aspect of the middle-third thigh. Some anaphylactic reactions require large doses of epinephrine that may be administered IV. • Cardiac arrest: If administered through an ET tube, follow with saline flush or dilute in isotonic saline flush (1 to 5 mL) based on patient length/weight. **Adverse Reactions:** Tachycardia, palpitations, cardiac dysrhythmias, diaphoresis, vomiting, headache, dizziness

Fentanyl

Use: Analgesic, anesthetic for intubation and maintenance	**Recommended Dose** IV: 1 μg/kg/dose every 30–60 minutes Intranasal: 1–2 μg/kg **Maximum Dose** 50 μg, titrate to effect	**Precautions:** There is an increased incidence of apnea when combined with other sedative agents, particularly benzodiazepines. Avoid rapid IV infusion; inject slowly over 3–5 minutes. If given rapidly IV, may cause chest wall or glottic rigidity, which may be reversed with a muscle relaxant. Intranasal administration: Give one-half in each nostril using atomizer device or drip into nostril with syringe. Maximum volume is 1 mL/nostril. **Adverse Reactions:** Apnea, bradycardia, nausea, vomiting

Flumazenil

Use: Reverse sedative effects of benzodiazepines, *except* those receiving benzodiazepines for seizures	**Recommended Dose** IV: 0.01–0.02 mg/kg over 15 seconds; repeat every 1 minute as needed When IV access is unavailable, may be given IM **Maximum Dose** 0.2 mg/dose and to cumulative total dose of 0.05 mg/kg or 1 mg	**Precaution:** May precipitate acute withdrawal in dependent patients. May precipitate seizures in high-risk patients receiving benzodiazepines over the long term, sedative/hypnotics, or other co-ingestants in an overdose. Observe for re-sedation. Avoid single-bolus injection. Do not give to patients receiving benzodiazepines for seizures. **Adverse Reactions:** Rebound sedation or respiratory depression owing to its short duration of action; rebound sedation especially common in children aged 1–5 years; flushing, nausea, blurred vision, agitation, thrombophlebitis, seizures

Fosphenytoin

Use: Seizures, status epilepticus	**Recommended Dose** 15–20 mg PE/kg IV, IM, or IO; do not administer faster than 2 mg PE/kg/min or a total of 150 mg PE/min **Maximum Dose** 1,500 mg PE	**Precautions:** Rate of infusion should not exceed 150 mg PE/min or 2 mg PE/kg/min. Reduce rate of infusion if HR decreases by 10 bpm or hypotension occurs. Dosages and concentrations are expressed as phenytoin sodium equivalents. Rapid IV administration may produce hypotension; may dilute in NS or D_5W. IM administration not preferred, but quadricep area may be used if needed. **Adverse Reactions:** Hypotension, bradycardia, central nervous system depression, ataxia, dizziness, headache, paresthesia, pruritus; itching is common and is controlled by reducing flow rate

Furosemide

Use: Fluid overload, congestive heart failure, diuresis, edema, pulmonary edema, hypertension	**Recommended Dose** 1–2 mg/kg IV, IO, or IM **Maximum Dose** 40 mg	**Precautions:** Do not give to child with hypovolemia. Contraindicated in anuria. **Adverse Reactions:** Hypotension, electrolyte depletion, alkalosis, tinnitus, ototoxic

Glucagon

Use: Calcium channel blocker overdose, hypoglycemia	**Recommended Dose** Hypoglycemia due to insulin excess: • For children <20 kg, 0.02–0.03 mg/kg • For children ≥20 kg, 1 mg IV, IO, or IM • Repeat every 15 minutes if needed for clinical effect; total of 3 doses Calcium channel blocker overdose: IV: 0.05 mg/kg load followed by 0.05–0.1 mg/kg/h infusion **Maximum Dose** Calcium channel blocker overdose: 5 mg/h Pediatric hypoglycemia: 1 mg	**Precautions:** Use immediately after reconstitution. Use caution in patients with pheochromocytoma. Supplemental carbohydrates (IV dextrose) should be given as soon as possible. **Adverse Reactions:** Nausea, vomiting, hypotension, tachycardia; nausea/vomiting incidence higher with rapid administration and higher doses

Glucose (Dextrose)

Use: Hypoglycemia	**Recommended Dose** Newborn: 2 mL/kg/dose 10% dextrose IV or IO Neonate: 5–10 mL/kg/dose 10% dextrose IV or IO <2 years: 5 mL/kg/dose 10% dextrose IV or IO ≥2 years: 2–4 mL/kg/dose 25% dextrose IV or IO or 5–10 mL/kg/dose of 10% dextrose IV or IO **Maximum Dose** Doses guided by repeated serum glucose level determinations	**Precautions:** Depending on situation, hypoglycemia may reoccur. Use caution in multiple concentrations. In emergency situations, 25% dextrose may be used peripherally in infants and adolescents. **Adverse Reactions:** Hyperglycemia, thrombophlebitis, extravasation, hyponatremia

Haloperidol

Use: Severe agitation	**Recommended Dose** 0.025–0.5 mg/kg IM/PO; may repeat every 20–30 minutes **Maximum Dose** ≤40 kg, 6 mg/d >40 kg, 15 mg/d	**Precautions:** Frequently given in same syringe with diphenhydramine. If dystonic reaction, give diphenhydramine. **Adverse Reactions:** Dystonic reaction, hypotension, decreased seizure threshold

Hydrocortisone

Use: Acute adrenal insufficiency/adrenal crisis, septic shock	**Recommended Dose** 1–2 mg/kg IV, IO, or IM **Maximum Dose** 100 mg	**Precautions:** Do not use for head injury. Use with caution in patients with hypertension, heart failure, or renal or hepatic impairment. If given IM, avoid deltoid muscle due to higher incidence of soft tissue atrophy. **Adverse Reactions:** Dysrhythmia, hypertension, adrenal suppression

Ibuprofen

Use: Analgesic, antipyretic	**Recommended Dose** 10 mg/kg/dose PO **Maximum Dose** 600 mg	**Precautions:** Cross-reacts with aspirin allergy, gastrointestinal bleeding. Liquid products may contain alcohol. Do not use in patients with kidney disease or in those who have a single kidney. Do not use in infants aged <6 months. Verify concentration of liquid products. **Adverse Reactions:** Vomiting, gastritis, ulcer formation, rash

Ipratropium

Use: Asthma	**Recommended Dose** Nebulized solution (0.5 mg/2.5 mL): • Children < 12 years: 0.25 mg nebulized every 20 minutes for 3 doses • Children ≥ 12 years: 0.5 mg nebulized every 20 minutes for 3 doses **Maximum Dose** 0.5 mg	**Precautions:** Use with albuterol every 20 minutes × 3. May be administered with or without further dilution. **Adverse Reactions:** Tachycardia, dry mouth, headache, cough, hoarseness, blurred vision

Ketamine

Use: Anesthesia for intubation, pain control, and agitation	**Recommended Dose** IV: 1–2 mg/kg for intubation and pain control IM: 4–5 mg/kg for intubation and pain, 4 mg/kg for agitation Intranasal: 5 mg/kg **Maximum Dose** 100 mg	**Precautions:** Administer slowly over 1 minute. Emergence reactions may occur up to 24 hours postoperatively: delirium, hallucinations, vivid dreams. Avoid use in patients with increased intraocular pressure or bowel obstruction. Hypersalivation/lacrimation common in pediatric patients; may be used in combination with anticholinergic drugs to decrease incidence. American College of Emergency Physicians considers the use of ketamine in those <3 months of age an absolute contraindication owing to high risk of airway complications. Several concentrations of products available. If giving intranasally, use 50 mg/mL or 100 mg/mL, dilute to concentration of 20 mg/mL and administer half in each nostril using atomizer device or needleless syringe. **Adverse Reactions:** Hallucinations, tonic-clonic movements, nausea, vomiting, decreased cough reflex, nystagmus, tachycardia, bronchospasm, hypertension, bradycardia, hypotension, apnea; may cause purposeless movements

Lidocaine

Use: VT, VF, wide-complex supraventricular tachycardia	**Recommended Dose** Shock-refractory VF or pulseless VT: • IV/IO loading dose: 1 mg/kg; repeat in 10–15 minutes for 2 doses if needed; • IV continuous infusion after loading dose: 20–50 µg/kg/min • ET: 2–3 mg/kg/dose Flush with 5 mL NS with IV/IO; flush with 2–5 mL for ET **Maximum Dose** IV/ET: 3 mg/kg	**Precautions:** Contraindicated in complete heart block and wide complex tachycardia due to accessory conduction pathways. Excessive dosage may result in myocardial depression, hypotension, agitation, or seizures. Hypersensitivity to amide anesthetics. If administered through an ET tube, follow the dose with saline flush or dilute in isotonic saline flush (1 to 5 mL) according to patient size. **Adverse Reactions:** Arrhythmias, seizures, respiratory depression or arrest

Lorazepam

Use	Recommended Dose	Precautions
Use: Anticonvulsant, anxiety, sedation	**Recommended Dose** Status epilepticus: 0.05–0.1 mg/kg IV or IO over 2–5 minutes; repeat 0.05 mg/kg second dose in 5–15 minutes if needed Sedation/anxiety: 0.05 mg/kg IV or IO over 2–5 minutes; repeat 0.05 mg/kg second dose in 5–15 minutes if needed **Maximum Dose** Status epilepticus: 4 mg/dose Sedation: 2 mg/dose	**Precautions:** Beware of respiratory depression. There is an increased incidence of apnea when combined with other sedative agents. Monitor oxygen saturation and be prepared to provide respiratory support. Do not reverse in patient with seizures. Dilute with equal volume of D_5W or NS. IV preparations contain alcohol. **Adverse Reactions:** Bradycardia, hypotension, apnea, confusion, hallucinations, myoclonic jerking in preterm infants

Magnesium Sulfate

Use	Recommended Dose	Precautions
Use: Asthma Eclampsia Torsades de pointes Documented hypomagnesemia	**Recommended Dose** 25–50 mg/kg IV/IO over 10–20 minutes 25–50 mg/kg IV/IO bolus if pulseless, over 10–20 minutes if pulse 50 mg/kg over 20 minutes 4 g over 20 minutes (may need to dilute in 100-mL saline) **Maximum Dose** 2 g	**Precautions:** Insufficient evidence to recommend magnesium administration during cardiac arrest. Use with caution in the presence of heart block. May cause hypotension in those taking nifedipine. **Adverse Reactions:** Vasodilation may produce hypotension if administered rapidly; flushing, hypermagnesemia

Mannitol

Use	Recommended Dose	Precautions
Use: Diuresis Reduces intercranial pressure	**Recommended Dose** IV: 0.25–1 g/kg over 20–60 minutes **Maximum Dose** 2 g/kg body weight	**Precautions:** Inspect vials for crystals; if present, redissolve by warming. Use 5-µm filter for 20% solutions or greater. Avoid excessive fluid loss with diuresis to prevent dehydration and electrolyte imbalance. Administer over 20–60 minutes. **Adverse Reactions:** Dehydration, fluid and electrolyte imbalance, headache, hypovolemia, seizures, water intoxication

Methylprednisolone

Use: Asthma, croup	**Recommended Dose** 1–2 mg/kg/dose IV or IO **Maximum Dose** 60 mg/d	**Precautions:** Rapid IV push of high doses ($>$ 250 mg) in $<$ 20 minutes may cause hypotension, arrhythmias, and sudden death. Use caution with multiple dosage forms; use methylprednisolone sodium succinate IV. May contain alcohol. **Adverse Reactions:** Edema, pituitary-adrenal suppression, hypokalemia, peptic ulcer, nausea, vomiting

Midazolam

Use: Anxiety, seizures, rapid-sequence intubation	**Recommended Dose** Status epilepticus: IV or IO: 0.1 mg/kg; IM or intranasal: 0.2 mg/kg; may repeat in 5–15 minutes as needed Sedation: IV, IO, or IM: 0.05–0.1 mg/kg Intranasal: 0.2 mg/kg **Maximum Dose** 6 months to 6 years: 6 mg $\geq$ 6 years: 10 mg	**Precautions:** Avoid rapid IV administration, which may produce respiratory arrest and seizures. There is an increased incidence of apnea when combined with other sedative agents, particularly benzodiazepines. Be prepared to provide respiratory support, regardless of route of administration. Monitor oxygen saturation. May be reversed with flumazenil. Myoclonus may occur in preterm infants. Paradoxical excitation may occur in children. May be reversed with flumazenil. Multiple-concentration parenteral products available. Use 5 mg/mL for intranasal administration, administer one-half dose in each nostril using atomizer or needleless syringe (maximum, 1 mL in each nostril). Administer IM injection undiluted into large muscle, preferably anterior-lateral aspect of thigh in pediatric patients. **Adverse Reactions:** Bradycardia, hypotension, cardiac arrest, apnea, respiratory depression

Morphine

Use	Dose	Precautions
Use: Severe acute and chronic pain	**Recommended Dose** • Neonates and infants aged ≤6 months: 0.05 mg/kg/dose IM, IV, IO • Infants aged >6 months and children: 0.05–0.1 mg/kg IM, IV, IO • Adolescents: 3–4 mg IV or IO, repeat in 5 minutes as needed **Maximum Dose** • Neonates and infants aged ≤6 months: 0.1 mg/kg • Infants aged >6 months, children, and adolescents: 5 mg	**Precautions:** Pediatric patients are more sensitive to effects of opiates. They may also have a hypersensitivity to similar opiates. Some products may contain sulfites. There is an increased incidence of apnea when combined with other sedative agents, particularly benzodiazepines. Be prepared to provide respiratory support, regardless of route of administration. Monitor oxygen saturation. May be reversed with naloxone. IM not preferred route of administration due to local tissue irritation, pain, variable absorption, and lag time to peak effect. **Adverse Reactions:** Respiratory depression, hypotension, rash, constipation

Naloxone

Use	Dose	Precautions
Use: Opiate intoxication	**Recommended Dose** Pediatric: 0.1 mg/kg/dose IV, IO, IM, ET, intranasal; repeat dose every 2–3 minutes if needed If given via ET tube, administer 2–3 times IV dose **Maximum Dose** 2 mg, but overdoses involving synthetic opioids may require considerably higher doses	**Precautions:** Dilute to 1–2 mL with NS for ET use. May induce acute withdrawal in opioid dependency. Patients who receive naloxone should be continuously observed for re-narcotization for at least 2 hours after last dose. Doses may be repeated as needed to maintain opiate reversal. IM absorption may be erratic. Do not administer naloxone to a newborn whose mother is suspected of recently abusing drugs, because there is a risk of acute withdrawal in the infant. If administered intranasally, alternate nostrils for repeated doses.

Nitrous Oxide, Dinitrogen Oxide, N_2O, Laughing Gas

Use: Analgesia, sedation	**Recommended Dose** 25%–50% with oxygen 50:50 **Maximum Dose** 70%	**Precaution:** Asphyxiation may occur. **Adverse Reactions:** Malignant hyperthermia, cardiac dysrhythmias, nausea, vomiting, delirium

Norepinephrine

Use: Shock	**Recommended Dose** 0.05–2.0 µg/kg/min IV, titrated to desired response **Maximum Dose** 2 µg/kg/min	**Precautions:** Double-check concentration and infusion rate. Avoid using scalp veins. Ensure adequate volume replacement before initiation. Central line preferred; extravasation may cause severe tissue necrosis. Do not abruptly stop the infusion; instead, gradually titrate down before discontinuing. **Adverse Reactions:** Bradycardia, hypertension, arrhythmias, palpitations, pallor, ischemic necrosis, organ ischemia

Olanzapine (Zyprexa)

Use: Agitation, psychosis	**Recommended Dose** Children aged <10 years: 1.25–2.5 mg PO/IM Children aged ≥10 years: 5–10 mg PO/IM **Maximum Dose** 10 mg	**Precaution:** Avoid use within 1 hour of benzodiazepine use. **Adverse Reactions:** Sedation, paradoxical reaction

Ondansetron

Use: Nausea/ vomiting	**Recommended Dose** IV: Aged 1 month - 12 years (or =/<40 kg) 0.15 mg/ kg; aged ≥12 years (>40 kg) 8 mg ODT: Aged ≥3 months and < 15 kg, 2 mg 15-30 kg, 4 mg >30 kg, 8 mg **Maximum Dose** IV, 16 mg ODT, 8 mg	**Precautions:** Do not use in patients with long QT syndrome. Serotonin syndrome may occur with 5-HT_3 receptor antagonist. **Adverse Reactions:** Headache, fatigue, dry mouth, malaise, constipation

Phenobarbital

Use: Status epilepticus, sedation	**Recommended Dose** 20 mg/kg IV or IO over 20 min (1 mg/kg/min); not to exceed 30 mg/min May repeat after 15 min if needed to maximum total dose of 40 mg/kg **Maximum Dose** 1,000 mg/dose	**Precautions:** There is an increased incidence of apnea when combined with other sedative agents. Be prepared to provide respiratory support. Monitor oxygen saturation. Avoid extravasation because parenteral solutions are very alkaline. Parenteral formulations may contain alcohol. **Adverse Reactions:** Drowsiness, hypotension, apnea, paradoxical excitation, respiratory depression, thrombophlebitis

Phenytoin

Use	Recommended Dose	Precautions
Use: Status epilepticus	**Recommended Dose** • Neonates: 15–20 mg/kg • Children: 20 mg/kg IV or IO over 20 min (1 mg/kg/min); not to exceed 50 mg/min **Maximum Dose** 1,000 mg/dose	**Precautions:** Incompatible with glucose solutions. Monitor HR and reduce infusion if rate decreases by 10 bpm. Rapid IV administration may trigger VF and cardiac arrest. Avoid extravasation. Injections may contain propylene glycol and benzyl alcohol. 0.22- to 0.55-µm in-line filter preferred for IV piggyback solutions. **Adverse Reactions:** Bradycardia, hypotension, arrhythmias, cardiovascular collapse, nystagmus, drowsiness, purple glove syndrome

Pralidoxime Chloride, 2-PAM, 2-Pyridine Aldoxime Methochloride

Use	Recommended Dose	Precautions
Use: Organophosphate poisoning, carbamate insecticide poisoning with nicotinic symptoms, anticholinesterase poisoning	**Recommended Dose** IV: 25–50 mg/kg over 5–30 minutes, then 10 mg/kg/h or repeat load after 1 hour IM: 15 mg/kg (up to 600 mg), repeat as needed every 15 minutes to a maximum of 45 mg/kg **Maximum Dose** 2 g/dose Severe signs and symptoms may require repeated dosing	**Precautions:** Rapid IV administration may cause tachycardia, laryngospasm, muscle rigidity, and transient neuromuscular blockade. Infuse IV loading dose over 15–30 minutes, not to exceed 200 mg/min. IV route preferred, but may be given IM when IV route is not immediately accessible. May be used in conjunction with atropine. **Adverse Reactions:** Nausea, headache, dizziness, diplopia, hyperventilation

Quetiapine (Seroquel)		
Use: Agitation, psychosis	**Recommended Dose** Aged <10 years: 6.25–12.5 mg PO Aged ≥10 years: 25 mg PO **Maximum Dose** 25 mg	**Precaution:** Can lower seizure threshold. **Adverse Reactions:** Hypotension, hypertension, QT prolongation

Rocuronium Bromide		
Use: Adjunct to general anesthesia to facilitate tracheal intubation and provide skeletal muscle relaxation during mechanical ventilation	**Recommended Dose** IV: 1 mg/kg **Maximum Dose** 1.2 mg/kg	**Precautions:** Ventilatory support is necessary. Prepare to respond with airway management. Do not mix with alkaline solutions. May interact with certain antibiotics that have neuromuscular blocking actions (eg, aminoglycosides) and enhance neuromuscular blockade. Toxicity may be increased in patients with pulmonary disease. **Adverse Reactions:** Muscle weakness, hypotension or hypertension, arrhythmias, tachycardia, bronchospasm, hiccoughs

Sodium Bicarbonate

Use	Recommended Dose	Precautions / Adverse Reactions
Use: Cyclic antidepressant overdose, hyperkalemia	**Recommended Dose** Pediatric: 1 mEq/kg IV or IO slowly **Maximum Dose** 50 mEq/dose	**Precautions:** Do not mix with calcium, dopamine, or epinephrine. May cause tissue necrosis owing to IV extravasation. Use caution with renal impairment. No more than 0.5 mEq/mL for neonatal use. **Adverse Reactions:** Cerebral hemorrhage, edema, hypernatremia, hypokalemia, hypocalcemia, metabolic alkalosis

Succinylcholine, Suxamethonium

Use	Recommended Dose	Precautions / Adverse Reactions
Use: Adjunct to general anesthesia, ET intubation, mechanical ventilation	**Recommended Dose** IV, IO, according to age: • <6 months, 2-3 mg/kg/dose • ≥6 months, 1-2 mg/kg/dose • Children, 1-2 mg/kg/dose • Adolescents, 1-1,5 mg/kg/dose IM: 4–5 mg/kg/dose	**Precautions:** Contraindicated in conditions associated with increased ICP, severe burns, spinal cord injury, neuromuscular disease, myopathy, or malignant hyperthermia. When these contraindications exist, use a nondepolarizing muscle relaxant such as rocuronium. Ventilatory support is necessary. If cardiac arrest occurs immediately after administration of succinylcholine, hyperkalemia must be suspected (particularly in boys aged <9 years). Toxicity is increased in patients with muscle injury, muscle myopathies, rhabdomyolysis, or low pseudocholinesterase levels. Children are more susceptible to developing bradycardia, cardiac arrest, and myoglobinemia. Atropine is recommended before administration of succinylcholine in children. **Adverse Reactions:** Bradycardia, hypotension, arrhythmias, apnea, cardiac arrest, hyperkalemia, malignant hyperthermia

Tranexamic Acid (TXA)

Use: Any sustained blunt or penetration trauma within 3 hours of injury and suspected hemorrhagic shock	**Recommended Dose** $<$ 12 years: 15 mg/kg IV over 10 minutes (maximum dose, 1 g) $\geq$ 12 years: 1 g IV over 10 minutes **Maximum Dose** 1 g	**Precautions:** Must be administered within 3 hours of injury. Not indicated for patients with known thrombophilia. Not indicated for isolated head injury. Not indicated for cervical spinal injury with motor deficit. Not indicated for traumatic arrest without return of spontaneous circulation. **Adverse Reactions:** Hypotension with rapid administration, nausea/vomiting, blurred vision, dizziness; patients with crush injury or those receiving TXA beyond the acute phase may have higher risk of disseminated intravascular coagulation

Vecuronium

Use: Adjunct to ET intubation, mechanical ventilation	**Recommended Dose** 0.08 -0.1 mg/kg IV/IO	**Precautions:** Airway management and ventilatory support are necessary. For intubated patient, should be used only when mechanical ventilation is available. **Adverse reaction:** Muscle weakness

Abbreviations: AV, atrioventricular; bpm, beats per minute; D_5W, dextrose 5% in water; ET, endotracheal; HR, heart rate; ICP, intracranial pressure; IM, intramuscular; IO, intraosseous; IV, intravenous; MDI, metered-dose inhaler; NG, nasogastric; NS, normal saline; ODT, oral dissolving tablet; PE, phenytoin equivalent; PO, per os (oral); PR, per rectum; VF, ventricular fibrillation; VT, ventricular tachycardia.

Glossary

A

abdomen The anatomical portion of the anterior trunk below the ribs and above the pelvis; it contains the stomach, lower part of the esophagus, small and large intestines, liver, gallbladder, spleen, pancreas, and bladder.

abdominal excursions The work of abdominal muscles in infants during the breathing cycle.

abrasion A portion of skin or of a mucous membrane scraped away as a result of injury.

absorb To take in or suck up.

abusive head trauma Seen in abused infants and children. The patient has been subjected to violent, whiplash-type shaking injuries inflicted by the abusing individual. This may cause coma, convulsions, and increased intracranial pressure due to tearing of the cerebral veins with consequent bleeding into the brain. (Old term: shaken baby/infant syndrome.)

acceleration-deceleration event A type of injury caused when a moving body part, such as the head, stops its forward motion suddenly.

acid A corrosive substance with low pH.

acidosis Excessive acidity of body fluids due to an accumulation of acids (as in diabetic acidosis or renal disease) or an excessive loss of bicarbonate (as in renal disease).

acrocyanosis Cyanosis of the extremities; acrocyanosis of the hands and feet may be normal in the infant within the first hour after birth.

acute Characterized by sharpness or severity, or having a sudden onset, sharp rise, and short course.

adenoidal Lymphoid tissue in the back of the mouth and oropharynx.

adrenaline Synonym for epinephrine. A hormone produced by the body that increases pulse rate and blood pressure; mediates the "fight-or-flight" response of the sympathetic nervous system when the body is under stress.

adrenergic agent A drug that mimics the effects of epinephrine (adrenaline) and norepinephrine.

adsorb Accumulation on the surface of another material, such as water clinging to a glass window.

afebrile seizure A seizure not accompanied by a fever.

agent Something that causes an effect; thus, bacteria that cause a disease are said to be agents of the specific disease. An injury agent is the energy causing the damage, such as thermal energy causing a burn. A drug is a pharmacological agent.

agonist A substance that stimulates or activates a specialized receptor on a cell and causes a response.

airway adjunct An artificial device used to maintain an open airway.

aldosterone A steroid hormone produced by the zona glomerulosa of the adrenal cortex in the adrenal gland.

alert, verbal, painful, unresponsive (AVPU) scale A standardized method of assessing the level of consciousness in all patients; categorizes motor response on the basis of responses to stimuli.

alkali A strong base with a high pH, usually corrosive to tissues.

alveoli The air sacs of the lungs in which the exchange of oxygen and carbon dioxide takes place.

amniotic fluid The liquid contained in the amnion, inside the uterus. This fluid is sterile, transparent, and almost colorless. The liquid surrounds and protects the fetus from injury and helps maintain an even temperature.

analgesia, analgesic A drug that relieves pain.

anaphylactic reaction An extreme, life-threatening systemic allergic reaction that may include shock and respiratory failure.

anaphylaxis A severe form of hypersensitivity reaction that produces dangerous physiological changes, such as bronchospasm, shock, and airway edema.

anatomical Relating to the anatomy or structure of an organism.

androgens A group of hormones that play a role in male traits and reproductive activity.

antecubital fossa The triangular area lying anterior to and below the elbow, bounded medially by the pronator teres muscle and laterally by the brachioradialis muscles.

anthrax A deadly bacterium (*Bacillus anthracis*) that lies dormant in a spore (protective shell); the germ is released from the spore when exposed to the optimal temperature and moisture. The route of entry is inhaled, cutaneous, or gastrointestinal (via consumption of food that contains spores).

antibiotics Any of a variety of natural or synthetic substances that inhibit growth of, or destroy, bacteria that are responsible for infectious diseases.

anticonvulsant Agent that prevents or stops convulsions.

antigen Protein recognized by the immune system that causes an allergic reaction.

antipyretic An agent that reduces fever.

antivenin A serum that counteracts the effect of venom from an animal or insect.

anxiolysis Reduction of anxiety, agitation, or tension.

apnea A temporary cessation of breathing.

apneic Characterized by absence of breathing.

asphyxia A condition caused by insufficient oxygen.

assessment Evaluation.

assisted ventilation To provide ventilation mechanically.

asthma A disease caused by increased responsiveness of the tracheobronchial tree to various stimuli. The result is paroxysmal constriction of the bronchial airways. Clinically, there is severe dyspnea accompanied by wheezing.

asymmetrical Without symmetry.

asystole Cardiac standstill; absence of contractions of the heart.

ataxia An abnormal gait.

atrioventricular (AV) heart block Blockage of the electrical impulse from the atrium of the heart to the ventricle.

atrium One of two (right and left) upper chambers of the heart. The right atrium receives blood from the vena cava and delivers it to the right ventricle, which, in turn, pumps blood into the blood vessels of the lungs. The left atrium receives blood from pulmonary veins and delivers it to the left ventricle, which, in turn, pumps blood into the body.

auscultation The process of listening for sounds within the body with a stethoscope.

avulsion A tearing away of a part or structure.

axial loading Vertical pressure on the spine.

axillary temperature The temperature taken in the armpit.

axonal shearing A tearing of axons or nerve sheaths, caused by sudden movement, to produce severe brain injury.

B

baseline A known or initial value with which subsequent observations can be compared.

basilar skull fracture A fracture into the base of the skull, sometimes associated with brain hemorrhage or brain injury.

Battle sign Bruising behind the ear; an indication of basilar skull fracture.

benzodiazepines A family of sedative-hypnotic drugs useful for treatment of seizures and agitation.

bezoar A hard mass of entangled material sometimes found in the stomach and intestines.

bilateral Pertaining to, affecting, or relating to 2 sides.

biological agent An organism that causes disease, including viruses, bacteria, and toxins.

biological pathogen A microorganism that can cause disease in a host.

blood pressure The perfusing pressure of blood.

brachial Pertaining to a main artery and vein of the arm.

bradycardia A slow heartbeat.

brain death Cessation of brain function.

brain perfusion Blood circulation in the brain.

brainstem The stemlike part of the brain that connects the cerebral hemispheres with the spinal cord.

brainstem functions Bodily functions controlled by the brain stem that are necessary for life, such as breathing.

brainstem herniation Bulging and compression of brain tissue; causes breathing to stop and the patient to die.

bronchiolitis Inflammation of the bronchioles by a virus.

bronchodilator A drug that helps open the airways to improve air movement and reduce wheezing.

bronchopulmonary dysplasia (BPD) Iatrogenic chronic lung disease that develops in premature infants after a period of oxygen therapy.

bronchovesicular Pertaining to the tree of pulmonary passages.

buccal Between the teeth and mucosa of the mouth.

buckle fracture A minor fracture only partially through the bone, in which the top layer of bone on one side is compressed, forming a slight angle or "buckle" in the surface.

bulging fontanelle An elevation of the immature opening of bone in the front of the skull; this sign may suggest increased intracranial pressure.

C

calcium channel blockers A family of drugs that helps reduce the speed of conduction through the heart and the overall work of the heart.

cannulating Introducing a catheter through a vein or passageway.

capillary refill time (CRT) A test that evaluates distal circulatory system function, performed by pushing on an area such as a nail bed and watching the speed of its return of pinkness after releasing the pressure.

capnometry The use of a capnometer, a device that measures the amount of expired carbon dioxide.

cardiac arrest The cessation of cardiac mechanical activity, determined by the inability to palpate a central pulse, unresponsiveness, and apnea.

cardiac dysrhythmia An abnormal cardiac rhythm.

cardiac medication Various medications used to treat for heart disease and cardiovascular conditions.

cardiogenic shock A reduced cardiac output secondary to abnormal cardiac function.

cardiomyopathy Disease of the myocardium, especially due to primary disease of the heart muscle.

cardiopulmonary compromise Acutely altered mental status, signs of shock, hypotension.

cartilage A specialized type of dense connective tissue, softer than bone, that is common in the skeletons of children.

cartilaginous growth plate The horizontal part of the bone that grows as the human body matures.

cathartic A purgative agent for the bowel.

caustic Corrosive and burning; destructive to living tissue.

central cyanosis Slightly bluish, grayish, or dark purple discoloration of the skin (on the trunk and face) due to presence of hypoxia.

central nervous system (CNS) The organ system that consists of the brain and spinal cord; it controls vital body functions.

central venous catheter (CVC) Catheter inserted into the vena cava to permit intermittent or continuous monitoring of central venous pressure and to facilitate obtaining blood samples for analysis.

cerebral cortex The higher brain; the source of the senses, thinking, feeling, and voluntary movement.

cerebral edema Swelling of the brain.

cerebral palsy A disorder of movement and tone that results from brain injury during fetal development or at birth.

cerebrospinal fluid (CSF) shunt Tube that allows fluid manufactured in the ventricles of the brain from the subarachnoid space to drain in another part of the anatomy outside of the brain, such as the peritoneum. This can lower pressure in the brain.

chest wall The musculoskeletal framework of the chest.

child maltreatment A general term applying to all forms of child abuse and neglect.

child neglect Failure by those responsible for caring for a child to provide for the child's nutritional, emotional, and physical needs.

child protective services (CPS) This agency is the community legal organization responsible for protection, rehabilitation, and prevention of child maltreatment and neglect. Child protective services has the legal authority temporarily to remove from their home any children at risk of experiencing injury or neglect and to secure foster placement.

child restraint system (CRS) A child safety device that is designed to secure an infant or child in motor vehicles, aircraft, and ambulances.

children and youth with special health care needs (CYSHCN) Those who have or are at increased risk of experiencing a chronic, physical, developmental, behavioral, or emotional condition and who also require health and related services of a type or amount beyond that required by children generally.

choanal atresia A narrowing or blockage of the nasal airway by membranous or bony tissue; a congenital condition (present at birth).

cholinergic crisis A crisis involving cholinergic drugs, pesticides, or "nerve gases" designed for chemical warfare. Cholinergic agents overstimulate normal body functions that are controlled by the parasympathetic nerves.

cholinergic impulse The transmission of nerve signals via the neurotransmitter acetylcholine.

circadian rhythm The regular recurrence, in cycles of about 24 hours, of biological processes or activities, such as sensitivity to drugs and stimuli, hormone secretion, sleeping, and feeding. This rhythm is set according to cycles of light and dark as well as to factors such as temperature, diet, social environment, and stress.

clavicle The collarbone; a bone, curved like the letter f, that articulates with the sternum and scapula.

coin rubbing A cultural ritual/traditional healing practice intended to treat an illness by rubbing hot coins on the body, often on the back, which produces rounded and oblong red, patchy, flat skin lesions.

colostomy The surgical establishment of an opening between the colon and the surface of the body to provide drainage of the bowel.

commotio cordis Sudden cardiac arrest resulting from a blunt, nonpenetrating blow to the chest. The basis of the cardiac arrest is ventricular fibrillation (a chaotically abnormal heart rhythm) triggered by chest wall impact immediately over the anatomical position of the heart.

compensated shock A clinical state in which the patient has clinical signs of inadequate tissue perfusion but a blood pressure in the normal range.

compensatory mechanisms Physiological responses initiated to help return the body's vital functions to normal after a severe insult to breathing, perfusion, or metabolic function.

complex febrile seizure A self-limited seizure in a previously healthy child between the ages of 6 months and 6 years that is associated with an elevated fever, lasts longer than 15 minutes, may involve focal motor activity, and occurs more than once in 24 hours.

complex partial seizure A seizure characterized by alteration of consciousness with or without complex focal motor activity.

compression A pressing or squeezing together.

concussion A brain injury causing any type of altered state of consciousness.

congenital Present at birth.

congenital anomaly An anatomical structure that is unusual or different at birth.

congenital dermal melanocytosis Blue-gray birthmark of the skin caused by abnormal pigment, rather than by trauma or bruising.

congenital diaphragmatic hernia A developmental defect of the diaphragm in which the abdominal organs herniate into the chest.

congenital heart disease (CHD) Heart disease that is present from birth.

congestive heart failure (CHF) A disorder in which the heart loses part of its ability to effectively pump blood, usually as a result of damage to the heart muscle and usually resulting in a backup of fluid into the lungs.

consent for care Permission to render care.

constipation Infrequent defecation with passage of unduly hard and dry fecal material.

contact burns A thermal burn caused by direct contact with a hot object, fluid, or gas.

contraindication A condition in which a medication or procedure should not be used because it may be harmful.

core perfusion Blood circulation in the core of the human body.

corrosive Producing corrosion or destruction of tissue.

cortical Pertaining to or of the outer layer of the brain.

cortisol A steroid hormone (a glucocorticoid) produced by the adrenal cortex that acts as the body's long-term stress responder and metabolic regulator. It is produced along with adrenaline during acute and chronic stress conditions.

crackles Rales; lung sounds that suggest fluid in alveoli.

cranium The area of the head above the ears and eyes; the skull. The cranium contains the brain.

crepitus The noise or feel of gas in soft tissues.

critical incident stress management (CISM) A comprehensive crisis intervention system that helps individuals and groups cope with the emotional and psychological impact of traumatic events.

crowning Stage in delivery at which the fetal head presents at the vaginal opening.

cupping The practice of placing warm cups on the skin to pull out illness from the body. This results in red, flat, rounded skin lesions that are often more intensely red at the borders.

Cushing triad The combination of hypertension, bradycardia, and irregular respirations that occurs with increased intracranial pressure.

cyanide A colorless gas used in many industrial processes that has an odor similar to that of almonds and is a chemical asphyxiant; exposure can occur from by-products of combustion at structure fires.

cyanosis Slightly bluish, grayish, slatelike, or dark purple discoloration of the skin due to hypoxia.

cyanotic heart disease A type of congenital heart disease with a right-to-left shunt resulting in partially oxygenated blood in the systemic circulation.

cyclic antidepressant A type of antidepressant drug that may cause coma, seizures, and conduction disturbances if taken in an overdose.

cystic fibrosis (CF) A congenital disorder that results in lung and digestive disorders due to improper functioning of mucus-producing or exocrine glands. Affected patients experience frequent lung infections, pneumothoraces, impaired digestion and absorption of nutrients, and poor growth.

D

decerebrate A posture characterized by rigid extension of the arms and legs; indicates pressure on the brain stem at the level of the pons and may appear in patients with severe brain swelling.

decompensated shock A shock state characterized by low blood pressure, which will rapidly progress to cardiac arrest if not rapidly corrected.

decontamination The process of removing a poison.

decorticate A posture characterized by flexion of the arms and extension of the legs; indicates pressure on the cerebral cortex and subcortical white matter with preservation of brainstem function and may appear in patients with severe brain trauma.

defibrillator An electrical device that shocks the heart; available in external and automatic implanted forms.

demarcated Defined or delimited, as an area in a boundary.

dendrite A projection from a neuron that makes connections with an adjacent cell.

dextrose A form of glucose (or sugar) found naturally in animal and plant tissue and derived synthetically from starch.

diabetes mellitus (DM) A metabolic disorder in which the ability to metabolize sugar is impaired, usually because of a lack of insulin.

diabetic ketoacidosis A form of acidosis in diabetes mellitus in which certain acids accumulate when sufficent insulin is not available.

diaphoretic A state of excessive perspiration caused by high physiological stress.

diaphragm The muscle separating the chest from the abdominal cavity, which allows breathing.

diaphysis The shaft of a long bone.

diastolic pressure The pressure that remains in the arteries during the relaxing phase of the heart's cycle (diastole) when the left ventricle is at rest.

diffuse axonal injury An injury to the brain, resulting in diffuse brain swelling.

dilated Widened.

direct medical control Physician instructions that are given directly by phone or radio.

dirty bomb Name given to a bomb that is used as a radiological dispersal device.

disaster A widespread event that disrupts community resources and functions, in turn threatening public safety, citizens' lives, and property.

distal Farthest from the center.

distal extremities Structures that are farther from the trunk or nearer to the free end of the extremity.

distension Inflation; enlargement.

distributive shock A clinical state characterized by maldistribution of blood volume and loss of vascular tone.

diving reflex Submersion of the face and nose in water to produce a vagal reaction; used to terminate an important dysrhythmia of childhood called supraventricular tachycardia.

do not resuscitate (DNR) Written documentation giving permission to medical personnel not to attempt resuscitation in the event of cardiac arrest.

Down syndrome A congenital disorder in which a person is born with 3 copies of chromosome 21 (trisomy 21). Clinical features include slanting eyes, a broad short skull, broad hands, and short fingers. Other congenital abnormalities include heart defects and esophageal atresia.

dressing Protective covering for diseased or injured parts.

drug-assisted intubation (DAI) A method of airway management that uses pharmacological agents to facilitate endotracheal intubation.

dysphagia Inability to swallow or difficulty in swallowing.

dysrhythmia Abnormal, disordered rhythm.

E

edema A local or generalized collection of tissue fluid.

effortless tachypnea Without the signs of increased work of breathing; this represents the child's attempt to exhale extra carbon dioxide to correct the acidosis generated by poor perfusion.

electrocardiogram (ECG) A 12-lead electrocardiographic recording used to evaluate the heart and its rhythm.

emancipated minor Person legally under age but recognized by the state as having the legal capacity to consent for self (usually older than 14 years).

emergency information form (EIF) A form that provides patient information to health care professionals.

emergency protective custody A child taken into a protective custody by a law enforcement officer if the legal guardian continues to refuse consent for lifesaving care.

emesis Vomiting.

emotional abuse The intentional infliction of emotional harm to a child.

emotional neglect The intentional omission of emotional support to a child.

empathy Awareness of and insight into the feelings, emotions, and behavior of another person.

EMS-EMSC continuum Emergency Medical Services–Emergency Medical Services for Children, the linked community services set up to prevent and treat childhood emergencies. The continuum includes prevention, the primary physician, out-of-hospital care, emergency department care, hospital care, and rehabilitation.

encephalitis Inflammation of the brain.

endotracheal intubation (ETI) A method of intubation in which an endotracheal tube is placed through a patient's mouth, directly through the larynx between the vocal cords, and into the trachea to open and maintain an airway.

enterovirus A species of virus that causes gastrointestinal or respiratory disease in children.

envenomation The act of injecting venom, such as by a snake or insect.

environment The surroundings, conditions, or influences that affect an organism or an injury.

environmental assessment Evaluation of the scene of an emergency to collect clues about what is wrong and the best route to take for treatment; gathering information by observing things such as damage to a vehicle or medication bottles in the patient's home.

epiglottis A leaf- or omega-shaped structure located immediately posterior to the root of the tongue that prevents food and secretions from entering the trachea.

epiglottitis Inflammation of the epiglottis.

epilepsy A condition of recurrent seizures.

epinephrine A substance produced by the body (commonly called adrenaline) that has a vital role in the function of the sympathetic nervous system; also a drug produced by pharmaceutical companies that increases blood pressure and causes bronchodilation; the drug of choice for an anaphylactic reaction.

epiphysis The end of the bone that is the secondary ossification center.

esophagus A muscular canal that carries food from the pharynx to the stomach.

etiology The cause and origin of disease.

evaporation The change from liquid to vapor.

exhalation The process of breathing out.

extensor posturing See **decerebrate**.

extraocular Movement of the eyes in various directions.

F

factitious disorder imposed on another (FDIA) A form of child abuse in which a caregiver fabricates or induces illness in a child to gain attention or sympathy.

family-centered care Involving the family in decisions about their child's treatment.

feeding tube A tube paced into the stomach through the mouth, nose, or skin.

fetus A human or mammal in an early form of intrauterine development.

flaccid Weak, lax, and soft.

flail chest An unstable condition of the chest wall due to 2 or more fractures of the ribs, resulting in ineffective breathing.

flexion The act of bending a limb or joint.

flexural creases The creases behind the knees or inside the elbows.

focal Limited to a particular part of the body.

fontanelle A soft spot of undeveloped bone lying between the cranial bones of the skull of a fetus or infant.

frenulum The skin between the upper lip and upper gum or the lower lip and lower gum or tissue connecting the tongue to the floor of the mouth.

fulminant pneumonia Sudden and intense inflammation of the lungs with infection.

G

gag reflex The protective reflex that keeps food, fluid, or secretions from getting into the trachea.

gastric decompression The removal of air and other contents from the stomach.

gastric feeding tube A tube that provides a channel directly into a patient's stomach, allowing removal of gas, blood, and toxins or insertion of medications and nutrition.

gastroenteritis Inflammation of the stomach and intestinal tract.

gastrointestinal (GI) decontamination The removal of poison from the stomach.

gastrostomy tube (G-tube or "button") A feeding tube placed directly through the wall of the abdomen.

generalized seizure Characterized by movements (often tonic-clonic) that indicate involvement of both cerebral hemispheres.

gestation The length of time from conception to birth.

glial cells Specialized cells that surround neurons, providing mechanical and physical support and electrical insulation between neurons.

glottis The sound-producing apparatus of the larynx, consisting of 2 vocal folds.

glucagon A hormone that has the property of increasing the concentration of sugar in the blood.

greenstick fracture A fracture involving only part of the outer layer or cortex of a bone.

grunting A short, low-pitched sound at the end of exhalation, present in children with moderate to severe hypoxia; it reflects poor gas exchange because of fluid in the lower airways and air sacs.

H

hazardous materials (hazmat) Any substance that is toxic, poisonous, radioactive, flammable, or explosive and causes injury or death with exposure.

head bobbing A movement in which the head lifts and tilts back during inspiration, then moves forward during expiration; a sign of increased work of breathing.

health information exchange (HIE) The sharing of health care information electronically across organizations within a region, community, or hospital system.

hematoma A swelling or mass of blood confined to an organ, a tissue, or a space and caused by a break in a blood vessel.

hemodialysis A form of dialysis in which the blood is removed from the patient through a catheter or fistula and then is returned to the body through another needle, removing various toxins, electrolytes, and fluid in the process.

hemodynamically stable Not changing or fluctuating in relation to the mechanics of blood circulation.

hemopericardium Accumulation of blood around the heart muscle in the pericardial sac.

hemophilia A congenital condition in which the patient lacks one or more of the blood's normal clotting factors.

hemostat Instrument clamp; in its closed position, it squeezes tissues or vessels and arrests the flow of blood.

hepatomegaly Enlargement of the liver.

hives Wheals; an itchy rash caused by contact with or ingestion of an allergic substance or food.

homeostasis The maintenance of a relatively stable internal physiological environment.

host The organism acted on in an injury or illness process.

hydrocarbon A basic organic compound made up of hydrogen and carbon.

hydrocephalus The increased accumulation of cerebrospinal fluid within the ventricles of the brain.

hydrochloric acid A powerful and corrosive aqueous solution of hydrogen chloride.

hyperalimentation The administration of nutrients by means of intravenous feeding.

hyperoxia Increased oxygen in the blood.

hyperthermia Unusually elevated body temperature.

hypertrophic cardiomyopathy (HCM) A condition in which the heart muscle is unusually thick, which means that the heart has to work harder to pump blood.

hypnotic drug Pertaining to sleep or sedation.

hypocarbia Decreased carbon dioxide in the blood, usually resulting from an excess rate of ventilation.

hypoglycemia Low blood glucose level.

hypoperfusion Inadequate circulation.

hypotension A decrease of systolic and diastolic blood pressure to limits below normal for age, representing decompensated shock/hypotensive shock.

hypotensive shock A shock state characterized by low blood pressure, which will rapidly progress to cardiac arrest if not rapidly corrected.

hypothermia A body temperature below normal range.

hypotonia Reduced muscular tension.

hypovolemia Diminished blood volume.

hypovolemic shock A clinical state of reduced intravascular volume.

hypoxemia A decreased oxygen saturation in blood detected by means of pulse oximetry or direct measurement of oxygen saturation in an arterial blood gas sample.

hypoxia A pathological condition in which the body as a whole (generalized hypoxia) or region of the body (tissue hypoxia) is deprived of an adequate oxygen supply.

hypoxic stress A subnormal concentration of oxygen.

I

ileostomy The surgical establishment of an opening between the small bowel and the surface of the body for the purpose of providing drainage of the bowel.

impending brainstem herniation A clinical state in which brain tissue, cerebrospinal fluid, and blood vessels are moved or pressed away from their usual position inside the skull.

impending herniation syndrome A clinical state in which there is severely abnormal brain pressure, just before the moment of tissue herniation and compression of brain tissue.

implantable cardioverter-defibrillator (ICD) A small device implanted in the chest to monitor and treat dangerous heart rhythms. An ICD can deliver electrical shocks and/or pace the heart to restore a normal rhythm.

implementation phase Second of the 3 phases in disaster response. Activities during this phase include search and rescue, victim triage, initial stabilization and transport, and definitive management of scene hazards and victims.

implied consent Permission for medical treatment for a patient who is unable to give consent under the legal assumption that they would want treatment if they were able to give permission.

in utero Within the uterus.

indirect medical control Existing or standing orders, written policies, procedures, and protocols.

indwelling central venous catheter Small, flexible plastic tube inserted into a large vein above the heart, usually the subclavian vein, through which access to the bloodstream can be gained. This catheter is left in place and allows drugs and blood products to be administered and blood samples withdrawn painlessly.

informed consent The legal and ethical requirement to obtain permission from a competent patient or a legal surrogate (such as a parent or guardian) before providing medical care or transport. In the context of minors, this generally means obtaining permission from a parent or legal guardian, because minors typically lack the legal authority to give consent.

in loco parentis This phrase means "in place of the parent." It refers to caregivers (such as grandparents, stepparents, or foster parents) who are not the legal parents but assume the responsibilities of a parent. These individuals have recognized rights to consent to medical care and perform other parental functions.

infusion A liquid substance introduced into the body for therapeutic or diagnostic purposes.

inspiratory The process of moving air into the lungs.

insulin A hormone produced by the islet of Langerhans (an exocrine gland in the pancreas) that enables sugar in the blood to enter the cells of the body; used in synthetic form to treat and control diabetes mellitus.

intercostal Between the ribs.

intercurrent Something that occurs during or in between other events, such as an illness that appears during the course of another.

intra-abdominal Within the abdomen.

intracranial Within the cranium or skull.

intracranial hypertension/increased intracranial pressure (ICP) Increased pressure of the cerebrospinal fluid that impairs brain function.

intramuscular (IM) Into a muscle; a medication delivery route.

intranasal (IN) Within the nasal cavity; a medication delivery route.

intraosseous (IO) Within the marrow cavity of a bone; intramedullary; a medication delivery route.

intravascular volume The water portion of the circulatory system surrounding the blood cells.

intravenous (IV) Within the vein; a medication delivery route.

ipecac An oral medicine to induce vomiting; this medicine is no longer recommended for use by prehospital professionals.

ischemia Deficiency of blood supply.

J

jaundice A condition characterized by yellowness of skin, whites of eyes, mucous membranes, and body fluids due to deposition of excess bilirubin in the blood (hyperbilirubinemia).

jugular venous distension A prominence of the jugular veins as they fill with blood; if patient is not supine, indication that the blood may be having difficulty flowing back into the right side of the heart. This can be caused by pericardial tamponade, tension pneumothorax, or right-sided heart failure.

K

ketogenic diet A diet that eliminates foods with glucose; may be used in children with severe, uncontrolled epilepsy to keep the child in a state of ketosis to help control seizures.

L

lactic acidosis The metabolic acidotic state resulting from the accumulation of lactic acid secondary to anaerobic cellular metabolism.

laryngoscope An instrument for examining the larynx.

laryngoscopy An examination of the interior of the larynx.

larynx The enlarged upper end of the trachea, below the root of the tongue, that contains the vocal cords.

lateral Pertaining to the side.

lateral decubitus position A position in which the patient lies on their side.

legal authority The ability to make medical decisions under the law.

lethargy Listlessness; weakness.

leukemia A cancerous condition in which certain cell lines begin to grow abnormally fast.

leukocyte (white blood cell) count Measured to determine whether an infectious process is present.

localize When a patient is able to pinpoint the site of a specific noxious or painful stimulus (eg, when a patient reaches for and pushes away the hand that is pinching them during a neurological examination).

long QT syndrome A condition characterized by a QT interval exceeding approximately 450 ms.

lordosis Forward curve of the lumbar spine.

lye Corrosive, alkaline cleaning liquid.

M

malaise Discomfort, uneasiness, or generalized ill feeling, often indicative of infection.

malposition An incorrect or abnormal position.

malrotation with volvulus An anatomical issue in which the small bowel is twisting and small-bowel obstruction results.

mandible The horseshoe-shaped bone forming the lower jaw.

mass-casualty incident (MCI) An emergency situation involving more than 1 patient, and one that can place such great demand on equipment or personnel that the system is stretched to its limit or beyond.

mature minor A person without the formal legal status of an emancipated minor but having similar characteristics: married, pregnant, on active-duty status in the armed service, or 15 years or older and living separate and apart from their guardians. This person has the legal right to give consent for treatment as well as the legal right to refuse it.

meconium The bowel contents of a fetus. The presence of meconium in amniotic fluid means the fetus may have suffered some type of stress, such as hypoxia, and may be depressed and need to be resuscitated.

mediastinum The space between the lungs, in the center of the chest, that contains the heart, trachea, mainstem bronchi, part of the esophagus, and large blood vessels.

medical control Physician instructions that are given directly by radio (online or direct) or indirectly by protocols or guidelines (offline or indirect), as authorized by the medical director of the service program.

medical home An approach to providing health care services in a high-quality and cost-effective manner. Children and their families who have a medical home receive the care they need from a pediatrician or family physician they know and trust. The pediatric health care professional and parents act as partners in a medical home to identify and access all the medical and nonmedical services needed to help children and their families achieve their maximum potential.

medical responsibility The moral and legal duty to provide medical care in an emergency.

meninges A set of 3 tough membranes—the dura mater, arachnoid, and pia mater—that encloses the entire brain and spinal cord.

meningitis Inflammation of the membranes of the spinal cord or brain.

meningococcal sepsis Bloodborne infection with the bacterium *Neisseria meningitidis,* leading to sepsis (fever or hypothermia, shock, and hypotension).

meningococcemia Infection of the blood stream by the bacterium *Neisseria meningitidis*. This is usually a severe infection characterized by fever, shock, and a characteristic purpuric rash (bruising of the skin) with or without meningitis.

metabolic acidosis A metabolic state of acidosis resulting from retention of hydrogen or other positively charged ions not related to respiratory compromise.

midaxillary line Imaginary vertical line drawn through the middle of the axilla (armpit), parallel to the midline.

minor A person not of legal age and thus requiring consent from a legal guardian to receive medical or surgical care.

minute ventilation The volume of air exchanged per minute [minute ventilation = tidal volume × respiratory rate].

miosis Abnormal contraction of pupils.

mortality Death.

motor activity Muscle use.

mottling A condition of abnormal skin circulation, caused by vasoconstriction or inadequate circulation.

multisystem trauma Injury involving more than 1 organ system, such as combined injury to the chest, abdomen, and brain.

muscular dystrophy A genetic muscle disorder that results in muscle weakness and wasting; patients are at risk of experiencing aspiration and pneumonia.

myocardial depression A clinical state in which the heart muscle is not working adequately.

myocardial function A measure of how well the heart is working.

myocardial infarction The death of part of the heart muscle, caused by partial or complete occlusion of one or more of the coronary arteries.

myocarditis Inflammation of the myocardium.

N

nasal cannula An oxygen delivery device in which oxygen flows through 2 small, tubelike prongs that fit into the patient's nostrils.

nasal flaring A spreading out of the nostrils, indicating increased work of breathing and hypoxia.

nasopharyngeal airway (NPA) Airway adjunct inserted into the nostril of a conscious patient who is not able to maintain a natural airway.

needle decompression The removal of air from a closed space, such as from the pleura.

neonatal seizure A seizure that occurs in newborn infants.

nerve agents A class of chemicals including organophosphates; they function by blocking an essential enzyme in the nervous system, which causes the body's organs to become overstimulated.

neurogenic shock Shock caused by paralysis of the nerves that control the size of the blood vessels, leading to widespread dilation and pooling of blood in the peripheral vessels to the extent that adequate perfusion cannot be maintained; seen in patients with spinal cord injuries.

neurovascular Concerning both the nervous and vascular systems.

nonblanching Not disappearing with pressure.

nonpulsatile fontanelle When the fontanelle or "soft spot" on an infant's head is full, usually tense, and does not seem to beat or pulse with each beat of the heart.

nuclear bomb A bomb that is extremely powerful owing to its use of atomic energy as a source of its explosive nature. In addition to the actual explosive force of the bomb, the radiation released by the explosion causes injury in a wider area.

O

obstetric Having to do with pregnancy and the delivery of a baby.

obstructive shock Shock or inadequate tissue perfusion that is caused by a restriction to blood flow out from the heart (eg, shock due to a critical coarctation or severe narrowing of the aorta, tension pneumothorax, or cardiac tamponade).

obturator An inner stabilizing structure that gives stiffness to a hollow tube, to allow insertion or clearing of an obstruction.

occlusion The closure of a passage.

occlusive dressing A dressing that covers a wound completely.

occult illness An illness that is not immediately obvious or is "hidden"; an illness that does not have obvious symptoms.

opioid A drug derived from opium or a synthetic variant that produces analgesia, sedation, and sometimes euphoria.

oral glucose A simple sugar that is readily absorbed by the bloodstream; it is carried on the emergency medical services unit.

organophosphate insecticide A type of poison with cholinergic properties, used as an insecticide.

oropharyngeal airway An airway adjunct inserted into the mouth to keep the tongue from blocking the upper airway and to make suctioning the airway easier.

oropharynx The part of the pharynx lying between the soft palate and the upper portion of the epiglottis.

ossification The formation of bone. An ossification center is an area in which cartilage is transformed through calcification into a new area of bone.

osteogenesis imperfecta A genetic disorder in which the bones are brittle and which results in fractures.

ostomy A surgical opening made in the skin as a passage through which waste products can leave the body.

otorrhea Any flow or discharge from the ear.

P

pallor Lack of color; paleness.

palpation Physical touching for the purpose of obtaining clinical information.

paradoxical irritability A marker for possible serious pediatric illness, a particular type of irritability in which attempts to console the child further distress them.

pathology The study and diagnosis of disease.

pathophysiology The study of how disease or injury affects the body.

pedal Related to the foot (eg, pedal pulses are pulses found in the foot).

Pediatric Assessment Triangle (PAT) Assessment tool that allows rapid formation of a general impression of the type and level of illness or injury in an infant or child without touching him or her; consists of assessing appearance, work of breathing, and circulation to the skin.

pediatric critical care center A type of specialized center for children with advanced resources (such as a pediatric intensive care unit) for care of the critically ill.

pediatric trauma center A type of specialized center for children that has advanced resources for care of critically injured children.

pelvic fracture A break through 1 or more bones of the pelvis (the hip bones and the sacrum and coccyx or lower parts of the spine).

percutaneous endoscopic gastrostomy (PEG) A procedure in which a tube is placed through the abdominal wall and into the stomach.

perfusion Blood circulation.

pericardial tamponade Compression of the heart due to a buildup of blood or other fluid in the pericardial sac.

periosteum The membrane, consisting of a double layer of connective tissue, that covers all bones except the articular surfaces.

peripheral cyanosis Slightly bluish or dark purple discoloration of the skin (on the hands and feet only).

peripheral vasoconstriction A decrease in size of the blood vessels in the outer extremities (hands and feet especially) through the contraction of the smooth muscle in the blood vessel walls that leads to a decrease in blood flow to those areas. This may produce peripheral cyanosis (bluish discoloration of the hands and feet) and prolonged capillary refill time.

peripherally inserted central catheter (PICC) An indwelling line that is partially implanted under the skin and partially exposed above the skin.

peritoneal dialysis A type of dialysis in which a special solution is instilled through a catheter into the patient's abdomen and that draws toxins, electrolytes, and other fluids from the body through the peritoneal membrane.

peritoneum The membrane lining the abdominal cavity (parietal peritoneum) and covering the abdominal organs (visceral peritoneum).

peritonsillar abscess A collection of pus adjacent to the tonsil.

petechiae Small, purplish, nonblanching spots on the skin that appear in certain severe fevers and may be indicative of possible sepsis.

petechial rash Inflammation containing petechiae, small areas of hemorrhage into the skin that do not blanch when they are subjected to pressure.

pharynx Passageway for air from the nasal cavity to the larynx and food from the mouth to the esophagus.

phencyclidine (PCP) A hallucinogen, referred to as PCP or angel dust. Moderate doses cause elevated blood pressure, rapid pulse, increased skeletal muscle tone, and sometimes myoclonic jerks.

physeal plate The segment of bone that is concerned with growth.

physical abuse See **child maltreatment**.

physical neglect See **child neglect**.

physician orders for life-sustaining treatment (POLST) A document outlining the treatment that is permitted when the patient still has a pulse and is breathing.

physiological Concerning body function.

Pierre Robin syndrome A condition present at birth marked by a small lower jaw (micrognathia). The tongue tends to fall back and downward (glossoptosis), and there is a cleft soft palate.

placenta The tissue attached to the uterine wall that nourishes the fetus through the umbilical cord.

plague An illness caused by infection with the bacterium *Yersinia pestis*. The disease is characterized by fever and chills followed by a severe illness with pneumonia, headache, and delirium. It is transmitted to humans via the bites of fleas from infected rodents and has a high fatality rate. It is an agent that could be used as a weapon of bioterrorism.

pleura The serous membrane that enfolds both lungs and is reflected on the walls of the thorax and diaphragm.

pleural space The space between the parietal and visceral layers of the pleura.

pneumomediastinum Air or gas in the mediastinal tissues.

pneumonia An inflammation of the lungs caused primarily by bacteria, viruses, and chemical irritants.

pneumothorax A collection of air in the pleural cavity, which if under pressure may cause severe physiological changes with poor venous return and inadequate cardiac output.

policy A medicolegal operational standard to guide prehospital professionals; intended to help with decision making in difficult or legally sensitive field situations.

polydipsia A condition in which a person has extreme thirst.

polyphagia Medical term for excessive or extreme hunger.

polyuria Excessive or abnormally large production or passage of urine.

posteriorly From the back, from behind, or from underneath.

postictal state Confusion a patient experiences after having a seizure.

postpartum After childbirth.

posturing Abnormal body positioning after a brain injury; it may occur in response to painful stimuli.

pre-eclampsia A condition during pregnancy characterized by gestational hypertension, typically accompanied by edema and proteinuria.

preterm labor Labor beginning before the 37th week of gestation.

primary brain injury Injury resulting from the direct biomechanical effects of impact forces on the brain that result in direct impact or sudden movement, causing shear stress of the brain.

procedure A medical intervention.

prone Lying horizontally with the face downward.

propylene glycol A solvent used in medicines.

protocol A step-by-step process for treatment.

proximal Nearest the point of attachment, center of the body, or point of reference; the opposite of distal.

pulmonary contusion A bruise of the lung.

pulmonary edema A build-up of fluid in the lungs.

pulmonary intoxicant A toxin or poison that may be absorbed through (eg, via inhalation) and cause harm to the respiratory system.

pulseless electrical activity (PEA) An organized cardiac rhythm on the cardiac monitor in absence of a palpable pulse.

purpura A rash that looks like bruising of the skin that is usually seen in overwhelming infections (sepsis) or when a patient has an inflammation of the blood vessels (vasculitis).

purpuric Pertaining to bruising of the skin.

pus The liquid product of inflammation, generally yellow in color.

Q

QRS complex The electrical shape of a major portion of the heart rhythm on the cardiac monitor, representing ventricular electrical activity.

quadriplegia Paralysis of all 4 extremities (both arms and both legs), usually due to an injury in the upper cervical portion of the spinal cord.

quality improvement (QI) A system of internal and external reviews and audits of all aspects of a system.

R

racemic Including all isomers of a drug, such as epinephrine.

radial Pertaining to the radius, the larger and more lateral of the 2 bones in the forearm.

reactivity The tendency of a substance to undergo chemical reaction, either by itself or with other materials, and to release energy.

recovery phase Final of 3 phases in disaster response. Activities include scene withdrawal, return to normal operations, and debriefing.

renal dialysis A technique for filtering the blood of its toxic wastes, removing excess fluids, and restoring the normal balance of electrolytes.

respiratory arrest The absence of respirations (ie, apnea) with detectable cardiac activity.

respiratory depression A condition in which there is a slowing of the respiratory rate and decreased respiratory effort, usually due to some effect on the respiratory center in the medulla of the brain. This may be caused by trauma, illness, or the effects of drugs (eg, morphine or diazepam) or toxins (eg, ethanol).

respiratory distress A clinical state characterized by increased respiratory rate, effort, and work of breathing.

respiratory failure A clinical state of inadequate oxygenation, ventilation, or both.

respiratory syncytial virus (RSV) A virus that commonly causes bronchiolitis.

retraction A physical drawing in of the chest wall between the ribs that occurs with increased work of breathing.

retropharyngeal abscess Swelling of the retropharyngeal nodes located between the cervical vertebrae and esophagus; can mimic the presentation of epiglottitis.

rhinorrhea Thin watery discharge from the nose.

ricin Neurotoxin derived from the castor bean. When introduced into the body, ricin causes pulmonary edema and respiratory and circulatory failure, leading to death.

Robin sequence See **Pierre Robin syndrome**.

S

salivation The act of secreting saliva.

saphenous veins Two superficial veins, the great and small, passing up the leg.

scald A burn to skin or flesh caused by moist heat and hot vapors (eg, steam).

scaphoid The wrist bone that is found just beyond the most distal portion of the radius.

scoliosis A lateral curvature of the spine.

scopolamine An anticholinergic agent with action similar to that of atropine.

secondary assessment A step in the patient assessment process in which a systematic physical examination of the patient is performed. The examination may be a systematic full-body evaluation or an assessment that focuses on a certain area or region of the body, often determined according to the chief complaint.

secondary brain injury Injury to the brain resulting from factors occurring after the initial biomechanical effects of the primary brain injury (such as hypoxia and hypotension).

secretion The process of producing liquid materials into the blood or body cavities.

sedative An agent that relaxes.

semi-Fowler position Lying in a bed in a supine position with the head of the bed at approximately 30°.

sepsis A pathological state, usually in a febrile patient, resulting from the presence of invading microorganisms or their poisonous products in the bloodstream.

septic shock Shock resulting from infection, involving hypotension and signs of inadequate organ perfusion.

serial examinations The act of repeatedly examining a patient to carefully watch and document the progression of signs or symptoms in an attempt to develop a diagnosis (eg, serial examinations of the abdomen to determine whether someone with abdominal trauma has a perforation of the intestine) or to watch for a change in their condition (eg, serial examinations of a child with a head injury to monitor their neurological status and watch for signs of increasing intracranial pressure).

serum glucose The level of glucose in the blood.

sexual abuse Rape, sexual assault, or sexual molestation.

shock A clinical syndrome in which the blood flow and oxygen delivery are inadequate for normal organ function.

sickle cell disease (SCD) A hereditary disease characterized by abnormal clumping together of deformed red blood cells. Affected patients experience painful crises, anemia, infection risks, strokes, and other serious complications.

simple febrile seizure A brief (less than 15 minutes), self-limited, generalized convulsion in a previously healthy child between the ages of 6 months and 6 years that is associated with an elevated fever. Children with simple febrile seizures have relatively short postictal periods, after which they return to their baseline with a nonfocal neurological examination result and the seizure does not recur within 24 hours.

simple partial seizure A focal (localized) seizure that involves a motor or sensory abnormality (eg, twitching of one hand or a visual disturbance) in a patient who remains conscious. In children, partial seizures are usually motor seizures and frequently progress to generalized seizures.

simple triage and rapid treatment (START) A triage system.

Sims position A semiprone position in labor with the patient on their side, with their opposite knee and thigh drawn well up, to facilitate delivery of a baby.

sinus arrhythmia A variation in the resting heart rate often seen in children and adolescents. As the child breathes in, the heart rate increases slightly; as they exhale, the heart rate decreases. This is a normal variation in children and not truly an arrhythmia. On electrocardiogram, each QRS complex is preceded by a P wave, and there are no missed or skipped beats.

sinus tachycardia Rapid heart rate in a child with normal conduction.

slurry A thin, watery mixture.

smallpox A rare, highly contagious viral disease; it is most contagious when blisters begin to form.

sniffing position An upright position in which the patient's head and chin are thrust slightly forward to keep the airway open; the child appears to be sniffing.

soft-tissue injuries Injuries to the skin, fat, muscles, ligaments, and tendons.

sort, assess, lifesaving interventions, and treatment and/or transport (SALT) A triage system.

spasticity Increased tone or contractions of muscles causing stiff and awkward movements.

spina bifida A congenital anomaly in which the posterior elements of the vertebrae have failed to fuse together. The spinal cord and its associated coverings (meninges) may protrude through this defect in the vertebrae, leading to a range of neurological impairment in the lower extremities that depends on the degree and level of the protrusion. When the defect is isolated to the bony structures without spinal cord or meningeal abnormality, this is termed spina bifida occulta.

spine The vertebral column.

spleen The major abdominal organ involved in the production and destruction of red blood cells and immune cells. It is filled with blood and can hemorrhage after injury.

splinting Fixation with a rigid material.

status epilepticus A state of continuous seizures or multiple seizures without an intervening return to consciousness.

sterile gauze Basic tool used to stop bleeding and keep wounds clean.

stress A force that disrupts equilibrium or produces strain.

stridor A harsh sound during inspiration, high-pitched owing to partial upper airway obstruction.

subcostal Beneath the ribs.

subdural hemorrhage Bleeding beneath the dura mater.

subglottic Beneath the glottis.

substernal Beneath the sternum.

sucking chest wound An open or penetrating chest-wall wound through which air passes during inspiration and expiration.

sudden unexpected infant death (SUID) The sudden death of an infant younger than 1 year in which the cause of death is not immediately obvious.

superior vena cava One of the two largest veins in the body; carries blood from the upper extremities, head, neck, and chest into the heart.

supine Lying on the back with the face upward.

supraclavicular Located above the clavicle.

supraglottic The area above the glottis or true vocal cords.

suprasternal Above the sternum.

suprasternal retractions A sign of increased breathing effort in which the muscles and skin above the sternum sink in above the manubrium as the patient attempts to breathe.

supraventricular tachycardia (SVT) An abnormal heart rhythm with a rapid rate and narrow QRS complex.

symmetry Correspondence in shape, size, and relative position of parts on opposite sides of a body.

sympathomimetic agent An adrenergic drug, producing effects resembling those resulting from stimulation of the sympathetic nervous system, such as effects following the injection of epinephrine.

symphysis pubis The junction of the pubic bones in the midline of the pelvis.

symptomatic ventricular dysrhythmias Abnormal ventricular electrical impulses (eg, ventricular tachycardia) that are associated with symptoms on the part of the patient.

synaptic connections Connections between 2 or more nerves (ie, synapses).

systemic inflammatory response syndrome (SIRS) An inflammatory state affecting the entire body.

T

tachycardia Rapid heart rate.

tachypnea Rapid respiration.

tamponade Compression of tissues.

tension pneumothorax An accumulation of air or gas in the pleural cavity that progressively increases and causes serious hemodynamic changes.

terrorism A violent act dangerous to human life, in violation of the criminal laws of the United States or of any state, to intimidate or coerce a government, the civilian population, or any segment thereof, in furtherance of political or social objectives.

thermoregulation Heat regulation.

thoracic Pertaining to the chest or thorax.

thoracic excursions The movements of the chest wall (rib cage and muscles) associated with respirations.

thoracostomy Opening of the chest wall to allow drainage of the chest cavity.

tidal volume The amount of air that is exchanged with each breath.

titratable The ability to adjust the desired effect of an agent by administering more or less of that agent as needed over time (eg, using an intravenous catheter to slowly administer more analgesic or sedative agents until a patient is just quiet enough to effectively complete a procedure).

tonic-clonic A seizure that features rhythmic back-and-forth motion of an extremity and body stiffness.

torticollis A tilting of the neck to one side.

totally implanted device A catheter totally implanted and not visible to the eye (mediport).

trachea A cylindrical cartilaginous tube from the larynx to the bronchial tubes. It extends from the 6th cervical vertebra to the 5th thoracic vertebra, where it divides at a point called the carina into 2 bronchi, one leading to each lung.

tracheitis An inflammation of the trachea.

tracheostomy Procedure in which the skin over the trachea is incised and a surgical wound is made in the trachea to permit an airway during tracheal obstruction.

tracheostomy tube A tube inserted into the trachea in children who cannot breathe or maintain a clear airway on their own.

transdermal Through the skin.

transient Not lasting; of brief duration.

transmucosal To pass across a mucous membrane (eg, the absorption of a toxin or pharmaceutical agent across the mucous membranes of the mouth).

traumatic brain injury (TBI) The preferred term for head trauma.

tripoding An abnormal position to keep the airway open; it involves leaning forward onto 2 arms stretched forward.

trismus Tonic contraction of the muscles of mastication (chewing).

tympanic temperature Body temperature measurement made by using a device that measures the reflectance of infrared light from the tympanic membrane (ear drum).

U

umbilical cord The attachment connecting the fetus with the placenta.

umbilical vein catheterization Placing a cannula into the umbilical artery or vein.

universal precautions Protective measures that have traditionally been developed by the Centers for Disease Control and Prevention for use in dealing with objects, blood, body fluids, or other vehicles for potential exposure to communicable disease.

universal standards for pediatric emergency care Standards of care agreed on and promoted by experts in pediatric emergency care and the organizations they represent for the management of children's care throughout the emergency medical system.

urostomy Surgical creation of a stoma to allow the elimination of urine.

V

vagal Pertaining to the vagus nerve.

vagal nerve stimulator (VNS) A small device implanted under the skin near the collarbone as a treatment for epilepsy.

vaginal introitus The vaginal opening.

vagus nerve The cranial nerve (X) that provides motor functions to the soft palate, pharynx, and larynx and carries taste bud fibers from the posterior tongue; sensory fibers from the inferior pharynx, larynx, and thoracic and abdominal organs; and parasympathetic fibers to thoracic and abdominal organs.

varicella (chicken pox) An acute viral disease with mild constitutional symptoms (headache, fever, malaise) followed by an eruption appearing in crops and characterized by macules, papules, and vesicles.

vascular tone The amount of constriction in a blood vessel or, more generally, the overall amount of constriction in the blood vessels of the body. Patients in shock often have marked vasoconstriction to increase vascular tone and blood pressure to maximize perfusion to vital organs. When there is a loss of vascular tone (eg, in sepsis or spinal shock), there is often generalized vasodilatation and severe hypotension.

vasculitis Inflammation of the blood vessels that usually is associated with pain, swelling, and often leakage of fluid and blood from the vessels into other organs. When this occurs in the skin, a purpuric rash often develops.

vasoactive agents A drug that increases vascular tone; used to increase blood pressure.

vasoconstriction Decrease in the caliber of blood vessels.

vasodilatation Dilation of blood vessels.

vasomotor Pertaining to the nerves having muscular control of the blood vessel walls.

ventilator A mechanical device for artificial ventilation of the lungs.

ventilation The process of delivering air into the lungs of a patient who is not breathing effectively or at all.

ventilation-perfusion mismatch A pathological state in which the oxygen going into the lungs is not mixing appropriately with the blood circulating through the lungs.

ventricle One of two (right and left) lower chambers of the heart. The left ventricle receives blood from the left atrium (upper chamber) and delivers blood to the aorta. The right ventricle receives blood from the right atrium and pumps it into the pulmonary artery.

ventricular fibrillation (VF) Disorganized, ineffective twitching of the ventricles, resulting in no blood flow and a state of cardiac arrest.

ventricular tachycardia (VT) A rapid heart rhythm in which the electrical impulse begins in the ventricle (instead of the atrium), which may result in inadequate blood flow and eventually deteriorate into cardiac arrest.

vertebral bodies The 33 bones that make up the spinal column.

vesicants Blister agents; the primary route of entry is through the skin.

viral myocarditis A viral infection of the heart that frequently leads to dysrhythmias, especially ventricular dysrhythmias, and poor muscle function, which produces congestive heart failure.

visual analog scores (VAS) Scales generated by asking a patient or research participant to quantify the amount of a sensation they are feeling (usually pain) by indicating a point on a line representing the level of their sensation. By measuring how far along the line the patient points, the clinician can gauge the patient's sensation. A frequently used technique for the measurement of pain in research studies.

vital signs The key signs that are used to evaluate the patient's overall condition, including respirations, pulse, blood pressure, level of consciousness, and skin characteristics.

vocal cords Two small folds of tissue in the larynx that vibrate as air moves across them to produce sound.

volume resuscitation Replenishing the blood volume.

W

wheezing Production of whistling sounds during expiration, such as occurs in asthma and bronchiolitis.

work of breathing An indicator of oxygenation and ventilation. Work of breathing reflects the child's attempt to compensate for hypoxia.

Index

Page numbers followed by *f* indicate a figure; by *t*, a table; and by *b*, an ALS box, Caution hexagon, Controversy feature, or Tip box.

A

B

C

D

E

F

G

J

K

L

M

N

O

P

Q

R

S

T

U

V

W

X

Y

Z